Atlas of
Wrist and Hand Fractures

Second Edition

Sigurd C. Sandzén, Jr., M.D.

Clinical Professor of Surgery
Division of Orthopedic Surgery
Southwestern Medical School
University of Texas Health Science Center

Director of Hand Surgery
Texas Scottish Rite Hospital for Crippled Children

Director of Hand Surgery
Division of Orthopedic Surgery
Parkland Memorial Hospital

Chief of Surgery
Medical Arts Hospital
Dallas, Texas

PSG Publishing Company, Inc.
Littleton, Massachusetts

Library of Congress Cataloging in Publication Data

Sandzén, Sigurd C. (Sigurd Carl), 1932–
   Atlas of wrist and hand fractures.

   Bibliography: p.
   Includes index.
   1. Hand—Fractures—Atlases. 2. Wrist—Fractures—
Atlases. I. Title. [DNLM: 1. Fractures—atlases.
2. Hand Injuries—atlases. 3. Wrist Injuries—
atlases. WE 17 S222a]
RD559.S26 1985   617′.157   85-3427
ISBN 0-88416-487-X

First Edition 1979
Second Edition 1986

Printed in the United States of America.

International Standard Book Number: 0-88416-487-X

Library of Congress Catalog Card Number: 85-3427

To Marcelle

Contents

Foreword to the First Edition

Primary recognition and correction of skeletal and articular derangement involving the distal forearm, wrist, and hand are fundamental to prevent overall functional impairment, especially when soft tissues and retinacular components are involved as well. Dr. Sandzén's timely and comprehensive coverage of this subject is a welcome addition to the many texts on the hand wherein fractures and joint injuries are often given but summary treatment.

The diversity and complexity of skeletal trauma demand careful analysis and precise reduction and fixation to minimize disability. This basic but detailed atlas is oriented toward the resident and the general orthopedic surgeon most responsible for this care. Accumulation of personal experience will naturally provoke some difference of opinion regarding the treatment of special problems and the specific uses of the image intensifier.

We are indebted to Dr. Sandzén for his dedicated effort in furthering our understanding of this difficult subject.

J. William Littler, M.D.
New York City

Foreword to the Second Edition

In this second edition, Dr. Sandzén has expanded the general format of his *Atlas of Wrist and Hand Fractures,* made more engaging through page and print enlargement and more appropriate placement of illustrations and legends and, in some pertinent cases, greater clarity of radiographic reproductions.

The entire text has been updated and a new chapter (16) added, which covers in depth internal fixation.

Chapter 3, "Injuries to the Distal Radius and Ulna," has been rewritten and emphasizes the need to differentiate distal metaphyseal fractures of the radius from the segmental articular ones for more effective treatment.

Chapters 4, "Wrist Injuries," 11, "Physeal Injuries," and 13, "Crush Injuries," are entirely reworked. Particular attention in Chapter 13 is focused on the diagnosis and treatment of the insidious closed compartment compression syndrome. A selected bibliography of pertinent references is included following each chapter.

The author's impressive clinical experience with this complex subject is elegantly expressed in this comprehensive work. It is a special tribute to his devotion for our benefit.

J. William Littler, M.D.
New York City

Acknowledgments

First Edition

Material from various sources has been freely incorporated. Particular thanks are due to Julio Taleisnik, M.D., for basic anatomy of the wrist, and to J. William Littler, M.D., and Richard G. Eaton, M.D., for anatomy of the digital joints. Michael Harty, F.R.C.S., and John W. Snow, M.D., reviewed the entire section on anatomy and made pertinent suggestions. The photographic technique used in Figures 1-1 and 1-2 was conceived by Dr. Snow.

James G. Boyes, Jr., M.D., and Francis M. Howard, M.D., were kind enough to review and offer constructive criticism on various sections in Chapter 4, Wrist Injuries. Members of the Orthopaedic Department of Abington Memorial Hospital and U.S. Walson Army Hospital provided many interesting cases. Special thanks for material are due to the following: Richard A. Cautilli, M.D., James G.T. Boyes, Jr., M.D., Richard G. Eaton, M.D., David P. Green, M.D., Stephen F. Gunther, M.D., David M. Junkin, M.D., Alan M. Larimer, M.D., Robert J. Neviaser, M.D., Samuel C. Santangelo, M.D., and John B. Webber, M.D.

I am grateful to Jo Bruck for help in research and to Joanne Williams and Wendy Jiminez for their secretarial efforts; Marie Goldstein, Editor, Margery Berube, Managing Editor, and William T. Strauss, Medical Advisor, PSG Publishing Company, Inc., for continued assistance and wholehearted support; and Norman Hauser, M.D., Radiologist, for his help in producing Figures 1-1 and 1-2.

I am particularly indebted to J. William Littler, M.D. for his basic teachings and sustained enthusiasm and support.

Second Edition

Special thanks to Peter Carter, M.D., Michael Doyle, M.D., Marybeth Ezaki, M.D., Ronald Linscheid, M.D., and Olayinka Ogunro, M.D., for use of their cases and for their valuable ideas and help, and to Lawrence Bone, M.D., for his review of and thoughtful comments on Chapter 16.

Thanks also to Cynthia Buchanan and Susan Stevens for their excellent secretarial and proofreading assistance.

Introduction

The purpose of this Atlas is to provide adequate information to enable the practicing physician to manage intelligently the spectrum of skeletal injuries involving the distal upper extremity. Skeletal, joint, and ligamentous injuries of the distal forearm, wrist, and hand are described and illustrated, and principles and recommended techniques of management are offered. Conservative treatment of closed reduction and external immobilization is emphasized for the vast majority of these injuries. Of equal importance is the proper selection of cases for which surgery is definitely recommended. These are clearly delineated. Although common injuries are emphasized, the majority of rare lesions are included.

The most common fractures of the upper extremity involve the long bones of the hand and digits (metacarpals and phalanges), and they are usually closed. The distal phalanges are those most often fractured and frequently are not treated with adequate thoroughness, thus resulting in prolonged morbidity. Metacarpal fractures are next in incidence, and the middle phalanges and carpals are injured least often.

The prime physiologic motions of the hand are thumb opposition, digital flexion and extension, and digital abduction from, and adduction to, the focal point of the hand, the central long finger. The goal of treatment is to restore the proper balance of skeletal stability and joint mobility for these physiologically coordinated digital functions. This requires normal reciprocal wrist function for maximum power and dexterity.

Malunion, nonunion, and chronic ligamentous avulsion impair function of the involved digit to a degree compatible with the severity of the lesion. However, the injured digit also hinders general function of the entire hand since the normal balance of coordinated digital synergism has been jeopardized.

The Atlas stresses the following points:

1. Precise evaluation of skeletal, joint, and ligamentous injuries for accurate diagnosis and proper initial treatment
2. Pathophysiology of these injuries
3. Techniques of fracture and joint reduction under appropriate anesthesia
4. Errors to be avoided and the management of complications
5. Effective physiologic immobilization
6. Early mobilization and rehabilitation

Diagnosis

The terms "jammed" or "sprained" finger and "strained" or "sprained" wrist must be avoided. Careful physical examination and radiographic evaluation usually provide an accurate diagnosis to enable proper treatment.

If the history and physical examination give reason to suspect skeletal (bone or joint) or ligamentous (avulsion or partial avulsion) injury, conservative treatment is the prudent course. Immobilization for a suspected fracture or dislocation should be instituted regardless of a negative initial radiographic evaluation. In this way a reduced dislocation, a physeal separation, or an occult fracture (e.g., occult

1

scaphoid fracture) will not be overlooked. Immobilization is indicated to treat soft tissue trauma whether or not a skeletal injury has been incurred. Radiographic reevaluation if symptoms persist (ten days to two or three weeks after injury) usually will reveal signs if any skeletal damage is present. These signs include bone resorption at the site of a fracture line, incipient callus deposits at a fracture site or physeal separation, and calcification at the site of ligamentous avulsion or periosteal elevation. A potentially serious situation will not be overlooked with this type of management.

The local signs and symptoms of musculoskeletal injuries include a variable degree of edema, congestion, hemorrhage, ecchymosis, pain, and point tenderness at the site of injury. Characteristic deformities may be evident depending upon the site of fracture or dislocation and the effect of adjacent muscles.

Radiographic evidence is important for documentation prior to providing specific anesthesia for the injury and before manipulation and reduction. Occasionally extreme vascular impairment distal to the site of injury requires that a fracture or dislocation, whether open or closed, be reduced prior to radiographic evaluation. If the injury is open, redislocation must be accomplished at the time of primary surgical debridement and cleansing of the wound before definitive reduction.

It is important to make a complete evaluation of the entire injured extremity in order to discover and diagnose other concurrent injuries. The contralateral upper extremity also should be meticulously examined, as should the entire skeletal system, including the spine and lower extremities if indicated by the type and severity of trauma sustained.

It is also important to consider the possibility of associated soft tissue injuries in closed wounds as well as open ones. For example, tendons and neurovascular structures may be penetrated by bone spicules, or nerves may suffer neurapraxia (external compression) from displaced bones, dislocated joints, or edematous soft tissue (e.g., median and/or ulnar nerve compression associated with carpal injuries).

Finally, circulatory compromise to structures distal to the site of injury must be accurately evaluated.

Pathophysiology

Fracture of a long bone introduces a "new joint," a false articulation, which is termed a pseudoarthrosis if nonunion results. This false articulation causes buckling or collapse of the long bone if the fracture is unstable.

Deformity (displacement, distraction, shortening, rotation, and angulation) at the site of fracture or dislocation can usually be predicted and is the result of:

1. The type of injury (e.g., crush, high-velocity through-and-through injury, etc.)
2. The mechanism of injury, including the degree, manner, and type of force applied
3. The contraction of muscles which originate proximal to the fracture or dislocation and insert distally and therefore cross the site of injury
4. The effect of synergistic and antagonistic actions of both extrinsic and intrinsic muscles

One problem in both the reduction and the maintenance of reduction of carpal, metacarpal, and phalangeal fractures is counteracting the distracting and compacting forces of the powerful extrinsic muscles of the forearm, which act directly on the relatively small bones or fracture fragments of the distal radius, the ulna, carpals, metacarpals, and phalanges, or at their insertions.

To avoid malalignment, malrotation, and angulation in long bone fractures and to reestablish proper length without distraction, it is necessary to achieve the best possible anatomic reduction. Anatomic length is an extremely important factor in both proximal and middle phalangeal fractures to restore proper balance of the extensor and flexor mechanisms, but some loss of length can be accepted in the metacarpals.

The inherent instability of some fractures and dislocations, combined with the potentially deforming forces of the muscles of the forearm on the site of injury, require that adequate radiographic evaluation be made at intervals during healing to be certain that fracture or joint reduction has been satisfactorily maintained.

Treatment

The most important factor in the immediate first aid of a fracture or dislocation is immobilization, usually with a splint, to prevent motion at the site of injury. No attempt should be made to correct the deformity unless vascular impairment is noted distal to the injury. If analgesia is necessary, medication may be administered intravenously, intramuscularly, or occasionally by mouth, depending upon the severity of injury and general condition of the patient.

Undisplaced and stable metacarpal and phalangeal fractures are initially immobilized for a few days before light active ranges of motion are allowed.

However, undisplaced articular fractures must be treated carefully with weekly radiographic evaluation for three to four weeks to be certain that the fracture does not become displaced.

It is important to strive for anatomic reduction of dislocations and displaced articular fractures. Fractures, dislocations, fracture dislocations, and ligamentous injuries of the carpals require meticulous attention to details of anatomic reduction, especially with respect to the head of the capitate, the lunate, and the scaphoid.

Adequate anesthesia must usually be administered before there is any attempt at manipulation and reduction of a fracture or dislocation.

A dislocation or fracture should usually be treated by primary closed manipulation, reduction, and physiologic immobilization. However, proper treatment may depend on the recognition of concurrent soft tissue injuries. Thus, marked swelling, such as that incurred in a severe crushing injury with or without fracture, is an indication to treat the injury initially by constant elevation and immobilization. After the swelling subsides, usually in five to seven days, definitive appropriate treatment of the fracture is then carried out. To prevent additional vascular impairment, a massively edematous and ecchymotic open wound should not be closed at the initial treatment. Instead, delayed primary closure is performed about five to seven days after the injury and after swelling has subsided.

Early diagnosis of Volkmann's ischemia of the muscles of the forearm secondary to closed trauma is vitally important. Only early surgical decompression of this retained pressure within a closed space will prevent the catastrophic sequence of prolonged ischemia, muscle necrosis, and ultimate contractures with impairment of nerve function.

A closed space compression injury may also be encountered in the dorsal (extensor) muscle mass of the forearm, in the hand (dorsally in the interossei and palmarly in the thenar, hypothenar and central compartments), and in the pulp of a distal phalanx, following a closed comminuted crush fracture of the tuft. Occasionally, incision and drainage are necessary to release the pressure of the retained hematoma and to prevent ischemic changes of vascularly impaired pulp tissue.

The effects of high-velocity missile injuries and high-voltage electrical burns on the surrounding soft tissue are well known. These injuries demand continuous reevaluation for the first few hours after injury to check the degree of soft tissue edema and consequent ischemia which often necessitate wide surgical release.

Though conservative treatment is adequate for the vast majority of the injuries considered in this Atlas, surgery is indicated for the following situations:

1. Open fractures, open fracture dislocations, and open dislocations—primarily for proper cleansing of the wound, including copious irrigation with a sterile isotonic solution and meticulous debridement of devitalized bone fragments, soft tissue, foreign material, and preservation of all viable tissue prior to reduction and, if indicated, primary wound closure
2. Displaced irreducible or unstable fractures of an articular surface, with or without joint subluxation or dislocation
3. Irreducible or unstable shaft fractures, particularly with malrotation, impingement on an adjacent joint, or marked shortening
4. Fracture avulsion of a collateral ligament which results in joint instability, particularly if the ligament is attached to a large segment of articular surface or if the fracture impinges on that joint
5. Complete avulsion of a collateral ligament insertion which results in joint instability, especially if the metacarpophalangeal joint of the thumb or the proximal interphalangeal joint of the index or little finger is involved
6. Irreducible or unstable dislocations or fracture dislocations
7. A retained foreign body or loose bone fragment either within a joint or which may act as a nidus for infection or impinge on a tendon or neurovascular structure and impair function
8. A closed space compression injury in which pressure must be relieved to prevent soft tissue ischemia and subsequent necrosis
9. Irreducible or unstable physeal separation
10. Pathologic fracture

Methods of reduction and fixation include closed reduction with percutaneous Kirschner wire fixation, open reduction with percutaneous Kirschner wire fixation, and open reduction with internal fixation.

Examples of closed reduction with percutaneous Kirschner wire fixation includes immobilization of a reduced metacarpal shaft fracture to adjacent normal metacarpals, balanced dynamic skeletal traction, and Kirschner wires placed longitudinally (intramedullary), obliquely, or crossed at the fracture site percutaneously.

The image intensifier aids greatly in closed manipulation and reduction of carpal trauma and long bone fractures and dislocations. It is *not* accurate enough to precisely evaluate closed reduction of displaced articular fractures of the wrist and hand.

If open reduction of a fracture or dislocation is necessary, it should not be performed in the average emergency room, but in a suitably prepared surgical suite. Such surgery is intricate and demands respect. A power drill, particularly the pistol-grip type, is indispensable for precise, meticulous fixation under tourniquet hemostasis.

Though tourniquet hemostasis may not be necessary, a pneumatic tourniquet should always be applied to the upper arm, just distal to the axilla, before treating a severe injury. Pressure for an adult is approximately 275–280 lb, and for a child, 175–200 lb. Continuous pneumatic hemostasis is safe up to two hours duration; if additional time is needed, the tourniquet should be released for 15 minutes before reinflation for one hour or less.

Often tourniquet inflation is unnecessary in treating an acute open injury since ligation or cauterization of damaged vessels will provide a satisfactory field for surgery. The extremity should be elevated at least five minutes before inflating the tourniquet; a Martin (often erroneously referred to as an Esmarch) bandage is not indicated.

Open reduction may be accompanied by either percutaneous or internal Kirschner wire fixation which is placed longitudinally (intramedullary), obliquely, or crossed at the exposed reduced fracture site or by pullout stainless steel wire fixation or by "pins-and-plaster," external fixator, or intraosseous wiring. Internal plate fixation is indicated in specific instances.

Skin traction is always contraindicated. Skeletal traction is occasionally helpful, but the vascular supply distal to the site of injury must be adequate.

A badly contaminated wound often limits primary treatment to gross repositioning of the fracture; definitive skeletal management is deferred until the soft tissues show no evidence of infection. Delayed primary care (five to seven days after injury) or secondary treatment may be necessary for an infected wound.

In general, the more severe the injury, the less indication there is for involved primary care. Usually the initial treatment of an acute injury should not include any complex reconstructive procedures, particularly if additional operative procedures are anticipated.

Immobilization

Prior to definitive immobilization normal anatomy should be restored. Proper rotational alignment, however, may be difficult to achieve. Anatomic alignment and rotation of the injured digit can be restored by comparing its configuration to adjacent normal digits and to corresponding digits of the contralateral normal hand in similar positions.

In general, the tips of the index, long, ring, and little fingers point to the tuberosity of the scaphoid when flexed. Since this is a generality, observation of the digital relationships in synergistic flexion and extension of both the injured and the contralateral normal hand is most important to provide proper immobilization. Observation of nail plate alignment is also helpful. The plane of the fractured digit's nail plate should correspond to those of its adjacent normal digits, just as that of the same digit on the opposite hand corresponds to its adjacent digits.

Provided anesthesia is adequate, examination of the injured digit actively and passively in extension and particularly in flexion is necessary to avoid rotational deformities.

Undisplaced and potentially stable fractures of the metacarpals and phalanges should be immobilized for a period of 12 to 14 days before light active ranges of motion are allowed. In a responsible patient early motion may be permitted after 7 to 10 days, particularly if the involved digit is taped to the adjacent digit or digits in a "buddy" fashion to provide some external stability. Immobilization of metacarpal and proximal phalangeal fractures should include the wrist and extend to the tip of the involved digit. Immobilization for middle and distal phalangeal fractures should incorporate the injured digit from the metacarpophalangeal joint distally to the fingertip.

Immobilization of a stable reduced fracture or dislocation should be continuous for approximately three weeks and should incorporate the normal digit on either side for the first two to two and one-half weeks after injury. Immobilization of a marginal digit (index or little finger) usually incorporates only a single adjacent digit.

Immobilization should always attempt to follow the pattern of physiologic positioning: wrist extension in slight ulnar deviation, metacarpophalangeal joint flexion, wide thumb abduction and opposition, and nearly complete extension of both proximal and distal interphalangeal joints.

Complications

Oversight and errors in the treatment of fractures, dislocations, and ligamentous injuries can be avoided by careful examination for, and attention to, associated injuries to the ipsilateral and contralateral extremities. By performing adequate physical examination and obtaining satisfactory radiographic evaluations, the correct diagnosis can be made and adequate appropriate and timely treatment initiated.

Mobilization and Rehabilitation

While one strives to achieve stability of a reduced fracture or joint dislocation, mobility of all uninvolved joints not incorporated in the immobilization should be stressed. It is extremely important to achieve a physiologic balance between immobilization and mobilization of the injured digit in order not to jeopardize the desired position of a reduced fracture or dislocation when early range of motion exercises are commenced. Early motion—dynamic use of the injured digit in synergistic flexion and extension with adjacent normal digits—is the key to physiologic rehabilitation.

General References

Beasley RW: *Hand Injuries*. Philadephia, W.B. Saunders, 1981.

Flatt AE: *The Care of Minor Hand Injuries*, ed 4. St. Louis, C.V. Mosby Co., 1979.

Green DP: *Operative Hand Surgery*. New York, Churchill Livingstone, 1982, vol 1.

Littler JW: The hand and upper extremity, vol 6, in Converse JM (ed): *Reconstructive Plastic Surgery*, ed 2. Philadelphia, W.B. Saunders, 1977.

Milford L: The hand, ed 2, in: *Campbell's Operative Orthopaedics*, ed 6. St. Louis, C.V. Mosby Co., 1982.

Moore DC: *Regional Block*, ed 4. Springfield, Ill, Charles C Thomas, 1965.

Rockwood CA Jr, Green DP: *Fractures in Adults*. Philadelphia, J.B. Lippincott Co., 1984, vol 1.

Sandzén SC Jr: *Current Management of Complications in Orthopedics: The Hand and Wrist*. Baltimore, Williams and Wilkins, 1985.

Weeks PM, Wray RC: *Management of Acute Hand Injuries: A Biological Approach*, ed 2. St. Louis, C.V. Mosby Co., 1978.

CHAPTER
1

Anatomy

Surface Anatomy of the
Wrist and Hand (Figures 1-1, 1-2)

The distal ulnar shaft which terminates in the ulnar head is easily palpated longitudinally along the dorsoulnar aspect of the distal forearm. The ulnar head is best palpated dorsally with pronation of the forearm, and palmarly with supination. The ulnar styloid process is the most distal protuberance projecting from the ulnar aspect of the head. The radial styloid process is palpated on the radial aspect of the distal forearm just beneath the tendons of the abductor pollicis longus and extensor pollicis brevis. The radial styloid process projects approximately 0.5 to 1.0 cm distal to the ulnar styloid process.

The distal radius may be palpated dorsally with the wrist either in neutral position or slight flexion. With more marked flexion of the wrist, the lunate is palpated as a dorsal protuberance slightly radial to the longitudinal midline of the forearm and wrist (i.e., slightly ulnar to the longitudinal midline of the distal radius). Distal to this protuberance is a slight hollow which represents the neck and body of the capitate.

On the dorsoradial aspect of the wrist, the "anatomic snuff box" is bounded radially by the abductor pollicis longus and the extensor pollicis brevis tendons and ulnarly by the extensor pollicis longus tendon. If the extensor pollicis longus tendon is followed proximally, it travels ulnarly, to a protuberance at about the midpoint of the dorsal distal radius (Lister's tubercle), and then angles radially.

In the hollow of the anatomic snuff box, the isthmus and distal third of the scaphoid and the trapezium are palpated. By passively moving the thumb metacarpal, the trapezium-thumb metacarpal joint (carpometacarpal joint of the thumb) can be felt. The metacarpal bases of the index, long, ring, and little fingers are recognized by the rather prominent flare of the metacarpal bases in the area of the carpometacarpal joints. Each metacarpal head is readily distinguished and palpated beneath its extensor apparatus but is particularly prominent with maximal metacarpophalangeal (MP) flexion. The proximal interphalangeal (PIP) joint articulation can be localized by passive flexion and extension, but the distal interphalangeal (DIP) joint is not as easily palpated because

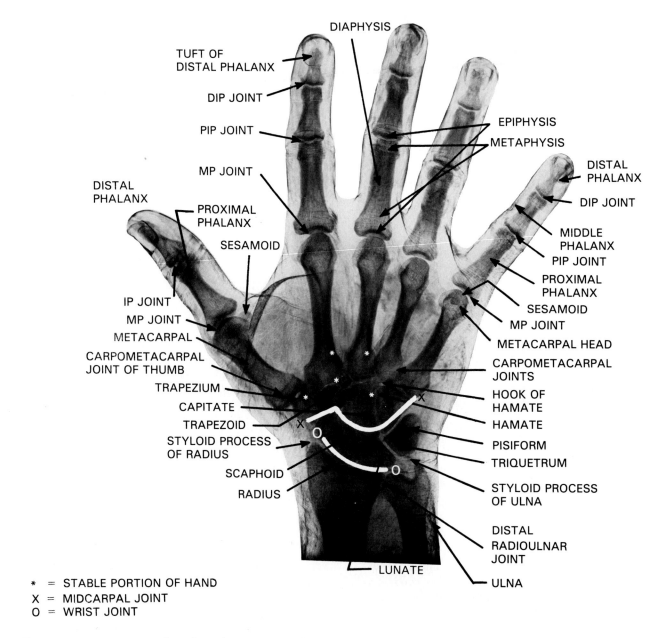

DIAPHYSIS

TUFT OF
DISTAL PHALANX

DIP JOINT

PIP JOINT

EPIPHYSIS

METAPHYSIS

MP JOINT

DISTAL
PHALANX

DISTAL
PHALANX

DIP JOINT

PROXIMAL
PHALANX

SESAMOID

MIDDLE
PHALANX

PIP JOINT

PROXIMAL
PHALANX

IP JOINT

MP JOINT

METACARPAL

CARPOMETACARPAL
JOINT OF THUMB

SESAMOID

MP JOINT

METACARPAL HEAD

CARPOMETACARPAL
JOINTS

TRAPEZIUM

CAPITATE

TRAPEZOID

STYLOID PROCESS
OF RADIUS

SCAPHOID

RADIUS

HOOK OF
HAMATE

HAMATE

PISIFORM

TRIQUETRUM

STYLOID PROCESS
OF ULNA

DISTAL
RADIOULNAR
JOINT

LUNATE

ULNA

* = STABLE PORTION OF HAND
X = MIDCARPAL JOINT
O = WRIST JOINT

Figure 1-1 Figures 1-1 and 1-2 have been prepared by painting and hand completely with barium paste and then obtaining PA (1-1) and lateral (1-2) radiographs. This method[1] illustrates the relationship of skin landmarks and soft tissue structures to the underlying skeletal system. The exact relationship of the digital joints to flexion creases, the distal phalanx and tuft of the distal phalanx in relation to the nail plate, and the exact location of the wrist joint and carpus are particularly noteworthy. On this PA view the wrist joint, or radiocarpal joint, between the distal radius proximally and the scaphoid and lunate distally, and the midcarpal joint—essentially a ball-and-socket articulation, with the scaphoid, lunate, and triquetrum proximally, forming the socket, and the capitate and hamate distally, forming the ball, extending radially between the scaphoid and trapezium and trapezoid—are well visualized.

The anatomic divisions of a long bone (metacarpal, proximal, middle, and distal phalanges) are seen outlined on the long finger proximal phalanx and include the diaphysis or shaft, the proximal and distal metaphysis, and the proximal and distal epiphysis.

For a thorough knowledge of the skeletal anatomy of the wrist and hand, Figures 1-1 and 1-2 should be studied and compared to routine normal radiographs; the reader also should locate and palpate the labeled skeletal landmarks on his or her own wrist and hand.

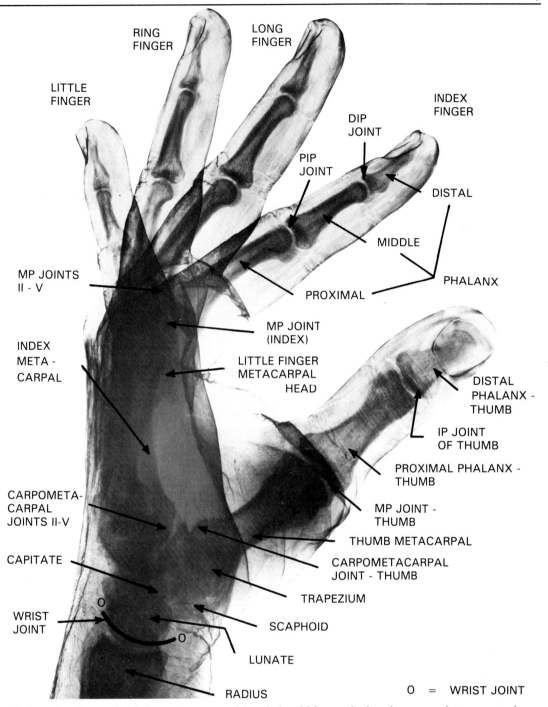

RING
FINGER

LONG
FINGER

LITTLE
FINGER

INDEX
FINGER

DIP
JOINT

PIP
JOINT

DISTAL

MIDDLE

PHALANX

PROXIMAL

MP JOINTS
II - V

MP JOINT
(INDEX)

INDEX
META -
CARPAL

LITTLE FINGER
METACARPAL
HEAD

DISTAL
PHALANX -
THUMB

IP JOINT
OF THUMB

PROXIMAL PHALANX -
THUMB

CARPOMETA-
CARPAL
JOINTS II-V

MP JOINT -
THUMB

CAPITATE

THUMB METACARPAL

CARPOMETACARPAL
JOINT - THUMB

TRAPEZIUM

WRIST
JOINT

O

O

SCAPHOID

LUNATE

RADIUS

O = WRIST JOINT

Figure 1-2 This lateral radiograph of the wrist area and hand should be studied and compared to a normal radiograph and to the surface anatomy of the reader's own wrist and hand as recommended for Figure 1-1. It is important to realize that this lateral radiograph demonstrates the PA configuration of the thumb ray (metacarpal, proximal, and distal phalanges). Similarly, in Figure 1-1, the PA view, the lateral (or oblique lateral) view of the thumb ray is depicted.

It is difficult to discern the index, long, ring, and little finger metacarpals in a true lateral view, but the digits usually can be recognized by their relative lengths and positions. For better study of individual metacarpals, oblique views of the hand should be made routinely.

In this lateral view the wrist joint and carpus may be localized in relation to surrounding soft tissue and surface anatomy. The digital skeleton, including the metacarpal, proximal, middle, and distal phalanges, is dorsally oriented in relation to the surrounding soft tissue structures. The mass of the palmar soft tissue includes the thick pulp on the tactile palmar surface of the digit and the two flexor tendons, flexor digitorum superficialis and flexor digitorum profundus.

of the proximity and mass of the extensor and the flexor profundus tendon insertions.

The flexor carpi radialis is clearly seen on the palmar aspect of the wrist extending longitudinally approximately 0.5 cm to the radial aspect of the midlongitudinal line of the forearm. The palmaris longus tendon, which is absent in about 15% of individuals, is noted just ulnar to this midlongitudinal line. Easily recognizable structures at the proximal wrist flexion crease include the pisiform, into which the flexor carpi ulnaris tendon inserts at the ulnar proximal aspect of the hypothenar muscle mass, and the tuberosity of the scaphoid, just radial to the tendon of the flexor carpi radialis. Approximately 1.0 cm distal to the scaphoid tuberosity, in line with the flexor carpi radialis tendon and concealed by the thenar muscle mass, is the crest or tuberosity of the trapezium. Two and one-half centimeters distally and somewhat radial to the pisiform, the hook of the hamate can be palpated through the hypothenar muscle mass.

The last four structures—the scaphoid tuberosity and crest of the trapezium laterally, and pisiform and hook of the hamate medially—form the lateral and medial osseous boundaries of the carpal canal. Respectively they afford attachment of the transverse carpal ligament which completes the boundaries of the carpal tunnel palmarly.

Functional Anatomy

Upper Extremity

The architecture of the entire upper extremity is designed to provide skeletal stability and physiologic mobility for optimal hand function.

Basically the upper extremity is a series of graduated lever arms, positioned by extrinsic muscles of the thorax, shoulder, arm, and forearm, and intrinsic muscles of the hand. These lever arms are long tubular bones progressively decreasing in size from the humerus to the distal phalanx. Each long bone has a diaphysis (body or shaft), two metaphyses, and two epiphyses (ends) which are covered by articular cartilage, except for the distal end of the distal phalanx. During growth each long bone posseses one or two physes or epiphyseal growth plates and may or may not have associated appositional growth areas or apophyses. The carpus (wrist bones) is located between the forearm and the hand and is composed of short bones which are modified cubes. These bones

have multiple articular surfaces and multiple ligamentous attachments but no tendon insertions except the pisiform. The scapula, a flat bone, and the clavicle, a long bone, complete the skeletal foundation of the upper extremity.

The strong, stable pillar which provides the foundation for the upper extremity skeleton is the humerus. Nearly unlimited motion of the humerus is possible proximally at the shoulder joint owing to the shallow ball-and-socket articulation of the humeral head with the glenoid fossa of the scapula. The scapula allows further mobility of the entire shoulder girdle on the chest wall. The clavicle, at the acromioclavicular joint, is the only skeletal connection between the upper extremity and the thorax. Stability, therefore, is compromised by this exceptional mobility, which accounts for the relative frequency of shoulder dislocations.

The elbow joint connecting the arm to the forearm is a ginglymus, or hinge-type joint, centered in the articulation of the trochlear notch of the ulna with the trochlea of the humerus. Proximally the head of the radius articulates with both the capitulum of the humerus and the radial notch of the proximal ulna, and distally the head of the ulna articulates with the ulnar notch of the distal radius.

The radius and ulna are held together at the proximal radioulnar joint primarily by the annular ligament. Through nearly their entire shaft lengths these bones are attached by the parallel, oblique fibers of the interosseous membrane which travels proximally from a point on the ulna, just proximal to the distal radioulnar joint, to a point just distal to the tuberosity of the radius. This interosseous attachment of the radius and the ulna is reinforced proximally by a band of fibrous tissue, the oblique cord, which runs in just the opposite direction of the interosseous membrane, i.e., it originates on the tuberosity of the ulna and travels distally and obliquely to attach to the radius at a point just distal to the radial tuberosity. Obviously the muscle mass surrounding the elbow and both bones of the forearm contributes to external stability. Distally the strongest connection is provided by the triangular fibrocartilage, which will be discussed under the Wrist in this chapter. Some additional strength is afforded by the anterior and posterior distal radioulnar ligaments, which are merely irregular thickenings of the joint capsule, and by the pronator quadratus muscle (particularly the deep head of this muscle.)[2]

Rotatory motions of pronation and supination of the forearm occur at these proximal and distal radioulnar joints. Supination is effected primarily by the supinator and also by the biceps brachiae. Pronation is effected primarily by the pronator teres and the pronator quadratus. The arc of pronation-supination centers on the long finger metacarpal and the head of the radius.

The distal articular surface of the radius is composed of two separate facets, a radial one for articulation with the scaphoid and an ulnar one for articulation with the lunate. This entire distal radial articular surface angles palmarly approximately 10° to 12° and ulnarly approximately 12° to 14°.

The synovial cavity of the distal radioulnar joint is L-shaped. The horizontal segment lies between the triangular fibrocartilage and the articular surface of the distal ulna. The vertical segment extends between the contiguous articular surfaces of the ulnar head and ulnar notch of the radius and extends somewhat proximally from the articular surfaces as a synovial pouch, the sacciform recess. The deeper the ulnar notch of the distal radius, the more secure is the distal radioulnar articulation.

Wrist Joint* (Figures 1-3, 1-4, 1-5)[3]

The wrist joint includes the distal articular surface of the radius proximally, and the proximal articular surfaces of the scaphoid and the lunate and the triangular fibrocartilage distally. The ulnocarpal meniscus (radiotriquetral ligament) lies between and is intimately attached to the triangular fibrocartilage and triquetrum. Therefore, the distal ulna does not participate in the wrist joint since it is separated from the triquetrum by the triangular fibrocartilage proximally and by the ulnocarpal meniscus distally. A pathologic, symptomatic false articulation between the distal ulnar articular surface abutting against the triquetrum may result from a relative lengthening of the ulna or shortening of the radius, with pathologic disruption of the triangular fibrocartilage and the meniscus (e.g., healed Colles' fracture with metaphyseal resorption and shortening of the radius, excision of the radial head, or congenital Madelung's deformity).

A synovial recess which surrounds the distal tip of the ulnar styloid process, which has no ligamentous attachment, is formed between the distal surface of the triangular fibrocartilage and the proximal surface of the meniscus. This space is called the prestyloid recess. It normally communicates with the wrist joint through an opening between these two structures, which form its proximal and distal boundaries. The prestyloid recess normally possesses abundant synovium and is therefore one of the earliest locations to be involved by rheumatoid arthritis.

One separate joint, the triquetral-pisiform joint, does not usually communicate with the wrist joint.

The anatomic wrist or carpus is composed of eight carpal bones, architecturally arranged roughly in a proximal and distal row, with the scaphoid serving as a connecting link between the two rows. The distal carpal row includes the trapezium, trapezoid, capitate, and hamate as a single osseoligamentous unit which functions as one complex bone. Strong, short intercarpal ligaments which connect the bones of this row prevent motion of each individual bone. The trapezoid is further immobilized by virtue of being completely embedded at its distal articulation in a concavity within the base of the second metacarpal. The base of the third metacarpal is firmly bound to the capitate and also to the adjacent index metacarpal base.

Centered in the distal carpal row is the capitate, the keystone of the carpus and the largest carpal bone. The focus of intercarpal articulations is a ball-and-socket type joint between the head of the capitate and a small segment of the hamate (ball) and the opposing concave surfaces of the scaphoid and lunate (socket), which will be discussed later. Motion of the entire distal carpal row centers primarily at the head of the capitate.

The trapezium, though firmly bound to the trapezoid, contributes to two mobile joints: distally it forms a double saddle-like joint with the base of the thumb metacarpal, permitting wide ranges of motion; proximally it articulates with the scaphoid in a gliding-type joint. The tendon of the flexor carpi radialis travels in a groove on the palmar surface of the trapezium just ulnar to a somewhat prominent ridge (the crest, or tubercule), to its points of insertion on the bases of the index and long metacarpals.

Just ulnar to the trapezium is the trapezoid, the smallest true carpal bone (excluding the pisiform), which is intimately associated with the base of the index metacarpal.

The hamate completes the ulnar aspect of the distal carpal row, articulating distally with the fourth and fifth metacarpal bases, and proximally with the triquetrum. The hamate-fifth metacarpal articulation is a modified saddle-type joint which somewhat resembles the trapezium-thumb metacarpal joint.

---

*The author thanks Julio Taleisnik, M.D., for much material included in this section on wrist anatomy.

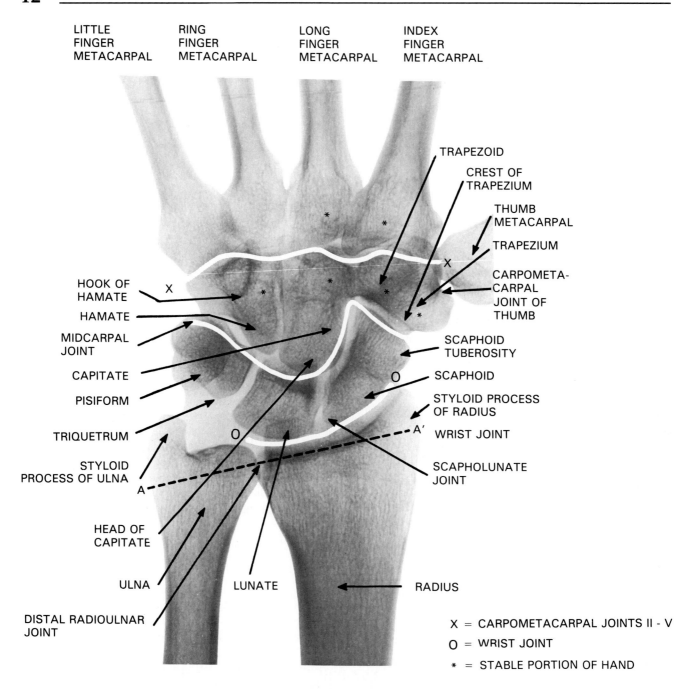

LITTLE FINGER METACARPAL

RING FINGER METACARPAL

LONG FINGER METACARPAL

INDEX FINGER METACARPAL

TRAPEZOID

CREST OF TRAPEZIUM

THUMB METACARPAL

TRAPEZIUM

CARPOMETA-CARPAL JOINT OF THUMB

HOOK OF HAMATE

HAMATE

MIDCARPAL JOINT

CAPITATE

PISIFORM

TRIQUETRUM

STYLOID PROCESS OF ULNA

HEAD OF CAPITATE

ULNA

LUNATE

DISTAL RADIOULNAR JOINT

SCAPHOID TUBEROSITY

SCAPHOID

STYLOID PROCESS OF RADIUS

WRIST JOINT

SCAPHOLUNATE JOINT

RADIUS

X = CARPOMETACARPAL JOINTS II - V

O = WRIST JOINT

* = STABLE PORTION OF HAND

Figure 1-3   (Enlargement of a PA radiograph of a normal wrist.) Individual carpal bones, their interrelationships with each other in carpal architecture, and the various joints described in the text can be studied. The ulnar angulation of the distal radial articular surface is denoted by line A–A'. Normally this angle is 12° to 14°.

Of particular importance are three areas: (1) The wrist joint, or radiocarpal joint, (radius proximally and scaphoid and lunate distally); (2) the midcarpal joint, the major portion of which is the ball-and-socket type articulation between the scaphoid, lunate, and triquetrum proximally, forming the socket, and the capitate and hamate distally, forming the ball, extending radially between the distal scaphoid and the trapezium and trapezoid; and (3) the carpometacarpal joints which demonstrate the extreme mobility of the thumb carpometacarpal joint, the intermediate mobility of the little finger and ring finger carpometacarpal joints, and the stability of the index and long finger carpometacarpal joints.

The stable portion of the hand is seen to include the entire distal carpal row (trapezium, trapezoid, capitate, and hamate) and the index and long metacarpals.

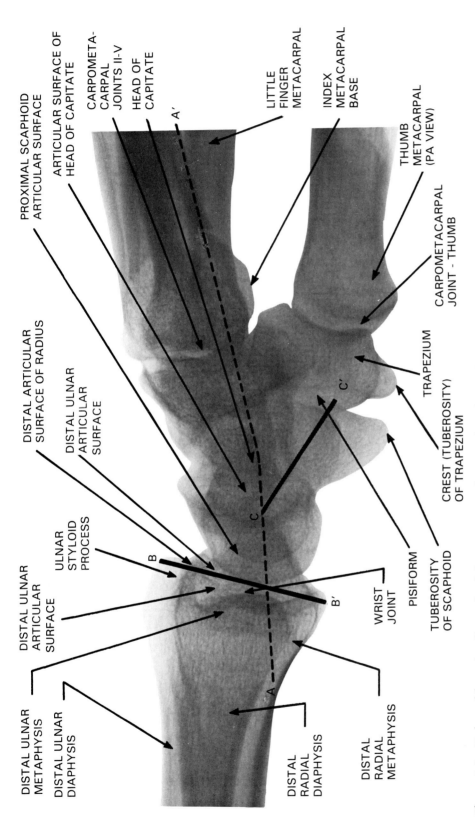

DISTAL ULNAR METAPHYSIS

DISTAL ULNAR DIAPHYSIS

DISTAL ULNAR ARTICULAR SURFACE

ULNAR STYLOID PROCESS

DISTAL ARTICULAR SURFACE OF RADIUS

PROXIMAL SCAPHOID ARTICULAR SURFACE

ARTICULAR SURFACE OF HEAD OF CAPITATE

CARPOMETA-CARPAL JOINTS II-V

HEAD OF CAPITATE

LITTLE FINGER METACARPAL

INDEX METACARPAL BASE

THUMB METACARPAL (PA VIEW)

CARPOMETACARPAL JOINT - THUMB

TRAPEZIUM

CREST (TUBEROSITY) OF TRAPEZIUM

TUBEROSITY OF SCAPHOID

PISIFORM

WRIST JOINT

DISTAL RADIAL DIAPHYSIS

DISTAL RADIAL METAPHYSIS

DISTAL ULNAR ARTICULAR SURFACE

Figure 1-4 (Enlarged lateral radiograph of the wrist area showing the relationship of the carpus to the distal radius and to the metacarpals.) The longitudinal axes of the distal radius, lunate, capitate, and long finger metacarpal coincide with the normal wrist in neutral flexion and extension. Here, slight extension of the wrist causes some dorsal angulation of the wrist, centered in the lunate and head of the capitate, noted in line A–A′.

The palmar tilt of the distal radial articular surface is noted in line B–B′ and normally averages 10° to 12°.

The palmar inclination of the scaphoid with its proximal pole dorsal and its distal pole palmar is seen in line C–C′ and averages 45° to 50°. The angle determined by the intersection of the longitudinal axis of the lunate (line A–A′) and the longitudinal axis of the scaphoid (line C–C′) is normally 30° to 60° (average 47°). Carpal instability involving rotational instability of the scaphoid with or without dorsal rotational instability of the lunate increases this angle (see section Rotational Instability in Chapter 4). The palmar position of the trapezium in relation to the remainder of the carpus can be appreciated in this lateral view because of the normal palmar tilt of the scaphoid connecting the proximal and distal carpal rows. From proximal to distal, the synchronous curves of the distal radial articular surface, the proximal articular surface of the lunate, the proximal articular surface of the scaphoid, and the articular surface of the head of the capitate also can be appreciated. As noted previously in Figure 1-2, the lateral view of the wrist and hand depicts the PA view of the thumb metacarpal. The biconcave "double saddle" configuration of the thumb carpometacarpal joint can be well visualized by studying Figures 1-3 and 1-4.

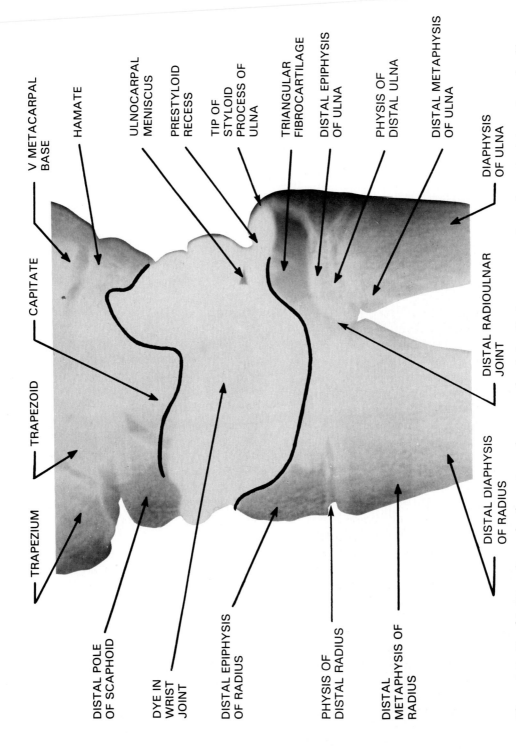

V METACARPAL BASE

HAMATE

ULNOCARPAL MENISCUS

PRESTYLOID RECESS

TIP OF STYLOID PROCESS OF ULNA

TRIANGULAR FIBROCARTILAGE

DISTAL EPIPHYSIS OF ULNA

PHYSIS OF DISTAL ULNA

DISTAL METAPHYSIS OF ULNA

DIAPHYSIS OF ULNA

CAPITATE

TRAPEZOID

TRAPEZIUM

DISTAL POLE OF SCAPHOID

DYE IN WRIST JOINT

DISTAL EPIPHYSIS OF RADIUS

PHYSIS OF DISTAL RADIUS

DISTAL METAPHYSIS OF RADIUS

DISTAL DIAPHYSIS OF RADIUS

DISTAL RADIOULNAR JOINT

Figure 1-5 On this PA radiograph of a wrist arthrogram of a skeletally immature patient, the wrist joint, triangular fibrocartilage, prestyloid recess, and ulnocarpal meniscus can be visualized. Only by such a study can the anatomy and interrelationship of these structures be appreciated. Clearly the distal ulna does not contribute to the wrist joint; the distal ulnar articular surface is in direct contact with the triangular fibrocartilage. The tip of the ulnar styloid process is seen within the prestyloid recess, whose proximal and distal boundaries are the triangular fibrocartilage and the ulnocarpal meniscus, respectively. The usual connection between the wrist joint and the prestyloid recess is well demonstrated. (Illustration courtesy of Julio Taleisnik, M.D.)

14

The hook of the hamate is the prominent palmar projection.

In the proximal carpal row the lunate, which is the only carpal that is larger palmarly than dorsally, provides a focal point owing to its articulation with the capitate head distally and with the radius proximally. Distally it also articulates with a small proximal portion of the hamate (an important functional consideration described in General Discussion in Chapter 4, Wrist Injuries). Radially and ulnarly it articulates with the scaphoid and the triquetrum, respectively.

The triquetrum completes the ulnar border of the proximal carpal row. It articulates radially and distally with the hamate and radially and proximally with the lunate.

The scaphoid is the most complex carpal bone, both in the motions at its various articulations and in its anatomic configuration. Interruption of its normal vascular supply may determine posttraumatic sequellae.[7] Distally it articulates with the trapezium and the trapezoid in a gliding-type motion. On its ulnar border distally it articulates with the capitate (as a portion of the socket which it forms with the distal lunate articular surface), and proximally, with the lunate, in a rotatory fashion. It articulates proximally with the radius, primarily in flexion and extension, but also in abduction and adduction and slight rotation. The scaphoid is the stable skeletal-connecting strut, or link, between the proximal and distal carpal rows. In this all-important function it is located in the most vulnerable area for injury, sustaining fractures far more frequently than any other carpal. The tubercule of the scaphoid lies just radial to, and acts as a pivoting point for, the tendon of the flexor carpi radialis. When viewed laterally on the radiograph, with the wrist in neutral position in regard to flexion and extension, the scaphoid is obliquely angulated in relation to the remainder of the carpus, at roughly 45° to 50°, palmarly from the dorsal position of its proximal pole to the palmar position of its distal pole.

The pisiform, though considered a carpal bone, is actually a sesamoid bone onto which the flexor carpi ulnaris tendon inserts. This is the only bone in the carpal configuration on which any tendon inserts. Distal ligamentous bands, including the pisohamate ligament and the pisometacarpal ligaments, tether the pisiform to the hamate and to the bases of the little and ring finger metacarpals, respectively.

The thick transverse carpal ligament which forms the superficial (palmar) boundary of the carpal canal is firmly inserted on four bony projections: radially it attaches to the tubercule of the scaphoid proximally and the crest of the trapezium distally, and ulnarly, to the pisiform proximally and the hook of the hamate distally.

Ligamentous Support of the Wrist (Figure 1-6)[4,5,8,9]

Because the ligamentous support of the wrist joint and carpus itself is so complex, only the basic anatomy will be discussed.

The carpus is literally suspended from the radius by ligaments radially and ulnarly (Figure 1-6). These ligaments, radially and palmarly (the palmar radiocarpal ligament) and ulnarly and dorsally (the ulnocarpal ligament complex), converge to attach primarily to the capitate, lunate, triquetrum, and scaphoid. The strongest ligaments are located on the palmar aspect and include the components of the palmar radiocarpal ligaments. There are two layers of these ligaments, but the superficial layer, though contributing somewhat to stability, is relatively unimportant. The deep layer is best seen from the interior of the joint surface and includes three definite structures: the radioscaphoid-capitate ligament, the radiolunate ligament, and the radioscaphoid-lunate ligament. The radioscaphoid-capitate ligament is most radial and has a weak central attachment to the concavity of the scaphoid. The radiolunate ligament is centrally located, and the radioscaphoid-lunate ligament is most ulnar. This latter ligament originates somewhat palmarly from the distal radial articular surface at the junction of the scaphoid and lunate facets and extends distally to attach to the scaphoid and the lunate at the proximal aspect of the radiocarpal joint.

The ulnocarpal complex completes the carpal suspension from the distal radius and includes the ulnocarpal meniscus, the triangular fibrocartilage, and the ulnolunate ligament. This complex structure actually originates from the ulnar aspect of the dorsal distal radius and should be considered functionally as a medial palmar radiocarpal ligamentous complex. The two most important ligamentous components of this complex include the triangular fibrocartilage and the ulnocarpal meniscus, or radiotriquetral ligament. Both these structures originate from a common origin on the dorsoulnar aspect of the distal radius. The triangular fibrocartilage, which is a strong, fibrous structure that runs parallel to the horizontal articular surface of the distal ulna, firmly joins the distal ulna

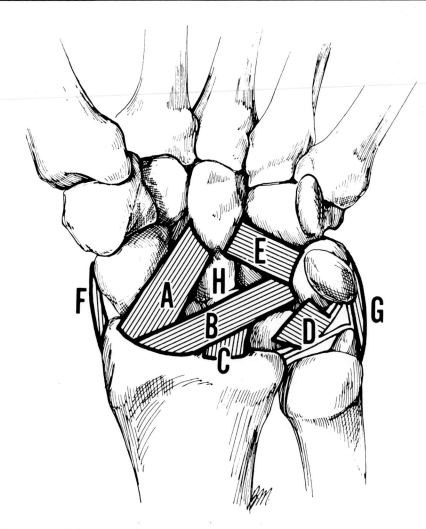

Figure 1-6 Palmar ligaments of the wrist. The major intracapsular ligaments on the palmar aspect of the wrist include: A. the radiocapitate or radioscaphocapitate ligament, B. the radiotriquetral or radiolunate-triquetral ligament, C. the radioscaphoid or radioscapholunate ligament, D. the ulnolunate ligament (originating from the meniscus), E. the capitotriquetral ligament, F. the radial collateral ligament, G. the ulnar collateral ligament, H. represents the space of Poirier, (Reprinted, by permission, from D.P. Green: Carpal Dislocations, in C.A. Rockwood Jr and D.P. Green (eds): *Fractures in Adults.* Philadelphia, J.B. Lippincott Co., 1984, vol 1, p 705).[8]

from the base of the ulnar styloid process to the distal radius and therefore separates the distal ulnar articular surface from the carpus. The ulnocarpal meniscus is a horizontal semilunar structure, distal and parallel to the triangular fibrocartilage, which swings palmarly around inside the joint capsule to insert deep on the ulnar aspect of the triquetrum. The ulnolunate ligament completes this complex and originates from the triangular fibrocartilage to insert on the lunate.

Though commonly referred to as important ligamentous structures, the radial and ulnar collateral ligaments are of only secondary importance. The radial collateral ligament is actually the radialmost portion of the superficial layer of the palmar radiocarpal ligament noted above. This ligament is actually more palmar than radial; it originates on the palmar margin of the radial styloid process and inserts onto the tuberosity of the scaphoid and walls of the flexor carpi radialis tunnel on the palmar aspect of the trapezium.

The ulnar collateral ligament is even less significant than the radial collateral ligament and is actually only a weak thickening of the joint capsule. It has little support value, originating on the ulnar aspect of the base of the ulnar styloid process and the wrist capsule and inserting on the triquetrum. It does not insert on the tip of the ulnar styloid process.

The dorsal ligaments of the wrist joint and carpus are much weaker than the palmar ligaments. The dorsal radiocarpal ligament originates from the radius and inserts on the lunate and triquetrum. It is weak over the proximal pole of the scaphoid and in the area of the capitate-lunate articulation. Some reinforcement is provided by the extensor tendon compartments.

Four carpal bones have particularly strong palmar intercarpal ligamentous attachments: the capitate, scaphoid, lunate, and triquetrum. V-shaped fibers originate from the radius, scaphoid, and triquetrum and converge distally to insert on the capitate. These fibers are referred to as the radiate, deltoid, or "V" ligament. If the central fibers of this ligament over the lunate are deficient or absent (space of Poirer-located palmar to the capitolunate joint) it is a V-shaped configuration comprising the radioscaphocapitate and the capitate triquetral ligaments and bounded proximally by the radiotriquetral ligament. If these fibers are present, the ligament is in a solid radiating or deltoid configuration.

A second "V" ligamentous configuration lies within the deltoid or "V" ligament. These fibers converge from the radius (radiolunate or radioscapholunate ligament) and from the triangular fibrocartilage (the ulnolunate ligament) to insert on the lunate.

Ligamentous attachments to the scaphoid involve three separate areas: the proximal pole, the distal pole and scaphoid tuberosity, and the central area of the scaphoid. Both the radioscaphoid-lunate ligament and the scapholunate interosseous ligaments (securing the scapholunate articulation) attach to the proximal pole of the scaphoid.

The radial collateral ligament attaches to the scaphoid tuberosity, and a portion of the deltoid or "V" ligament attaches to the distal pole connecting it to the capitate.

Centrally the deep radioscaphoid-capitate ligament forms a sling beneath the scaphoid, which is loosely attached. Therefore, rotatory subluxation of the scaphoid is impossible if both the radioscaphoid-lunate ligament and the radioscaphoid-capitate ligaments are intact.

Inserting at the base of the pisiform facet of the triquetrum are portions of the deltoid or "V" ligament (capitate-triquetral portion), the lunate-triquetral ligament from the lunate, the radio-triquetral ligament from the radius and the ulnocarpal meniscus from the dorsoulnar aspect of the distal radius.

All these strong ligamentous connections to these four carpals are located on the palmar aspect. Dorsal ligaments are present in these various areas but are much less defined and much less critical for carpal stability.

Midcarpal Joint

The midcarpal joint is located primarily between the scaphoid, lunate, and triquetrum in the proximal carpal row and the capitate and hamate in the distal row. However, it does extend radially between the distal scaphoid and the trapezium and trapezoid.

What must be remembered in any concept of intercarpal function is that *all bones of the entire distal carpal row are firmly bound together as a single functioning osseoligamentous structure.* There is no independent motion of any single bone in the distal carpal row. This distal row is intimately bound to the hand, particularly at the bases of the index and long metacarpals *(stable portion of the hand)*, and therefore "moves with the hand."

Skeletal stability of the carpus is afforded by the scaphoid, which integrates the motions of the proximal and distal carpal rows as a connecting skeletal strut. A stable scapholunate articulation with intact scapholunate interosseous, radioscaphoid-capitate, and radioscaphoid-lunate ligaments is necessary to provide scaphoid stability in this role.

The proximal carpal row acts as a middle link in a three-link system of the radius, the proximal carpal row, and the distal carpal row. The movements of the proximal carpal row are thus governed by the connecting link of the scaphoid, the longitudinal pressure of the hand centered at the head of the capitate in its articulation with the lunate and the scaphoid at this all-important joint, and by the distal radius.

Intercarpal Motion

Functionally the carpus can be divided into three relatively distinct areas:

1. The central flexion-extension area
2. The radial mobile area
3. The ulnar rotational area (as explained in Taleisnik's modification of the Navarro columnar theory)

The central flexion-extension area is comprised of the midcarpal joint and includes the entire distal carpal row and hand centered at the head of the capitate. In this area the midcarpal joint is a condyloid or ball-and-socket type configuration. This central joint of the head of the capitate articulating with the scaphoid and lunate is the focal point of intercarpal flexion and extension, radial and ulnar deviation, and rotation. However, since the entire distal carpal row acts in unison, the usual concept of the condyloid joint must be expanded. The capitate and the hamate form the "ball," and the proximal articulation of the "socket" is formed by the scaphoid, the lunate, and the triquetrum. This concept can be better appreciated in cases of congenital lack of segmentation of the capitate and hamate where this expanded view of the condyloid articulation is more evident (Figures 4-2, under Chapter 4, Wrist Injuries). Certainly there is a rotational component to the hamate-triquetral articulation which somewhat tethers the ulnar aspect of this expanded condyloid joint.

The radial mobile area includes only the scaphoid. The scaphoid forms an integral part of four separate and distinct functional articulations. Proximally it articulates with the distal radius, which involves radial and ulnar gliding, flexion and extension, and minimal rotation. Its ulnar articulation with the lunate allows some rotation, but normally the proximal scaphoid and the lunate function together as a single unit, flexing with radial deviation of the wrist and extending with ulnar deviation. The scaphoid must flex with radial deviation to prevent impingement of the scaphoid tuberosity on the styloid process of the radius. Although scaphoid and lunate flexion and extension are normally simultaneous, the arc of scaphoid motion is greater than that of the lunate. From neutral position to full extension, both the lunate and the scaphoid rotate approximately 30°. However, from neutral position to full flexion the lunate rotates 30°, and the scaphoid rotates approximately 60°. Therefore, some rotation must occur at the scapholunate articulation to account for this discrepancy. Medially there is a distinct rotation of the capitate head on the scaphoid in this condyloid articulation. Distally flexion and extension gliding of the combined trapezium and trapezoid occurs on the distal scaphoid articular surface. Because of significant motion occurring at both the trapezium-thumb metacarpal joint and at the scaphoid-trapezium joint, degenerative arthritic changes are prone to occur at these locations.

The strong radioscaphoid-capitate ligament loosely attached on the palmar aspect of the central scaphoid provides a strong sling which acts as a fulcrum on which the scaphoid rotates.

The ulnar area of rotation between the triquetrum and the hamate is also a portion of the expanded concept of the condyloid joint noted above.

In flexion and extension the proximal and distal carpal rows move in unison. In flexion the proximal carpal row and particularly the lunate slide dorsally to impinge on the dorsal articular lip of the distal radius. The converse occurs with extension.

It must be remembered that the distal carpal row always moves in the direction of the hand because of the intimate connections at the carpometacarpal joints, particularly the index and long fingers. With radial deviation of the hand the distal carpal row deviates radially; however, the proximal carpal row deviates ulnarly. Conversely, with ulnar deviation of the hand and the distal carpal row, the proximal carpal row deviates radially. These reciprocal motions appear to be produced by pressure of the capitate head as it slides on the lunate and also by flexion and extension of the scaphoid.

Wrist and Intercarpal Motion

Normally, wrist and midcarpal joint motions occur simultaneously and synergistically. Flexion, extension, abduction and adduction (radial and ulnar deviation), and rotation occur in both the wrist and midcarpal joints.

Extension and ulnar deviation are primarily functions of the wrist joint, whereas palmar flexion and radial deviation are primarily functions of the midcarpal joint. Though some rotation occurs at the midcarpal joint, it is primarily a function of the wrist joint. The prime plane of motion of the wrist and intercarpal joints is extension and radial deviation combined with flexion and ulnar deviation.

The prime wrist flexors and extensors travel across the wrist and midcarpal joints radially and ulnarly to the central point of the carpus (articulation of the head of the capitate with the scaphoid and lunate). The eccentric insertions of these strong motors work favorably in powerful lever actions for flexion and extension, and radial and ulnar deviation.

All the prime wrist flexors and extensors insert into the bases of metacarpals except for the flexor carpi ulnaris. The extensor carpi radialis longus inserts on the dorsal aspect of the index metacarpal base, the extensor carpi radialis brevis inserts primarily on the long finger metacarpal base dorsally, and the flexor carpi radialis inserts primarily on the palmar aspect of the index metacarpal base. Thus the stable portion of the hand is generously endowed with strong motor power. The extensor carpi ulnaris inserts on the dorsal aspect of the little finger metacarpal base, and the flexor carpi ulnaris is the only wrist motor which inserts into a carpal bone, the pisiform. Distal prolongations of this insertion, however, continue onto the bases of the little finger and ring finger metacarpals by the pisometacarpal ligaments and onto the hook of the hamate by the pisohamate ligament. The rather inconsequential palmaris longus tendon inserts primarily into the palmar fascia and also into the transverse carpal ligament.

Carpometacarpal Joints

In the carpometacarpal joint area there exist two of the most stable joints which permit no motion, the carpometacarpal joints of the index and long finger metacarpal bases; there are also two very mobile joints, the carpometacarpal joints of the thumb and the little finger.

The thumb metacarpal base articulates with the trapezium in a double saddle-shaped configuration which is the most mobile carpometacarpal joint (discussed under the Thumb in this chapter).

The trapezoid, as noted, is mortised into the base of the index metacarpal base, affording a very secure fixation. The radial aspect of the index metacarpal base articulates with the trapezium, and the ulnar aspect, with the capitate. Therefore, even if the entire trapezoid were excised, or traumatically avulsed, the base of the index metacarpal still remains fixed firmly to the distal carpal row (refer to Figure 4-34A under Chapter 4, Wrist Injuries).

The long finger metacarpal is firmly bound to the capitate and to the adjacent index finger metacarpal base. Therefore all the carpals in the distal carpal row and the index and long metacarpal bases are firmly joined and function together as a single osseoligamentous unit, the fixed stable portion of the hand.

The little finger metacarpal base articulates with the hamate in a saddlelike joint which somewhat resembles that of the thumb carpometacarpal joint but is not as mobile.

The ring finger metacarpal base articulates with the hamate, primarily in a joint similar to that of the little finger but with even less motion permitted. The radial aspect of its metacarpal base articulates with the capitate.

The mobile portion of the hand consists, therefore, of the radial and ulnar bordering digits, the thumb, and the little and ring fingers combined unit, respectively.

Functional Arches of the Hand

Structurally the hand and wrist conform to two basic physiologic functional arches which are both concave palmarly. These arches allow coordinated synergistic digital flexion and thumb-little finger opposition. Usually the distal phalanges flex toward the scaphoid tuberosity with digital flexion (index-little finger). Full thumb-little finger opposition usually achieves parallel pulp-to-pulp contact of the distal phalanges of these two digits.

The longitudinal arch (or arches, since each ray—digit with its corresponding metacarpal—and contiguous carpal forms its own separate arch) is centered about the metacarpophalangeal joints. The long finger ray and the capitate are the focal point.

The transverse arch originates basically at the central carpus and specifically at the capitate. The trapezium and trapezoid are located more palmarly than the capitate and hamate since they must articulate with the distal scaphoid, which is obliquely and palmarly oriented about 45°. The transverse arch radiates distally from this central carpal arch, flaring out in a cone shape which is open palmarly. The secondary transverse arch is located at the metacarpophalangeal joints and is centered specifically in the area of the index and long metacarpal heads. Though this distal transverse arch may be relatively flat when the hand is at rest, both strong thumb-little finger opposition and strong clenching of a fist best demonstrate its maximum curvature.

The functional anatomy of extrinsic digital flexors and extensors and intrinsic hand musculature will be discussed briefly. The ulnar nerve innervates the flexor carpi ulnaris and flexor digitorum profundus to the little and ring fingers and occasionally to the long finger. This nerve also innervates the hypothenar muscles; all the true intrinsic muscles of the hand (interossei and lumbricals), except for the first and second lumbricals; and the muscles of the thenar eminence which lie ulnar to the flexor pollicis longus tendon (adductor pollicis and the deep head of the flexor pollicis brevis). Strong grasp of the hand (e.g., grasping a hammer handle) is concentrated in the ulnar area of the hand; the combination of these powerful ulnar nerve-innervated extrinsic flexors and intrinsic hypothenar muscles physiologically coordinates with the mobile little and ring finger rays and synergistic wrist and intercarpal joint extension, with radial deviation and flexion, and with ulnar deviation.

The median nerve innervates extrinsic muscles used for power in grasping and intrinsic muscles of the hand concerned primarily with fine motion. These include the flexor carpi radialis, the flexor digitorum profundus to the index and long fingers, the flexor pollicis longus, the flexor digitorum superficialis, and those intrinsic muscles concerned with the extremely important function of thumb abduction and opposition (abductor pollicis brevis, opponens pollicis, and the superficial head of the flexor pollicis brevis), and the first and second lumbricals.

The radial nerve innervates the extensors, including the abductor pollicis longus, extensor pollicis brevis, extensor pollicis longus, extensor digitorum communis, extensor indicis proprius, extensor digiti minimi, and extensor carpi ulnaris.

Obviously, sensory innervation of the hand and fingers by median and ulnar nerves is indispensable for physiologic hand function, but radial nerve sensory innervation is usually insignificant.

The complex functions of the intrinsic muscles of the hand, including the interossei, lumbricals, and muscles contained in the thenar and hypothenar compartments, will be discussed in the section on the MP joint and also in the section on the MP joint of the thumb, both in this chapter. Basically the interossei abduct, and the palmar interossei adduct, the index, ring, and little fingers from the central pillar of the long finger metacarpal. They also flex the MP joints, extend the DIP joints, and aid in extension of the PIP joints. The lumbricals coordinate synergistic activity between the deep flexors (flexor digitorum profundi) and the extensor mechanisms. In addition, as components of the lateral bands they aid in DIP and PIP extension; they aid only questionably in MP flexion. The thenar and hypothenar intrinsic muscles act on the thumb and little finger, respectively.

Pathologic conditions may destroy the arches of the hand and cause severe functional disability by flattening the transverse arch and flattening or reversing the longitudinal arch. This results in loss of thumb and little finger opposition and flattening or recurvatum deformities at the MP joints with hyperflexion of the interphalangeal joints (e.g., combined median-ulnar nerve palsy).

The synergistic action of carpal, intercarpal, and digital motion permits maximum digital function. Digital flexion is synergistic with wrist and intercarpal extension; conversely, digital extension is synergistic with wrist and intercarpal flexion.

The extrinsic digital flexors and extensors are centrally oriented as they cross the wrist and intercarpal joints; therefore their influence on radial and ulnar deviation is minimal, except for those involved with the thumb, particularly the abductor pollicis longus, which can be an effective radial deviator in certain situations.

Digital Joints * (Figure 1-7)

Similarities of the Ligamentous Support of all Digital Joints. The ligamentous support of the MP, PIP, and DIP joints is basically similar. Each joint possesses two strong lateral collateral ligaments, two thin accessory collateral ligaments, and a thick, strong palmar plate. The lateral collateral and accessory collateral ligaments actually comprise a single inseparable structure; they are artificially designated as separate entities because of their discrete anatomic functions.

These structures suspend the base of each phalanx from a condyle or condyles of the more proximal bone at the articulation. The lateral collateral and accessory collateral ligaments attach to and form the lateral boundaries of the palmar plate at each joint. The palmar plate supports and forms an integral part of the flexor sheath at each joint level. The deep transverse intermetacarpal ligaments add substantial support to the palmar plates at the MP joints.

The behavior of the lateral collateral ligaments of the MP joint is different from that at both interphalangeal joints and is discussed specifically in relation to each joint.

Because of the more tenuous attachment of the palmar plate of the MP and DIP joints proximally, avulsion is more likely to occur at these areas. However, because of the two strong lateral check ligaments firmly attaching the PIP joint palmar plate proximally, avulsion or fracture avulsion of this joint occurs distally at the base of the middle phalanx.

Metacarpophalangeal Joint. The digital metacarpophalangeal joints are condyloid and primarily allow flexion and extension but also abduction, adduction, and some rotation. The average flexion is 90° to 95° but hyperextension of 20° to 30° and even as much

---

*The author thanks Richard G. Eaton, M.D., and J. William Littler, M.D., for much material included in the sections on anatomy of the digital and thumb joints.

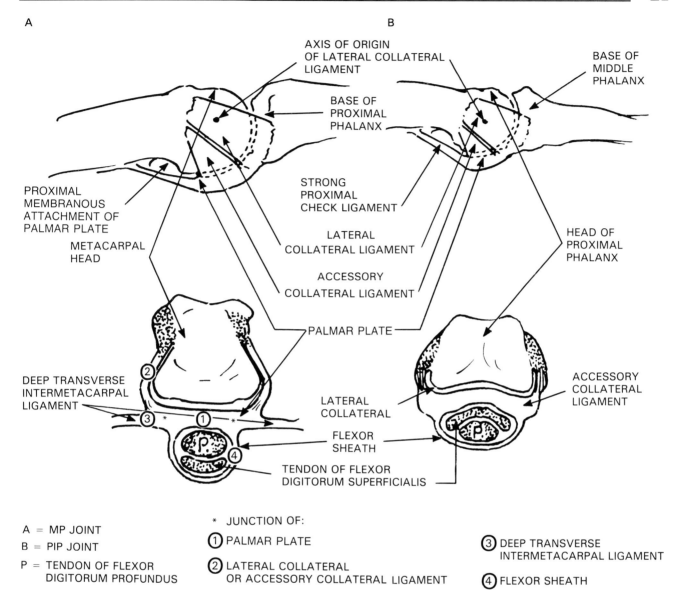

A
B

AXIS OF ORIGIN
OF LATERAL COLLATERAL
LIGAMENT

BASE OF
MIDDLE
PHALANX

BASE OF
PROXIMAL
PHALANX

STRONG
PROXIMAL
CHECK LIGAMENT

PROXIMAL
MEMBRANOUS
ATTACHMENT OF
PALMAR PLATE

METACARPAL
HEAD

LATERAL
COLLATERAL LIGAMENT

ACCESSORY
COLLATERAL LIGAMENT

HEAD OF
PROXIMAL
PHALANX

PALMAR PLATE

DEEP TRANSVERSE
INTERMETACARPAL
LIGAMENT

ACCESSORY
COLLATERAL
LIGAMENT

LATERAL
COLLATERAL

FLEXOR
SHEATH

TENDON OF FLEXOR
DIGITORUM SUPERFICIALIS

A = MP JOINT
B = PIP JOINT
P = TENDON OF FLEXOR
    DIGITORUM PROFUNDUS

* JUNCTION OF:
① PALMAR PLATE
② LATERAL COLLATERAL
  OR ACCESSORY COLLATERAL LIGAMENT

③ DEEP TRANSVERSE
  INTERMETACARPAL LIGAMENT
④ FLEXOR SHEATH

Figure 1-7 Diagrammatic representation of the ligamentous support of the metacarpophalangeal (MP) joint, A, compared to that of the proximal interphalangeal (PIP) joint, B.

The general format of the ligaments is similar, except that in the MP joint the deep transverse intermetacarpal ligaments are seen on each side in direct continuity with the palmar plate, the lateral collateral ligaments, the accessory collateral ligaments, and the flexor sheath. The lateral view of both joints illustrates the lateral collateral ligament superiorly and the accessory collateral ligament inferiorly. In A, the origin of the lateral collateral ligament is seen to be dorsal and eccentric to the arc of motion of the metacarpal condyle, whereas in B, the lateral collateral ligament origin is centered on the axis of rotation of the proximal phalangeal head.

In the cross-sectional views a contrast is seen between the articular surface of the metacarpal head and that of the proximal phalangeal head: the metacarpal head is seen to flare out palmarly rather significantly, whereas the proximal phalangeal condyles flare minimally.

In both joints the palmar plate and the flexor tendons within the flexor sheath are suspended from the condyles of the proximal bone of each joint by the accessory collateral ligaments.

The more tenuous proximal attachment of the MP joint palmar plate is seen in comparison to the two strong check ligaments of the PIP joint. (Reprinted, by permission, from Richard G. Eaton, M.D. and J. William Littler, M.D., *Joint Injuries of the Hand*, Fig. 6, 1971, Springfield, Ill., Charles C Thomas, Publisher.)

as 45° is common. The articular surface of the metacarpal head is rounded dorsally and rather flat palmarly and presents a greater surface area inferiorly. The metacarpal head also flares out from the dorsal to the palmar aspect. The articular surface of the proximal phalangeal base is concave to fit the convex metacarpal head congruously.

As mentioned previously, the primary ligament support of the MP joint includes two lateral collateral ligaments, two accessory collateral ligaments, and the palmar plate.

Each collateral ligament originates dorsally on the lateral aspect of the metacarpal head dorsal to the flexion-extension axis of the MP joint. It travels obliquely across that joint and inserts on the palmar aspect of the proximal phalangeal base and into the distal portion of the palmar plate laterally.

Each accessory collateral ligament originates from the metacarpal head near the axis of extension-flexion inferior to the origin of the lateral collateral ligament. It is flat and thin and flares out in a fan shape to insert on the lateral border of the palmar plate and also blends into the deep transverse intermetacarpal ligament, which, in turn, is continuous with the flexor sheath inferiorly.

The palmar plate is a thick, tough structure distally at its insertion on the base of the proximal phalanx. Proximally it thins out to become nearly membranous at its metacarpal attachment. This thin proximal portion folds in like the bellows of an accordian or a telephone booth door as the MP joint flexes. Hyperextension of the MP joint is possible because the thin proximal portion of the palmar plate stretches. Distally and laterally the palmar plate on both sides is attached to a lateral collateral ligament, and in its midportion laterally, to an accessory collateral ligament. The adjacent lateral borders of the index, long, ring, and little finger palmar plates are connected by the deep transverse metacarpal ligaments. Therefore the proximal phalanx is suspended by the palmar plate, the lateral collateral ligaments, the accessory collateral ligaments, and the deep transverse metacarpal ligaments.

The MP joint is most stable in maximal flexion since the lateral collateral ligaments are stretched tautly in this position. The eccentric origin of the collateral ligament dorsal to the flexion-extension axis, the broader, flatter palmar surface of the metacarpal head, and the bilateral flaring of the metacarpal head palmarly all contribute to this effect of collateral ligament stretching. Particularly in flexion the accessory collateral ligaments offer additional stability by firmly holding the palmar plate against the palmar surface of the metacarpal head.

In extension the lateral collateral ligaments are lax and the MP joint is relatively mobile, permitting ulnar and radial deviation and some rotation by the intrinsic muscles.

Extrinsic support of the MP joint includes the deep transverse metacarpal ligaments, tendons of the long flexors (flexor digitorum profundus and superficialis), the common extensor tendons, the proper extensors to the index and little fingers, and ramifications of the intrinsic muscles.

There are three deep transverse metacarpal ligaments which connect the adjacent lateral aspects of the palmar plates of the index, long, ring, and little finger MP joints. Since these ligaments actually insert into the palmar plates, they might be better called interpalmar plate ligaments rather than metacarpal ligaments. These ligaments are also intimately associated with both the lateral collateral ligaments and the accessory collateral ligaments of the MP joints as well as the flexor sheaths.

A portion of the first dorsal interosseous tendon of insertion, on the radial aspect of the index finger MP joint palmar plate, and of the abductor digiti minimi tendon, on the ulnar aspect of the little finger MP joint palmar plate, help stabilize the exposed areas of these marginal rays, which are devoid of the deep transverse metacarpal ligamentous support.

The common extensors have a limited insertion on the periosteum of the base of the proximal phalanges or into the dorsal capsule of the MP joints. The proper extensor tendons to the index finger (extensor indicis proprius) and to the little finger (extensor digiti minimi) travel ulnar to their appropriate common extensor tendons. They have a similar variable insertion and provide particularly independent extension of those two digits. The sagittal bands of the extensor apparatus extend from the extensor digitorum communis (and proprius of the index and little fingers) to the palmar plate on each side at the MP joint level and therefore secure the extensor tendon(s) dorsally in the midline.

At the level of the MP joint the profundus tendon is just commencing to enter the decussation of the superficialis tendon in the flexor sheath, which itself is firmly bound to, and is actually an integral portion of, the palmar plate. Tendon support from the intrinsic muscles includes that of the lumbricals and the interossei as well as the abductor digiti minimi and flexor digiti minimi.

Each lumbrical muscle originates from its profundus tendon in the palm, travels through the lumbrical canal radial to its MP joint and palmar to the deep transverse metacarpal ligament, which acts as a fulcrum. Each lumbrical inserts into the radial aspect of the lateral band of the extensor apparatus of its particular digit.

The four dorsal interossei insert variably into bone, ligamentous structures, and the extensor apparatus. The first dorsal interosseous inserts virtually completely onto the radial aspect of the index finger proximal phalangeal base and into the palmar plate. A very few fibers continue and insert into the radial aspect of the extensor apparatus. The second dorsal interosseous inserts roughly 60% onto the radial aspect of the long finger proximal phalangeal base and 40% into the extensor apparatus. The third dorsal interosseous inserts nearly completely into the ulnar aspect of the long finger extensor apparatus, with only a few fibers inserting onto the ulnar aspect of the proximal phalangeal base. The fourth dorsal interosseous inserts about 40% onto the ulnar aspect of the ring finger proximal phalangeal base and 60% into the extensor apparatus.

The three palmar interosseous muscles insert into the extensor apparatus of three digits. The first interosseous inserts into the ulnar aspect of the index finger; the second, into the radial aspect of the ring finger; and the third, into the radial aspect of the little finger.

The abductor digiti minimi inserts into the ulnar aspect of the little finger MP joint palmar plate and onto the ulnar aspect of the proximal phalangeal base; it contributes some fibers into the extensor apparatus also. Therefore, this muscle tendon unit actually performs functionally as a fifth dorsal interosseous muscle.

The flexor digiti minimi joins the abductor in a common insertion onto the ulnar aspect of the proximal phalangeal base of the little finger and into the palmar plate. This muscle does not contribute fibers to the extensor apparatus.

The primary function of the interossei (both dorsal and palmar) and the abductor digiti minimi, via the lateral bands, is to flex the MP joints and, aided by the lumbricals, to extend the DIP joints. By contributions from the lateral bands to the central extensor tendons these same muscles aid in extending the PIP joints. (It is questionable whether the lumbricals actively aid the MP flexion.)

In addition, the dorsal interossei and the abductor digiti minimi abduct the index, ring, and little fingers from the central long finger, and the palmar interossei adduct these same digits toward that central ray.

Proximal Interphalangeal Joint. The proximal interphalangeal joint is a ginglymus or hinge-type joint. It has the greatest range of flexion and extension of any digital joint, with an average of 105°. The head of the proximal phalanx, divided into two condyles separated by a cleft, fits the contiguous articular surface of the middle phalangeal base and articulates in a tongue-in-groove configuration. The base of the middle phalanx is 10% wider transversely than the condyles of the opposing proximal phalanx.

The intrinsic ligamentous support of the PIP joint resembles that of the MP joint in general and includes two lateral collateral ligaments, two accessory collateral ligaments, and a palmar plate. The PIP joint collateral ligaments, however, are broad and stout and originate from an indentation on the lateral aspect of the proximal phalangeal condyle approximately on the flexion-extension axis. Each ligament runs obliquely to insert on the palmar aspect of the middle phalangeal base and the lateral margins of the distal aspect of the palmar plate. Thus it must diverge laterally and distally because of the wider transverse diameter of the middle phalangeal base.

The fibers of the lateral collateral ligaments are parallel, but the dorsal and palmar portions function differently. In flexion the entire collateral ligament is taut; in extension only the palmar portion and the palmar plate are taut.

The accessory collateral ligaments originate in the area of the condylar origin of the collateral ligaments, are triangular in shape, and flare out palmarly. Each inserts into the lateral aspect of the palmar plate and is continuous with the lateral collateral ligament to complete both lateral walls of the proximal interphalangeal joint capsule.

The palmar plate is thick distally at its insertion on the palmar base of the middle phalanx and proximally projects as two very strong check ligaments laterally, which attach to the lateral-palmar aspects of the proximal phalanx. Centrally the proximal border of the palmar plate is a free edge, enabling the palmar synovial pouch to protrude through this area. These check ligaments are formed by reflected fibers from the dorsal portion of the flexor sheath, the horizontal reflection of the accessory collateral ligaments insertion, and the lateral margin of the palmar plate, all contributing their inherent strength.

Because of the strength of the palmar plate, including its broad, thick distal insertion and its two strong proximal lateral check ligaments, little hyperextension of this joint is possible in contrast to the MP joint. The palmar plate (and the flexor sheath beneath) is suspended bilaterally by the collateral and accessory collateral ligaments.

In complete flexion the base of the middle phalanx impinges on the area immediately behind the condyles (retrocondylar recess) of the proximal phalanx. This, plus the tongue-in-groove configuration of the joint and the fact that the entire collateral ligament is taut in complete flexion, insures PIP joint stability in that attitude.

Extrinsic or extracapsular support is provided dorsally, palmarly, and bilaterally. Dorsally the extensor apparatus is composed of the common extensor tendon (augmented by the proper extensor in the index and little fingers) and fibers from the lumbrical and interosseous muscles. The conjoined lateral bands dorsal to the PIP joint are stabilized by the transverse retinacular ligaments which attach to the flexor sheath bilaterally. The transverse retinacular ligaments function at the PIP joint as the sagittal bands function at the MP joint. The flexor digitorum superficialis is deep to the flexor digitorum profundus tendon in the flexor sheath palmarly at this level, and bilaterally the oblique retinacular ligaments and the lateral bands offer support.

The flexor digitorum superficialis tendon inserts several millimeters distal to the insertion of the palmar plate on the middle phalanx. This insertion extends distally to the distal third of that phalanx. Because of this extensive insertion, the superficialis tendon exerts excellent leverage action for powerful PIP joint flexion; also, because of its insertion somewhat distal to the palmar plate insertion, it does not impinge upon that joint in maximum flexion.

Distal Interphalangeal Joint. The distal interphalangeal joint resembles the proximal interphalangeal joint in function and in ligamentous support.

The middle phalangeal head possesses two condyles separated by a shallow cleft and, as in the PIP joint, there is essentially the same amount of articular surface in contact in both flexion and extension.

DIP joint flexion rarely exceeds 80°, but hyperextension is greater than at the PIP joint because the DIP joint palmar plate does not possess the two strong check ligaments proximally. Extrinsic support includes the tendon insertions of the common extensor

(primarily the lateral bands) and the flexor digitorum profundus on the distal phalanx.

The flexor digitorum profundus tendon inserts just distal to the insertion of the palmar plate on the distal phalanx and therefore has less power for leverage action on the DIP joint than the superficial flexor exerts on the PIP joint. The profundus tendon also has a much less extensive insertion on the distal phalanx than the superficialis tendon has on the middle phalanx. Because of the proximity of the profundus tendon insertion to the palmar plate insertion on the distal phalanx, DIP joint flexion is somewhat hindered by the tendon mass.

The extensor tendon (composed primarily of the lateral bands) inserts on the dorsal aspect of the distal phalangeal base and is intimately associated with the articular cartilage there.

The Thumb

Carpometacarpal Joint. Since the trapezium is firmly bound to the trapezoid and indeed to the entire distal carpal row, it has virtually no independent motion. In contrast, the carpometacarpal joint or trapezium-thumb metacarpal joint is a very mobile articulation. Though described as a saddle-type joint, it is actually a reciprocally biconcave joint resembling two saddles whose concave surfaces are opposed to each other at right angles, or 90° rotation. All motions are possible, including abduction, adduction, flexion, extension, and the combination of these motions, circumduction. This wide range of motion at a joint which is subjected to the stresses of repetitive thumb pinch makes it particularly susceptible to the changes of degenerative and posttraumatic arthritis.

The strongest carpometacarpal joint ligament is the deep ulnar or anterior oblique carpometacarpal ligament connecting the palmar beak of the thumb metacarpal to the deep intercarpal ligaments and the crest of the trapezium. This ligament is lax on joint flexion and taut on hyperextension. The corresponding radial or posterior oblique carpometacarpal ligament is a much weaker structure, and therefore stability on the dorsal aspect of the joint is not great, despite added strength provided by the insertion of the abductor pollicis longus tendon and the passage of the extensor pollicis brevis tendon.

Additional extrinsic support is provided by the extensor pollicis longus tendon dorsally, the flexor pollicis longus tendon palmarly, and the origins of the thenar muscles palmarly, including the abductor pollicis brevis, the flexor pollicis brevis, and the adductor pollicis.

Metacarpophalangeal Joint. The metacarpophalangeal joint of the thumb is a semicondyloid type articulation which permits flexion, extension, abduction, adduction, and limited rotation. Flexion ranges from 5° to 100°, with an average of about 75°. The degree of flexion depends upon the anatomic configuration of the single broad condyle of the metacarpal head. If the head is round (the majority of cases), 90° to 100° of flexion is achieved. If it is flat (about 10% to 15% of cases), little flexion is possible, and the MP joint actually "opens like a book" on the dorsal aspect rather than as a gliding of the joint surfaces.[6]

Intrinsic ligament support includes two collateral ligaments, two accessory collateral ligaments, and the palmar plate. Each lateral collateral ligament arises from the midpoint of the metacarpal head and travels palmarly, obliquely, and distally to insert on the palmar-lateral side of the proximal phalangeal base and to the distal-lateral aspect of the palmar plate. Each accessory collateral ligament originates palmar to the lateral collateral ligament origin from the metacarpal head, fans out, and inserts laterally into the palmar plate at the level of the sesamoids.

The palmar plate is a broad, thick ligamentous structure inserting on the base of the proximal phalanx, which is thinner at its proximal metacarpal attachment. Two sesamoid bones, lateral and medial, are incorporated within the distal third of the palmar plate at the level of the accessory collateral ligament insertions.

Both extrinsic and intrinsic tendons add external support to the joint. The extrinsic tendons include the extensor pollicis longus and brevis on the dorsal aspect and the flexor pollicis longus on the palmar aspect. The extensor pollicis longus tendon inserts partially into the capsule of the MP joint and/or the periosteum of the base of the proximal phalanx, but the majority of the tendon runs distally to insert on the base of the distal phalanx. The extensor pollicis brevis runs parallel and on the radial aspect of the extensor pollicis longus to insert primarily into the base of the proximal phalanx but contributes some fibers which travel with the extensor pollicis longus to insert on the distal phalanx. The flexor pollicis longus runs in its sheath, which is intimately associated with the palmar plate on its palmar aspect, and continues distally to insert on the base of the distal phalanx.

The intrinsic muscles contributing to MP joint support include the adductor pollicis, the abductor pollicis brevis, and the flexor pollicis brevis. The opponens pollicis has no influence on the MP joint.

The adductor pollicis tendon inserts into the medial or ulnar sesamoid and the proximal phalangeal base, contributing fibers to the extensor apparatus.

The abductor pollicis brevis inserts into the lateral capsule and into the extensor apparatus.

The flexor pollicis brevis inserts into the lateral or radial sesamoid and into the base of the proximal phalanx.

Therefore, through their insertions into the extensor apparatus of the thumb, both the adductor pollicis and abductor pollicis brevis act as lateral bands and function in the thumb similarly to the function of the lateral bands at the PIP joint levels of all the other digits.[10] These lateral bands of the thenar intrinsics obliquely cross the MP joint dorsal to the flexor-extensor axis to insert into the extensor apparatus; they therefore aid the extensor pollicis brevis and extensor pollicis longus to extend the proximal phalanx at the MP joint and the distal phalanx at the IP joint. If palmar migration of these lateral bands occurs (e.g., rheumatoid arthritis), a boutonniere deformity of the thumb results with flexion (inability to extend) of the MP joint and hyperextension of the IP joint.

Without this intrinsic dynamic thenar muscle support for the thumb MP joint, significant chronic collateral ligament attenuation and weakening occurs. An example of this occurs in ulnar nerve palsy in which the adductor pollicis and deep head of the flexor pollicis brevis muscles cannot function. The ulnar collateral ligament of the MP joint attenuates due to repetitive pinch between the ulnar aspect of the thumb distal phalanx and adjacent digits.

Interphalangeal Joint. The interphalangeal joint of the thumb is a hinge-type joint which permits little motion other than flexion and extension. The broad head of the proximal phalanx distal articular surface possesses two condyles which articulate synchronously with two concave surfaces on the base of the distal phalanx.

The intrinsic ligament structure of this joint is similar to that of the MP joint. The lateral collateral ligaments, however, are shorter and thicker and not as obliquely oriented.

The palmar plate is essentially similar to that of the MP joint, and stability of the IP joint is augmented by the broad insertions of the extensor pollicis longus and flexor pollicis longus onto the distal phalangeal base.

References

1. Snow JW, Switzer H: Method of studying the relationships between the finger joints and the flexor and extensor mechanisms. *Plast Reconstr Surg* 1975;55:242–243.
2. Johnson RK, Shrewsbury MM: The pronator quadratus in motions and in stabilization of the radius and ulna at the distal radioulnar joint. *J Hand Surg* 1976;1:205–209.
3. Lewis OJ, Hamshere RJ, Bucknill TM: The anatomy of the wrist joint. *J Anat* 1970; 106:539–552.
4. Taleisnik J: The ligaments of the wrist. *J Hand Surg* 1976;1:110–118.
5. Taleisnik J: Wrist: Anatomy, function and injury, in *AAOS Instructional Course Lectures.* St. Louis, C.V. Mosby Co., 1978, vol 27, pp 61–87.
6. Coonrad RW, Goldner JL: A study of the pathological findings and treatment in soft-tissue injury of the thumb metacarpophalangeal joint. *J Bone Joint Surg (Am)* 1968;50-A(3):439–451.
7. Taleisnik J, Kelly P: The extraosseous and intraosseous blood supply of the scaphoid bone. *J Bone Joint Surg (Am)* 1966;48:1125–1137.
8. Green DP: Carpal dislocations, in Rockwood CA Jr, Green DP (eds): *Fractures in Adults.* Philadelphia, J.B. Lippincott Co., 1984, vol 1, pp 703–742.
9. Mayfield JK, Johnson RP, Kilcoyne RF: The ligaments of the human wrist and their functional significance. *Anat Rec* 1976;186:417–428.
10. McFarlane RM: Observations on the functional anatomy of the intrinsic muscles of the thumb. *J Bone Joint Surg* 1962;44-A:1073–1088.

General References

Basmajian JV: *Grant's Method of Anatomy,* ed 10. Baltimore, Williams and Wilkins, 1980.
Gelberman RH, Menon J: The vascularity of the scaphoid bone. *J Hand Surg* 1980;5(5):508–513.
Hollinshead WH: *Anatomy for Surgeons: Volume 3 The Back and Limbs,* ed 3. New York, Harper Medical, 1982.
Spinner M: *Kaplan's Functional and Surgical Anatomy of the Hand,* ed 3. Philadelphia, J.B. Lippincott Co., 1984.

CHAPTER 2

General Principles of Management

Radiographic Evaluation

Accurate radiographic documentation and evaluation is imperative for a definitive diagnosis prior to treatment of a fracture or dislocation. Multiple views centered on the area of injury, localized by symptoms and physical examination, are often necessary for accurate diagnosis.

In addition to the routine posterior-anterior (PA) and lateral films (Figures 1-1 through 1-4), diagnosis may be aided by two oblique views and perhaps other special ones, particularly in cases of wrist injuries (e.g., scaphoid and carpal tunnel views). Special procedures such as laminagraphy and polydirectional computerized tomography occasionally may be of assistance in evaluating carpal injuries, especially fractures of the lunate. Supplementary radiographs of the injured wrist with the application of distraction forces also may be helpful.

It should be remembered that the apparent space seen on radiographs between articular surfaces at a joint is not a true space but is occupied by the articular cartilage overlying the involved bones. Comparison of the cartilage space of the involved joint to adjacent normal joints and to the comparable joint of the contralateral extremity may be helpful.

There are two important considerations in the skeletally immature patient: the presence of physes (epiphyseal growth plates) in the digital long bones and the different times of ossification of the carpal bones.

Physes are located proximally in all the phalanges and distally in all the metacarpals except the thumb, where it is located proximally. These epiphyseal growth plates become obvious with ossification of the epiphyses of the long bones beginning at the second or third year of life. The epiphyses become fused to the diaphyses in the 17th to 19th year and obliterate the physes. Either the thumb or index metacarpal, or both, and occasionally the remaining metacarpals, may possess proximal and distal physes (refer to figure 2-11).

Ossification of the individual carpal bones occurs differently for each specific bone in a fairly predictable time sequence and order. The capitate is the first to ossify at age six months to one year. The hamate ossifies at approximately the same time. Progressive ossification of the other carpals occurs in a spiral fashion from the ulnar aspect to the radial aspect of the proximal carpal row, then the radial aspect of the distal carpal row, and finally the pisiform.

The triquetrum ossifies at age 2 to 3 years, the lunate at about 4 years, the scaphoid at 5 years, the trapezium at 6 years, the trapezoid at 6 to 7 years, and the pisiform at 12 years of age.

Occasionally extra ossicles are found in the carpus; the most frequent is the os styloideum which is located between the capitate and trapezoid and may be likened to a styloid process of the long finger metacarpal base. The next most frequently occurring extra ossicle is the paratrapezium located between the trapezium and the thumb metacarpal on the radial aspect of the trapezium. This extra ossicle is integrated into the carpometacarpal joint of the thumb.

Probably the most frequently and usually erroneously diagnosed wrist abnormality is a bipartite scaphoid. This abnormality is actually quite rare, and the vast majority of such diagnoses in reality represent old fractures of the scaphoid (see section on Scaphoid Fractures in Chapter 4, Wrist Injuries).

If congenital variances or abnormalities are found on radiographic examination of the wrist, the contralateral "normal" wrist should also be examined by radiograph. Often such variations are present bilaterally.

The clinical differentiation between an acute or old fracture and a congenital variant in carpal anatomy is obviously important. Symptoms and physical findings usually are not helpful for differentiation except that the patient with an acute fracture generally has more symptoms and exhibits tenderness to gentle palpation.

A congenital variation has rounded contours and normal-appearing joints between adjacent bones. In contrast, an acute fracture is seen as a sharp linear or comminuted separation with little similarity to a joint. An old fracture exhibits a widened space due to bone resorption but does not usually resemble a normal joint. The opposing bone surfaces do not show the distinct linear or comminuted findings of an acute fracture, nor do they show the gently rounded contours of the congenital abnormality. A major aid in the diagnosis of an old fracture is the finding of post-traumatic arthritic changes in adjacent joints often accompanied by hypertrophic osteophytic formations (see section Scaphoid Fractures in Chapter 4, Wrist Injuries).

Carpal coalition, or actually lack of segmentation of a portion of the carpus, is often found associated with various obvious congenital abnormalities—complex syndactyly, central defect of the hand, radial hemimelia (radial club hand)—but is rarely found in the "normal" hand and then only as an incidental finding.

The most common lack of segmentation is between the triquetrum and the lunate (the lunequate figure 4-3), but isolated abnormalities in segmentation have been noted between almost all the carpals.

Multiple radiographic views are usually necessary for accurate diagnosis of these rare abnormalities. Isolated carpal lack of segmentation generally involves two bones in the same carpal row (proximal or distal carpal row), and function is not impaired.

If symptoms and the findings of physical examination indicate skeletal trauma, then appropriate conservative immobilization should be carried out despite initial negative radiographs. Repeat radiographs after 10 to 14 days or sometimes three weeks will usually disclose a fracture line following bone resorption (see section on errors and complications in this chapter and section Scaphoid Fractures in Chapter 4, Wrist Injuries).

Postreduction radiographs are essential prior to cast immobilization, particularly in wrist injuries. A residual scapholunate dissociation must always be suspected after successful closed reduction of a dorsal perilunate dislocation or subluxation and a palmar lunate dislocation or subluxation. Details of a scapholunate dissociation or rotatory instability of the wrist may be obscured if radiographs are taken through plaster immobilization, thus delaying early recognition and treatment of this lesion.

Follow-up radiographic evaluation is necessary at periodic intervals, particularly with undisplaced or reduced articular fractures, in order to diagnose possible position loss early enough to provide proper treatment to prevent malunion and irreversible joint changes.

Periodic radiographic evaluation is also necessary to be certain that satisfactory reduction is maintained at a fracture site which is inherently unstable.

Radiographs of diaphyseal fractures of the long bones (metacarpals and phalanges) are taken to check the position at the fracture site rather than to determine the amount of callus formation which is insignificant in these areas of predominantly cortical bone.

Radiographic reevaluation after reduction of a joint subluxation or dislocation is imperative to diagnose redislocation or resubluxation if instability is suspected.

In general, new radiographic studies should be performed for an injury in a patient initially treated elsewhere and referred for consultation. Even if the patient brings recent radiographs, the accurate status of the injury at the precise time of consultation and evaluation can only be verified by new studies.

Xerography generally provides no additional information about skeletal trauma. However, this procedure is helpful in visualizing details of bone structure, particularly in the arthritides (e.g., rheumatoid arthritis) and to reveal foreign bodies in soft tissue.

It is strongly recommended that every opportunity be taken to study in detail radiographs of normal wrists. One should have readily available a series of normal wrist radiographs for comparison with current cases of trauma. There is no substitute for a good understanding of normal anatomy, especially in the complex area of the wrist.

Anesthesia

To permit pain-free manipulation for definitive reduction of a fracture or dislocation, adequate anesthesia usually must be provided. Prior to anesthesia, however, accurate evaluation of sensory and motor innervation, vascular status, and musculotendinous function distal to the site of injury should be determined and recorded as accurately as possible, even though such determinations may be difficult because of patient anxiety or pain.

The type of anesthesia used depends on the area of injury, the physician's preference, and the particular patient. Anesthesia of the peripheral nerves may be performed in the area of the brachial plexus, in the large major nerves themselves (median, ulnar, and radial), or peripherally in the individual common and proper digital nerves of the distal palm. Local infiltrative anesthesia may be preferred in some areas, particularly in the dorsum of the hand. Injection of an anesthetic into a fracture hematoma, particularly in fractures involving the distal radial metaphysis (Colles' and Smith's fractures), is effective. Intravenous regional anesthesia (Bier's block) is an excellent alternative with certain restrictions. Finally, general anesthesia may be preferred in certain cases of massive trauma, and in infants and children.

Peripheral Nerve Block

The easiest and most effective form of anesthesia for digital fractures and dislocations, particularly acute fingertip injuries, is to block the common and proper

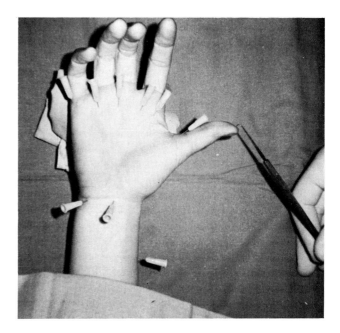

Figure 2-1 No. 25 needles placed in palm of hand and palmar aspect of wrist illustrate good locations at which to anesthetize peripheral nerves. Note injection sites for palmar proper digital nerves to radial aspect of index finger and to ulnar aspect of little finger. Also note site at which to block both proper digital nerves to thumb.

palmar digital nerves, augmented by infiltrative dorsal anesthesia (Figure 2-1). From 2.5 to 5.0 ml of 1.5% to 2.0% lidocaine is injected with a No. 25 short needle at a point approximately midway between the distal palmar flexion crease and the web between the proximal phalanges. The needle is angled proximally. At this level the two proper digital nerves have bifurcated from the common palmar digital nerve and anesthesia of all three structures is achieved. (Care should be taken to note accurately the anatomic course of the two proper digital nerves to the thumb, the proper digital nerve to the radial aspect of the index finger, and the proper digital nerve to the ulnar aspect of the little finger.) Two such injections must be performed to block the palmar aspect of each individual digit. Anesthesia of the entire digit is completed by dorsal infiltrative anesthesia, achieved by subcutaneous injection in a proximally radiating fashion in the area of the metacarpophalangeal (MP) joints (Figure 2-2).

In order to avoid possible irreversible ischemia, epinephrine should never be used in any injection distal to the wrist. This is particularly important in digits which have already suffered the insult of severe traumatic ischemia.

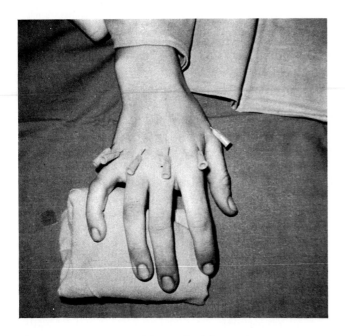

Figure 2-2 An acceptable method for performing dorsal infiltrative anesthesia for dorsum of hand and digits. In this area peripheral sensory branches are too small for individual nerve block type anesthesia. Again, note proximal direction of needles.

Anesthetic block within a digit itself—particularly in conjunction with a circumferential, rubber band type hemostatic tourniquet at the base of the digit—is not recommended. The additional insult of an anesthetic agent, regardless of the amount injected into the digit, can occlude vessels in the constricted area beneath Cleland's ligament and result in peripheral ischemia. This "digital block" anesthesia may result in irreversible ischemic changes, especially in the severely damaged digit which has already sustained impaired vascularity in the initial trauma.

Peripheral nerve block of the median, ulnar, and radial nerves provides excellent anesthesia for larger areas. Such peripheral nerve blocks also may be used to potentiate incomplete nerve blocks of the brachial plexus.

Injection of 5 to 10 ml of 1.5% to 2.0% lidocaine will anesthetize the ulnar nerve at the elbow just anterior to the olecranon process and posterior to the medial epicondyle of the humerus, where it is easily palpated.

Excellent anesthesia for the median and radial nerves can be performed at the wrist in similar fashion. The median nerve is anesthetized on the palmar aspect of the wrist just ulnar to the flexor carpi radialis tendon of insertion and just at the radialmost aspect of the palmaris longus tendon insertion (if that latter tendon is present) in the area of the wrist-flexion crease. The radial nerve is blocked approximately four finger breadths proximal to the radial styloid process on the radial aspect of the distal radius, where it can be palpated.

Blocking the ulnar nerve at the wrist is excellent, but the dorsal cutaneous branch of the ulnar nerve must also be blocked dorsally at the base of the little finger metacarpal and the carpo-metacarpal joint. This cutaneous branch of the ulnar nerve originates roughly at the junction of the middle and distal thirds of the forearm and provides sensation to the major portion of the dorsum of the little finger and to the ulnar half of the ring finger.

Brachial Plexus Block

Anesthesia of the brachial plexus provides excellent anesthesia for upper extremity trauma, including the area of the elbow. The axillary approach is recommended since the supraclavicular approach occasionally results in a pneumothorax.

For the axillary approach the area is prepared and draped as for surgery, and the axillary artery is palpated as cephalad as possible, with the shoulder abducted 90° and the upper extremity supinated. Lidocaine 1.5% is preferred, since 25 to 30 ml can be administered to the average adult without fear of toxicity. A 10-ml, three-ring syringe with a No. 25 short needle offers the best control with the least trauma. With the shoulder abducted 90°, the median nerve distribution is anesthetized just lateral, or cephalad, to the artery, and the ulnar nerve distribution, just medial, or caudal, to the artery. Paresthesias elicited in the sensory distribution of the particular nerve may be of help. The needle is then angled to the posterior of the artery from both sides to anesthetize the radial nerve. Roughly 5 to 10 ml of anesthetic agent are infiltrated at each site. To complement or augment a brachial plexus block, block of appropriate peripheral nerves supplying sensory innervation to the injured area may be performed simultaneously or later, as necessary.

Infiltrative Anesthesia

Infiltrative anesthesia is used primarily on the dorsum of the hand (Figure 2-2) but also may be used in any area of the forearm or arm for which peripheral nerve block anesthesia is not suited. The anesthetic agent should be administered either proximal to or at the circumference of the wound and should not be injected into the wound itself. If the wound should be contaminated, direct injection of an anesthetic agent into the wound would carry the contamination into adjacent normal tissue.

In infants and young children and in the elderly patient a solution of 1.0% to 1.5% lidocaine should be used for all types of infiltrative and peripheral nerve block anesthesia. Epinephrine may be introduced proximal to the palm to prolong anesthesia, when necessary, in the healthy adult. It should never be injected distal to the palm, however, as this may cause vasoconstriction and possible irreversible ischemia.

Anesthetic Injection of Fracture Hematomas

Injection of local anesthetic agents into a hematoma at the site of a fracture or joint dislocation in a closed injury is acceptable practice. Theoretically a closed wound is converted into an open wound by this method, but there is little opportunity for introduction of bacteria if sterile precautions are observed prior to injection and an aseptic technique is used.

Intravenous Regional Anesthesia

Intravenous regional anesthesia (Bier's block) is very effective for closed manipulation and reduction of upper extremity fractures and dislocations and for some surgery. (For meticulous surgery, usually not effected at the initial treatment of skeletal trauma, this method may not be preferred because the operative field is "wet" due to the edema from the amount of injected anesthetic agent.) A No. 20 needle or venous catheter is inserted into a superficial vein, the upper extremity is exsanguinated with the use of a Martin rubber bandage, and the proximal tourniquet of a double-tourniquet arrangement on the upper arm is inflated; 20 to 40 ml of 0.5% lidocaine is injected intravenously (maximum dosage in a healthy adult is 400 to 450 mg). When tourniquet pain due to ischemia becomes severe—about 20 to 30 minutes after inflation—the distal tourniquet is inflated and pain is completely relieved since this area has been previously anesthetized. If the tourniquet is released or spontaneously deflates less than 20 minutes after the intravenous injection of the anesthetic, however, toxic effects and even death can result from the large quantity of local anesthetic which suddenly enters the general circulation.

This technique, therefore, is contraindicated in the care of open wounds for which the tourniquet must be deflated to evaluate hemostasis and soft tissue viability.

General Anesthesia

General anesthesia is indicated in various situations which include a particularly apprehensive patient, children under the age of five, and patients with massive injuries usually involving multiple digits, wrist and hand, forearm or arm. It is also indicated in severe infections of the finger (tendon sheath infection), the hand (potential fascial space infection), or the forearm or arm, particularly if complicated by ascending lymphangitis and lymphadenitis involving the epitrochlear and/or axillary nodes. Again, general anesthesia is indicated if distant sites are utilized for donor resurfacing (distant pedicle or large split-thickness skin graft) or skeletal augmentation (iliac or rib bone graft).

Open Fractures and Dislocations

The most important factor in the treatment of open fractures and dislocations is the provision of meticulous wound cleansing, irrigation, and debridement of all foreign material and nonviable soft tissue and bone. (Refer to Figures 13-5A–D in Chapter 13.) Care must be taken to debride any exposed contaminated bone using sharp rongeur excision "down to the clean bleeding bone" before definitive fracture or joint reduction. Appropriate tetanus prophylaxis is mandatory. If a patient has received a tetanus toxoid booster within five years of the current open injury, no further treatment is necessary. If the time interval is longer than five years, 0.5 cc of tetanus toxoid and usually 250 units of tetanus immune globulin (human) should be given, particularly in massive wounds.*

If the extremity or digit distal to the open injury is severely compromised vascularly, reduction should be accomplished as soon as possible. However, at definitive primary treatment the fracture or joint must be redisplaced to permit proper cleansing, debridement, and removal of all foreign matter.

---

*For general principles of tetanus prophylaxis and immunization the reader is referred to *Early Care of the Injured Patient* by the Committee on Trauma of the American College of Surgeons, pp 48–52, 2nd ed, 1976, Philadelphia, W. B. Saunders Co.

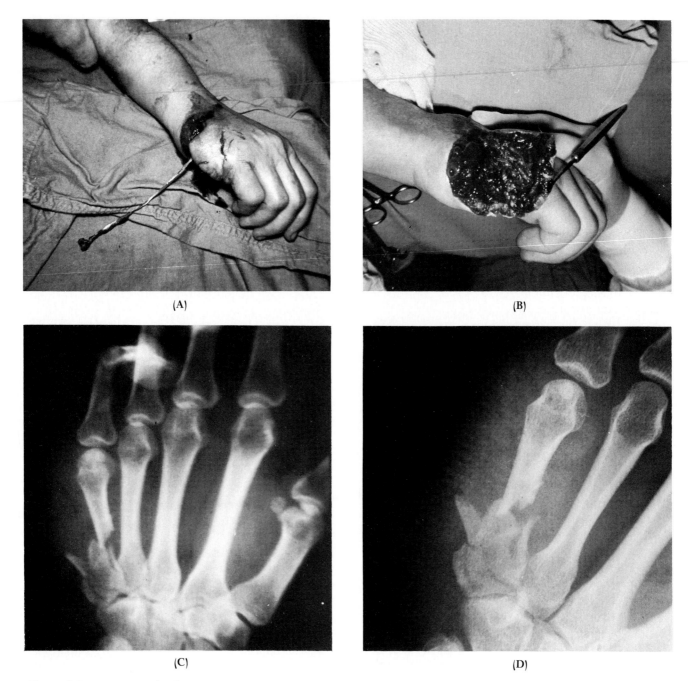

(A)

(B)

(C)

(D)

Figure 2-3 **(A)** Severe dog bite injury to ulnar aspect of hand causing partial avulsion of hypothenar muscle mass, a large distally based pedicle of skin, open comminuted displaced fracture of little finger metacarpal in its proximal metaphysis, and avulsion of proper extensor to little finger. Initial treatment was meticulous cleansing, irrigation, and wound debridement, including large segment of exposed extensor tendon. Wound packed open; all digits and wrist immobilized in palmar splint. **(B)** Retraction of large distally based segment of skin and subcutaneous tissue on dorsal aspect of hand at time of delayed primary closure 4 days after injury shows a clean wound with no evidence of further tissue necrosis or infection. Skin closure was effected after manipulation of fracture, with no attempt at deeper soft tissue reconstructions. **(C)** Radiograph of initial injury shows comminuted displaced fracture of proximal metaphysis of little finger metacarpal. **(D)** Acceptable position after manipulation and reduction at time of delayed primary skin closure with no internal fixation. No further reconstruction necessary; normal function after healing with complete extension by common extensor. This case demonstrates the necessity of open treatment of any bite wound, particularly a human bite wound.

Internal skeletal fixation should be used only when absolutely necessary to avoid a possible foreign body nidus for an infection (Figures 2-3A–D).

Open physeal injuries must be treated in a similar manner with meticulous wound toilet (refer to Figures 11-28A–C and 11-33A–C in Chapter 11, Physeal Injuries). Care should be taken to be as gentle as possible to try to prevent cessation of growth. Parents of these patients must be informed that after such severe trauma to the growth area, either a growth disturbance or cessation of growth is a distinct possibility.

The type and site of an open injury determine whether a wound should be treated by primary closure, open treatment, delayed primary closure, or free or pedicled skin resurfacing (Figures 2-3A–D). Primary soft tissue and/or skeletal reconstruction requires a meticulously clean wound with no danger of contamination or tissue necrosis. A human bite injury of the hand should never be primarily closed, and, generally, animal bites should be packed open initially. Specific types of open injuries (e.g., crush, projectile injuries, etc.) are discussed in the appropriate sections of this Atlas.

Immobilization

The proper balance between adequate physiologic immobilization and early mobilization, combined with rehabilitation and physical therapy, holds the key to restoration of skeletal and ligamentous function to as near normal as possible.

The physiologic position for immobilization of the wrist, hand, and digits includes: (1) wrist extension of 30° to 45° with slight ulnar deviation; (2) metacarpophalangeal joint maximum flexion; (3) proximal and distal interphalangeal joint extension (either complete, in the "clam digger" position, or minimal flexion, with increasing flexion from the index to the little finger of 5°, 10°, 15°, and 20°, respectively); and (4) wide thumb abduction and opposition (Figure 2-4).

The injured digit must be accurately aligned with its neighboring digits to prevent malrotation. Proper alignment and rotation of the injured digit is achieved by comparing it to adjacent normal digits and to the corresponding digits of the contralateral normal hand in similar positions. In general, upon digital flexion the tips of the index, long, ring, and little fingers point to the tuberosity of the scaphoid. Because this is a generality, however, observation of digital relationships in synergistic flexion and extension

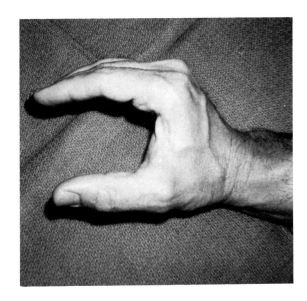

Figure 2-4 Position of immobilization of the hand: wrist extension, MP joint flexion, PIP and DIP joint extension, and wide thumb abduction and opposition.

of the contralateral normal hand is very important. Observation of nail plate alignment is also helpful since the plane of the fractured digit's nail plate should correspond to those of its adjacent normal digits, just as the nail plate of the same digit on the opposite hand corresponds to those of its adjacent digits. The physician must always be aware of possible individual variations of the normal by examining the contralateral normal hand.

Immobilization must be continued long enough to guarantee maintenance of fracture reduction or joint relocation once light activity is commenced. The majority of diaphyseal fractures involve predominantly cortical bone, which may be unstable and therefore should be immobilized for three and one-half to four weeks. Metaphyseal fractures involve cancellus bone and require immobilization for about three weeks.

In the responsible patient an undisplaced or stable reduced fracture may be subjected to light activity after five to ten days of immobilization to allow subsidence of edema. Such immobilized digits may be taped to an adjacent digit or digits in a "buddy" system to provide additional protection in this early phase of healing.

Immobilization of a reduced unstable fracture of the metacarpal, proximal, or middle phalanges should include the adjacent normal digit on either side. If the injured digit is a border digit (index or little finger), at least one adjacent digit should be incorporated.

The thumb must always be considered a separate entity and should be immobilized in wide abduction and opposition.

Soft Compressive Dressing

In injuries with severe soft tissue trauma or multiple fractures, a bulky, layered, compressive, non-constrictive soft dressing is often temporarily employed, in conjunction with plaster splint immobilization and constant elevation, for three to five days following trauma to reduce edema and congestion prior to manipulation and reduction. If ace bandages are used, they should be loosely wrapped and never applied under stretch to avoid constriction and peripheral edema. Bias-cut stockinette, which is not constrictive, is the safest material for a soft circumferential dressing. A large compressive dressing is often used postoperatively to allow subsidence of edema prior to applying a definitive well-molded plaster splint or cast.

Splint Immobilization

"Sugar tong" splint immobilization is excellent treatment for a distal metaphyseal fracture of the distal radius. A variant of the sugar tong provides good immobilization for metacarpal fractures only if care is taken to avoid pressure during application. The sugar tong splint is applied first to the palmar aspect of the hand or wrist, extends proximally along the palmar aspect of the forearm around the olecranon process and distal humerus, and terminates on the dorsal aspect of the forearm, wrist, and hand. This immobilization allows some elbow motion, yet provides more restriction than a short arm cast would. Allowing for increase or decrease in swelling is an important aspect of this immobilization since the plaster is not circumferential.

Palmar or dorsal splints may provide either temporary or permanent immobilization for wrist or hand fractures (Figure 2-5). The advantages of splint immobilization are that a possibly constrictive circumferential plaster cast is avoided and the soft dressing portion of the splint immobilization conforms to the surface anatomy when edema subsides. One should generally avoid single-digit metal splint immobilization for primary fracture treatment because (1) this method of immobilization does not effectively prevent motion at the fracture site and thus causes unnecessary pain and (2) circumferential constriction

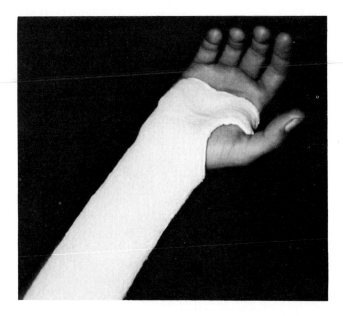

Figure 2-5   Palmar splint immobilization for minor wrist trauma. Palmar splint should be molded to correspond to both transverse and longitudinal axes of hand and should allow full motion of thumb and MP joints of the other digits, if indicated.

may easily occur and result in peripheral edema and additional pain and vascular impairment.

Individual digit splint immobilization is fine after subsidence of the initial edema of trauma and manipulation, but the importance of maintaining constant dryness must be stressed.

Night splints and splints to avoid accidental injury from strenuous activity are good adjunctive measures once physical therapy and light activity have been commenced.

Plaster Cast Immobilization

The two primary arches of the hand (longitudinal and transverse) must be properly molded in the physiologic position while applying a cast which incorporates the hand and the wrist.

Long arm cast immobilization is necessary for any fracture of the forearm involving either or both bones, except for distal metaphyseal and stable articular distal radial fractures. Long arm cast immobilization with incorporation of the thumb, index, and long fingers is advised in the treatment of delayed union of a fractured scaphoid or after bone graft for nonunion of a scaphoid fracture.

A long arm cast is imperative to immobilize any digital injury in an infant or young child to prevent possible contamination of an open injury or displacement at any fracture or dislocation site. This long arm cast should be incorporated into a sling with Velpeau-type immobilization of the entire upper extremity to the chest wall, particularly in the active or uncooperative infant or child.

The short arm cast is preferred by some to treat distal radial fractures. It is particularly advantageous if pins-and-plaster immobilization is used.

The short arm-thumb spica cast is used for any fracture or dislocation of the thumb unit (trapezium, metacarpal, or proximal phalanx) and for scaphoid fractures (Figures 2-6A,B). The thumb is maintained in wide abduction and full opposition, and motion of the MP joints of all other digits is allowed.

Traction

Dynamic skeletal traction immobilization is rarely necessary and should be undertaken with extreme caution. Meticulous follow-up care is necessary to avoid distraction and vascular impairment, or loss of position of the fracture. Those situations for which skeletal traction is indicated are unstable fractures of the proximal thumb metacarpal and extremely comminuted, unstable proximal phalangeal fractures and extremely comminuted articular fractures of the metacarpophalangeal or proximal interphalangeal joints. The rubber band traction is applied to a transverse Kirschner wire fixation through the middle phalanx. Moberg traction (Kirschner wire fixation through the nail plate and distal phalanx) is acceptable, but both skin and pulp traction alone are definitely contraindicated. "Banjo" traction is also contraindicated since the MP joints are completely extended in this type of immobilization.

Internal Immobilization

Percutaneous Kirschner wire fixation may be used with either closed or open manipulation and reduction. Kirschner wire fixation of unstable articular fractures is particularly necessary to maintain anatomic reduction of the articular surface. Percutaneous Kirschner wire fixation may transversely fix a reduced metacarpal fracture to adjacent intact metacarpals to maintain satisfactory position and length.

Kirschner wires for immobilization of metacarpal and phalangeal fractures may be longitudinal, transverse, or oblique depending upon the surgeon's choice and the type and position of the fracture. Usually, parallel Kirschner wires are preferred and

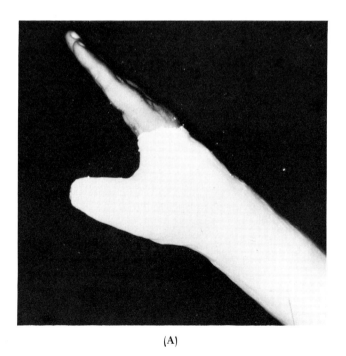
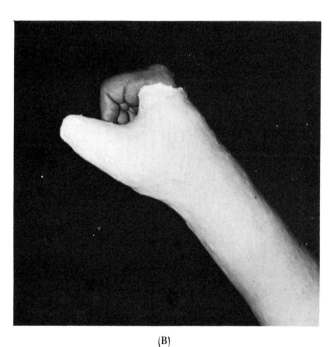

(A)   (B)

Figure 2-6 **(A)** Thumb spica cast immobilization should extend to tip of thumb but should not restrict MP joint motion of other digits (unless incorporation of index and long finger is desired—see text). Complete digital extension is seen here. **(B)** Nearly complete digital flexion emphasizes preservation of good MP joint flexion.

crossed Kirschner wires are to be avoided at the fracture site since distraction may result.

Internal distraction devices may be used temporarily to maintain metacarpal length when there is significant bone loss, but usually transverse Kirschner wire fixation achieves the same result more easily.

Small plates have been used to fix metacarpal and phalangeal fractures primarily, but generally this represents overtreatment of these injuries.

Immobilization should be sufficient to maintain reduction of a fracture or dislocation and should incorporate any other digits necessary for maintenance and protection of the reduction. Those joints not included in the immobilization, however, should not be restricted.

In general, the physiologic position of wrist and digits should be employed for immobilization. The MP joints should not be immobilized in extension, nor should the interphalangeal (IP) joints be immobilized in significant flexion. Immobilization of the digits over a roll of gauze in the palm, immobilization of the tip of the digit to the palm, or immobilization of a digit on a tongue depressor is not physiologic functional immobilization and should be avoided.

If cast immobilization is provided, it is important to check at roughly 8 to 10 hours to make sure that circulation in the digits is adequate. Occasionally application of a soft compression dressing which includes all the digits prevents undue digital edema during the first 24 to 48 hours after application of either a long arm or short arm cast. At the end of this period, the compressive immobilization is removed and digital motion permitted.

If circulation of the digits appears to be impaired at any time, cast immobilization must be split bilaterally and all padding must be separated *down to the skin*. If splint immobilization has been used, the soft dressing should be cut down to the skin and rewrapped.

Immobilization must be properly carried out in order to promote physiologic healing and to permit as much motion as possible of all uninvolved digits. Early motion—synergistic flexion and extension with adjacent normal digits—is paramount to the physiologic rehabilitation of the injured digit(s).

Hand Therapy and Dynamic Rehabilitation

The patient must be convinced that the role he plays in his therapy, as specifically instructed by his physician, is the key to his rehabilitation. Prescribed exercises should be performed at specific intervals all through the waking hours, not just once or twice a day or during a daily visit to the therapist. The patient must cooperate and help himself energetically, intelligently, and with determination.

Basic rehabilitation exercises for the upper extremity should stress:

1. Shoulder circumduction
2. Active elbow flexion and extension
3. Wrist extension and flexion
4. MP joint flexion and extension
5. PIP and DIP joint flexion and extension (both independently for each separate joint and in synergism with other digits and wrist extension and flexion)
6. Thumb abduction and opposition

It is important that the shoulder and elbow be exercised and used regularly if they are not incorporated in the immobilization. A simple circumduction exercise is enough to maintain completely normal shoulder motion. As previously noted, all joints not immobilized should be allowed free ranges of motion. Disuse of uninvolved joints of the injured extremity is both dangerous and avoidable.

Rehabilitative exercise of the injured part should begin as soon as healing has progressed sufficiently to prevent loss of position at the fracture site or dislocation.

Aggressive-passive range-of-motion exercises of joints are to be avoided since they rupture adhesions, and the resulting hemorrhage and edema often hinder rehabilitation irrevocably. Rather, adhesions should be gently stretched only to the point of causing minimal, if any, pain.

Exercise to regain active and passive ranges of joint motion should emphasize synergism of wrist extension and digital flexion and, conversely, wrist flexion and digital extension. The key to physiologic positioning of the wrist, hand, and digits is wrist extension. This is the "strength position" for powerful digital grasp and maximal digital flexion.

Both general, coordinated activity of all joints of the involved extremity—particularly the hand—and specific active and passive range of motion exercises for each separate joint are important in the overall rehabilitation. Each joint should be actively flexed and extended "to the count of ten." A small piece of wood may be used to block joint activity proximally, or the involved digit may be held at a point just proximal to the individual joint to concentrate active motion at that specific area.

Active flexion of digits on a sponge rubber ball or loose roll of yarn, or molding of Silly Putty or modeling clay, aids in general active physical rehabilitation, strengthens muscles, and aids in increasing ranges of joint motion. A hard rubber ball is not useful because MP flexion is hindered in attempting to grasp any such incompressible round object.

Active and passive abduction of the thumb metacarpal from the index metacarpal and active thumb opposition to the tip of every other digit should also be stressed.

Whirlpool or warm, moist soaks, combined with exercise, also help regain both active and passive ranges of motion. *Dependence of the hand must be avoided* during such treatment, however, to prevent dependent edema.

Dynamic splints which employ rubber bands or spring steel may be used adjunctively to regain motion. Knuckle-bender dynamic splints for MP joint flexion and knuckle-benders and reverse knuckle-benders for PIP joint flexion and extension are particularly useful.

Static splints such as the "safety pin" splint and strap help to relieve flexion contractures of the PIP joint. Both MP and IP joint flexion can be increased passively by mild progressive force exerted by padded straps or wide rubber bands.

The primary concern of the hand therapist is to instruct the patient in the precise exercises prescribed by the attending physician and to re-evaluate the patient periodically to determine his progress and to be certain that he is carrying out the exercises properly.

Possibilities for Error in Diagnosis and Treatment, and Complications

Physical Examination

If a fracture is suspected either by subjective symptoms or physical examination or both, the injury should be treated as a fracture regardless of an essentially negative initial radiographic examination. After conservative immobilization for approximately two to three weeks new radiographs will usually verify the presence or absence of an originally occult fracture (e.g., occult scaphoid fracture or physeal separation without displacement—Salter undisplaced Type I injury—refer to section on Scaphoid Fractures in Chapter 4 and to Chapter 11, Physeal Injuries). The case in Figures 2-7A,B is an example of this and illustrates the importance of "listening to the patient." A 42-year-old man sustained a crushing injury to the area of the ring finger DIP joint. Radiographic study showed no evidence of fracture or dislocation (Figure

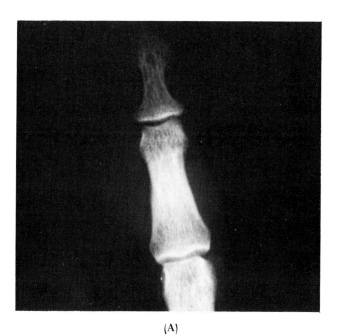

(A)

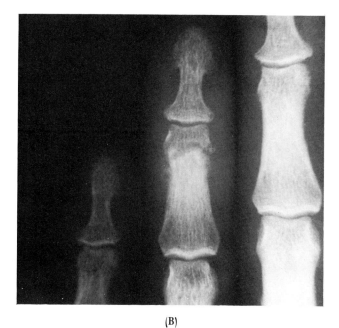

(B)

Figure 2-7 **(A)** Radiograph shows no evidence of fracture or dislocation. No treatment instituted and patient returned to work. **(B)** Six weeks after injury PA radiograph shows rarefaction transversely in area of junction of diaphysis and distal metaphysis of ring finger middle phalanx. Area of delayed union is visible, with excessive calcified new bone in soft tissues due to continued periosteal irritation owing to lack of immobilization.

2-7A). No treatment was instituted, and the patient returned to work. Five weeks later the patient requested reevaluation because of continued pain and limited motion, accompanied by diffuse, moderate swelling of the entire digit. Despite the patient's repeated complaints, no radiographic studies had been made since the time of injury. Six weeks after injury, a PA radiograph showed rarefaction transversely in the area of the junction of the diaphysis and distal metaphysis of the ring finger middle phalanx (Figure 2-7B).

Digits with suspected fractures require initial immobilization to allow the initial effects of trauma to subside. Radiographic reevaluation two to two and one-half weeks postinjury is indicated if the patient remains symptomatic. In this case, such reevaluation clearly would have demonstrated this fracture, owing to rarefaction at the fracture site. At reevaluation six weeks after injury the digit was immobilized by aluminum splint during periods of strenuous activity to relieve pain. Three weeks later the patient was asymptomatic, with normal ranges of MP, PIP, and DIP joints, indicating complete healing of the fracture.

Also, if it is strongly suspected from history and physical findings that a joint dislocation has occurred even though the joint is in normal position at initial examination and treatment, appropriate immobilization of the suspected dislocation should be carried out (refer to section General Considerations in Chapter 9). Occasionally a small avulsion fracture seen on radiographs may aid in the diagnosis.

It is extremely difficult, and sometimes impossible for many weeks postinjury, to differentiate nerve malfunction due to external compression (neurapraxia), from partial nerve avulsion or transsection when a portion of the sensory and motor modalities remains intact. The most important single diagnostic aid is examination of motor and sensory function distal to the site of injury or fracture prior to anesthesia and reduction. Although this examination often will not be accurate because of pain, anxiety, and other extraneous factors, documentation is essential. The nerve may be compressed by hemorrhage and edema, obscuring an accurate diagnosis, but at least the findings will be documented prior to any manipulation attempts. Only in this way can nerve damage or partial laceration from bony spicules incurred at the time of injury be differentiated from nerve damage inflicted at the time of manipulation and reduction. The case described in Figures 2-8A–I is a good example of such a situation.

Hemostasis should be achieved by compressive dressing, elevation, and immobilization; a tourniquet is rarely necessary. Probing of an open wound in an attempt to establish hemostasis or to diagnose injured structures is definitely contraindicated. Accurate diagnosis of injured structures is made at wound exploration only after appropriate anesthesia and meticulous wound toilet have been carried out.

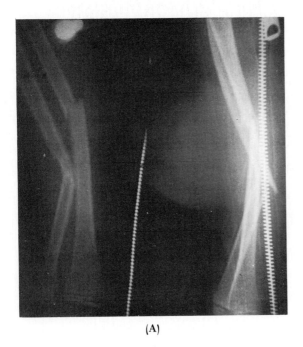

(A)

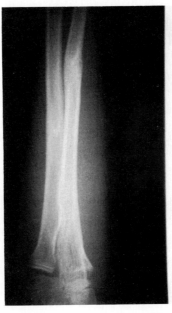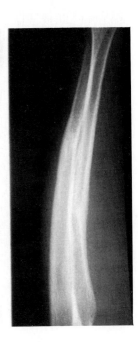

(B)

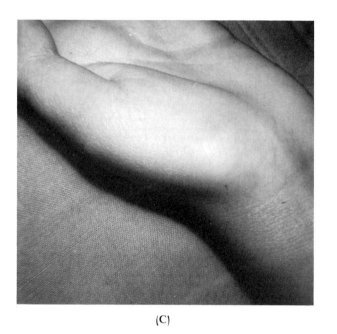

(C)

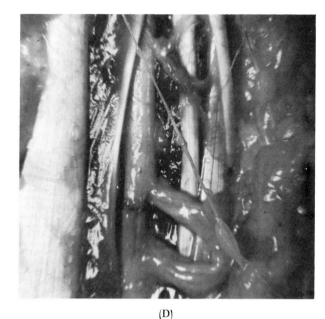

(D)

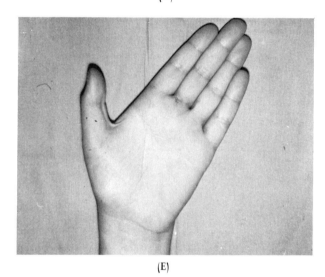

(E)

Figure 2-8 (A) *Facing page.* Both bone fractures of forearm in a 14-year-old male, sustained in a fall, can be seen in both views: the ulna fractured at midshaft and the radius approximately at junction of proximal and middle thirds of shaft, with 30° to 35° angulation. (B) *Facing page.* Radiographs 7 months postinjury show acceptable healing at both fracture sites. (C) Physical findings at that time showed mild thumb-index web contracture and atrophy of median innervated thenar musculature. Patient noted hypesthesia in pulp of thumb distal phalanx and most of index finger. Oblique view accentuates atrophy of thenar musculature. (D) Exploration of median nerve at site of healed fracture showed abundant cicatrix involving profundus musculature and nerve. Intact fibers of median nerve were separated carefully from neuroma in continuity binding down this partially lacerated median nerve at fracture site. Close-up view illustrates partial neurorrhaphy following excision of neuroma in continuity while normal portion of nerve at right is maintained and protected. Interposition of nerve graft at site of neuroma excision may be preferred. (E) Acceptable sensation postoperatively in median nerve distribution, but no improvement of thenar muscle atrophy. Palmar view shows mild to moderate thumb-index web contracture and thenar muscle atrophy. (F) Attempt at opposition poor due to absence of motor power of abductor pollicis brevis, superficial head of flexor pollicis brevis, and opponens pollicis.

(continued)

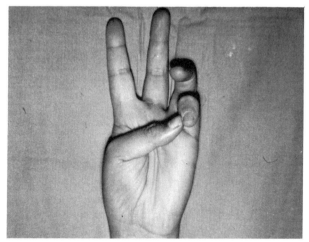

(F)

Figure 2-8 *(continued)*
(G) Operative view shows tendon transfer of superficialis tendon of ring finger through a pulley in transverse carpal ligament into thumb metacarpal and proximal phalanx to provide thumb opposition. Z-plasty deepening of the thumb web accomplished simultaneously. **(H)** Excellent opposition restored following opponensplasty. **(I)** Correction of thumb-index web contracture and excellent thumb abduction are illustrated here.

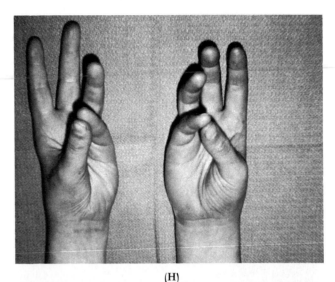

(H)

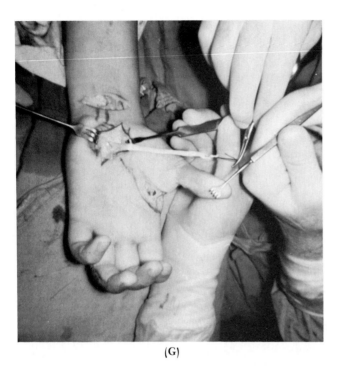

(G)

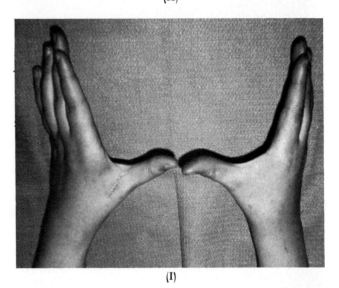

(I)

Radiographs

Inadequate radiographs because of improper technique or insufficient, unsatisfactory views are a primary cause for misdiagnosis and/or mismanagement. *The specific area* of fracture or dislocation diagnosed by history and/or physical examination *must be centered on the film.* Routine PA and lateral views should be supplemented by oblique and special views and studies. Overlap of a marker (Figures 2-9A–D) or of adjacent normal digits (Figures 2-10A–D) will obscure details of the pertinent injury. Dislocations, fracture dislocation, and individual carpal fractures of the wrist as well as malalignment, malrotation, angulation, and displacement of digital fractures can be diagnosed accurately only by *true* PA, lateral and two oblique views, supplemented by additional radiographs as necessary.

Physical examination of a fracture discloses specific tenderness upon gentle palpation in the area of injury; edema, ecchymosis, and abnormal configuration are usually obvious. Radiographs show sharp edges at the site of fracture rather than the smooth contours of a congenital abnormality (e.g., differentiation between bipartite scaphoid and scaphoid fracture, or the smooth contours of the adjacent bone at the epiphysis and diaphysis at an epiphyseal growth plate in an abnormal location, Figure 2-11). An accessory or abnormal phalanx (e.g., Delta phalanx, Figure 2-12) is differentiated from trauma by similar criteria.

Congenital Abnormalities. In a young child with obvious congenital abnormalities such as short digits (Figure 2-13), syndactylies, missing digits, etc., one

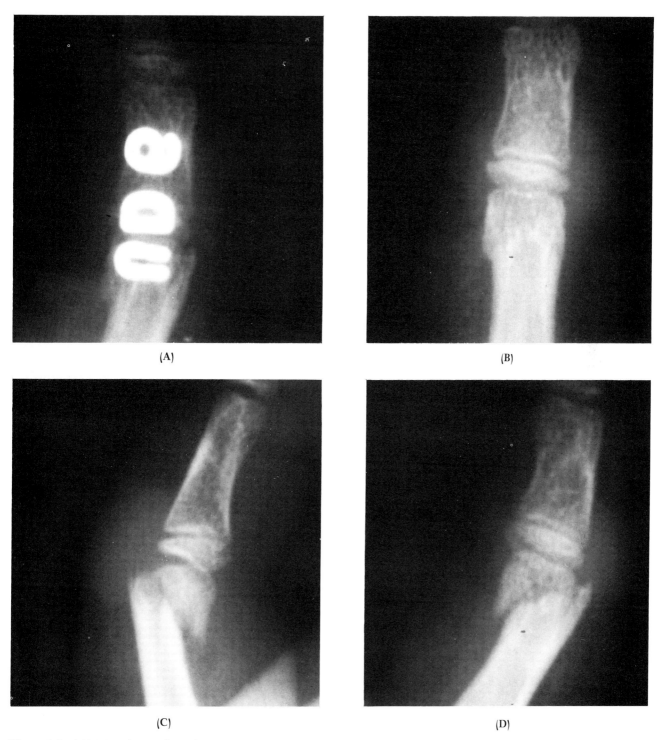

(A)

(B)

(C)

(D)

Figure 2-9 (A) PA radiograph to diagnose possible fracture of proximal phalanx. Film is completely useless since technician placed marker directly over part to be studied. (B) Repeat PA radiograph shows essentially no abnormality. (C) Lateral radiograph shows a displaced oblique fracture through distal metaphysis of proximal phalanx. (D) Oblique view also demonstrates displaced fracture. Case represents two important points: (1) physician cannot accept inadequate radiographs and (2) multiple radiographic views are mandatory in many cases to demonstrate lesion and to provide accurate diagnosis and treatment.

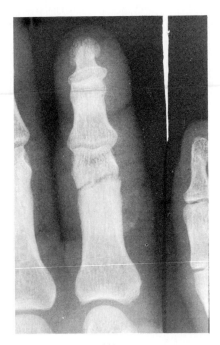

(A)

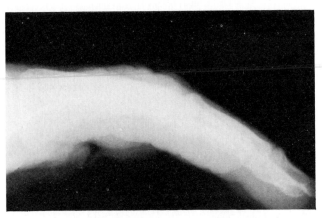

(B)

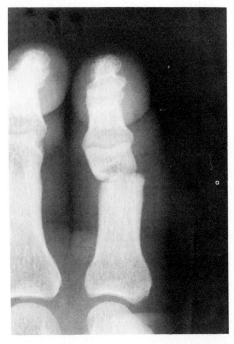

(C)

Figure 2-10 **(A)** PA radiograph shows an apparently acceptable position of transverse proximal phalangeal fracture through distal shaft or distal metaphysis. **(B)** Superimposition of adjacent digits on lateral radiograph obscures details of specific digit to be examined. **(C)** Four weeks after initial examination, PA radiograph discloses delayed union with angulation and displacement at site of fracture. **(D)** True lateral radiograph discloses a 90° dorsal rotation of proximal phalangeal condyles at fracture site. Condyles are protruding dorsally or superiorly. Case demonstrates importance of obtaining precise radiographs of fracture without obscuring details by overlying digits. Arthrodesis of PIP joint was finally necessary. *(Illustrations 2-10A–D courtesy of S. R. Shaffer, M.D.)*

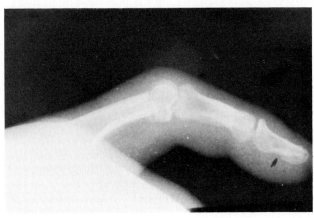

(D)

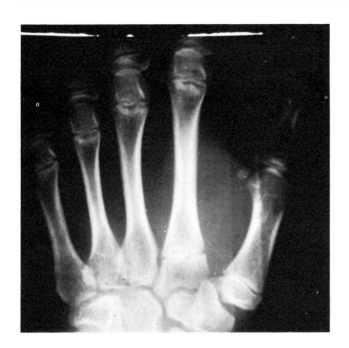

Figure 2-11 A proximal physis can be seen in index metacarpal. Contours of contiguous areas of diaphysis and proximal metaphysis of index finger are rounded and do not resemble an acute fracture.

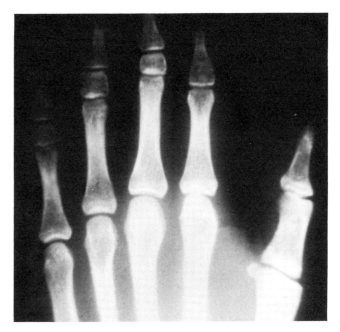

Figure 2-13 Close-up PA view shows abnormally short digits with multiple other abnormalities. Proximal phalanges are unusually long and middle phalanges unusually short in long, ring, and little fingers; also, middle phalanx is absent in index finger. These congenital abnormalities should not be mistaken for trauma.

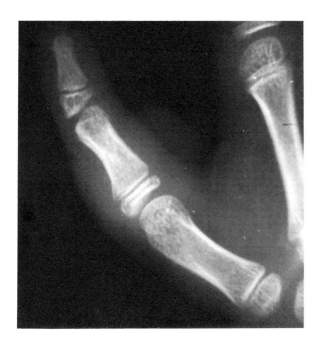

Figure 2-12 PA view demonstrates an extra ossicle, a Delta phalanx, in thumb. Cortical surfaces of such a bone, which are in contact with other bones at joints, are rounded, and there is no evidence of characteristic findings of an acute fracture. Case demonstrates importance of differentiation of certain congenital abnormalities from fractures. Certainly gross examination of digit should help.

can expect to find other skeletal abnormalities which may be quite apparent (refer to Figure 4-1 in Chapter 4, Wrist Injuries). However, congenital skeletal abnormalities may be very confusing in an adult whose hand appears to be normal and functions so (refer to Figures 4-2 and 4-3 in Chapter 4).

If a radiograph of a wrist is confusing and leads one to suspect congenital abnormalities or old injuries, the contralateral normal wrist should be evaluated with comparable views. However, similar findings noted in both wrists do not rule out the possibility of bilateral trauma (e.g., bilateral scaphoid fractures).

Calcific deposits, particularly in relation to flexor tendons at the wrist (Figures 2-14A–C) and occasionally in the digits (Figure 2-15), may resemble separate ossicles. The rounded contours of the calcific deposits and the unlikely location in soft tissues should aid in correct diagnosis.

Tumors. Abundant callus at the site of an undiagnosed or untreated fracture (Figure 2-16), an osteochondroma (Figure 2-17), or a growth

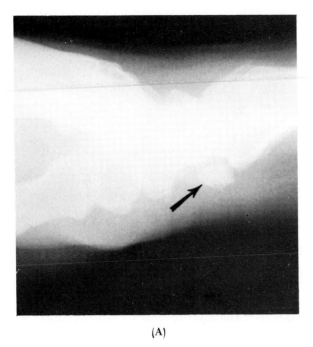

(A)

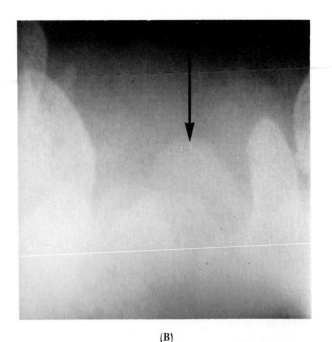

(B)

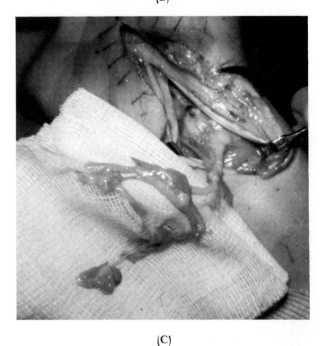

(C)

Figure 2-14 **(A)** Lateral radiograph shows large radiopacity palmar to carpus which resembles an extra carpal ossicle. **(B)** "Carpal tunnel" view shows pisiform and hook of hamate on right, crest of trapezium and tuberosity of scaphoid on left, and large radiopacity at base of carpal tunnel toward ulnar aspect. **(C)** At surgery, median neurolysis and flexor tenosynovectomies permitted removal of large calcific deposit noted deep to flexor tendons and superficial layer of palmar capsule of wrist. Symptoms of median nerve compression were relieved by above procedures combined with partial excision of transverse carpal ligament.

disturbance of an epiphysis (dysplasia epiphysalis hemimelica) should not be confused with a tumor, which may or may not have an associated pathologic fracture. It is important to make a distinction between different types of tumors, with or without pathologic fractures, and tumorlike conditions, although at times it is difficult to do so without biopsy and histological examination of the tissue.

The most common primary bone tumor encountered in the hand and digits is an enchondroma (Figures 2-21–2-24). Rarer lesions include osteoid-osteoma (Figure 2-18), glomus tumor (Figures 2-19A,B), intraosseous inclusion cyst, metastatic tumor, rare primary malignancies, periosteal reaction to trauma and surgery (Figures 2-20A,B), etc. The most important diagnostic feature of the common en-

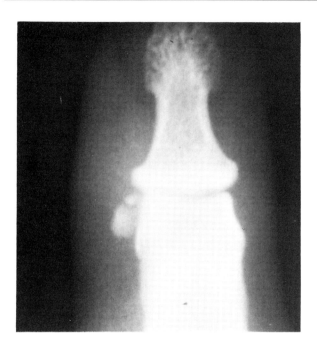

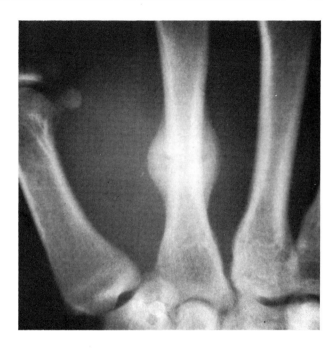

Figure 2-15 A calcific deposit is noted on lateral aspect of middle phalangeal condyles just proximal to DIP joint in area of origin of collateral ligament of DIP joint. Finding must be differentiated from a possible ossicle, aberrant sesamoid, or tumor.

Figure 2-16 Exuberant callus seen at site of healing index metacarpal shaft fracture sustained 3 weeks previously and treated without immobilization. The history helped in distinguishing this finding from a tumor or pathologic fracture.

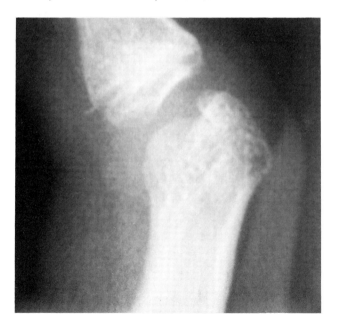

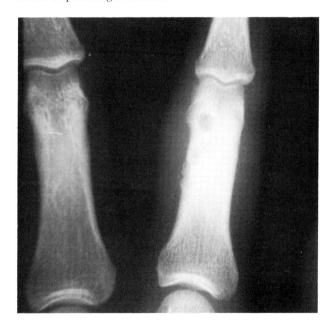

Figure 2-17 Radiograph shows radial angulation at PIP joint of index finger combined with irregularity of distal end of proximal phalanx. Large osteochondroma is seen extending from articular surface of ulnar condyle of proximal phalanx. Radiograph has all the findings applicable to malunion of a large displaced articular fracture of the proximal phalanx distal articular surface.

Figure 2-18 PA view of index finger proximal phalanx shows radiolucent round lesion in distal diaphysis surrounded by sclerosis and thickening of surrounding diaphysis. Lesion was diagnosed as an osteoid-osteoma both clinically, prior to surgery, and at histological examination of lesion after removal. Differential diagnosis initially must include abscess (Brodie's) of proximal phalanx.

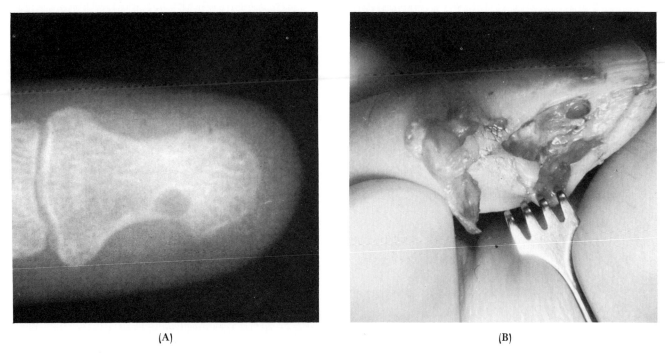

(A)   (B)

Figure 2-19 **(A)** Radiograph showing rounded radiolucency in distal phalanx on its lateral aspect just proximal to base of tuft. **(B)** Photograph at surgery shows both bony defect in distal phalanx from which a portion of soft tissue mass was removed and that mass located proximally on the finger. Pre- and postoperatively after histological examination lesion was diagnosed as a glomus tumor, a portion of which had eroded into the distal phalanx. Symptoms of lesion had been present for four years prior to surgery.

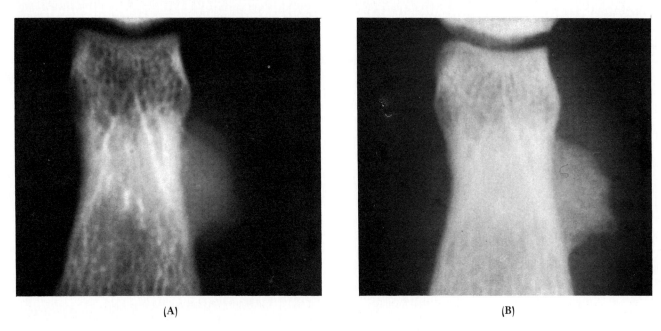

(A)   (B)

Figure 2-20 **(A)** Light calcification of a lesion extending from cortex of middle phalangeal lateral aspect 4 weeks after crushing trauma to this area and subsequent surgical exploration. **(B)** Same lesion noted 4 weeks later shows increased calcification and definite bone formation. Dorsal exposure of site revealed periosteal new bone formation resulting both from initial trauma and from surgical stimulation of periosteum. Saucerization to remove this mass resulted in minimal recurrence, not significant enough to warrant additional surgery.

chondroma is an associated pathologic fracture (Figure 2-21). A pathologic fracture occurs in a bone which is either generally (osteogenesis imperfecta) or locally (enchondroma) abnormal and is caused usually by rather insignificant trauma which would not cause fracture in the normal bone. Usually the diagnosis of enchondroma follows a pathologic fracture through a lesion which previously has been completely asymptomatic and unrecognized (Figures 2-21, 2-22B, 2-23A, 2-24).

Preferred initial treatment of a large lesion is curettage of the tumor with insertion of an autogenous bone graft (iliac crest or rib) to provide stability (Figures 2-22A–E). If necessary, internal fixation may be employed in an unstable situation (Figure 2-23A–C). It does not make sense to allow the fracture to heal first and then to perform excision of the enchondroma and bone graft secondarily as a reconstructive procedure. Immobilization necessary to heal a pathologic fracture is usually longer than normal because of the scarcity of normal bone in the area of the lesion. This prolonged immobilization is compounded by immobilization following the reconstructive bone graft, which additionally impairs ranges of motion of joints of the involved digit needlessly.

A small enchondroma may be curetted and allowed to fill in with fibrous tissue. In Figure 2-24 surgery was elected to prevent recurrence of a pathologic fracture and included complete removal of the enchondroma, but no bone graft. Digital function was normal postoperatively.

If histologic study reveals a rare malignant primary or metastatic tumor, radical resection or possibly deletion may be indicated. Appropriate studies are mandatory to discover the primary site of a metastatic lesion.

Primary Treatment

After the initial examination, adequate anesthesia by an appropriate method is mandatory prior to wound toilet in an open injury and is usually necessary prior to any attempt at reduction in the closed wound.

Meticulous wound toilet is by far the most important part of the initial care of an open wound. Specimens for culture and sensitivity and for tissue cell count precede wound toilet. Gentle cleansing to the full depth of the lesion and copious irrigation with a sterile physiologic solution are mandatory. Debride-

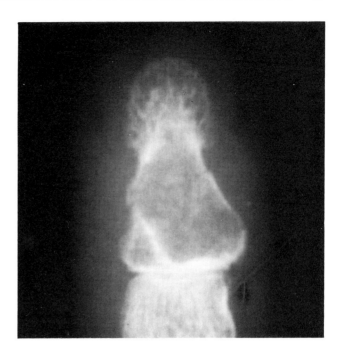

Figure 2-21   PA view shows replacement of roughly 80% of distal phalanx by enchondroma with markedly attenuated cortices and calcific stippling within lesion. A pathologic fracture sustained by minimal trauma (typing) is noted.

ment of only nonviable tissue, with no sacrifice of viable structures, completes the wound toilet. A particularly dirty wound should be cleansed and irrigated twice with sterile glove changes in between.

Proper cleansing, debridement, and irrigation are vitally important in all open injuries to prevent infection and are especially important in two particular wounds: open physeal separations (Figures 2-25A–E) and injuries complicated by severe vascular impairment. Meticulous cleansing, debridement, and irrigation of an open physeal separation (e.g., open traumatic physeal separation of the distal phalanx with avulsion of the nail plate base) are extremely important. Reduction of such a separation without adequate cleansing may result in infection and osteomyelitis and cessation or aberrant growth of that physis. In the digit or extremity which has suffered severe distal vascular impairment, this ischemia may progress to gangrene if infection supervenes. The massive edema accompanying the infection may completely occlude the already compromised circulation.

Extensive cicatrix following infection hinders later attempts to restore joint motion and tendon and nerve function.

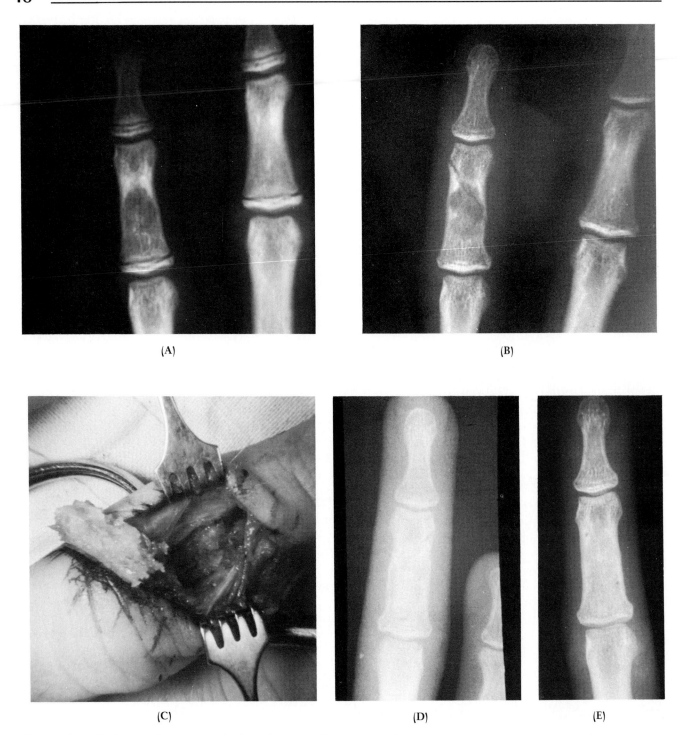

(A)

(B)

(C)

(D)

(E)

Figure 2-22 (A) Torsional injury to the long finger, (right) on PA radiograph, sustained by a 14-year-old boy. No skeletal injury was found, and lesion in adjacent ring finger middle phalanx, left, was *not* diagnosed. (B) PA view of same ring finger middle phalanx 3 years later shows pathologic fracture through large enchondroma now occupying approximately 75% of digit's middle phalanx. (C) Photograph at surgery shows removal of cortical segment of middle phalanx and illustrates gross appearance of tissue of enchondroma, both on internal surface of removed bone fragment and in depth of wound. (D) PA radiograph of middle phalanx 2 weeks after surgery shows acceptable position of autogenous iliac graft after excision of tumor. (E) PA radiograph 1 year after surgery shows good incorporation of iliac bone graft and no evidence of residual tumor. Complete digital extension and flexion with normal function resulted 1 year after surgery.

Figure 2-23 (A) Pathologic fracture through ring finger proximal phalanx is oblique, somewhat displaced, rotated, and unstable. An enchondroma occupies approximately 50% of proximal phalanx. (B) Treatment involved excision of lesion, autogenous iliac graft, and temporary Kirschner wire fixation to stabilize minimal proximal phalangeal bone remaining at fracture site after complete removal of lesion. (C) PA radiograph 8 months after surgery shows good incorporation of iliac graft and good healing of fracture site, with anatomic alignment and rotation of proximal phalanx. Case illustrates the necessity of internal fixation in treatment of such a fracture if iliac bone graft does not afford required stability for fracture healing.

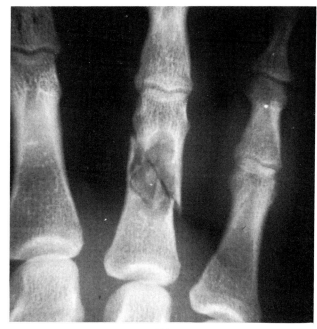

(A)

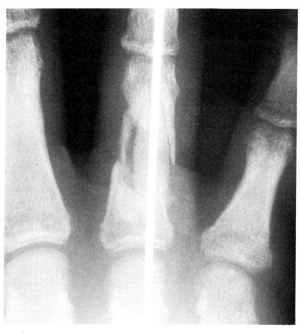

(B)

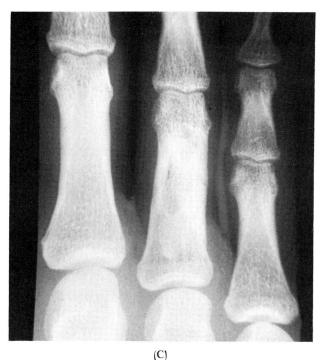

(C)

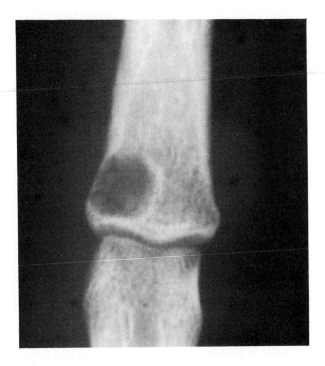

Figure 2-24 Rounded radiolucency on lateral aspect of middle phalanx close to its base is noted. Some calcification can be seen within lesion as well as sclerotic borders and pathologic fracture of cortex. Fracture was sustained by a relatively minor injury.

Initial open treatment of the wound is strongly advocated if gross contamination is suspected, particularly in human bites, after extensive initial wound toilet and debridement, supplemented by antibiotics, tetanus toxoid booster, and usually tetanus immune globulin. If infection develops, immediate wide surgical exploration and further debridement are necessary to avoid osteomyelitis.

In a human bite wound, if the extensor tendon has been lacerated and particularly if a joint has been violated (usually MP or PIP joint) this is a true surgical emergency mandating hospitalization, radical surgical debridement with open wound treatment, intravenous antibiotics, appropriate tetanus prophylaxis, immobilization and elevation (Figures 2-26A–D).

Significant functional impairment usually results if treatment is delayed more than eight hours after this type of wound.

Anatomic reduction of shaft fractures will prevent malunion, including angulation, displacement, shortening, and malrotation. Anatomic reduction of dislocations, fractures, and fracture dislocations of the wrist is necessary to restore normal carpal anatomy required for stability and asymptomatic physiologic ranges of motion. Anatomic reduction of a large displaced articular fracture involving a significant portion (usually 25% or more) of the articular surface is mandatory to restore joint surface congruity as well as possible.

In open crush injuries proper recognition of the severity of soft tissue damage will require either open treatment initially or a very loose wound closure because of the anticipation of subsequent massive edema with its inherent complication of ischemia and possible closed space or closed compartment compression syndrome. As shown in Figures 2-27A,B, it is of extreme importance to recognize severe soft tissue trauma, regardless of how innocuous the fracture may appear on radiographic evaluation. The wound must be cleansed meticulously, regardless of the size of the open area, particularly when it is in relation to a fracture, again, no matter how innocuous that fracture might seem.

Always suspect concurrent injury to areas other than the site of primary trauma in both the contralateral (refer to Figures 5-5A–E) and ipsilateral extremities (refer to Figure 8-11B). The patient in Figures 2-28A–D sustained an elbow fracture dislocation when he had fallen forcibly onto his outstretched right upper extremity. Closed manipulation and reduction of the fracture dislocation was followed by eventual excision of the radial head four weeks after the initial injury. During this time the patient had minimal complaints regarding his right wrist; he was, however, a stoic individual and actually complained of little pain in the severely injured elbow. Radiographs of the ipsilateral (right) wrist six weeks after injury showed gross distortion of carpal architecture due to palmar lunate dislocation. A later radiograph showed even greater relative lengthening of the ulna due to both elbow and wrist injuries and excision of the radial head. At this time the patient had increasing symptoms of pain and limitation of pronation and supination of the wrist. When last examined the patient had pronation to neutral and supination to 35°. Reconstruction of the wrist could be done to improve motion and to relieve pain but would be complicated by the relative disparity in length of the radius and the ulna.

Thorough repetitive examinations of all areas of a severely traumatized extremity, therefore, are extremely important. In this case the wrist lesion was completely missed because of the patient's high pain threshold and because all attention was directed to the severe fracture dislocation of the elbow.

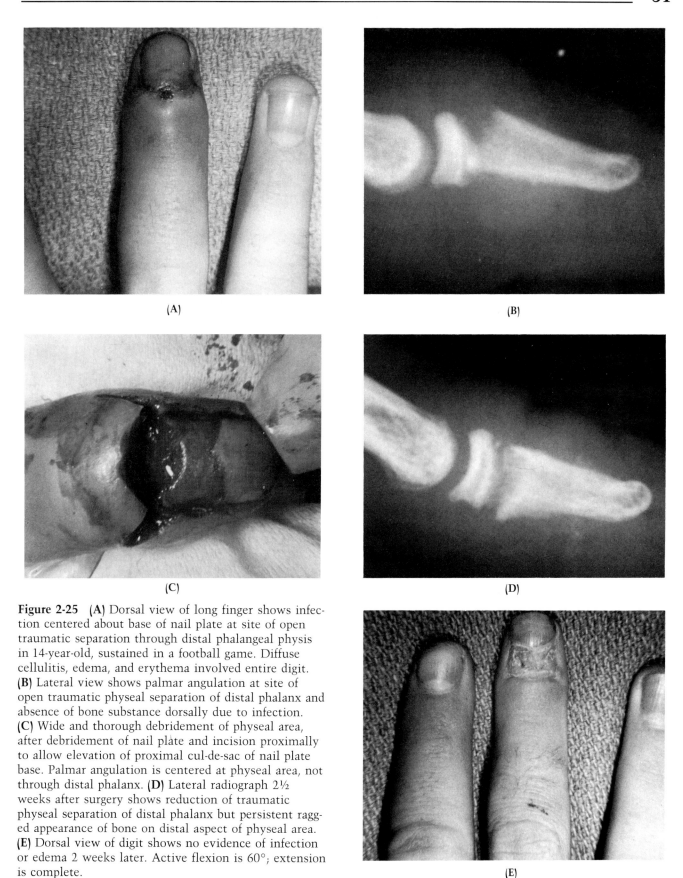

Figure 2-25 (A) Dorsal view of long finger shows infection centered about base of nail plate at site of open traumatic separation through distal phalangeal physis in 14-year-old, sustained in a football game. Diffuse cellulitis, edema, and erythema involved entire digit. (B) Lateral view shows palmar angulation at site of open traumatic physeal separation of distal phalanx and absence of bone substance dorsally due to infection. (C) Wide and thorough debridement of physeal area, after debridement of nail plate and incision proximally to allow elevation of proximal cul-de-sac of nail plate base. Palmar angulation is centered at physeal area, not through distal phalanx. (D) Lateral radiograph 2½ weeks after surgery shows reduction of traumatic physeal separation of distal phalanx but persistent ragged appearance of bone on distal aspect of physeal area. (E) Dorsal view of digit shows no evidence of infection or edema 2 weeks later. Active flexion is 60°; extension is complete.

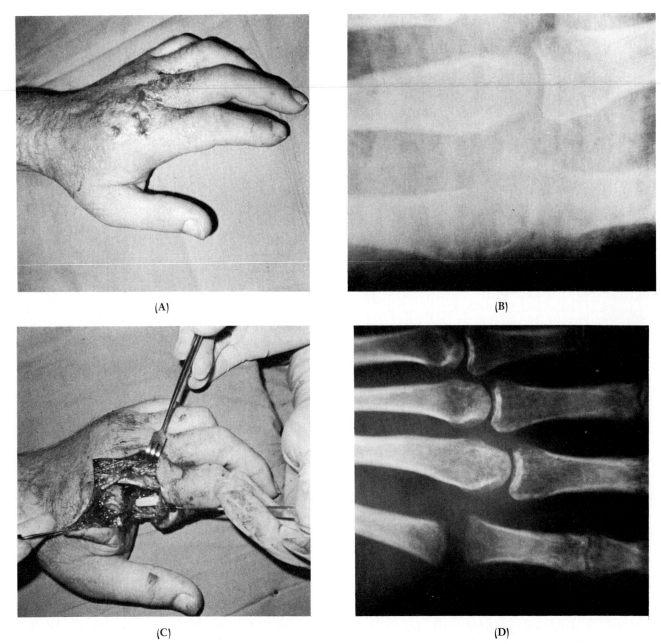

(A)

(B)

(C)

(D)

Figure 2-26 **(A)** Oblique view of hand of a 26-year-old male shows excoriations and abrasions on dorsoradial aspect of MP joint area centered on MP joint of index finger. Moderate swelling of entire dorsum of hand and digits is noted. Patient sustained a human bite injury 10 days previously and was treated initially by cleansing of wound with primary skin closure. **(B)** PA view of index and long finger MP joint in plaster immobilization shows incongruity of index finger MP joint and obvious osteomyelitis of index metacarpal distal metaphysis and head and base of proximal phalanx. **(C)** Oblique view shows extent of debridement necessary to eradicate necrotic and grossly infected tissue from wound. Distal metaphysis and head of index metacarpal, base of proximal phalanx, extensor indicis proprius and common extensor tendons to index finger, a large segment of first dorsal interosseous, adductor pollicis, first palmar, and second dorsal interosseous muscles were excised. View shows flexor tendons of index finger (flexor digitorum profundus and superficialis) which were not sacrificed. Wound was treated open and healed from within out in approximately 6 weeks. Reconstruction will entail arthroplasty of MP joint area and restoration of index finger extension by tendon transfer. **(D)** PA radiograph following surgery shows absence of base of index finger proximal phalanx and distal metacarpal metaphysis and metacarpal head.

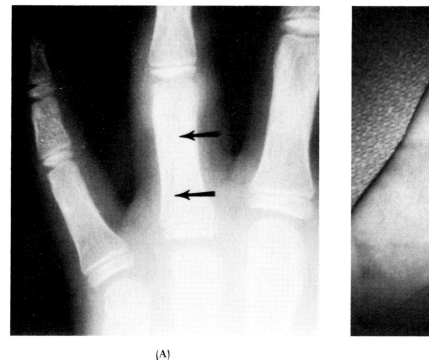

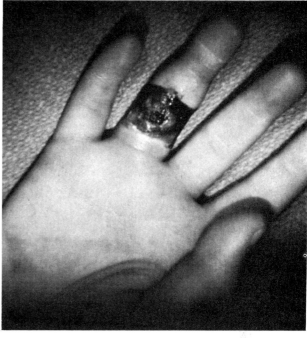

(A)
(B)

Figure 2-27 (A) PA radiograph shows a barely discernible undisplaced fracture of distal end of ring finger proximal phalanx. (B) Palmar view of injured digit shows necrosis of palmar tissues at site of crushing injury compounded by infection of a small open wound, which produced severe compromise of digit's vascularity. Though viability was precarious in this digit, it persisted.

Follow-up Care and Immobilization

Periodic radiographic reevaluation is necessary after satisfactory manipulation, reduction, and immobilization, particularly with a reduced articular fracture dislocation, or carpal instability so that a redisplacement can be diagnosed in time to permit re-reduction and internal fixation, if necessary, before malunion occurs.

Adequate physiologic external and/or internal immobilization is most important to prevent thumb-index web contracture, and in digits index through little fingers, extension contractures of the MP joints and flexion contractures of the PIP joints. Initial immobilization of a fracture or dislocation prevents motion in general, and specifically at the fracture site, with maximal symptomatic relief. It is vitally important to maintain constant elevation to relieve edema (Figures 2-29A,B) and to keep the dressing or cast dry. Maceration between immobilized adjacent digits is prevented by adequate soft tissue interposition, preventing contact at contiguous skin surfaces (Figure 2-30).

Therapy

Another most important aspect in the care of musculoskeletal injuries of the upper extremity is early motion and intelligent therapy. The role of the therapist in rehabilitation of an upper extremity injury is to teach the patient the proper basic exercises prescribed by the physician to regain physiologic active motion. It is extremely important to stress to the patient (1) that it is his or her responsibility to do the exercises at definitely prescribed intervals throughout the entire waking day and (2) that after the initial instruction the role of the therapist is one of periodic evaluation and encouragement i.e., to reinforce that these exercises are properly carried out as often as prescribed and to record progressive restoration of joint motion.

Motion of uninvolved joints and digits not essential for effective immobilization should be maintained throughout the entire period of immobilization of injured structures. Mobilization of the injured structure should be commenced as soon as healing has provided enough stability to prevent redis-

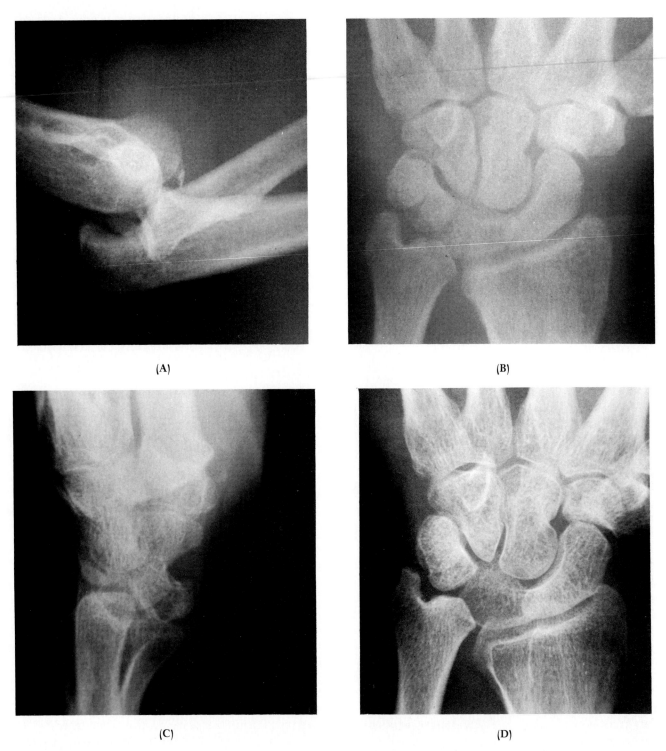

(A)

(B)

(C)

(D)

Figure 2-28 **(A)** Lateral radiograph discloses a posterior fracture dislocation of right elbow, including posterior dislocation of ulna and posterior fracture dislocation of radial head. **(B)** PA view of ipsilateral right wrist taken 7 weeks after injury shows rarefaction of lunate and indistinct articulations of lunate with adjacent carpals and distal radius. **(C)** Lateral view shows complete anterior dislocation of lunate with palmar tilt of approximately 65°. **(D)** PA view 3 weeks later shows similar findings in lunate with increased deossification of that bone and greater relative lengthening of ulna. Distal ulnar articular surface actually impinges on the triquetrum.

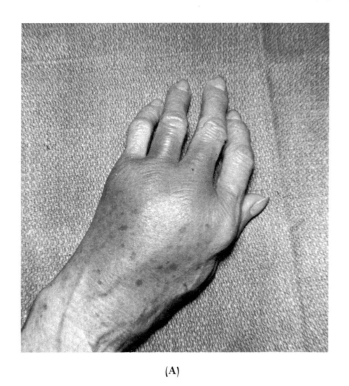

(A)

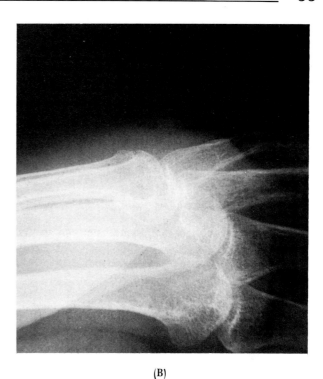

(B)

Figure 2-29 (A) Massive dorsal edema and ecchymosis due to inadvised sustained dependency following a rather minor fracture. (B) Radiograph illustrates fracture of ring finger metacarpal neck which is minimally palmarly angulated.

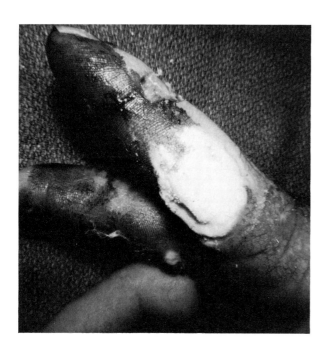

Figure 2-30 Extensive maceration noted 2 days after application of immobilization because patient allowed dressing to become wet. Such extensive maceration of skin can progress to gross infection and even loss of digit.

placement, angulation, rotation, shortening, or redislocation.

Complications

If delayed union (Figures 2-31A–E, 2-32A–D) or non-union (Figures 2-33A,B) occurs because of soft tissue interposition, surgical exposure and extraction of this soft tissue is indicated. If delayed union or nonunion is due either to fracture displacement or angulation, (e.g., displaced or angulated scaphoid fracture) or to motion at the fracture site, open reduction and autogenous bone grafting with internal fixation for stability, if necessary, should be considered. A bone graft is also indicated to replace a large segmental loss of bone.

Delayed union and nonunion of digital fractures are uncommon and usually result from severe trauma with extensive periosteal stripping and injury or from soft tissue interposition at the fracture site.

If balanced skeletal traction is used to maintain reduction, it is essential to avoid undue traction at the fracture site which may result in distraction, causing delayed union or nonunion.

Figure 2-31 (A) PA view illustrates oblique, rotated, proximally displaced proximal phalangeal shaft fracture 4 weeks after injury. Neither physical findings nor radiographic evidence indicated fracture healing. (B) Lateral radiograph shows a characteristic dorsal angulation at fracture site and no evidence of healing callus. (C) Palmar view in relaxed position prior to surgery shows significant crossover of ring finger beneath long finger due to rotational deformity. (D) Dorsal exposure of fracture site showed interposition of soft tissue including periosteum and lateral band at site of fracture nonunion. PA radiograph 2½ weeks after surgery shows anatomic reduction and internal fixation of fracture. (E) Lateral view shows similar findings. Complete normal digital flexion and extension regained 5 months after injury. Case illustrates a rather uncommon finding of proximal phalangeal fracture nonunion due to soft tissue interposition, necessitating surgical extraction of that tissue, open reduction, and internal fixation of fracture site, but no bone graft.

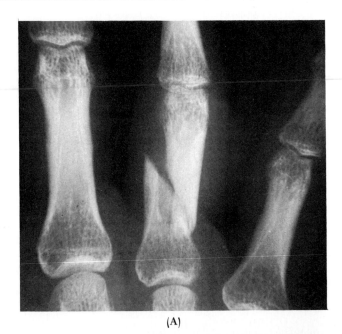

(A)

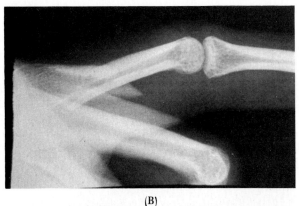

(B)

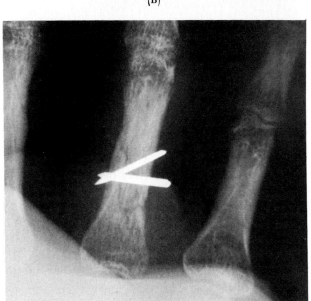

(D)

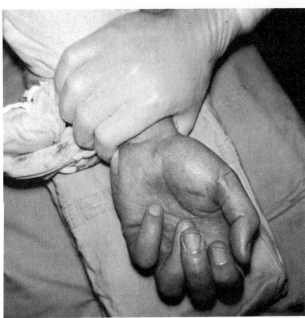

(C)

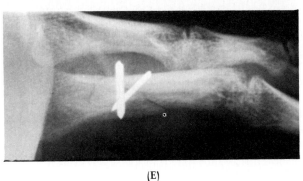

(E)

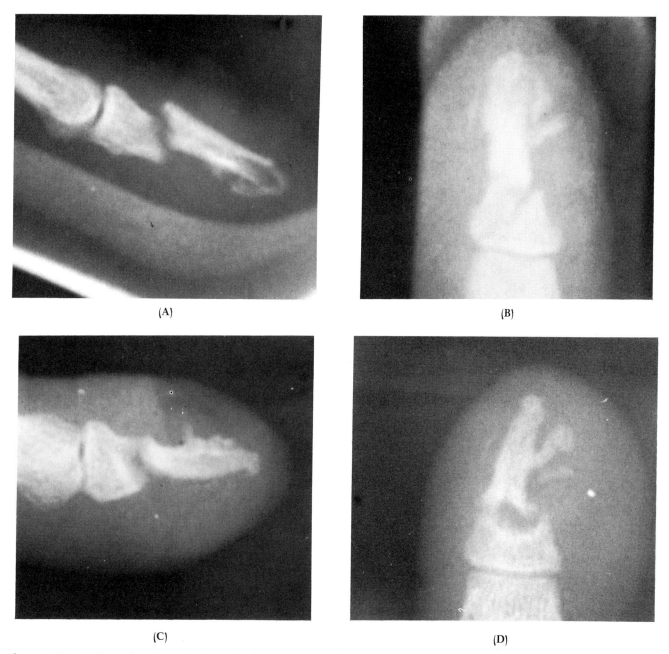

(A)

(B)

(C)

(D)

Figure 2-32 (A) Lateral radiograph 1 week after severe crush injury shows aluminum splint immobilization and acceptable alignment of distal phalangeal fracture, with correction of initial palmar angulation but considerable gap between proximal and distal bone fragments. (B) PA radiograph shows acceptable position and alignment of fracture. (C) Lateral radiograph 5½ months after injury shows tenuous healing at fracture site with sclerosis of distal segment. (D) PA view shows similar findings. Case illustrates the rather unusual findings of prolonged delayed union of a distal phalangeal fracture due to severity of crush injury, which produced excessive periosteal damage.

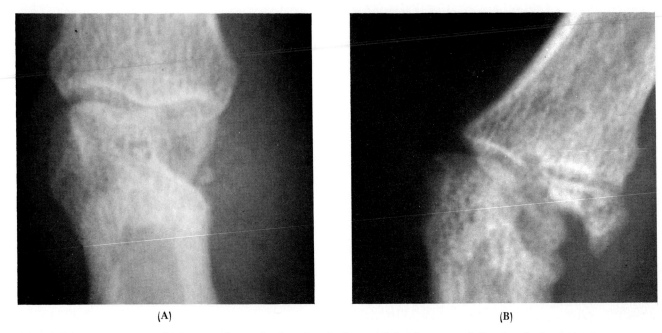

(A)   (B)

Figure 2-33 **(A)** PA view of PIP joint shows displaced articular condylar fracture of distal end of proximal phalanx. **(B)** Close-up view 3 months after initial trauma shows loss of position and complete instability at fracture site with bone resorption, angulation, and nonunion. Arthrodesis was performed. Case illustrates necessity of anatomic reduction and stable fixation of a large displaced articular fracture fragment and maintenance of reduction to avoid malunion or nonunion.

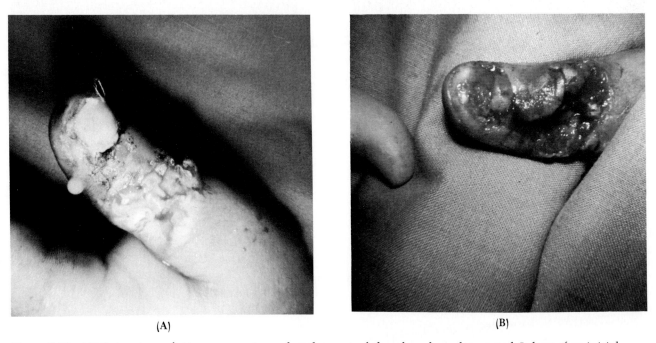

(A)   (B)

Figure 2-34 **(A)** Extensive soft tissue necrosis on dorsal aspect of thumb and exudate noted 5 days after initial treatment of open IP joint fracture of thumb by closure of capsule and primary extensor pollicis longus tenorrhaphy. Initial injury inflicted by a contaminated saw. Inadequate primary wound toilet combined with inadvised primary reconstructive procedures resulted in extensive severe infection. Preferred initial treatment would be meticulous wound toilet and open treatment. **(B)** Same wound after extensive debridement of necrotic tissue, including nail plate, and all infected material.

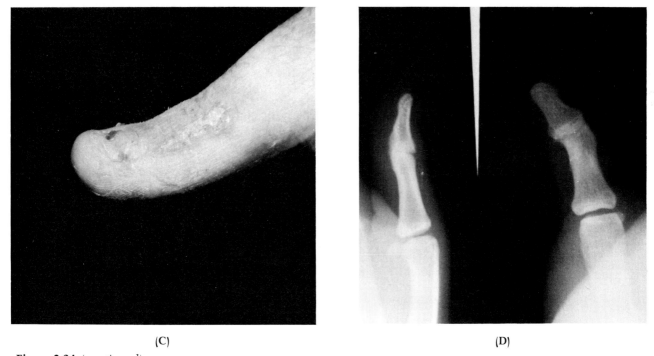

(C)   (D)

Figure 2-34 *(continued)*
(C) Autofusion of thumb IP joint occurred in malposition, as noted 3 months after injury. **(D)** Lateral and oblique views show hyperextension and radial angulation at site of IP joint spontaneous fusion. Patient did not desire osteotomy for a more physiologic position.

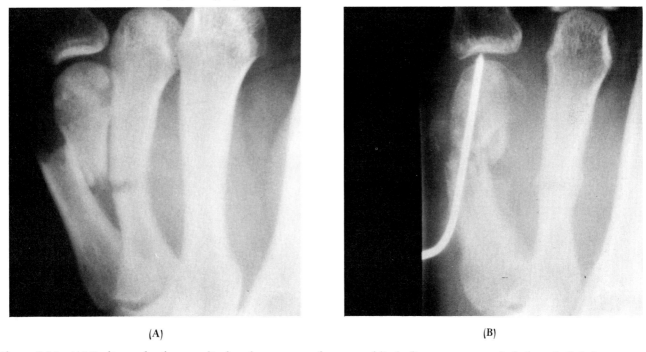

(A)   (B)

Figure 2-35   **(A)** Radiograph of open, displaced transverse fracture of little finger metacarpal shaft and slightly angulated incomplete fracture of ring finger metacarpal shaft. **(B)** Radiograph 1 month after open reduction and Kirschner wire fixation of little finger metacarpal fracture. Fracture site is unstable, and radiographic changes of osteomyelitis are noted, including blunting and rounding of bone edges at fracture site, calcification in soft tissues, and no evidence of union. Physical examination showed both local and systemic findings of infection. Fracture of ring finger metacarpal is healing well.

(continued)

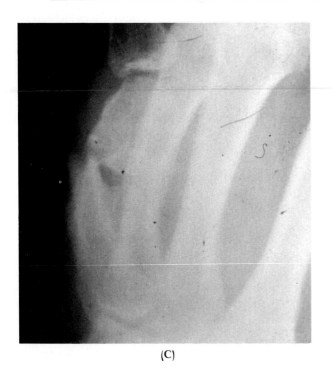

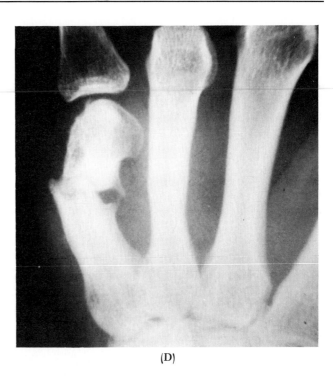

(C)   (D)

Figure 2-35 *(continued)*
(C) Radiograph 1 month later after removal of internal fixation shows nonunion with persistent chronic osteomyelitis. **(D)** PA radiograph 2½ months later shows no evidence of infection but nonunion at the fracture site of little finger metacarpal metaphysis. *(Illustrations 2-35A–D courtesy of H.A. Yocum, M.D.)*

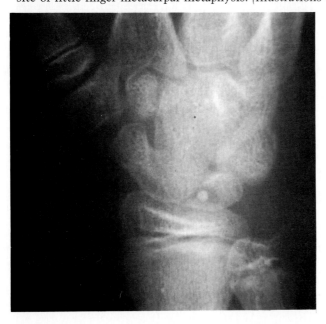

Figure 2-36   PA view of 10-year-old girl who fell on a lead pencil 3 weeks previously shows protrusion of a radiopaque foreign body palmarly from lunate. At exploration a piece of lead pencil and wood fragments were removed from lunate. Associated abscess and osteomyelitis were debrided and wound packed open. *(Illustration courtesy of A.M. Larimer, M.D.)*

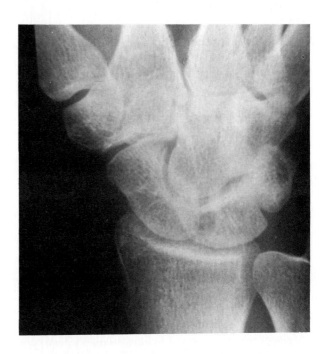

Figure 2-37   Somewhat oblique view of wrist illustrates a radiolucent lesion in lunate which was an enchondroma, not an abscess.

If infection is the cause of delayed union or nonunion, surgical exposure, radical debridement, and saucerization of the site should precede any attempt at bone graft or internal fixation (Figures 2-34A–D). Generally no reconstructive work should be carried out in a previously infected or potentially infected area until one is as certain as possible that the infection has been eradicated (Figures 2-35A–D). Antibiotic therapy is indicated at the time of reconstructive surgery and should begin prior to the actual surgical procedure. Exploration of the site of nonunion with debridement of all cicatrix down to normal-appearing bleeding bone should be effected. Specimens should be obtained for routine culture and sensitivities and the wound packed open. If cultures prove negative and there is no evidence of infection after loose primary closure of the skin, seven to ten days later an autogenous iliac bone graft combined with secure internal fixation may be carried out in an attempt to heal this nonunion.

If infection does develop, wide surgical debridement and open treatment is often necessary, as noted above for delayed union and nonunion. If pyarthrosis develops (Figures 2-26A–D), similar wide surgical debridement, if necessary, is usually preferred to tube irrigation because of the small area involved in digital joints. Early effective eradication of the infection is necessary to achieve the best functional results of maximum joint range of motion, tendon gliding, and nerve function with minimal cicatrix formation.

It is important to differentiate between a bone infection (osteomyelitis) (Figure 2-36) and a tumor or other conditions (Figure 2-37).

Posttraumatic and degenerative arthritis will be more severe if anatomic repositioning of an articular fracture is not accomplished primarily. If malunion of a large displaced articular fracture has occurred, osteotomy is usually necessary at a later time to reestablish the best possible articular surface and to minimize arthritic changes. Ligamentous reconstruction is necessary to restore normal anatomy if initial conservative treatment has resulted in marked ligamentous laxity or malposition of osseous elements (e.g., Gamekeeper's thumb and scapholunate dissociation).

If a large nerve such as the median, ulnar, or radial becomes entrapped, either in the area of fracture reduction or by callus formation, causing functional impairment, the nerve should be surgically explored and freed.

Sympathetic dystrophy and/or Sudek's atrophy occur in a small percentage of cases following upper extremity trauma. These conditions are quite refractory to treatment since there is often a marked overlay of associated anxiety in an apprehensive person. Treatment consists primarily of three to five stellate ganglion blocks performed on consecutive or alternate days. If necessary, the series may be repeated. A dynamic, very closely regulated program of medication and therapy is carried out concurrently. Early recognition of this complication and initiation of therapy provide the best result.

The "shoulder-hand syndrome" with a "frozen shoulder" (capsulitis) may result from prolonged external immobilization or because of patient inability, misunderstanding, or actual intention not to use the involved upper extremity. Aggressive therapy is the best treatment for this lesion, the basic fundamental exercise being that of pendulum circumduction. Rarely should manipulation of the involved joint be necessary since virtually all these lesions respond well to an intelligent, aggressive, self-administered therapy program. Examination of the shoulder one to two years after the initial diagnosis of chronic capsulitis reveals essentially normal function of that joint in the vast majority of cases.

General References

Adams J, Kenmore PJ, Russel PH, et al: regional anesthesia in the upper limb, in Adams JP (ed): *Current Practice in Orthopaedic Surgery*. St. Louis, C.V. Mosby Co., 1969, vol 4.

Flatt AE: *The Care of Minor Hand Injuries*, ed 3. St. Louis, C.V. Mosby Co., 1972.

Sandzén SC Jr: Treating acute hand and finger injuries Part 1. *Am Fam Physician* 1974;9:74–97.

Sandzén SC Jr: Treating acute hand and finger injuries Part 2. *Am Fam Physician* 1974;9:100–117.

Sandzén SC Jr: *Atlas of Acute Hand Injuries*. New York, McGraw-Hill and PSG Publishing Co., Inc., 1980.

CHAPTER
3

Injuries to the Distal Radius and Ulna

Although this Atlas is designed to provide information on the proper diagnosis and treatment of fractures and dislocations of the distal radius, ulna, wrist, and hand, discussion would be incomplete without a brief reference to the forearm in general.

The stability of the radius and ulna is a definite prerequisite to strong muscular use of the wrist and digits. Therefore, following significant trauma, the entire upper extremity must be reconstructed as anatomically as possible to provide the necessary stability, mobility, muscle power, and innervation, both motor and sensory, to position and power the hand correctly for physiologic movement and sensibility (Figures 3-1A–D).

Dynamic compression plate (DCP) fixation is recommended for irreducible and/or unstable both bone fractures of the forearm.

An undisplaced solitary fracture of the distal third of the radial diaphysis (Piedmont fracture) occasionally may be treated conservatively. However, displacement and/or angulation usually occurs because of the pull of the brachioradialis at its inser-

tion on the radial styloid process which necessitates open reduction and internal plate fixation.

The same fixation is applicable for an irreducible Piedmont fracture and for the Galeazzi injury complex (Figures 3-2A,B).

The Galeazzi fracture (Figures 3-2A,B) includes displacement or angulation of a fracture of the distal third of the radius, combined with dissociation (subluxation or dislocation) of the distal radioulnar articulation and dorsal or palmar subluxation or dislocation of the distal ulna. The radial shaft fracture is usually unstable, and open reduction is generally necessary to establish stability by internal plate fixation. After reduction of the fracture of the radial shaft, reduction of the distal radioulnar articulation follows spontaneously. There is no necessity for any ligamentous reconstruction if treated within three weeks of injury.

Though solitary fracture of the distal shaft of the ulna usually does not require internal fixation, should it be necessary, dynamic compression plate fixation is best.

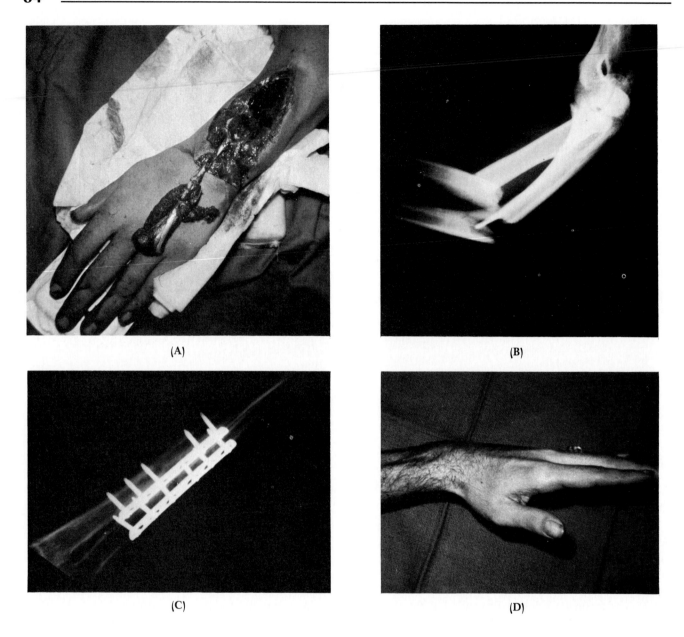

Figure 3-1 **(A)** Forearm caught in rotary mechanism of dough-making machine. Injuries included: open mid-shaft fractures of radius and ulna; diastasis of distal radioulnar articulation with open dorsal dislocation of distal ulna; and extensive soft tissue trauma to dorsum of forearm, including avulsion of most of extensor musculature. Photograph taken after meticulous cleansing and irrigation prior to debridement of devitalized tissue, including avulsed muscle and tendons on dorsum of hand. **(B)** Lateral radiograph shows dorsal angulation and displacement of both midshaft fractures. Note diastasis of distal radioulnar articulation due to divergence of radial and ulnar shafts distally. Initial therapy included delayed primary skin closure and external long arm cast immobilization. No attempt made of initial reconstruction or internal immobilization because of gross wound contamination. **(C)** Oblique radiograph 3 weeks after injury shows compression plate (Bagby) fixation of both reduced forearm fractures. Autogenous bone grafts were not included in open reduction and internal fixation, although preferred by some surgeons. **(D)** Complete digital but incomplete wrist extension following second and final reconstructive procedure, which included tendon transfers of flexor carpi ulnaris around distal ulna into common extensors and rerouting of palmaris longus tendon into rerouted extensor pollicis longus tendon distally to provide thumb extension and abduction. Complete digital flexion was also achieved (not shown).

Figure 3-2 **(A)** PA view shows Galeazzi fracture dislocation of forearm (fracture in distal third of radius and dislocation of distal ulna). **(B)** Lateral view shows dorsal angulation at fracture of radius and palmar dislocation of distal ulna. *(Illustrations 3-2A,B courtesy of R.A. Cautilli, M.D.)*

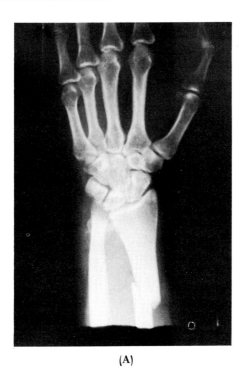

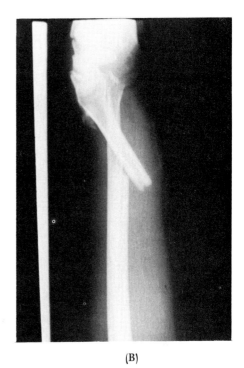

(A)

(B)

Metaphyseal and Segmental Articular Fractures of the Distal Radius

Fractures of the distal radius are very common, particularly in the older age groups, and in most cases are sustained by a fall on the outstretched hand.

Initial diagnosis must differentiate between a distal metaphyseal fracture, which may or may not extend into the distal radial articular cartilage (Figure 3-3), and isolated segmental articular fractures with or without subluxation of the carpus (Figure 3-4).

Differentiation of these fractures by their anatomic location rather than by eponym helps to understand these lesions and their care.

Metaphyseal fractures include:

1. Fracture of the distal radial metaphysis with dorsal angulation and/or displacement distal to the fracture site (distal radius carpus and hand)— resembling a "silver fork" deformity—Colles' fracture (Figures 3-5A–C)
2. Fracture of the distal radial metaphysis with palmar angulation and/or displacement—Smith's fracture (Figures 3-17A,B)

Colles' and Smith's fractures usually occur in middle-aged and elderly persons.

3. Salter I and II physeal separations, occurring in the skeletally immature

Fracture of the ulnar styloid process usually occurs in association with these distal radial metaphyseal and physeal fractures.

A distal metaphyseal fracture may be complicated by:

1. Involvement of the distal radial articular surface (Figure 3-7) and/or
2. Involvement of the distal radioulnar joint (Figure 3-18 and 3-20)

Segmental articular fractures of the distal radius include:

1. Dorsal segmental fracture of the distal radial articular surface usually with dorsal, proximal displacement of that articular fragment, associated with dorsal subluxation or dislocation of the carpus—dorsal Barton's fracture (Figures 3-21, 3-22)

METAPHYSEAL FRACTURES

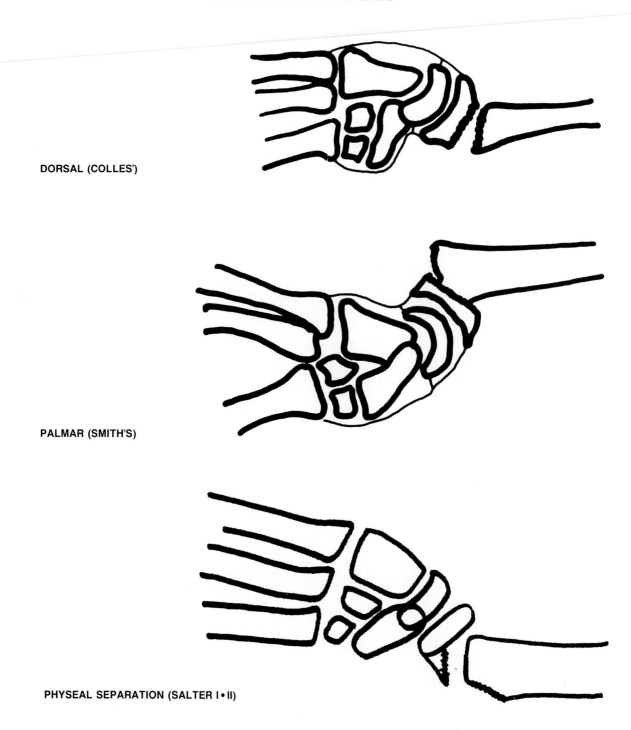

DORSAL (COLLES')

PALMAR (SMITH'S)

PHYSEAL SEPARATION (SALTER I • II)

Figure 3-3 Classification of fractures of the distal radius—metaphyseal fractures: dorsal (Colles') and palmar (Smith's) fractures involve the metaphysis of the distal radius but may have articular components extending into the wrist, the distal radioulnar joint, or both. Salter I and II physeal separations are the equivalent injuries in the skeletally immature. *(Reprinted, by permission, from Richard A. Cautilli, M.D., et al., Classifications of fractures of the distal radius, The Jefferson Orthopaedic Journal, 3:48, 1974.)*

ARTICULAR FRACTURES

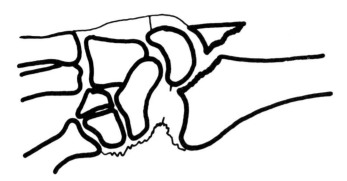

DORSAL (DORSAL BARTON'S)

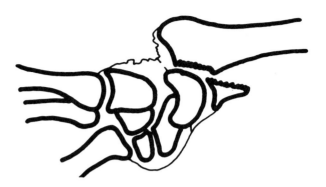

PALMAR (PALMAR BARTON'S)

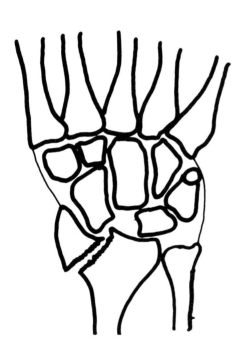

RADIAL (CHAUFFEUR'S)

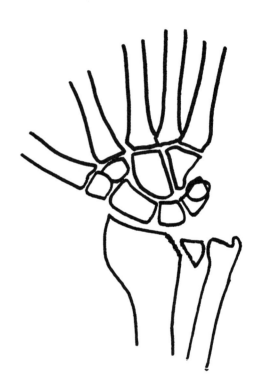

**ULNAR
(ULNAR VARIANT OF
CHAUFFEUR'S FRACTURE)**

Figure 3-4 Classification of segmental articular fractures of the distal radius—includes dorsal and palmar, radial and ulnar segmental articular fractures. Each injury consists of an articular fracture of a portion of the distal radial articular surface combined with subluxation or dislocation of the wrist. These injuries are basically unstable and must be differentiated from the more common Colles' and Smith's fractures to ensure proper treatment (not included are Salter III and IV physeal injuries discussed in Chapter 11). *(Reprinted, by permission, from Richard A. Cautilli, M.D., et al., Classifications of fractures of the distal radius. The Jefferson Orthopaedic Journal, 3:48, 1974.)*

2. Palmar segmental fracture of the distal radial articular surface usually with palmar, proximal displacement of that fragment, associated with palmar subluxation or dislocation of the carpus—palmar Barton's fracture (Figures 3-23, 3-24)
3. Fracture of the radial styloid process usually with radial, proximal displacement of that articular fragment, associated with radial subluxation or dislocation of the carpus—chauffeur's fracture (Figures 3-25, 3-26A–C, 3-27A,B)
4. Fracture of the ulnar aspect of the distal radial articular surface usually with injury to the distal ulna and distal radioulnar joint—ulnar variant of chauffeur's fracture (Figures 3-30–3-32)
5. Salter III and IV physeal separations

Fracture of the ulnar styloid process often occurs in association with distal radial segmental articular fractures also.

A segmental articular fracture of the distal radius, particularly the radial variant (chauffeur's fracture) may have associated scapho lunate dissociation and/or fractured scaphoid.

Differentiation between distal metaphyseal or nonarticular and segmental articular fractures of the distal radius is extremely important with respect to treatment.

Distal Metaphyseal Fractures

Colles' fracture (Figures 3-5A–E, 3-6A–F, 3-7A,B), the most common upper extremity fracture in the middle-aged or elderly person, is characterized by dorsal angulation and/or displacement of the distal radius distal to the fracture site and is usually caused by a fall on the palmar aspect of the outstretched hand (Figure 3-5A). Radiographs show a shortening of the radius, a silver fork deformity due to the displacement of the fracture, and a fracture of the styloid process of the ulna (Figures 3-5B,C). In addition to loss of normal radial length, there is loss of the normal palmar tilt and often of the ulnar angulation of the distal radial articular surface. The amount of shortening and loss of tilt depends on the severity of comminution and the amount of displacement. Instead of an ulnar styloid fracture, fracture of the distal ulnar shaft may sometimes occur (Figure 3-16A). Whether or not there is some type of ulnar fracture present, variable disruption of the distal radioulnar joint usually occurs.

Excellent anesthesia prior to reduction can be obtained by injection of 10 ml of 1.5% lidocaine into the fracture hematoma and 3 to 5 ml of the same substance into the area of the ulnar styloid process fracture.

Reduction of a Colles' fracture is achieved by disimpacting the fracture (if necessary), followed by longitudinal distal traction on the hand ("shaking hands with the patient") as the assistant exerts proximal traction and immobilizes the forearm proximal to the fracture. Forceful pressure on the dorsal aspect of the distal radius aided by countertraction or palmar pressure proximal to the fracture effects reduction. A sandbag or firmly rolled sheet placed proximal to the fracture site affords a good fulcrum to counteract the pressure applied dorsally distal to the fracture site. Some pronation of the distal radius and hand aids in reduction, but immobilization is effected with the wrist in neutral position or slight pronation. Some palmar flexion and ulnar deviation of the wrist is essential to maintain reduction, but the "Cotton-Loder" position of marked palmar flexion and ulnar deviation is *definitely contraindicated* as it causes impaired vascular supply, excessive edema, impaired digital motion, and often results in median nerve compression. The resultant impairment of wrist and finger motion and function due to such improper immobilization all too often results in flexion contractures of the wrist and digits which are quite refractory to prolonged aggressive physical therapy.

Methods of immobilization after reduction vary from a short arm cast to a long arm cast, depending on the clinician's preference. If a circular cast is used, one should be prepared to split the cast longitudinally "down to the skin" to relieve edema which may occur within the first 8 to 24 hours after manipulation and reduction.

A sugar tong splint immobilization offers an excellent alternative to either of the above types. After reduction the splint is applied from the dorsum of the distal metacarpus, proximally around the distal humerus and olecranon process of the ulna at the elbow, and to the palmar forearm out to the distal metacarpus. The palmar portion of the splint should not impinge on the MP joints of index through little fingers in order to allow physiologic digital flexion and extension. The thumb metacarpal should be maintained in wide abduction and thumb MP and IP joint motions permitted. With this type of immobilization relative elbow immobility is achieved, and there is no danger of complications such as vascular impairment or edema due to circular cast immobilization. If complications should develop, simply

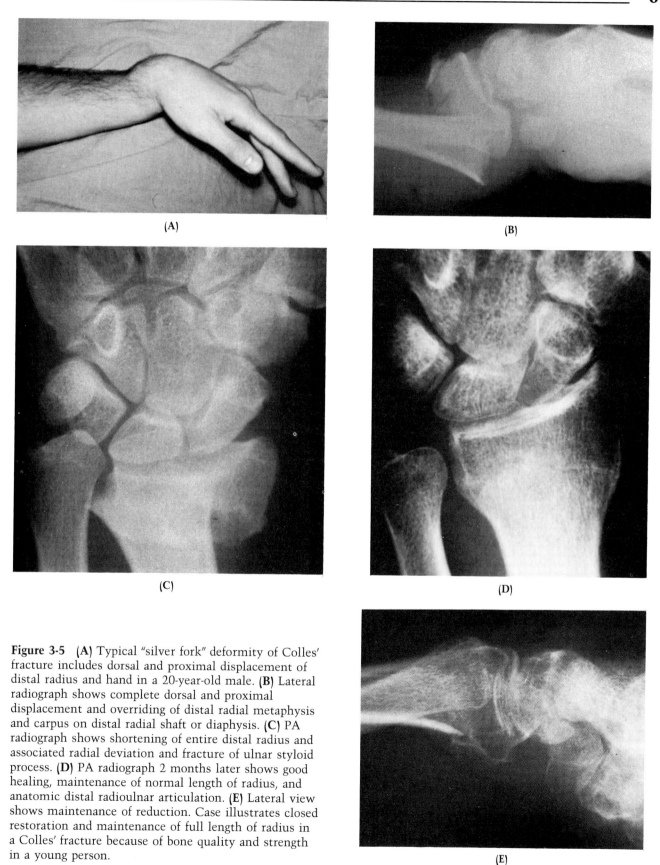

Figure 3-5 (A) Typical "silver fork" deformity of Colles' fracture includes dorsal and proximal displacement of distal radius and hand in a 20-year-old male. (B) Lateral radiograph shows complete dorsal and proximal displacement and overriding of distal radial metaphysis and carpus on distal radial shaft or diaphysis. (C) PA radiograph shows shortening of entire distal radius and associated radial deviation and fracture of ulnar styloid process. (D) PA radiograph 2 months later shows good healing, maintenance of normal length of radius, and anatomic distal radioulnar articulation. (E) Lateral view shows maintenance of reduction. Case illustrates closed restoration and maintenance of full length of radius in a Colles' fracture because of bone quality and strength in a young person.

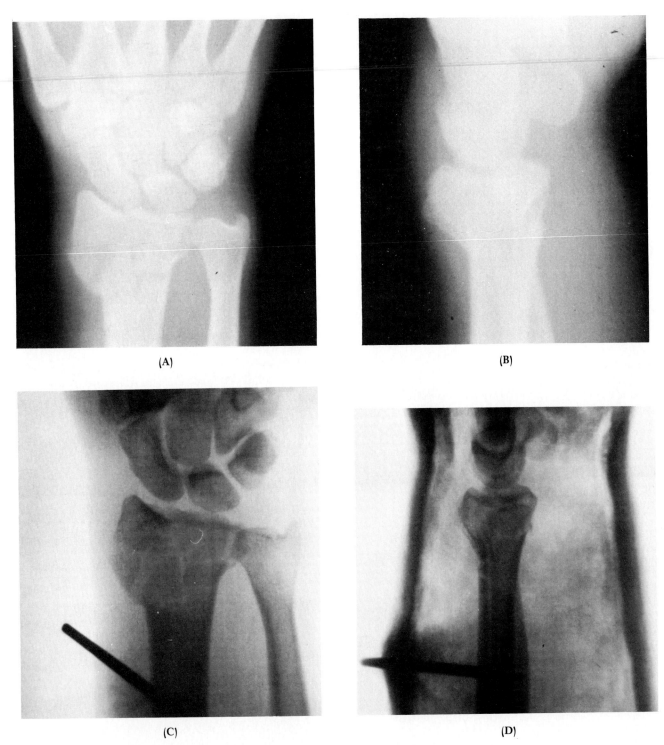

(A)

(B)

(C)

(D)

Figure 3-6 (A) PA radiograph shows comminuted Colles' fracture with some shortening of distal radius in a 45-year-old healthy male. (B) Lateral radiograph shows loss of normal palmar tilt of distal radius and comminution of fracture. (C) PA view illustrates restoration of good length of radius and acceptable position of comminuted fracture fragments following closed manipulation, reduction, and insertion of Steinmann pin transversely through bases of index and long finger metacarpals, and of modified Haggie pin in shaft of radius proximal to fracture site, for pins-and-plaster immobilization. (D) Lateral radiograph after immobilization shows modified Haggie pin extending dorsally into shaft of radius to avoid damage to radial nerve. Note that distal radial articular surface does not have normal palmar angulation of 12°. This method of treatment does not reestablish palmar tilt.

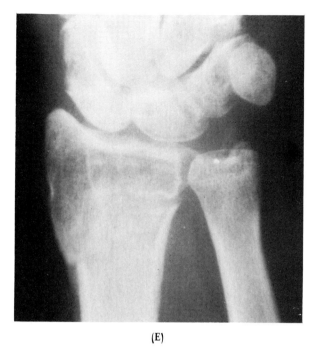

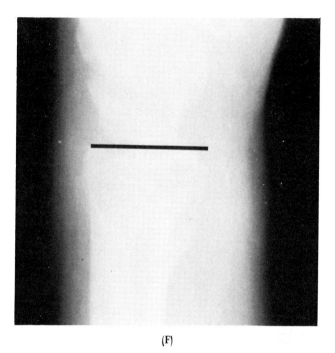

(E) (F)

Figure 3-6 *(continued)*
(E) Three months later PA view shows normal length of distal radius, good distal radioulnar articulation, and good articular surface of distal radius. Case illustrates the most appropriate patient and type of injury for this particular technique of immobilization. **(F)** Lateral radiograph shows excellent healing, but not restoration, of normal distal radial palmar angulation.

cutting the soft compression dressing on the radial or ulnar aspect of the sugar tong splint will relieve the difficulty.

An excellent method for treating an unstable distal radial metaphyseal fracture is to drill a modified Haggie pin (Figures 3-6A–F) transversely or from dorsal to palmar aspect across the shaft of the radius, just proximal to the fracture site at the approximate junction of the middle and distal thirds of that bone. A modified Haggie pin is preferable to a Kirschner wire since its bone fixation is more stable. A large Kirschner wire or small unthreaded Steinmann pin is then driven transversely across the metacarpals of the index and long finger (stable portion of the hand), preferably near to their bases in the proximal third of the shaft. Insertion of these pins obviously should be carried out under sterile surgical conditions. Care must be taken in placing the proximal pin to avoid damage to the superficial radial nerve and, with respect to the distal pin, to avoid impingement on the thumb-index web space. Bending the portion of the distal pin which protrudes from the skin should relieve any such web impingement.

After the fracture has been disimpacted, the thumb, index, and long fingers are secured by Chinese finger traps, and a padded 10-lb weight is hung from the arm with the elbow flexed 90°. The entire upper extremity is then suspended by the Chinese finger traps applied to the index and long fingers and the thumb. A repeat radiograph with the weight applied to the fracture should show suitable reduction and maintenance thereof on both PA and lateral views. The portions of both the proximal and distal pins protruding from the skin (the distal pin protruding from both points of entrance and exit) are incorporated into a short arm cast immobilization after application of a small sterile sponge over each pin. This method regains length of the distal radius but does not restore the palmar tilt to the distal radius (Figures 3-6D,F).

This pins-and-plaster immobilization is an extremely valuable procedure for treating unstable distal metaphyseal fractures in the physiologically younger patient. Disadvantages of this technique include prolonged immobilization, a minimum of eight to ten weeks to insure sufficient fracture healing prior to pin removal, and exertion of traction across multiple joints, including the wrist, intercarpal, and carpometacarpal joints.

An external fixator may be preferred rather than pins and plaster treatment and is particularly useful with concurrent soft tissue injuries necessitating consecutive dressing changes. Meticulous atten-

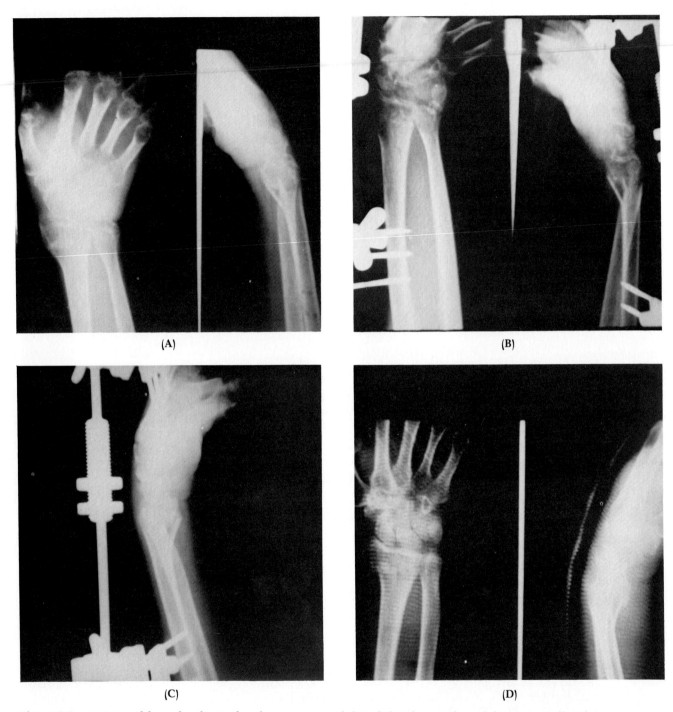

(A)

(B)

(C)

(D)

Figure 3-7   (A) PA and lateral radiographs of a comminuted dorsal distal metaphyseal fracture (Colles' fracture) involving the distal radial articular surface after reduction and immobilization in a long arm cast. (B) Because of the extensive comminution and involvement of the distal radial articular surface an external fixator was employed with reduction maintained in PA and lateral radiographs. (C) True lateral radiograph shows excellent position of the fracture achieved with approximately 5° palmar angulation of the distal radial articular surface maintained. (D) The result eight weeks after initiation of external immobilizer treatment shows good length of the radius and palmar tilt of approximately 5° on PA and lateral radiographs.

tion to details of technique are necessary whichever type external fixator is used (Figures 3-7A–D).

If the distal radius is not severely comminuted and a large intact segment of the radial styloid persists, a Steinmann pin may be inserted obliquely through the distal ulnar shaft into the distal radius, terminating just proximal to the external cortex of the radial styloid (DePalma method). This procedure is generally not as satisfactory as the pins-and-plaster technique or open reduction with internal or percutaneous fixation.

In the elderly patient the preponderance of osteoporotic medullary (spongy) bone in the distal radial metaphysis makes these methods less desirable because of the prolonged time for healing. *It should be remembered that the single most important goal in the treatment of a Colles' type fracture in the elderly patient is to insure as far as possible the best ultimate function of the hand.* Therefore the majority of such fractures in the elderly should probably be treated by closed manipulation and reduction. Despite a shortened radius, which results in some cosmetic unacceptability after healing has occurred, hand function should be normal. If the protruding distal ulna impinges on the carpus (triquetrum) enough to cause pain and limitation of motion (pronation and supination and ulnar deviation) (Figures 3-8A,B), a reconstructive procedure involving excision of the distal ulna may be carried out with excellent results (Darrach procedure) if properly executed (Figures 3-9A,B and 3-10A–C). There is no reason whatever to perform primary excision of the distal ulna in the initial treatment of Colles' fracture (Figure 3-11).

Regardless of the type of immobilization, complete digital and shoulder ranges of motion should be maintained and stressed during the entire treatment.

Complications inherent in the pathology and treatment of Colles' type fractures include:[1]

1. Malunion of the distal radius with shortening and loss of the normal palmar and/or ulnar tilt of the distal radial articular surface (Figures 3-8A,B, 3-12C,D)
2. Compression of the median nerve by protruding bone spicules (Figures 3-13A,B)
3. Incomplete reduction
4. Spontaneous rupture of common extensor tendons by constant friction during their continuous motion over an abnormal distal radioulnar articulation, combined with posttraumatic and degenerative arthritic changes (Figures 3-14A–G)

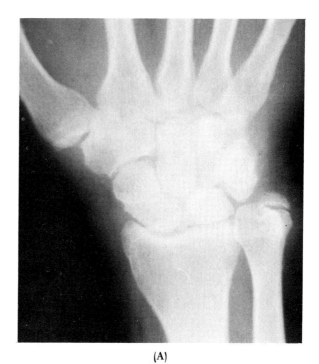

(A)

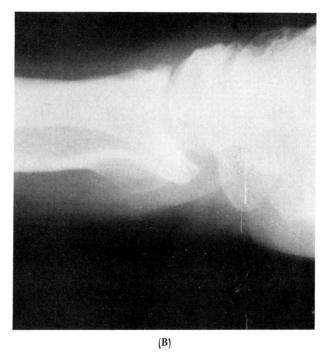

(B)

Figure 3-8 **(A)** PA radiograph shows healed Colles' fracture sustained 8 years previously. Note shortening of distal radius and impingement of relatively longer ulna upon wrist, abutting against lunate and triquetrum. Blunting of distal ulna and ununited fracture of the ulnar styloid process also evident. **(B)** Lateral view shows 15° reversal of normal 12° to 14° palmar tilt of distal radius with secondary dorsal subluxation of carpus.

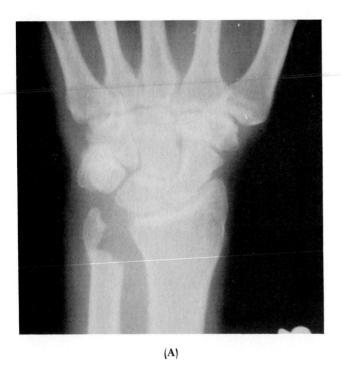

(A)

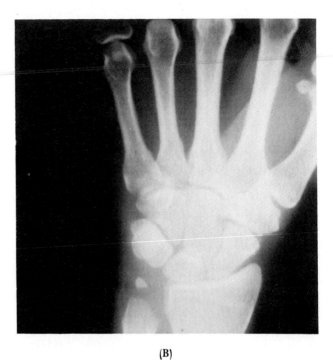

(B)

Figure 3-9 **(A)** One technique of a modified Darrach procedure is to leave the external cortex of the ulna and excise only the radial aspect of the distal ulna. **(B)** Another technique of a modified Darrach procedure is to subperiosteally excise a small segment of the distal ulna with care to maintain periosteum and the ulnar collateral ligament of the wrist.

5. Rupture of the extensor pollicis longus tendon, usually in the area of Lister's tubercle (Figures 3-15A–D)
6. Nonunion (Figures 3-16A–C)

The mirror image of the Colles' fracture involves palmar angulation or displacement of the distal radius and hand. This is usually caused by a fall on the flexed wrist (Smith's fracture, Figures 3-17A,B, 3-18A,B, 3-19). Reduction and maintenance of reduction are just opposite that for Colles' fracture. Immobilization should incorporate moderate wrist extension, ulnar deviation, and essentially neutral pronation and supination. With extensive comminution and/or instability, the pins-and-plaster technique may be equally well utilized in the appropriate patient.

Complications with Smith's fracture are similar to those with Colles' fracture.

A severely comminuted distal metaphyseal fracture of the radius with involvement of the distal radial articular surface is probably best treated by the pins-and-plaster technique of immobilization to restore the anatomy of the distal radius as well as possible (Figures 3-18A,B).

Involvement of the distal radioulnar joint by fracture comminution or dislocation naturally increases the severity of injury (Figures 3-20A,B) and increases also the ultimate disability with decrease of motion, primarily pronation and supination.

For a discussion of physeal separations—Salter I and II, see Chapter 11.

Segmental Articular Fractures of the Distal Radius[2,3,4,5]

Included in this discussion are dorsal (dorsal Barton's fracture), palmar (palmar Barton's fracture), radial (chauffeur's fracture) and ulnar (ulnar variant of chauffeur's fracture) segmental articular fractures and Salter III and IV physeal injuries (discussed in Chapter 11) (Figure 3-4).

Dorsal Segmental Articular Fracture (Dorsal Barton's fracture). A hyperextension injury, consists of a dorsal articular fracture of the distal radius, usually proximally displaced, associated with dorsal subluxation

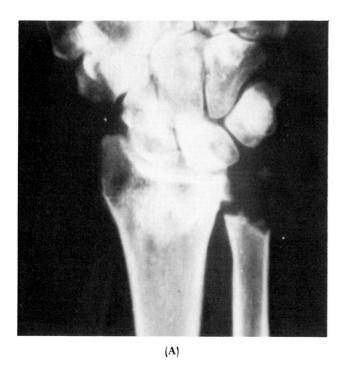

(A)

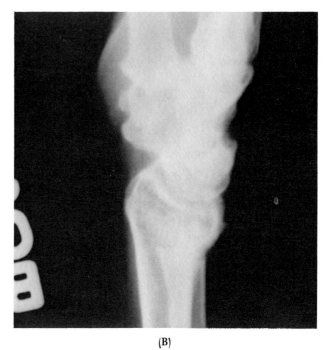

(B)

Figure 3-10 **(A)** An incorrectly performed Darrach procedure with excision of too large a segment of the distal ulna followed malunion of a Colles' fracture. **(B)** Lateral view shows 40° dorsal angulation of the malunion. **(C)** Because of chronic persistent dysesthesia on the dorsoulnar aspect of the wrist and hand, exploration revealed a neuroma of a large dorsal cutaneous branch of the ulnar nerve severed at the time of resection of the distal ulna.

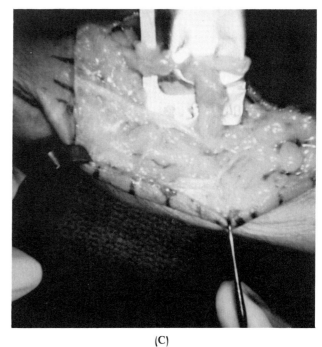

(C)

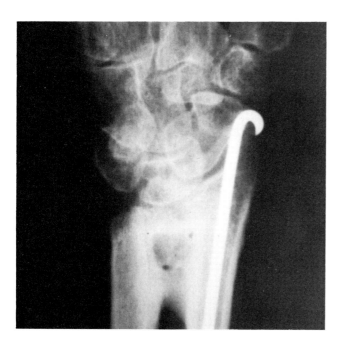

Figure 3-11 *(At left)* Oblique view illustrates result of improper initial treatment of Colles' fracture, which included primary Darrach procedure of distal ulna with Rush rod fixation of the radius. Synostosis of distal radius and ulna is seen with retention of Rush rod 14 months after injury. *(Illustration courtesy of H.A. Yocum, M.D.)*

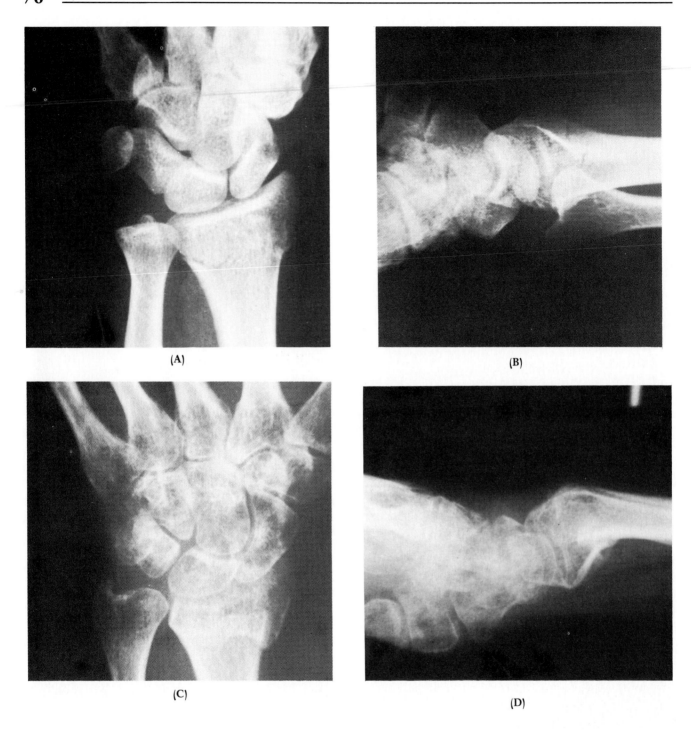

(A)

(B)

(C)

(D)

Figure 3-12 (A) PA radiograph of essentially undisplaced fracture of distal radial metaphysis. Carpal architecture is normal. (B) Lateral radiograph shows no displacement of distal metaphyseal fracture. Carpal architecture is normal. (C) PA radiograph 4 months after injury shows malunion of fracture with shortening of radius following complete loss of position in plaster immobilization. (D) Lateral view shows malunion with severe palmar displacement of carpus. Case illustrates importance of radiographic follow-up, even of an innocuous appearing fracture, to insure maintenance of proper position. Early diagnosis of displacement to allow manipulation and reduction and pins-and-plaster fixation, if necessary, will prevent malunion. *(Illustrations 3-12A–D courtesy of J.H. Wolf, M.D.)*

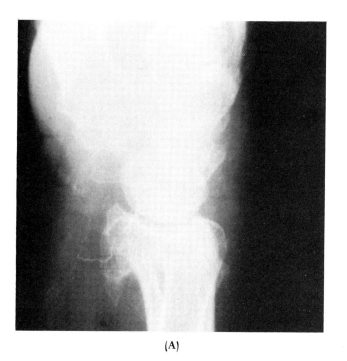

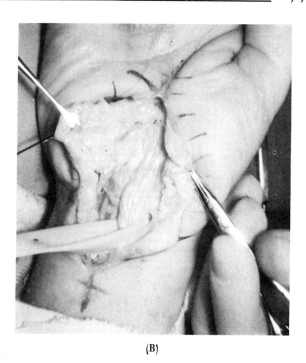

(A)   (B)

Figure 3-13 **(A)** Lateral radiograph of healed Colles' fracture in 72-year-old male shows palmar protrusion of healed bony spicule at site of healing combined with loss of normal palmar tilt of distal radius. **(B)** Excision of transverse carpal ligament and median neurolysis to relieve chronic median nerve compression exerted by bone spicule protruding into flexor area. No attempt made to remove spicule since pressure on median nerve was released following excision of portion of transverse carpal ligament and external neurolysis.

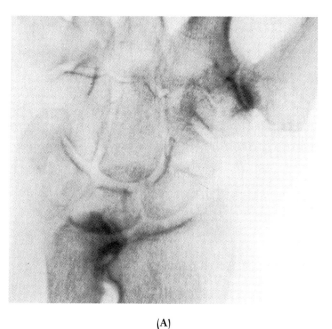

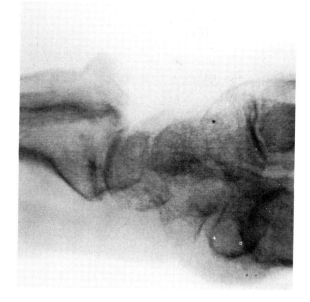

(A)   (B)

Figure 3-14 **(A)** PA radiograph of healed Colles' fracture 2½ years after injury in 78-year-old female shows incongruity of distal radioulnar articulation and shortening of distal radius, with abnormal increase of the radioulnar inclination of distal radial articular surface. **(B)** Lateral radiograph shows dorsal protrusion of distal ulna with degenerative and posttraumatic changes. Because of irregularity and bone spurs in area of distal radioulnar articulation following healing, spontaneous attrition and rupture of common extensors to ring and little fingers and extensor digiti minimi tendon to little finger occurred.

(continued)

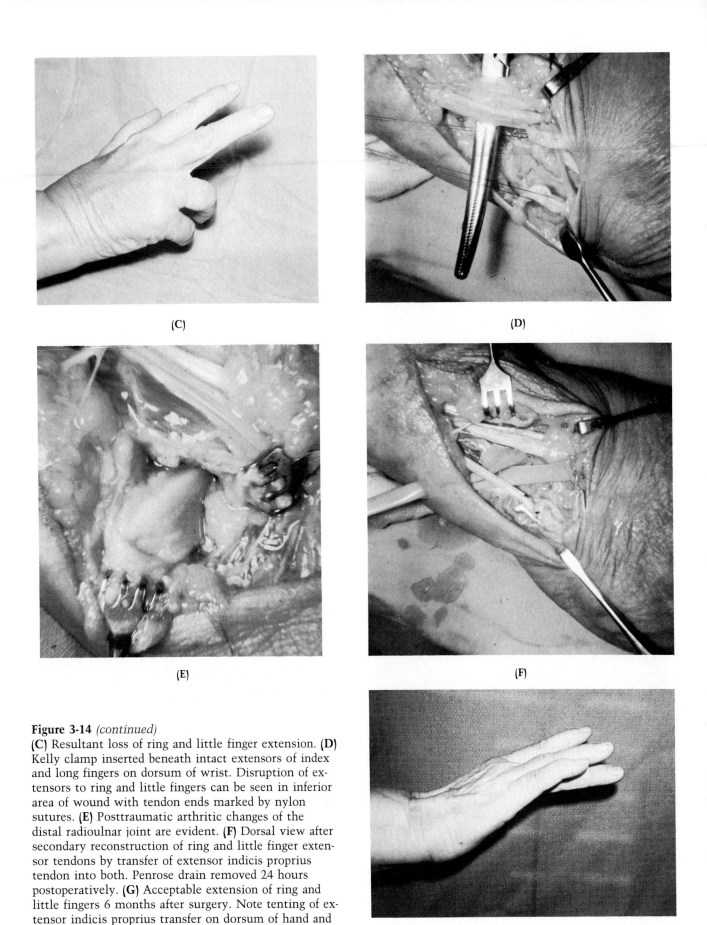

Figure 3-14 *(continued)*
(C) Resultant loss of ring and little finger extension. **(D)** Kelly clamp inserted beneath intact extensors of index and long fingers on dorsum of wrist. Disruption of extensors to ring and little fingers can be seen in inferior area of wound with tendon ends marked by nylon sutures. **(E)** Posttraumatic arthritic changes of the distal radioulnar joint are evident. **(F)** Dorsal view after secondary reconstruction of ring and little finger extensor tendons by transfer of extensor indicis proprius tendon into both. Penrose drain removed 24 hours postoperatively. **(G)** Acceptable extension of ring and little fingers 6 months after surgery. Note tenting of extensor indicis proprius transfer on dorsum of hand and wrist. Almost complete digital flexion also achieved.

78

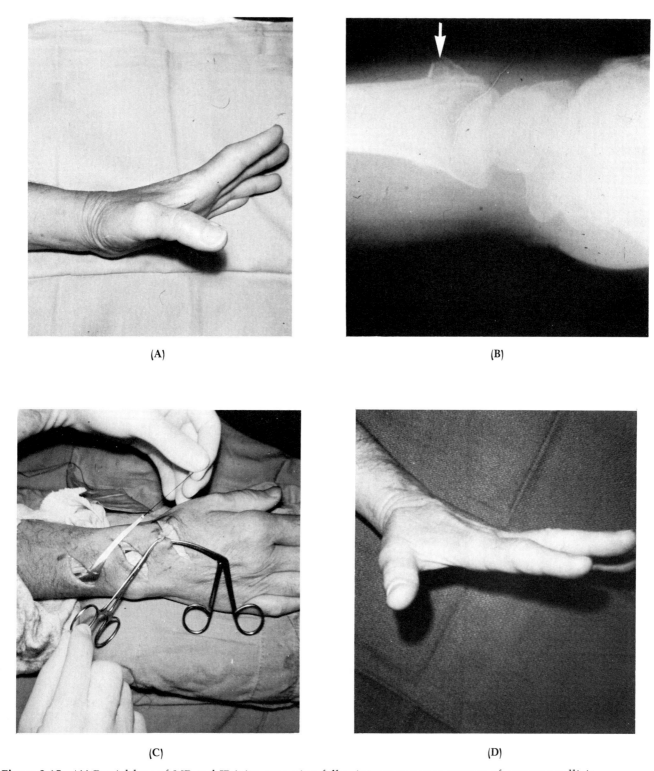

(A)　　　　　　　　　　　　　　　　(B)

(C)　　　　　　　　　　　　　　　　(D)

Figure 3-15 **(A)** Partial loss of MP and IP joint extension following spontaneous rupture of extensor pollicis longus tendon eroded by bony spur at site of healed Colles' fracture (68-year-old female). **(B)** Lateral view shows protruding bone spicule in area of Lister's tubercle. **(C)** Dorsal view shows transfer of extensor indicis proprius tendon into distal end of ruptured extensor pollicis longus tendon. **(D)** Three months after surgery extension of thumb acceptable and flexion (not shown) normal.

Figure 3-16 **(A)** Close-up PA radiograph shows an extremely comminuted open Colles' fracture associated with fracture of distal ulnar shaft in a 75-year-old woman. Shortening of radius and angulation of ulna at respective fracture sites are obvious. Initial treatment was meticulous cleansing, debridement, and irrigation, followed by pins-and-plaster fixation incorporated in a short arm cast. Radial length was restored. **(B)** PA radiograph 10 weeks after injury shows nonunion of Colles' fracture and union of ulnar shaft fracture. **(C)** Lateral radiograph does not illustrate well nonunion of Colles' fracture which occurred owing to massive injury sustained by radius and to loss of bone substance at fracture site, although there was no infection. Advanced age of patient precluded bone graft of nonunion. *(Illustrations 3-16A–C courtesy of D.C. Brown, M.D.)*

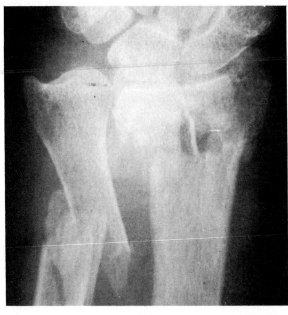

(A)

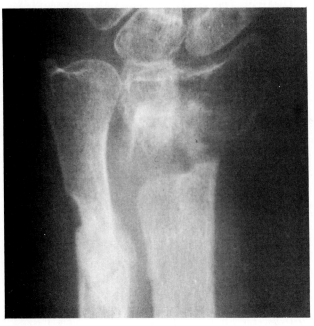

(B)

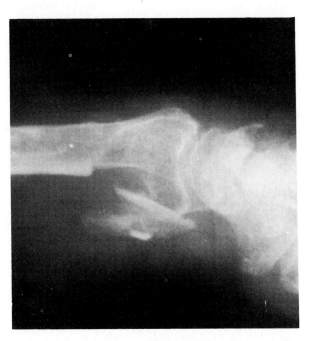

(C)

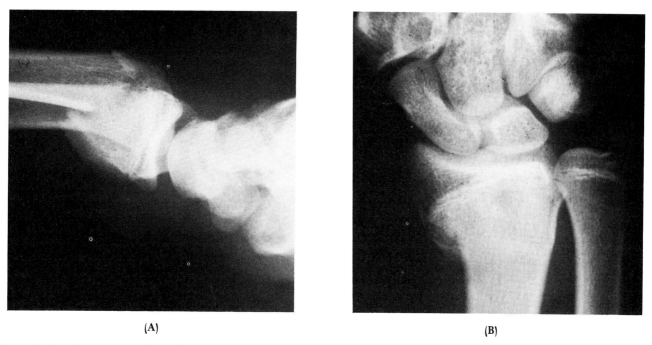

(A)

(B)

Figure 3-17 **(A)** Lateral radiograph of Smith's fracture of distal radius in a 16-year-old male showing palmar angulation and displacement at fracture site. **(B)** PA view shows shortening and radial deviation of distal radius. *(Illustrations 3-17A,B courtesy of D.M. Junkin, M.D.)*

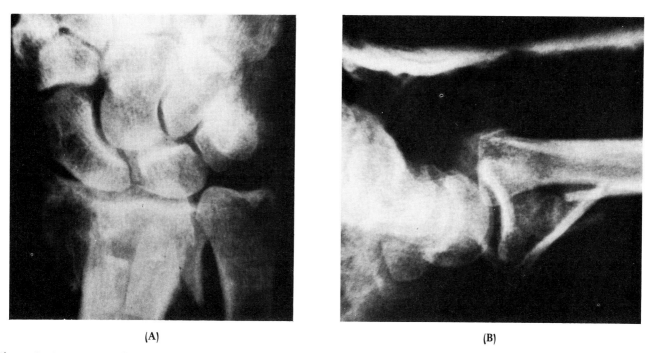

(A)

(B)

Figure 3-18 **(A)** PA radiograph illustrates grossly comminuted fracture of distal radial metaphysis with shortening of radius. **(B)** Corresponding lateral radiograph shows palmar and proximal displacement at fracture site. Diagnosis is comminuted unstable Smith's fracture of distal radial metaphysis. Treatment included closed manipulation and reduction with pins-and-plaster fixation. *(Illustrations 3-18A,B courtesy of B.I. Rambach, M.D.)*

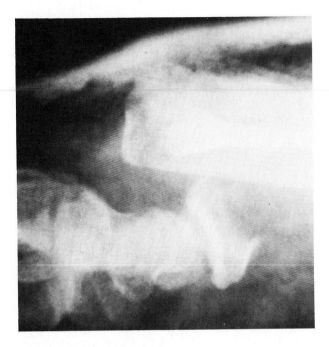

Figure 3-19   Lateral view shows a severe Smith's fracture with complete palmar and proximal displacement of distal radius and hand.

or dislocation of the carpus. The palmar portion of the distal radial articular surface remains intact (Figures 3-21, 3-22).

The method of reduction and maintenance thereof is exactly opposite that for Colles' fracture, *with which it may be easily confused.* Inherent in the pathology of dorsal Barton's fracture is disruption of the ligamentous structure on the contralateral (palmar) surface of the fracture subluxation. The intact ligament on the ipsilateral side of the fracture subluxation maintains its normal anatomic connection between the displaced articular fragment and the carpus. This connection is an integral factor in achieving and maintaining reduction of the fracture subluxation or dislocation. Dorsal fracture subluxation is reduced by mild extension of the wrist to reduce the dorsal articular fracture fragment of the radius. If palmar flexion is attempted, the intact dorsal ligament will prevent reduction of the fragment, and traction on that intact ligament actually "flips out" the articular fracture fragment. Carpal instability may be an associated finding.

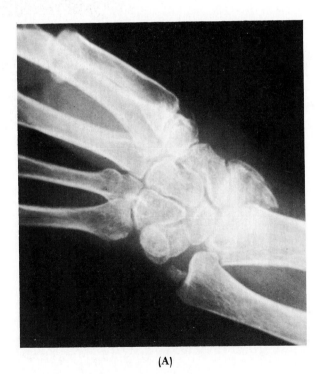

(A)

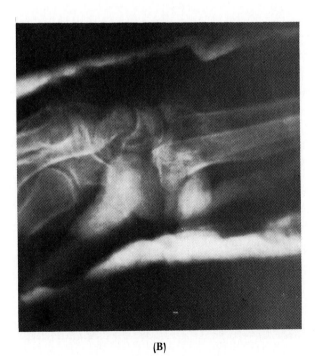

(B)

Figure 3-20   (A) PA view of comminuted Colles' fracture. Because of involvement of distal radioulnar articulation, prognosis is for poor functional result. (B) Lateral view in plaster immobilization shows palmar dislocation of distal ulna and DISI carpal instability following manipulation and reduction of Colles' fracture. Reduction of fracture and distal ulnar dislocation achieved by manipulation followed by pins-and-plaster immobilization. *(Illustrations 3-20A,B courtesy of J.R. Rubin, M.D.)*

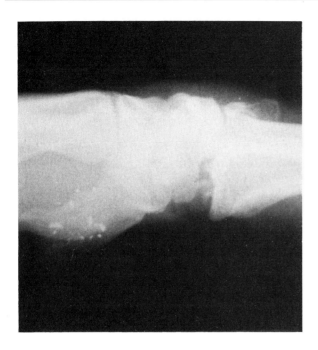

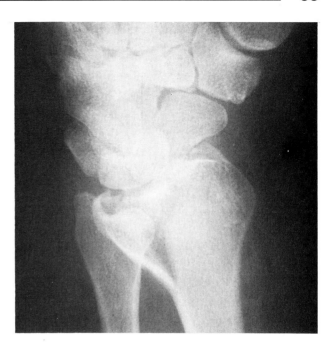

Figure 3-21 Lateral radiograph illustrates dorsal Barton's fracture subluxation of distal radius. Note displaced articular fracture of dorsal aspect of distal radial articular surface, with dorsal and proximal displacement of fracture fragment in close association with carpus, which is dorsally and proximally subluxed. *(Reprinted, by permission, from R.A. Cautilli, M.D., et al., Classifications of fractures of the distal radius, The Jefferson Orthopaedic Journal 3:47, 1974.)*

Figure 3-22 Oblique radiograph shows dorsal Barton's fracture involving oblique segment of ulnar aspect of distal radial articular surface. Dorsal and proximal displacement of fracture fragment is combined with dorsal subluxation of carpus.

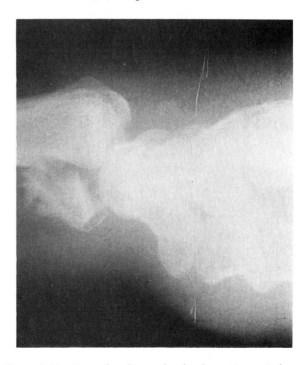

Pins-and-plaster or external fixator technique may be used to maintain a satisfactory reduction of the fracture subluxation.

Percutaneous Kirschner wire fixation or open reduction and internal fixation of a large articular segment, if necessary, may be preferred in the young individual to guarantee the best possible articular surface.

Buttress plate fixation may be preferred occasionally (see Chapter 16) but is more frequently used in the palmar type.

Palmar Segmental Articular Fracture (Palmar Barton's fracture). A palmar flexion injury, includes an articular fracture of the palmar aspect of the distal radial articular surface, usually with palmar proximal displacement, combined with palmar subluxation or dislocation of the carpus (Figures 3-23, 3-24A–C). The dorsal distal radial articular surface remains intact.

Figure 3-23 Lateral radiograph of palmar Barton's fracture subluxation. Note large palmar articular segment of distal radius displaced palmarly and proximally in close association with palmar subluxation of carpus. *(Illustration courtesy of E.J. Resnick, M.D.)*

Figure 3-24 (A) Lateral radiograph of palmar Barton's fracture subluxation of distal radius. Note comminution of dorsal articular segment. (B) Lateral radiograph following reduction and internal plate fixation of fracture shows marked comminution of dorsal fracture fragment. (C) PA view shows reduction of fracture with internal palmar plate fixation. Dorsal fragment was not secure enough to maintain stable reduction and required internal plate fixation to prevent redisplacement. *(Illustrations 3-24A–C courtesy of R.G. Eaton, M.D.)*

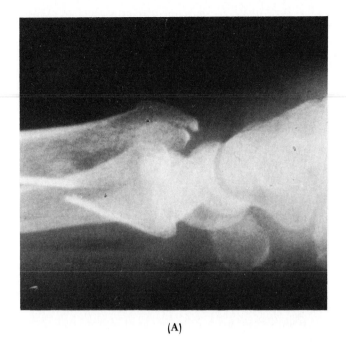

(A)

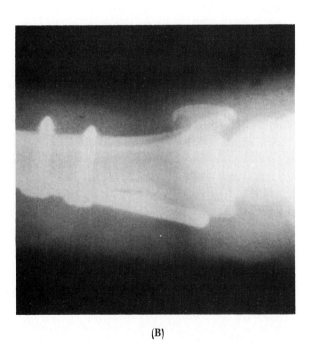

(B)

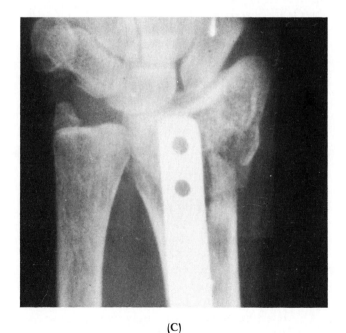

(C)

It is extremely important to realize this lesion is a *palmar segmental articular fracture* not a variant of a palmar metaphyseal fracture (Smith's fracture) as erroneously described in Thomas' classification.[6] Reduction involves slight palmar flexion which is necessary to reduce and maintain reduction of the fracture fragment. This is exactly the opposite of the maneuver used to reduce Smith's fracture with which palmar Barton's fracture may easily be confused. Carpal instability may also be associated with this condition.

Other methods of treatment include the same procedures previously described for the dorsal fracture, including internal fixation.

Palmar buttress plate fixation may be preferred (Figures 3-24A–C).

Radial Segmental Articular Fracture (chauffeur's fracture). Consists of fracture of the radial styloid or radial aspect of the distal radial articular surface, usually with radial proximal displacement, associated with radial or radial and palmar or dorsal subluxation or dislocation of the carpus (Figures 3-25, 3-26A–E, 3-27A–E). The ulnar portion of the distal radial articular surface remains intact. Thus either merely the radial styloid process itself (Figure 3-25), a significant portion of the radial aspect of the distal radial articular surface (Figure 3-26B), or any degree of severity of injury between (Figure 3-27A) may be involved.

A significant segment of either palmar or dorsal articular surface of the distal radius may be in continuity with the radial articular fragment (Figures 3-26B,C).

Any undisplaced articular fracture must be closely followed radiographically to diagnose displacement (Figures 3-28, 3-29).

Ulnar Segmental Articular Fracture (ulnar variant of chauffeur's fracture). Segmental fracture of the ulnar aspect of the distal radial articular surface (ulnar variant of chauffeur's fracture) referred to elsewhere as a medial cuneiform fracture,[7] rarely is an isolated lesion (Figure 3-30) but usually occurs with massive trauma to the ulnar aspect of the distal forearm and wrist, often with significant injury to the distal ulna and distal radioulnar joint (eg, diastasis of the distal radioulnar joint with or without dorsal or palmar dislocation of the ulna (Figure 3-31) or massive penetrating or through-and-through wound (Figure 3-32)). Open reduction is necessary to treat the articular fracture and the distal radioulnar joint diastasis and/or injury to the distal ulna.

A displaced Salter-Harris III or IV physeal separation of the distal radius also may be confused with the above lesion depending upon the location of displacement but naturally occurs in the skeletally immature.

Open reduction and internal fixation is necessary if closed reduction cannot provide a satisfactory articular surface of the distal radius.

The key to proper diagnosis of the segmental articular fractures of the distal radius is accurate radiographs focused specifically on the central point of injury and including four views minimally (PA, lateral and two obliques).

Scaphoid fracture or scapholunate dissociation may be associated with either dorsal or palmar Barton's fracture and is quite frequently associated with a chauffeur's fracture (Figure 3-25). Fracture of the

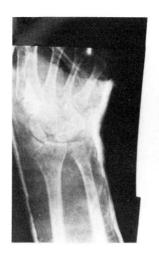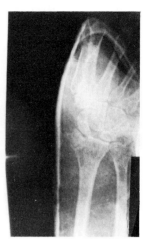

Figure 3-25 PA radiograph shows displacement of radial styloid articular fracture fragment, dissociation of scapholunate articulation, and subluxation of scaphoid. Force of injury traveled obliquely through carpus causing avulsion of scapholunate articulation and subluxation of scaphoid; it continued through radius to produce chauffeur's fracture of radial styloid process. *(Reprinted, by permission, from R.A. Cautilli, M.D., et al. Classifications of fractures of the distal radius, The Jefferson Orthopaedic Journal 3:47, 1974.)*

scaphoid with or without displacement (Figure 3-27A) or rupture of the scapholunate ligament occurs as a direct extension of the force which causes fracture and displacement of the radial styloid, or vice versa (Figure 3-25). If this complication occurs, reduction of the scaphoid fracture or reestablishment of proper anatomic relationship of the scaphoid and lunate must be accomplished and maintained, in addition to reduction of the articular fracture (see Chapter 4, Wrist Injuries, specifically Scaphoid Fractures and Scapholunate Dissociation).

Any severity of carpal instability may be found with this injury (Figures 3-27A,B). If necessary, surgical exposure from the palmar aspect and internal reduction of the scaphoid and any other fractures should be carried out with or without internal fixation and/or ligament reconstruction as indicated (Figures 3-27C–E). This severe open contaminated injury was treated initially by proper wound toilet and pins-and-plaster immobilization of the reduced chauffeur's fracture. Delayed soft tissue healing necessitated delayed open reduction of the lunate. Wrist disability will be moderate or severe due to the absence of the proximal third of the scaphoid. Sufficient stability and motion may be obtained by anatomic reduction to avoid proximal row carpectomy or wrist arthrodesis (Figures 3-27D,E).

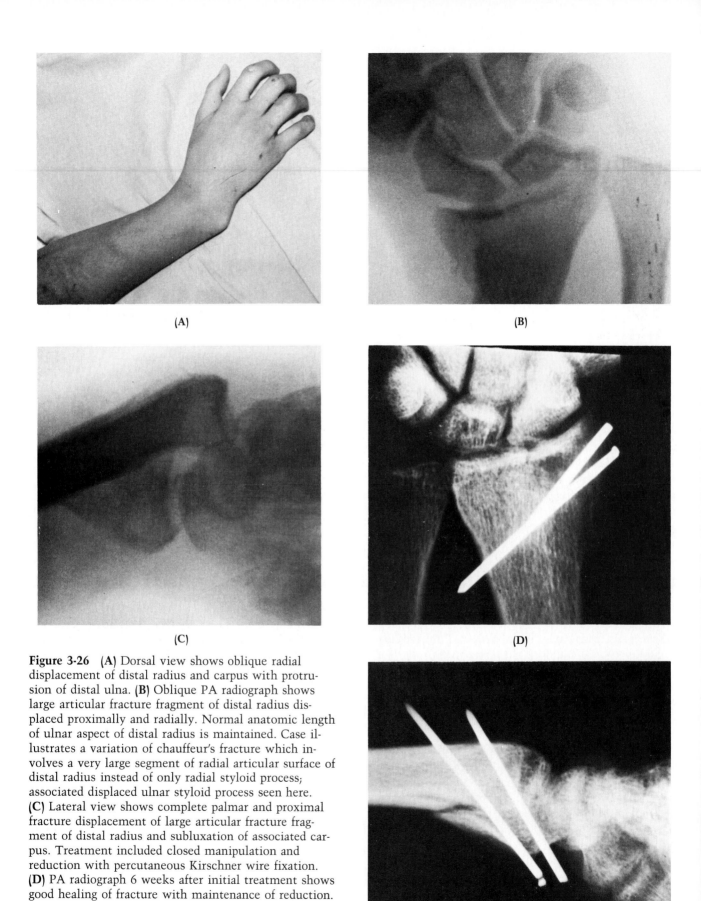

(A)

(B)

(C)

(D)

(E)

Figure 3-26 **(A)** Dorsal view shows oblique radial displacement of distal radius and carpus with protrusion of distal ulna. **(B)** Oblique PA radiograph shows large articular fracture fragment of distal radius displaced proximally and radially. Normal anatomic length of ulnar aspect of distal radius is maintained. Case illustrates a variation of chauffeur's fracture which involves a very large segment of radial articular surface of distal radius instead of only radial styloid process; associated displaced ulnar styloid process seen here. **(C)** Lateral view shows complete palmar and proximal fracture displacement of large articular fracture fragment of distal radius and subluxation of associated carpus. Treatment included closed manipulation and reduction with percutaneous Kirschner wire fixation. **(D)** PA radiograph 6 weeks after initial treatment shows good healing of fracture with maintenance of reduction. **(E)** Lateral view shows similar findings. Temporary Kirschner wire fixation was removed at this time.

86

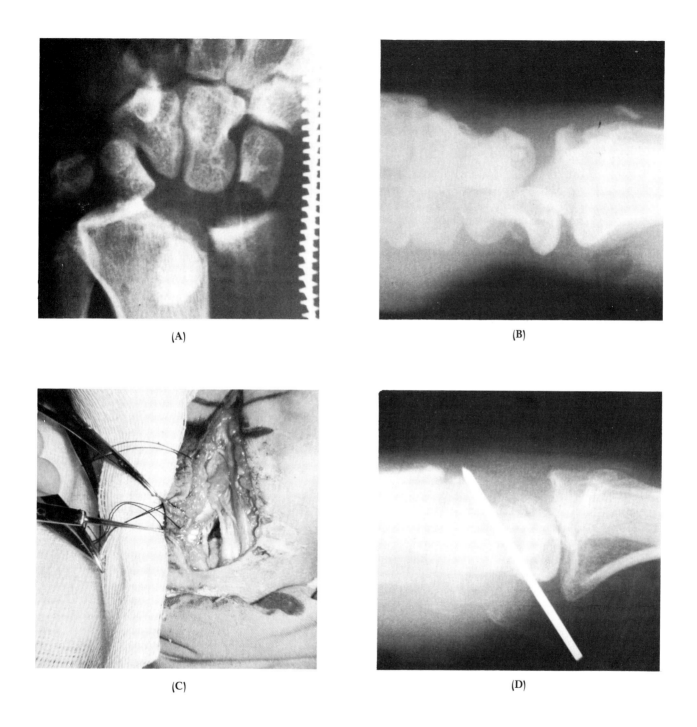

(A)

(B)

(C)

(D)

Figure 3-27 **(A)** PA radiograph illustrates severe open fracture dislocation of wrist, including displaced chauffeur's fracture of distal radius, complete anterior and ulnar dislocation of lunate, palmar and proximal displaced fracture of proximal third of scaphoid, and dorsal subluxation of distal ulna. The proximal scaphoid segment, devoid of any soft tissue attachment, was removed from open wound at time of initial debridement. Initial diagnosis is: open anterior transscaphoid perilunate fracture dislocation, combined with complete palmar ulnar dislocation of lunate, dorsal subluxation of distal ulna, and open displaced chauffeur's fracture of distal radius. **(B)** Lateral radiograph after application of traction shows palmar displacement of the lunate. **(C)** Palmar approach to carpus to reduce anterior dislocation of lunate included sectioning of transverse carpal ligament and Guyon's fascia as patient demonstrated persistent findings of ulnar neurapraxia. View shows median nerve centrally in operative field and palmarly dislocated lunate just to its left. **(D)** Lateral view after open reduction and temporary Kirschner wire fixation of lunate shows acceptable carpal anatomy.

(continued)

Figure 3-27 *(continued)*
(E) PA view shows the best possible reestablishment of carpal anatomy. Proximal portion of scaphoid is absent and decreased vascularity of the lunate noted. Ulnar nerve function returned completely and patient demonstrated limited but acceptable painless wrist motion. Proximal carpectomy or arthrodesis of wrist were avoided by early anatomical fracture and joint reduction.

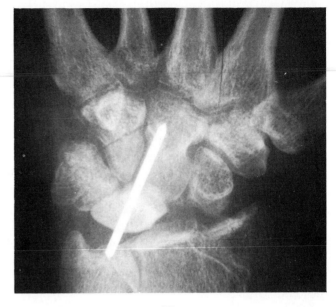

(E)

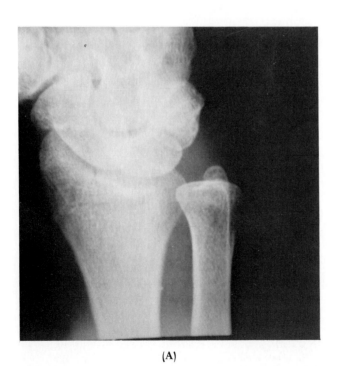

(A)

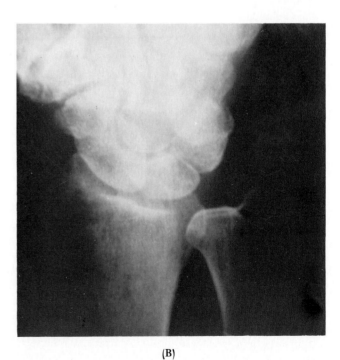

(B)

Figure 3-28   **(A)** Undisplaced segmental articular fracture of the radial aspect of the distal radius. (chauffeur's fracture) **(B)** Healed fracture with no loss of position six weeks after injury.

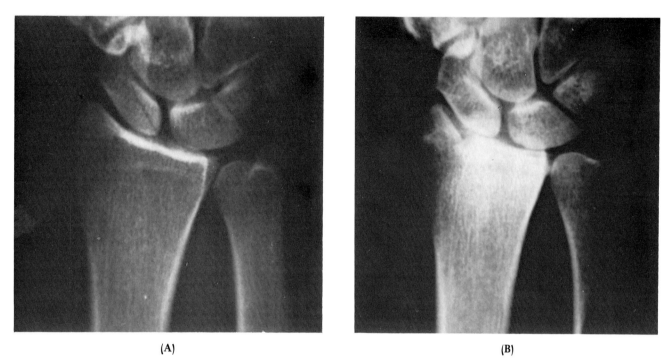

(A)   (B)

Figure 3-29 **(A)** An undisplaced segmental articular fracture of the radial aspect of the distal radius similar to that in Figure 3-28A. (chauffeur's fracture) **(B)** Five months later, malunion of that displaced segmental articular fracture is seen. Inattention to careful radiographic reevaluation at seven to 10 day intervals prevented timely anatomic open reduction and fixation.

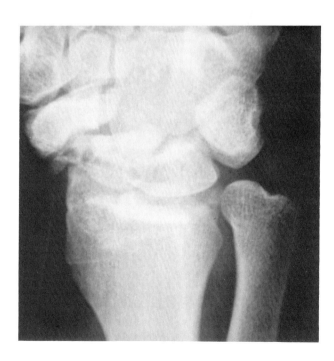

Figure 3-30 Small segmental articular fracture of the ulnar aspect of the distal radius (ulnar variant of chauffeur's fracture).

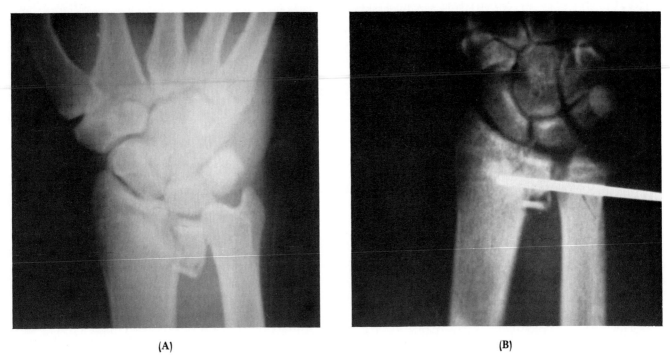

(A)

(B)

Figure 3-31 **(A)** Displaced segmental articular fracture of the ulnar aspect of the distal radius (ulnar variant of chauffeur's fracture) with diastasis of the distal radioulnar joint). **(B)** Treatment was open reduction of both the fracture and the distal radioulnar diastasis and fixation with a single transverse Kirschner wire.

Fracture of the Head of the Ulna

Fractures of the distal end (distal epiphysis) of the ulna (ulnar head) are uncommon except for those of the ulnar styloid which occur discretely or in association with a distal radial metaphyseal fracture (Colles' or Smith's fracture—see section on ulnar styloid fractures, Chapter 4, Wrist Injuries).

Traumatic Physeal Separation of the Distal Radius and Ulna

Physeal injury of the distal radius may involve the distal metaphysis (Salter Type II) or may be a segmental articular fracture (Salter Types III and IV).

Traumatic physeal separation of the distal radius (Figures 3-33A,B) usually occurs in a dorsal direction because the very strong palmar radiocarpal ligament is attached on the metaphysis proximal to the physeal growth plate. This strong anatomical structure prevents palmar physeal separation, a condition not encountered by this author.

Treatment of the dorsal physeal separation is similar to the maneuvers performed to reduce a Colles' fracture; reduction should not be difficult. If closed reduction is impossible due to soft tissue interposition, surgical exposure and extraction of the interposed soft tissue with care to avoid damage to the physeal plate are necessary to obtain anatomic reduction. Incomplete reduction is acceptable if digital extension and flexion are essentially normal.

Occasionally open reduction and fixation are necessary to restore normal articular anatomy in Salter III and IV lesions.

Distal ulnar physeal separation is rare and usually is encountered only from extensive trauma in an open injury (Figures 3-34A–D). In any open injury involving a physeal plate, meticulous wound toilet is particularly important prior to reduction and appropriate immobilization to prevent infection and premature closure of the physeal growth line. The latter, however, may occur in the absence of infection because of effects of trauma per se.

Figure 3-32 (A) Massive injury to the ulnar aspect of distal forearm and wrist from a shotgun blast. (B) After meticulous wound toilet, the distal ulna has been debrided and a displaced articular fracture of the ulnar aspect of the distal radius (ulnar variant of chauffeur's fracture) is seen. (C) Reduction and Kirschner wire fixation of that articular fragment followed meticulous wound toilet.

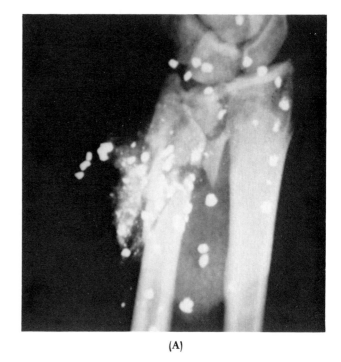

(A)

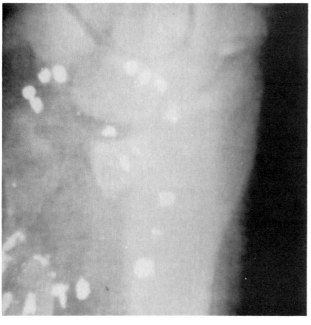

(B)

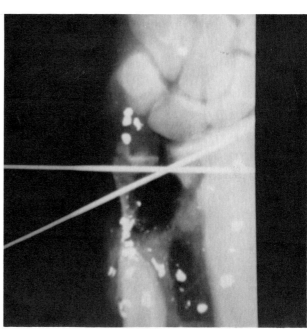

(C)

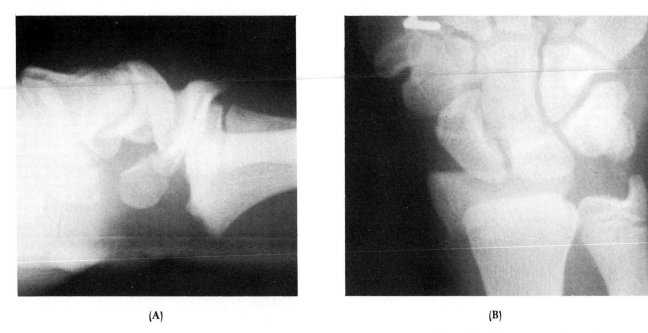

(A)   (B)

Figure 3-33 **(A)** Lateral radiograph shows dorsal angulation and displacement through Salter Type I physeal separation of distal radius. **(B)** PA view shows shortening of distal radius and radial displacement of epiphysis, with accentuation of distal radial metaphysis at area of distal radial physis. There is also superimposition of distal radial epiphysis upon carpus. On physical examination injury resembles configuration of Colles' fracture in an adult. Closed manipulation and reduction are effected as in treatment of Colles' fracture.

Distal Radioulnar Dissociation[8]

Dislocation of the distal ulna or distal radioulnar dissociation is associated with rupture of the triangular fibrocartilage and may occur either with a displaced or markedly angulated fracture of the radial shaft (Galeazzi fracture) or radial head (Essex-Lopresti fracture), or as a solitary injury.

Palmar dislocation of the distal ulna occurs less frequently than its dorsal counterpart. However, palmar dislocation is a more serious injury because of impingement of the distal ulna on the median and/or ulnar nerve (Figures 3-20B, 3-35A–C, 3-36A). A palmar protrusion proximal to the wrist in the central area of the distal forearm may be noted on physical examination. Radiographs show a double density shadow (PA view), which is indicative of a superimposition of the distal radius over the distal ulna associated with palmar dislocation (Figure 3-35A). Lateral view shows an abnormal location of the distal ulna palmar to the distal radius (Figure 3-36A).

Closed or, if necessary, open reduction should be achieved as soon as possible after diagnosis, fol-

lowed by four weeks of immobilization in a long arm cast, with the elbow flexed 90° and the wrist in the neutral position or slight pronation to prevent redislocation.

If closed reduction is unsuccessful, the distal ulna should be surgically reduced, bearing in mind its correct relationship to the ulnar groove of the distal radius (Figure 3-35B). No reconstruction of ligaments is necessary at this time. However, if palmar dislocation is found to be present some weeks after injury, it may be necessary to perform a Darrach procedure combined with tethering of the distal ulna to the radius by means of a tendon transfer (extensor carpi ulnaris) or a free tendon graft or fascial sling.

Dorsal dislocation of the distal ulna is much more common than palmar dislocation (Figures 3-36B,C) and often may become recurrent, particularly if treatment is delayed or inadequate. The PA radiograph shows a diastasis of the distal radioulnar joint (Figure 3-36C), and lateral view, a dorsal displacement of the distal ulna (Figure 3-36B). Reduction must be accomplished as soon as possible for the best result. Immobilization is effected in the neutral position or in slight supination in a long arm cast as described above for palmar dislocation.

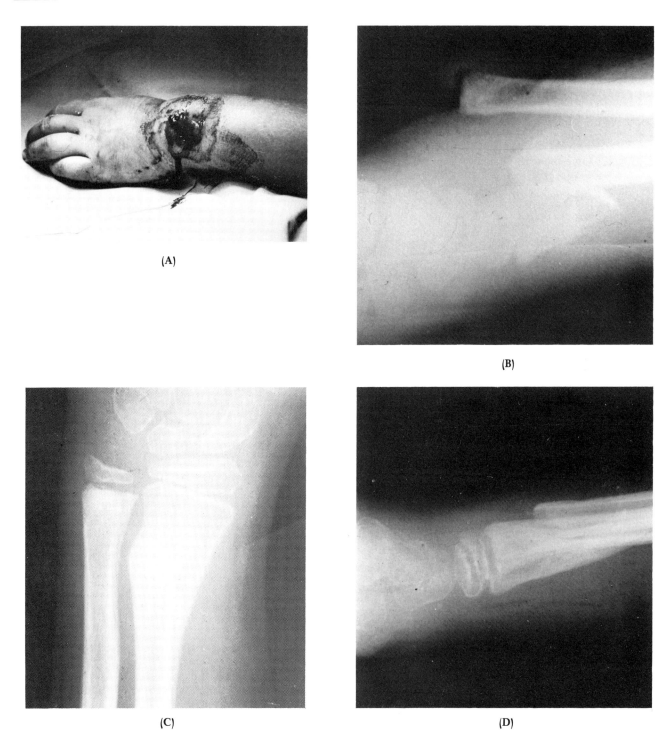

(A)

(B)

(C)   (D)

Figure 3-34 (A) Traumatic open physeal separation through distal ulna with distal ulnar shaft protruding from skin. (B) Lateral radiograph shows a traumatic physeal separation through distal ulna with protrusion of ulnar diaphysis dorsally through skin in open injury, with associated comminuted palmar and proximally displaced fracture through distal radius. (C) PA view 12 weeks after injury. Primary treatment consisted of meticulous wound toilet, open reduction, and delayed primary skin closure. Note restoration of acceptable anatomy of distal radius and ulna with maintenance of physis of ulna. (D) Lateral view shows good position at healed fracture site of distal radius and acceptable anatomy of distal radioulnar articulation. *(Illustrations 3-34A–D courtesy of D.M. Junkin, M.D.)*

Figure 3-35 (A) PA radiograph shows incongruity of distal radioulnar articulation and superimposition of ulna on radius. (B) Surgical exposure after unsuccessful attempt at closed reduction shows exposed head of distal ulna palmarly dislocated centrally in distal forearm. Majority of digital flexors are retracted radially (to the left) for exposure. Open reduction was necessary since closed reduction proved impossible. (C) Oblique and PA radiographs show anatomic position restored after open reduction with no attempt at ligamentous reconstruction. Normal motion followed continuous immobilization for 4 weeks in long arm cast with wrist in neutral position of pronation and supination.

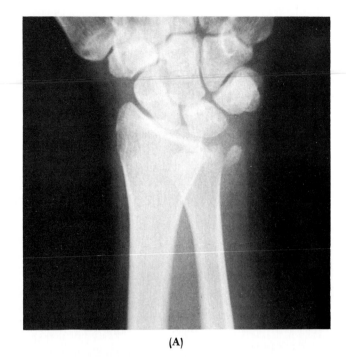

(A)

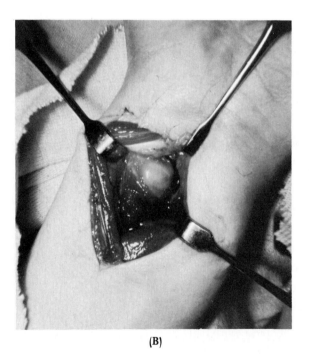

(B)

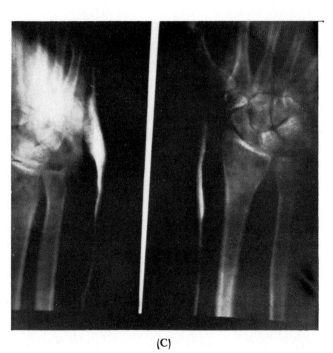

(C)

Figure 3-36 (A) Lateral radiograph of case in Figures 3-35A–C shows palmar protrusion of the subluxed distal ulna. (B) Dorsal ulnar subluxation in this case may be compared to palmar ulna subluxation in Figure 3-36A. (C) PA view of case in Figure 3-36B (dorsal ulnar subluxation) shows abnormal space or diastasis between distal ulna and radius.

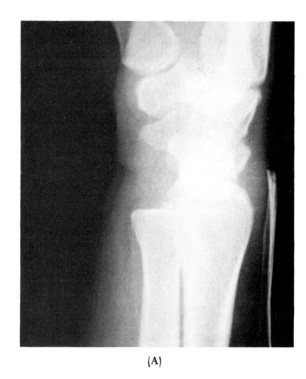

(A)

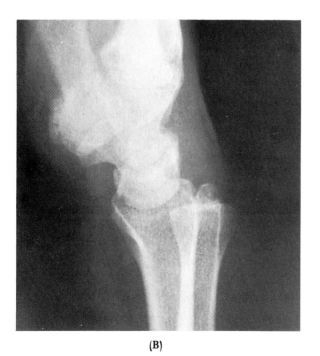

(B)

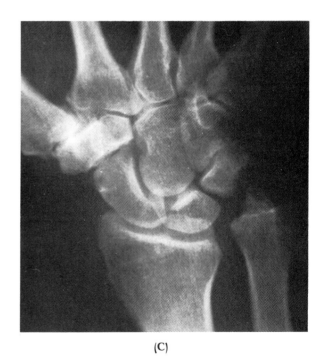

(C)

In undiagnosed or untreated cases of dorsal dislocation, secondary degenerative or posttraumatic arthritis develops. Often no reconstructive procedure is indicated. The Darrach procedure may at times be indicated as described previously, and occasionally ligament reconstruction or a "tethering" type of procedure using the flexor carpi ulnaris can be considered.

Essex-Lopresti fracture is a fracture of the radial head with angulation or displacement signifi-cant enough to produce an associated dissociation of the distal radioulnar joint. Restoration of the prox-imal radioulnar articulation by treatment of the fractured radial head, either by closed or open manipulation and reduction or by excision and re-placement with a silastic implant, is necessary to restore proper length of the radius. Only then is acceptable, stable reduction and restoration of a distal radioulnar articulation achieved.

References

1. Cooney WP, Dobyns JH, Linscheid RL: Complications of Colles' Fractures. *J Bone Joint Surg* 1980;62-A:614–619.
2. Cautilli RA, Joyce MF, Gordon E, et al: Classifications of fractures of the distal radius. *Jefferson Orthop J* 1974;3:46–56.
3. Cautilli RA, Joyce MF, Gordon E, et al: Classifications of fractures of the distal radius. *Clin Orthop* 1974;103:163–166.
4. King RE: Barton's fracture—dislocation of the wrist. *Curr Pract Orthop Surg* 1975;6:133–144.
5. Thompson GH, Grant TT: Barton's fractures, reverse Barton's fractures-confusing eponyms. *Clin Orthop* 1977;122:210–221.
6. Dobyns JH, Linscheid RL: Fractures and dislocations of the wrist, in Rockwood CA, Green DP (eds): *Fractures in Adults*, ed 2. Philadelphia, J.B. Lippincott Co., 1984.
7. Saito H, Shibata M: Classification of fractures at the distal end of the radius with reference to treatment of comminuted fractures, in Boswick JA (ed): *Current Concepts in Hand Surgery*. Philadelphia, Lea & Febiger, 1983, pp 129–145.
8. Bowers WH: Distal radioulnar joint, in Green DP (ed): *Operative Hand Surgery*. New York, Churchill Livingston, 1982, vol 1, pp 743–769.

CHAPTER
4

Wrist Injuries

General Discussion

The usual mechanism responsible for the majority of carpal injuries is direct force on the palmar aspect of the hand or the wrist with the wrist extended, such as occurs from a blow to, or a fall on, the outstretched hand.

Wrist stability depends primarily on the integrity of the scaphoid bone itself and that of the normal scapholunate articulation and of the components of the palmar radiocarpal ligament. The most stable attitude of the wrist is flexion and radial deviation, which protects the scaphoid and especially the lunate. Since injury is usually sustained with the wrist in extension or hyperextension, causing palmar distraction and dorsal compression, the carpals are in jeopardy, particularly the scaphoid since it is the single stable skeletal connection between the proximal and distal carpal rows. The brunt of the hyperextension injury is sustained at the midcarpal joint level; therefore the scaphoid is particularly vulnerable at its waist or at its articulation with the lunate. Thus fracture of the waist or middle third of the scaphoid is the most common isolated fracture of the carpus, with the exception of minor dorsal avulsion fractures.

When subjected to severe trauma the wrist usually divides into two segments, the lunate segment with or without the proximal scaphoid (transscaphoid perilunate fracture dislocation and perilunate dislocation, respectively) and the remainder of the carpus. This common division is primarily due to the great strength of the palmar radiocarpal ligament augmented by the ulnocarpal ligament complex.

"Dislocation" in all general discussions infers "and/or subluxation" but not vice versa.

Carpal trauma should be regarded as an entire spectrum of injuries and the lunate is the focal point (refer to Figures 1-3 and 1-4).

Damage to the radial aspect of the lunate in the area of the scapholunate joint may cause scaphoid fracture or scapholunate dissociation, usually along with a rotational deformity of the scaphoid and/or the lunate. If trauma also involves the distal border of the lunate, which articulates with the capitate, then fracture through the capitate neck with or without displacement and with or without an associated scaphoid fracture (scaphocapitate syndrome); perilunate or transscaphoid perilunate fracture dislocation, or rotation, dorsal subluxation or dislocation of the lunate may occur. If, in addition, trauma includes the third border of the lunate, its articulation with the triquetrum, the result may be complete dorsal perilunate dislocation, complete dorsal transscaphoid perilunate fracture dislocation, or fracture of the triquetrum associated with either of the above. Finally, if the fourth border of the lunate, its proximal aspect, also is included in the injury along with avulsion of the dorsal ligamentous attachments, palmar dislocation of the lunate may result.

Different positions of the wrist at the time of impact, different angles of the force externally applied to different areas of the carpus or hand and severity of injury account for various pathologic entities.

Impact on the thenar area of the hand with the wrist in extension and radial or ulnar deviation usually produces fracture of the scaphoid. However, if trauma is more severe, the result may be a dorsal transscaphoid perilunate fracture or dislocation.

Impact on the hypothenar area, particularly if a cylindrical object had been held in the hand at the time of impact, often results in rotatory subluxation of the scaphoid with or without scapholunate dissociation.

If impact is sustained centrally on the hand, the result may be dorsal perilunate dislocation, dorsal transscaphoid perilunate fracture dislocation, or palmar dislocation of the lunate.

Any isolated carpal bone can be fractured, dislocated, or suffer fracture dislocation or subluxation, and any combination of multiple carpal fractures, dislocations, or fracture dislocations may be encountered. *The physician should be aware that multiple injuries are common in severe trauma to the wrist.*

Age may be a significant factor due to the inherent stability of various structures and anatomic areas. A child or adolescent in whom the physes are still functioning will often sustain a traumatic dorsal physeal separation of the distal radius. A healthy adult may sustain a fracture of the scaphoid and/or rotational instability of the scaphoid or lunate, scapholunate dissociation, lunate dislocation, dorsal perilunate dislocation, or dorsal transscaphoid perilunate fracture dislocation. A comminuted Colles' fracture will often occur in an elderly individual with diffuse osteoporosis.

Obviously general factors such as local and systemic pathology (e.g., enchondroma and osteoporosis respectively), congenital abnormalities (e.g., ligamentous laxity or absence of the central portion of the deltoid ligament), general muscle tone and nutrition, and many other conditions will influence the type and severity of injury.

Physical findings vary from almost no swelling and minimal symptoms to excessive swelling and severe pain. Deformities may or may not be localized, but there is often a diffuse broadening or thickening of the wrist, particularly if some time has elapsed since the injury. Point tenderness, if elicited, aids in the diagnosis.

Accurate diagnosis is possible only by adequate radiographic examination with multiple views of good quality centered on the pathology. The lateral view is the most important. However, this should be supplemented by PA (often both in ulnar and radial deviation) and two oblique views. *The key to radiographic interpretation of the lateral view is proper identification of the lunate.* After this cornerstone has been identified all other carpals can be related to it and to the distal radius.

In addition to routine radiographic views, the carpal tunnel view, lateral view in neutral, extension and flexion, AP (supination) views in neutral, maximal radial and ulnar deviation and clenched fist position, a distraction radiograph of the wrist both in PA and lateral (to attempt to separate the various carpal components) and laminographs (tomographs) may be of help for diagnosis in specific instances. The image intensifier may be particularly valuable for correct interpretation of carpal pathology and arthrography may sometimes be indicated.[1,2] An associated fracture of the ulnar styloid, often encountered, should be searched for.

Confusion in radiographic interpretation may be due to congenital variances in carpal segmentation (Figures 4-1, 4-2, 4-3), accessory carpal bones,[3,4] old injuries, and in children, unawareness of the specific chronological sequence of ossification of the carpal cartilage anlages (refer to Figure 4-80).

Of particular importance are differentiation of the dorsal perilunate dislocation from a palmar dislocation of the lunate and recognition of a residual postreduction scapholunate dissociation with or without rotational deformity of the scaphoid and/or lunate (see Wrist and Carpal Instability in this chapter).

Only after accurate diagnosis can proper treatment for the specific injury or injuries be provided. Too often carpal injuries go unrecognized or are misinterpreted because of insufficient or inaccurate radiographic evaluation at the initial examination, resulting in no treatment or incorrect and/or inadequate treatment.

As normal anatomy as possible must be restored to the carpus and distal radius to ensure proper stability and mobility with minimal incidence and severity of posttraumatic and degenerative arthritic

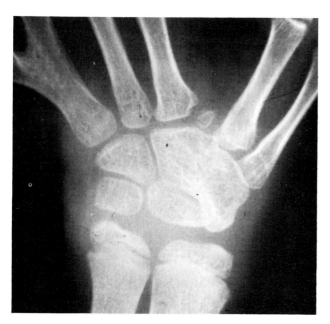

Figure 4-1 Multiple congenital abnormalities of distal radius and ulna, carpus, and hand. Note lack of segmentation of scaphoid, trapezium, trapezoid, and capitate, probably also associated with lack of segmentation of lunate. Multiple carpal defects, including lack of segmentation of numerous carpals, in an extremity with multiple severe congenital defects are common, as in this case of Apert's syndrome with multiple complex syndactylies.

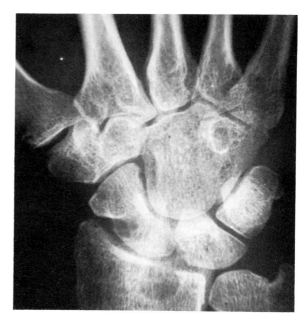

Figure 4-2 PA radiograph shows complete lack of segmentation of capitate and hamate in an otherwise normal hand with normal physiologic motion. It is virtually impossible to diagnose lack of carpal segmentation without radiographs in a normal appearing and functioning adult wrist.

changes. The majority of carpal injuries, including displaced fractures, subluxations, and dislocations, can be treated by closed manipulation and reduction if treated within a few hours of injury. However, if closed manipulation and reduction are impossible, or if instability persists with recurrence of the original deformity particularly found in multiple carpal injuries, and particularly if associated with distal radial pathology, fixation must be provided. The easiest alternative is to provide percutaneous Kirschner wire fixation after successful closed manipulation and reduction. If this is unsuccessful, open reduction either with internal or percutaneous fixation is strongly recommended. Exposure should be as limited as possible to achieve the desired reduction and fixation in order to prevent needless soft tissue dissection and periosteal, ligamentous, and capsular elevation. Unnecessary soft tissue elevation decreases vascularity to the bone and may be an important cause for avascular changes and delayed union or nonunion. If possible, a palmar surgical approach to the carpus is recommended to avoid damage to the more important blood supply entering from the dorsum.

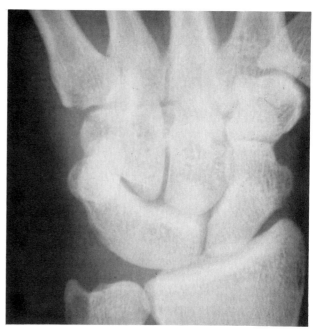

Figure 4-3 Lunequate—lack of segmentation of lunate and triquetrum.

Four to six weeks of plaster immobilization (long or short arm cast) suffice in the majority of instances, except for scaphoid fractures (discussed under Scaphoid Fractures in this chapter). Should delayed healing become evident with or without avascular necrosis, which is more common in the more severe injuries, additional immobilization should be provided until either fracture healing results or a decision is made to bone graft the fracture site.

Wrist motion is an integral part of the entire upper extremity motion. There is no reason to disregard this important joint and merely "fuse the wrist" to provide a stable, painless result. Such treatment is both old-fashioned and unphysiologic and is somewhat like recommending arthrodesis of the hip rather than arthroplasty reconstruction. There is no indication for wrist arthrodesis if relatively painless, stable motion can be preserved. Only by precise diagnosis and adequate treatment of the acute injury to reestablish normal carpal anatomy can this objective be attained.

Fractures of the Ulnar Styloid

Fracture of the ulnar styloid process usually occurs as a component of Colles' fracture or Smith's fracture and occurs less frequently as an isolated injury. Diagnosis includes point tenderness over the ulnar styloid process, usually with some concurrent edema. For the solitary lesion treatment is conservative immobilization of the undisplaced fracture until symptoms of acute trauma have subsided (about two to three weeks posttrauma) (Figure 4-4A). Treatment of a relatively undisplaced ulnar styloid fracture is conservative immobilization of the wrist for about three weeks to allow satisfactory asymptomatic healing (Figure 4-5). Closed manipulation and reduction under suitable anesthesia should be attempted for moderate or marked displacement of an ulnar styloid process fracture. If fracture union is not achieved, however, usually no functional impairment results from the pseudoarthrosis (Figures 4-4B, 4-6A,B).

Rarely (less than 1%) an isolated basilar ulnar styloid process fracture is associated with wrist joint instability indicating severe concomitant ligament injuries. In this instance, surgical exploration, fracture reduction and fixation, and appropriate ligament repairs are necessary.

Rarely, after displaced fracture of an ulnar styloid process in a skeletally immature person, the detached styloid process grows progressively, mimicking an extra carpal bone at skeletal maturity. If on comparison radiographs (Figures 4-6A,B) a similar bone is noted in the contralateral carpus with an essentially normal styloid process, a diagnosis of

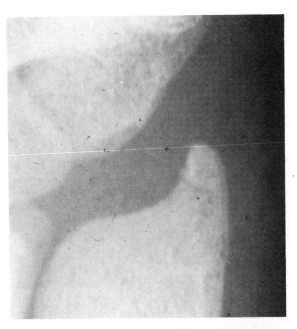

(A)

(B)

Figure 4-4 (A) PA view of undisplaced fracture of ulnar styloid process treated by immobilization for 3½ weeks in short arm cast. (B) PA radiograph 3 months later shows nonunion of undisplaced ulnar styloid fracture. Note bone resorption at site of nonunion. No indication for further treatment since patient was asymptomatic.

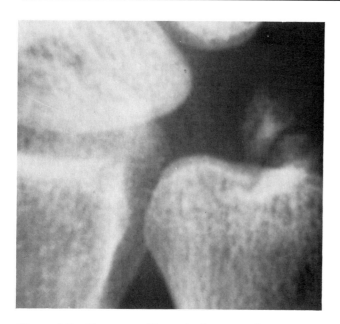

Figure 4-5 Close-up radiograph shows moderate displacement of fractured ulnar styloid process.

either an accessory carpal or a bony lunula (intrameniscal ossification) should be considered. If the finding is unilateral and the styloid process itself is atrophic, the separate ossicle represents dissociated growth of an original portion of the styloid process.

A displaced articular fracture fragment of the distal ulna should be excised (Figures 4-7A, 4-8A), particularly if it is symptomatic, to prevent posttraumatic and degenerative arthritic changes (Figures 4-7A,B) due to impingement of the fragment on the distal ulnar articular surface, which may necessitate resection of the distal ulna at a later date (Darrach procedure) (Figures 4-8A–C).

In performing resection of the distal ulna care should be taken to excise only the portion articulating with the distal radius and impinging on the carpus. The styloid process and all attached ligaments, including the ulnar collateral ligament, should be protected. Too aggressive resection of the distal ulna results in instability and dorsal subluxation of the distal ulnar shaft due to sacrifice of ligamentous

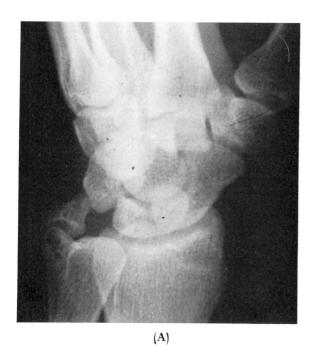

(A)

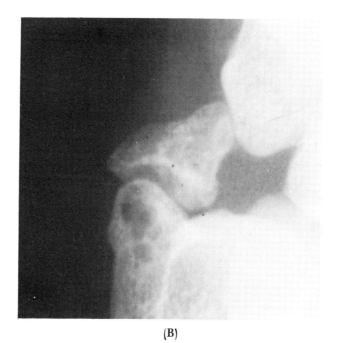

(B)

Figure 4-6 **(A)** Oblique view of "wrist fracture" sustained 45 years previous to radiograph, probably a displaced fracture of ulnar styloid process which grew as a separate ossicle until patient's skeletal maturity. Articulation of large separate bone fragment with atrophic remnant of base of ulnar styloid process exhibiting cystic changes. (Contralateral ulnar styloid process normal.) Enlarged separate ulnar styloid process could be mistaken easily for an extra carpal bone. **(B)** Close-up of Figure 4-6A. Note distinct articulation between atrophic remnant of ulnar styloid base and large separate ossicle.

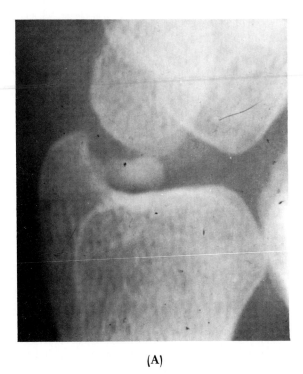

(A)

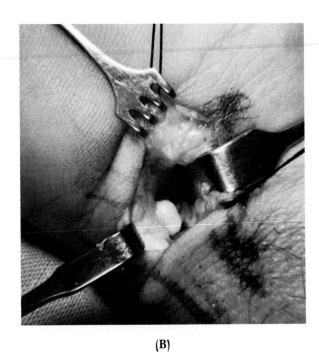

(B)

Figure 4-7 **(A)** Close-up oblique view of wrist showing intraarticular bony fragment just distal to ulnar styloid process. Note irregularity of ulnar styloid articular surface. Defect represents area from which free fragment was traumatically displaced. **(B)** Palmar surgical approach was used to remove free osteocartilaginous displaced intraarticular fracture fragment, seen centrally in the wound. Close-up view shows smooth, shiny cartilaginous articular surface of fragment.

restraints (Figures 4-9A,B). Any reconstructive tethering procedure using either a free tendon graft or a tendon transfer (flexor or extensor carpi ulnaris) to secure the distal ulnar shaft to the radius is only reasonably successful at best.

Wrist Dislocation

Radiographic documentation of isolated carpal dislocation at the radial carpal joint is rare. However, dislocation of the carpus (wrist dislocation) may not be as uncommon as generally believed. The majority of carpal dislocations must reduce spontaneously because very few are seen clinically or radiographically (Figures 4-10A,B). Only by complete avulsion of the very strong palmar radial carpal ligament complex and the ulnocarpal ligament complex dorsal dislocation of the carpus is possible. The radial and ulnar collateral ligaments of the wrist and the dorsal radiocarpal ligament, however, may remain intact. Reduction by gentle traction and manipulation should not

be difficult, but avascular necrosis of the lunate and/or the proximal portion of the scaphoid may occur. The mechanism of injury is an extremely severe blow on the palmar aspect of the carpus or hand. Conservative immobilization of the hand and wrist (neutral pronation-supination) in a long arm cast should be continued for six weeks postreduction for satisfactory soft tissue healing.

Dorsal subluxation of the scaphoid or the lunate at the radiocarpal joint is usually associated with rotational instability and may accompany an articular fracture of the distal radius. (See section on Wrist and Carpal Instability in this chapter.)

Dorsal Avulsion Fractures of the Carpus

These fractures are quite common and are sustained both by extension and palmar flexion injuries. They result from avulsion of ligaments or portions of ten-

Figure 4-8 **(A)** Close-up of PA radiograph of wrist shows a free irregular osseous fragment just distal to ulnar articular surface. **(B)** Close-up of same wrist 6 months later shows fragmentation and comminution of small bone fragment with irregularities of distal ulnar articular surface. **(C)** Same case after Darrach excision of distal ulna, with preservation of ulnar styloid process and ulnar collateral ligament. Surgery necessary due to chronic pain and limitation of motion by impingement of free irregular segment of bone on distal ulnar articular surface causing posttraumatic arthritic changes. Postoperatively normal asymptomatic wrist motion resulted. Initial removal of free fragment would have prevented joint damage.

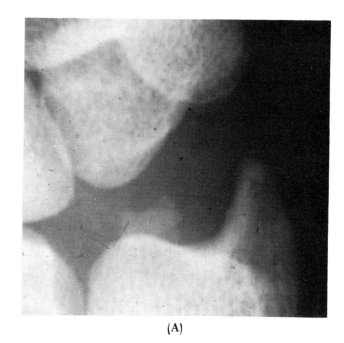

(A)

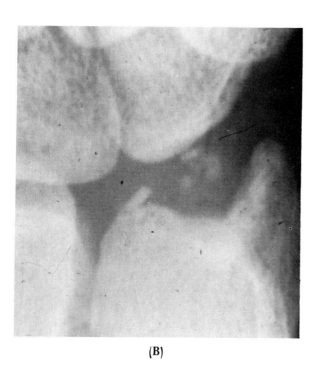

(B)

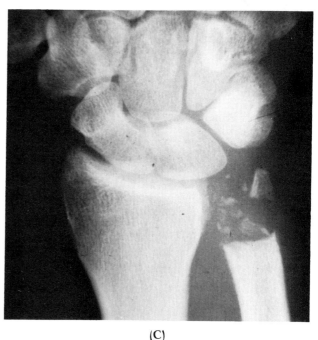

(C)

don insertions, usually wrist extensors. The triquetrum is generally involved (refer to Figure 4-75), but virtually any carpal may sustain this injury.

Treatment consists of immobilization for two to three weeks or until symptoms subside. It is important to have the initial diagnosis verified by specific point tenderness localized at the site of avulsion and documented by satisfactory radiographs, particularly the lateral view which shows the displaced avulsion fracture. If the diagnosis is not made and no support for the wrist is supplied (palmar plaster splint), pain and swelling will be markedly prolonged and occasionally a carpal instability pattern may develop.[5]

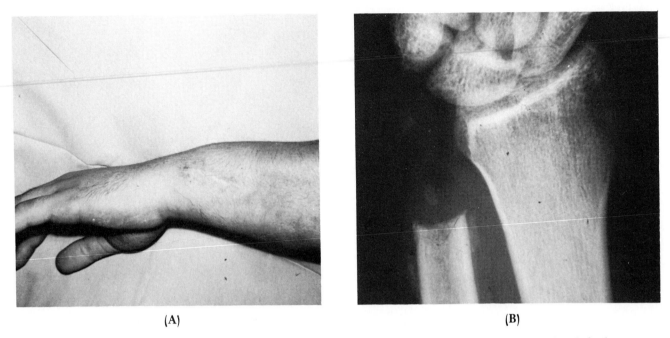

(A)   (B)

Figure 4-9 **(A)** Ulnar view shows dorsal ulnar mass protruding just proximal to wrist and generalized thickening of wrist. **(B)** PA radiograph demonstrates cause of dorsal ulnar soft tissue mass protrusion. Approximately 2½ to 3 cm of distal ulna had been incorrectly excised previously in a too-aggressive Darrach procedure, causing instability of distal radioulnar joint and dorsal protrusion of distal ulnar shaft.

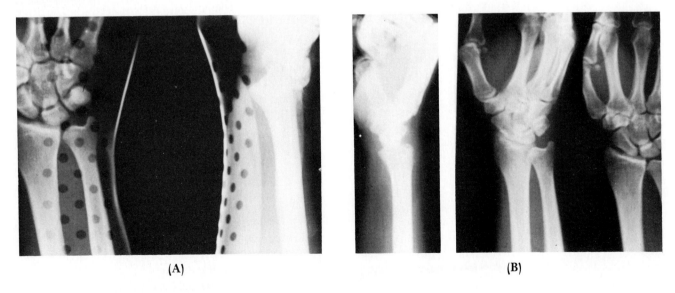

(A)   (B)

Figure 4-10 **(A)** Wrist, left, in PA view does not appear too abnormal. Lateral view, right, illustrates a complete dorsal dislocation of carpus (scaphoid and lunate) from distal radius. **(B)** Lateral, oblique, and PA views 2½ months after injury and closed reduction show essentially normal configuration of wrist joint and carpus. Physical examination disclosed excellent motion. *(Illustrations 4-10A,B courtesy of R.A. Cautilli, M.D.)*

Scaphoid Fractures

Fracture of the scaphoid is the most common isolated fracture of the wrist except for small dorsal avulsion fractures. To provide the necessary stability, the scaphoid anatomically serves as the skeletal bridge or strut between the proximal and distal carpal rows and is responsible for coordinated synergistic action of the carpus. The intimate association of the scaphoid with the distal radius, the lunate, the capitate, the trapezium, and the trapezoid denotes its multiple roles in relation to each specific joint with which it articulates (see Chapter 1, Anatomy). The scaphoid, though well protected in wrist flexion and radial deviation, is particularly susceptible to trauma in wrist extension, the usual position of injury.

The majority of scaphoid fractures occur in young males by a fall on the outstretched hand. Symptoms may be mild discomfort and swelling, with some limitation of extension and radial deviation and pain with strenuous use and on lifting. Often no medical aid is sought for many days or weeks because of limited symptoms and the notion that the wrist is merely "sprained."

On physical examination there is tenderness with discrete palpation of the scaphoid dorsally in or near the anatomic "snuff box" and palmarly in the area

of the tuberosity, or just proximal to it. Pain is elicited on radial deviation and extension of the wrist and upon applying longitudinal pressure on, or compression to, the thumb metacarpal.

Radiographic evaluation should include close scrutiny of routine PA and lateral views, augmented by oblique views and a scaphoid view of the wrist, *which is an A-P view with the hand in supination and marked ulnar deviation.* With this particular view the long axis of the scaphoid is most nearly horizontal, and distraction at the site of fracture may be seen.

If physical findings are positive but initial radiographs fail to show evidence of a fracture, the patient should be treated by two to three weeks of immobilization in a short arm-thumb spica cast. At the end of that time the cast should be removed and radiographs taken again. A fracture which is initially occult usually will be noticeable after two weeks, due to osteoporosis with bone resorption at the fracture line. If, however, symptoms and findings of a scaphoid fracture persist with a negative radiographic evaluation at the end of two to three weeks, this entire regimen is repeated.

The scaphoid may be fractured through its tubercule (Figures 4-11A,B, 4-12), through the distal third (Figure 4-13), through the waist or central

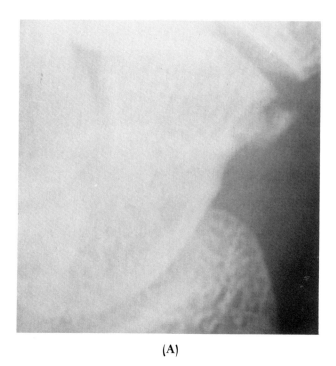

(A)

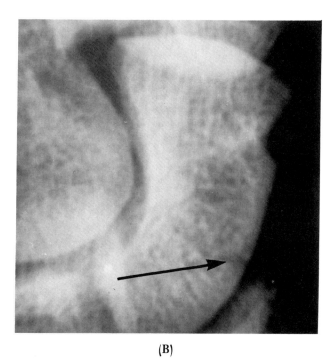

(B)

Figure 4-11 **(A)** Discrete fracture of scaphoid tuberosity **(B)** Radiograph 2 years later. Tuberosity fracture has healed, but note, in addition, recent undisplaced fracture at junction of proximal and middle thirds of scaphoid at lateral aspect.

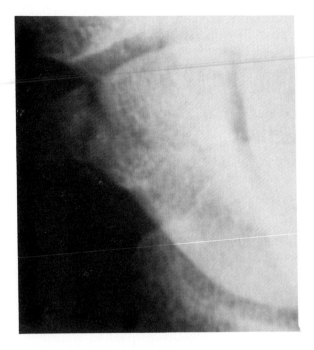

Figure 4-12 Comminuted articular fracture of scaphoid tuberosity. *(Illustration courtesy of J.H. Wolf, Jr., M.D.)*

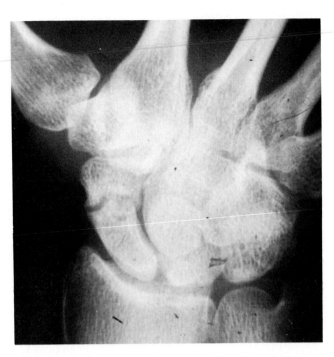

Figure 4-13 Transverse fracture of distal third of scaphoid.

portion (Figure 4-14), through the proximal portion (Figure 4-15), or it may be extensively comminuted (Figure 4-16). The specific point of fracture is probably determined by multiple factors, the most important being the position of the wrist at the time of initial trauma, which includes the variables of pronation and supination, flexion and extension, and radial and ulnar deviation. In extension or hyperextension and radial deviation the scaphoid is particularly vulnerable to massive blunt trauma by impingement of the radial styloid process, resulting from external force applied to the palmar aspect of the hand or wrist.

Roughly 10% of fractures occur in the distal third of the scaphoid, 50% to 70% in the waist, 20% to 40% in the proximal third, and 1% to 5% involve the tuberosity.

Since the majority of blood supply to the scaphoid enters dorsally and distally, avascular changes following fracture occur most frequently in the proximal third and least frequently in the distal third. Since fracture to the waist of the scaphoid is most common and the blood supply is generally adequate for satisfactory healing, there is usually no problem with an undisplaced fracture in this area as long as it is treated adequately.

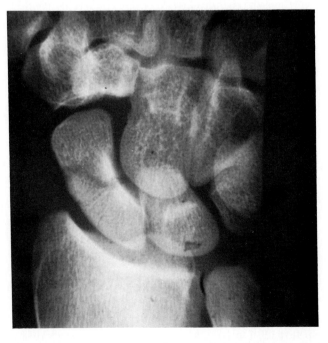

Figure 4-14 Oblique fracture of middle third of scaphoid.

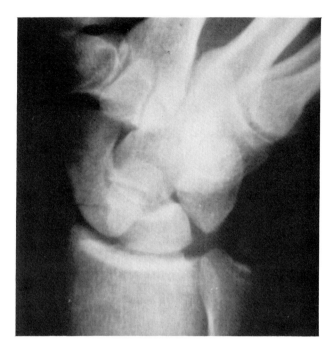

Figure 4-15 Transverse fracture in proximal third of scaphoid.

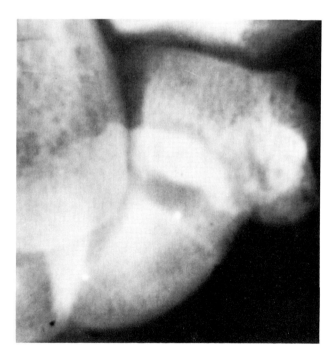

Figure 4-16 Comminuted fracture of scaphoid, including transverse fracture through middle third and fracture of scaphoid tuberosity involving scaphotrapezium articulation. *(Illustration courtesy of H.A. Yocum, M.D.)*

An unpredictable amount of avascular change in the proximal segment follows roughly 20% to 30% of fractures through the middle third of the scaphoid and a much higher percentage in a fracture in the proximal third (Figure 4-17). Fracture in the proximal third inherently involves interruption of the vascularity since this area has no independent blood supply, and temporary avascularity often occurs, although it may not progress to avascular necrosis.

If the patient is first seen weeks or months after trauma, vacuolization at the fracture site may be noted in addition to the bone resorption.

The diagnosis of a bipartite scaphoid is made with discretion, particularly if arthritic changes of surrounding joints (wrist, scapholunate, scaphocapitate, and scaphotrapezium-trapezoid) are seen radiographically. In a bipartite scaphoid the adjacent surfaces of the segments of that bone are smooth because each is covered by articular cartilage, and there are no findings indicative of a recent fracture

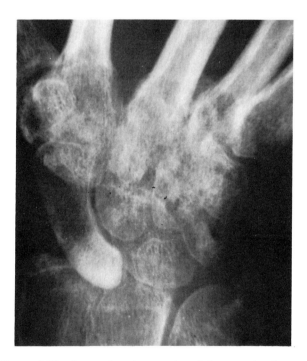

Figure 4-17 Avascular changes involving proximal third of scaphoid following union of fracture at junction of proximal and middle thirds of scaphoid. Osteoporotic appearance of distal two-thirds of scaphoid is due to normal circulation and represents disuse osteoporosis similar to that in all other carpals and distal radius and ulna. Proximal scaphoid segment does not appear osteoporotic because impaired circulation to this fragment prevents normal deossification.

unless superimposed injury has occurred. The contralateral wrist should be radiographically studied since a bipartite scaphoid is usually found bilaterally. However, despite findings of a segmented scaphoid bilaterally, the occurrence of bilateral scaphoid fractures is far more common and is usually the correct diagnosis.

The only fracture not involving an articular surface is a very specific discrete fracture of the scaphoid tuberosity, such as might occur in an avulsion type of injury (Figures 4-11A,B). Usually, however, the fracture of the tuberosity does extend into the most radial and palmar aspect of the scaphotrapezial articulation (Figure 4-12). The tuberosity has its own periosteal blood supply, and healing normally occurs well since there is usually no significant displacement.

Treatment for fracture of the scaphoid tuberosity is immobilization in a short arm-thumb spica cast for four weeks.

Scaphoid fracture may be displaced or undisplaced.

For an undisplaced fracture through the body of the scaphoid, there are various opinions as to the correct immobilization which includes short arm-thumb spica cast immobilization, long arm-thumb spica cast immobilization, and long arm-thumb spica cast immobilization incorporating both the index and long fingers with the MPs flexed.

Usually swelling is not a problem with fracture of the scaphoid, but if moderate edema is present, immobilization may be initially provided by a short arm molded plaster splint incorporating the thumb. A cast is then applied about five to seven days later following continued elevation to reduce edema and congestion; this allows a snug, well-molded fit of the definitive cast for necessary immobility.

Regardless of the type of immobilization preferred, it should incorporate the thumb out to its tip in wide metacarpal abduction and opposition. The wrist position should be neutral regarding flexion and extension, with a very slight radial deviation of 5° to 10°. It appears that this position will best approximate the fracture fragments (as determined at surgical explorations).

Immobilization for eight to ten weeks in a short arm-thumb spica cast is generally adequate for fractures in the middle and distal thirds of the scaphoid. Fractures of the proximal third, however, often require prolonged immobilization due to the impaired vascularity and delayed union, often with avascular changes. In severe injuries avascular changes of the proximal pole of the scaphoid, but not

necessarily aseptic necrosis, can be expected. It is important to change casts as seldom as possible. Radiographs may be obtained through a window in the cast, so there is no reason to remove a well-fitted plaster cast until indicated by adequate healing.

If at the time of cast removal and radiographic reevaluation, six to eight weeks posttrauma, healing is not progressing and osteoporosis is increasing with cystic changes noted at the fracture site, it is advisable to immobilize the upper extremity in a long arm-thumb spica cast incorporating the index and long fingers to their tips, with MP flexion and IP extension. Nearly total immobilization of the scaphoid is rendered by incorporation of these two additional digits and by lengthening the cast above the elbow. This method of immobilization is recommended for undiagnosed scaphoid fractures discovered some weeks or months after the initial trauma (Figures 4-18A–E, 4-19A–D), often with radiographic findings of a wide line of osteoporosis at the fracture site.

In general, displacement or rotation of a scaphoid fracture indicates more severe trauma than mere fracture of the scaphoid (Figures 4-20A–L, 4-46A–D).

An unstable or displaced scaphoid fracture results in carpal instability; as a corollary, if carpal

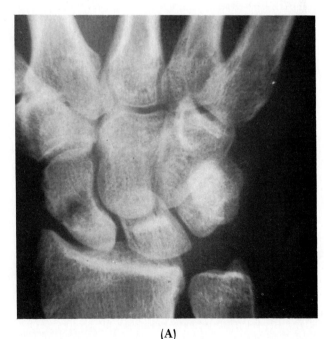

(A)

Figure 4-18 **(A)** Jagged transverse fracture of scaphoid through middle third or neck was not recognized on this original radiograph of 18-year-old male who sustained a wrist injury in football practice.

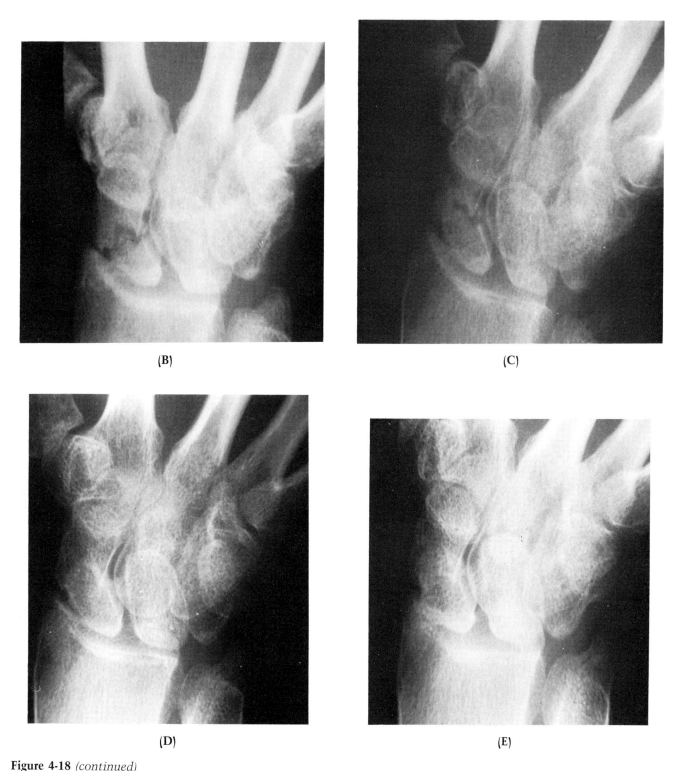

(B)

(C)

(D)

(E)

Figure 4-18 *(continued)*
(B) Six weeks later scaphoid view shows definite fracture through middle third. Short arm-thumb spica cast immobilization was provided at that time. **(C)** Scaphoid view 3 months after initiation of treatment illustrates definite persistence of delayed union of this fracture. At this time a long arm-thumb spica cast was applied incorporating index and long fingers with their MP joints in flexion. **(D)** Scaphoid view 4 months after application of long arm cast immobilization shows good healing of scaphoid fracture. **(E)** Scaphoid view 2 months after discontinuation of immobilization shows good contour of scaphoid and its adjacent joints.

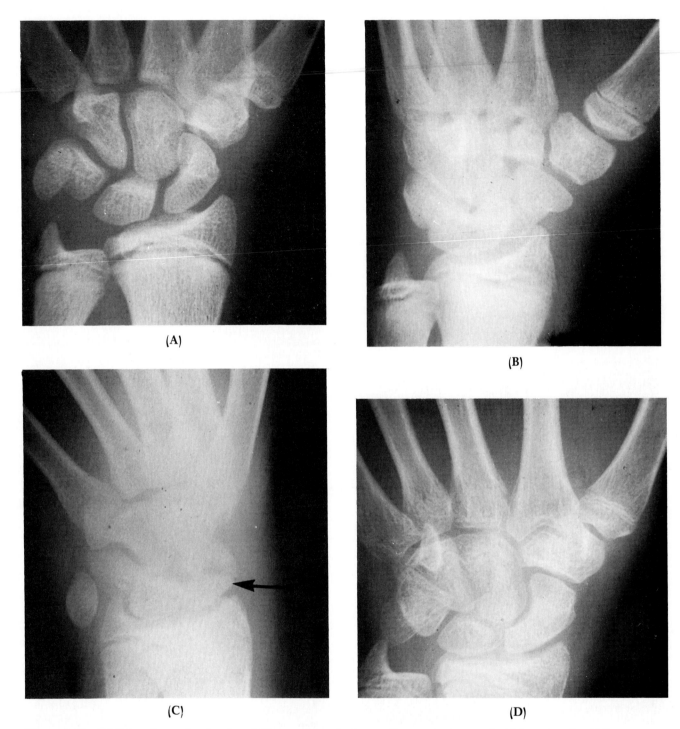

(A)

(B)

(C)

(D)

Figure 4-19 (A) PA radiograph of wrist of 12-year-old male is not diagnostic for scaphoid fracture. (B) Oblique view shows questionable fracture line through middle third of scaphoid. Case emphasizes importance of primary treatment of 3 weeks immobilization of an injured wrist which initially demonstrates physical findings of scaphoid fracture, after which time repeat radiographs should reveal an originally occult scaphoid fracture. (C) No treatment instituted primarily in this case, but symptoms warranted radiographic reevaluation 2 months after original injury. Oblique view taken then shows definite transverse fracture through middle third of scaphoid and wide area of osteoporosis at fracture site. (D) PA view 3 months later after discontinuation of a long arm-thumb spica cast immobilization with incorporation of index and long fingers demonstrates complete healing of originally occult scaphoid fracture.

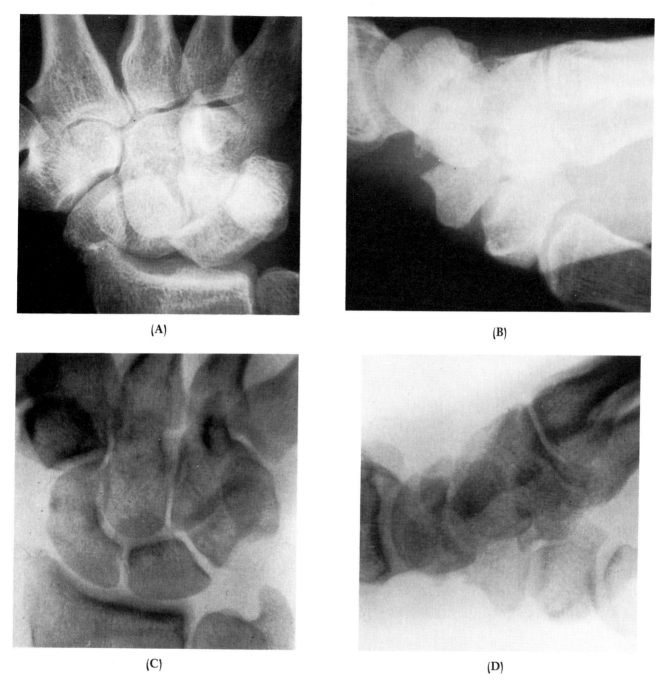

(A)

(B)

(C)

(D)

Figure 4-20 **(A)** PA radiograph of injury sustained in fall from a horse shows obvious distortion of proximal carpal row with large gap between lunate and distal portion of scaphoid. Capitate appears to be displaced proximally into a diastasis between scaphoid and lunate. Note bony superimposition in area of capitate and distal scaphoid segment. **(B)** Lateral view shows completely displaced transverse fracture of scaphoid with palmar angulation of lunate. **(C)** PA radiograph following successful closed manipulation and reduction of displaced scaphoid fracture. **(D)** Lateral radiograph shows anatomic reduction.

(continued)

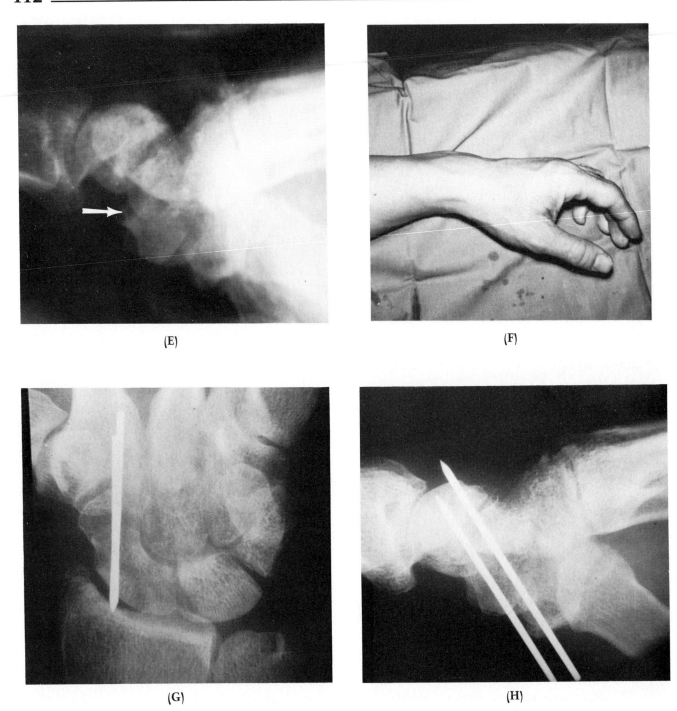

(E)

(F)

(G)

(H)

Figure 4-20 *(continued)*
(E) Lateral radiograph in plaster cast immobilization 3 days after manipulation and reduction shows redisplacement of unstable scaphoid fracture. **(F)** Obvious thickening of wrist and palmar subluxation of metacarpus noted prior to surgical exploration. Transverse dorsal incision was utilized to explore and perform open reduction and internal fixation of displaced unstable scaphoid fracture. **(G)** Large transverse rent in the dorsal capsule of wrist was observed. Capsular avulsion, combined with marked wrist instability, classifies this injury as an unstable palmar transscaphoid perilunate fracture dislocation of the wrist with spontaneous reduction of all carpal elements except for the displaced unstable scaphoid fracture. Oblique radiograph after open reduction and internal Kirschner wire fixation of reduced scaphoid fracture shows acceptable position. **(H)** Lateral view shows similar findings.

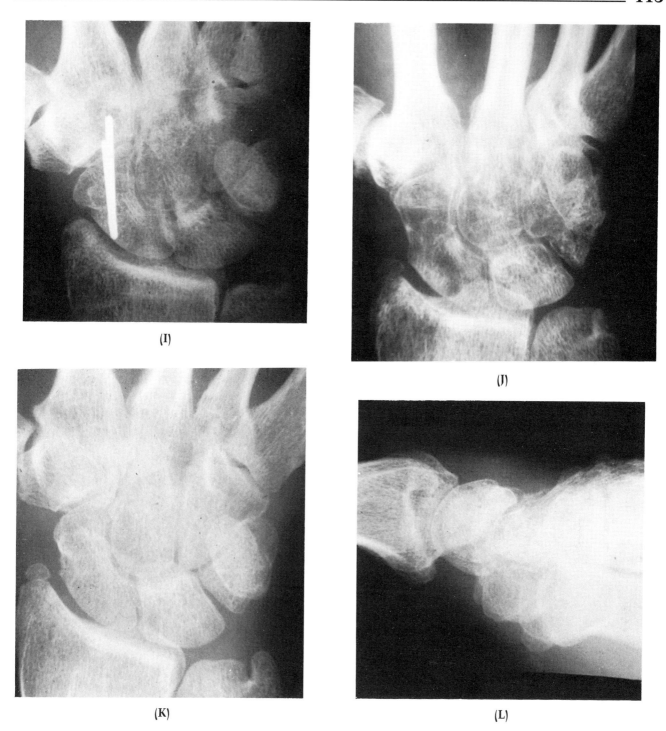

(I)

(J)

(K)

(L)

Figure 4-20 *(continued)*
(I) In PA view normal carpal architecture is seen. **(J)** Oblique view 5 months after surgery and 6 weeks after removal of temporary Kirschner wire fixation shows healing of scaphoid fracture and essentially normal architecture of wrist. Osteoporosis is noted in all carpals with no evidence of avascular necrosis in proximal portion of scaphoid. **(K)** PA radiograph 8 months after surgery shows complete healing of scaphoid fracture, normal architecture of carpus, and no osteoporosis of carpals. Of interest is irregularity of radial styloid process which undoubtedly impinged on scaphoid at time of injury, causing fracture of scaphoid. **(L)** Lateral radiograph shows normal anatomy. Physical examination of injured wrist was essentially normal except for approximately 15° diminished wrist extension.

instability is present, a fractured scaphoid rarely unites. Functionally the distal scaphoid segment moves with, and is a part of, the distal carpal row, and the proximal segment acts with the proximal row.

In the displaced, irreducible or unstable scaphoid fracture with or without rotation of the proximal segment, open reduction, usually with Kirschner wire fixation, is mandatory to achieve and maintain anatomic position (Figures 4-20A–L). Of extreme importance is the diagnosis of any concomitant abnormal intercarpal or radiocarpal relationship signifying additional pathology (e.g., lunate dislocation or subluxation, transscaphoid perilunate fracture dislocation, articular displaced fracture of the distal radius, etc.).

It should be remembered that a displaced or rotated scaphoid fracture may be the only persistent evidence of a dorsal or palmar transscaphoid perilunate fracture dislocation originally sustained, with spontaneous reduction of the carpus. Disruption of the scapholunate articulation with rotation of the proximal portion of the scaphoid and scapholunate dissociation may occur with dorsal transscaphoid perilunate fracture dislocation, and less frequently with solitary fracture of the scaphoid. These findings should be diagnosed early to afford the best proper initial treatment. (See section on Wrist and Carpal Instability in this chapter.)

In occasional specific instances, the primary treatment of a scaphoid fracture may involve screw fixation (eg, ASIF or Herbert screw) (Figures 4-21A,B, 4-22), but generally these techniques should be reserved for cases of delayed or nonunion. These methods allow light use of the wrist during healing with essentially no external immobilization. Great care must be taken not to drill too large a cavity in the proximal scaphoid segment prior to insertion of the ASIF screw. If this detail is disregarded, the screw will not fix the proximal fragment and immobilization will not be achieved (Figure 4-22). The only recourse is primary bone graft and Kirschner wire internal fixation. Also, to achieve the lag effect, the screw threads should not cross the fracture line.

The most frequent causes for delayed union or nonunion of a scaphoid fracture are missed or erroneous diagnosis (Figures 4-18A–E, 4-19A–D), failure to recognize concurrent unreduced dislocations or fracture dislocations of the carpus, improperly or inadequately reduced or unstable scaphoid fractures (Figures 4-46A–D), and failure to immobilize the fracture properly.

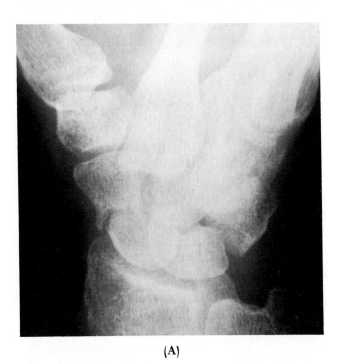

(A)

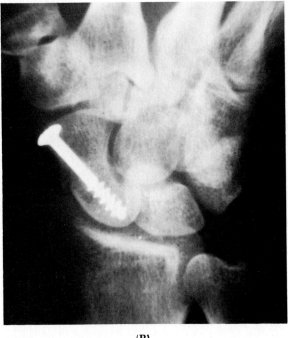

(B)

Figure 4-21 **(A)** Oblique radiograph illustrates transverse fracture through isthmus or middle third of scaphoid. **(B)** Oblique radiograph 6 weeks after screw fixation of acute scaphoid fracture shows good progress in healing. *(Illustrations 4-21A,B courtesy of T.E. DuPuy, M.D.)*

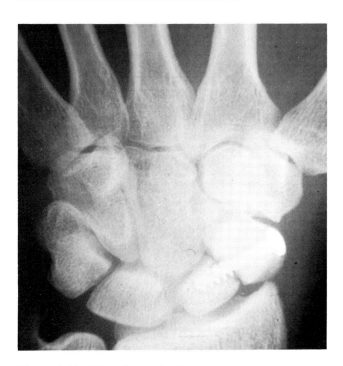

Figure 4-22 PA radiograph illustrates osteoporosis around screw in proximal scaphoid fragment with obvious inadequate fixation of fracture. Figures 4-21A,B and 4-22 illustrate importance of anatomic reduction and stable fixation if such fixation is used to treat a scaphoid fracture. *(Illustration courtesy of T.E. DuPuy, M.D.)*

For delayed union of a scaphoid fracture, particularly in the proximal third, the long arm cast immobilization noted above should be continued for four months. At this time serious consideration should be given to inserting an autogenous bone graft, augmented by Kirschner wire fixation if necessary (Figures 4-23A–D, 4-24A–G).

The above conservative treatment (or operative treatment, if indicated) is recommended for scaphoid fractures diagnosed up to six to eight months post-trauma. Occasionally a patient is seen six months to one and one-half or two years after injury with an undiagnosed (Figure 4-24A–G), untreated, or inadequately treated scaphoid fracture. A wide line of osteoporosis at the fracture site may be complicated by large cystic changes on each side of the fracture site and actual shortening of the scaphoid length. Though prolonged immobilization in the manner described previously may result in fracture union, autogenous iliac bone graft (Figures 4-23A–D) with internal immobilization (Figures 4-24A–G), if indicated, offers a more certain prognosis for healing.[6]

Iliac or rib bone is preferred to bone from any other site (eg, distal radius) since this bone is com-

posed of a good ratio of cortical to cancellous components. The technique is not discussed here, but the palmar Russe approach and technique[7] is advocated because of good exposure and less trauma to scaphoid vascularity. Simultaneous radial styloidectomy is indicated if impingement on the scaphoid inhibits motion. It must be remembered that radiographic localization at surgery is extremely important (Figure 4-23B) to be certain of proper placement of the bone graft (Figures 4-25A,B), and care must be taken to avoid damage to adjacent articular surfaces. The case illustrated in Figures 4-25A,B demonstrates the importance of radiographic localization of the site of nonunion at the time of iliac bone graft if there is any doubt at all concerning the precise location of the nonunion. Kirschner wire temporary fixation should be used if necessary to provide satisfactory immobilization and stability (Figure 4-24F).

The principle of the Herbert screw is fracture fixation by a screw which has threads at both ends with a pitch difference so that there is impaction of the two fragments with compression across the fracture site (Figure 4-26A–F). Technically, no screw threads should cross the fracture site and anatomic reduction is necessary to prevent malunion[8,9] (Figure 4-27A,B). One fault with this technique is the necessary violation of scaphoid-trapezium joint which may cause later ligamentous instability or post-traumatic arthritic changes.

The AO screw by design has a very prominent head on the lag screw (see Figure 4-21B). Technically, the threads of this screw also should not cross the fracture line and should remain only in the proximal fragment to provide impaction fixation of the fracture (see Figure 4-22). A technique of compression plate fixation (Ender) which has a 96% rate of union in the designer's hands, has been introduced recently and may prove to be valuable in the treatment of delayed and nonunion of the scaphoid.

Obviously a nonunion which has healed after a successful bone graft will not eliminate symptoms if adjacent carpal joints and/or the wrist joint have arthritic changes.

Occasionally, fusion of a small proximal scaphoid fragment to the lunate by autogenous bone graft might be considered rather than fusing that fragment to the large distal scaphoid segment.

Failure of a scaphoid fracture to heal after bone graft may be due to continued displacement (failure to reduce the fracture adequately) or instability of the fracture, sclerosis at the fracture line, carpal instability, or unrecognized or untreated concomitant carpal injuries.

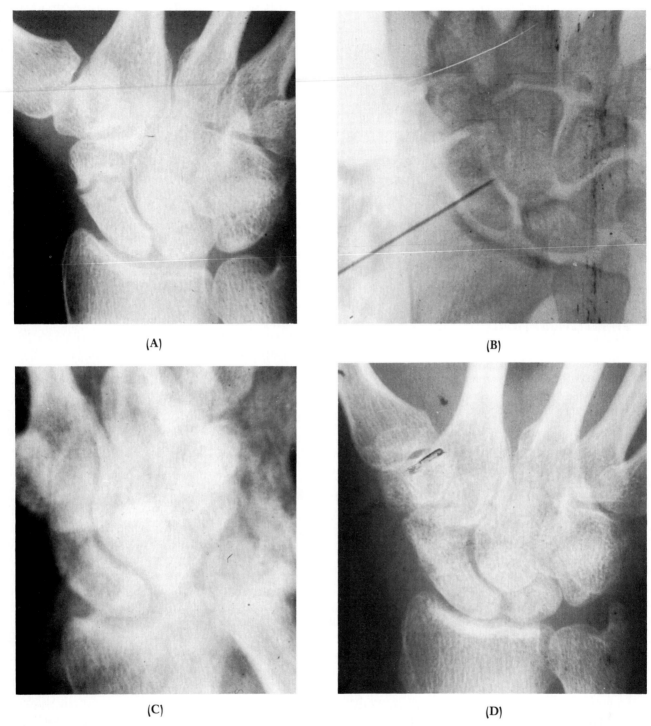

(A)

(B)

(C)

(D)

Figure 4-23 (**A**) Fracture through distal third of scaphoid is noted on AP radiograph of wrist in ulnar deviation (scaphoid view). Original fracture, sustained in hyperextension injury one year before, was treated initially with a short arm-thumb spica cast for 8 weeks and reimmobilized because of apparent nonunion for 4 more months in long arm-thumb spica cast 8 months after trauma. (**B**) Radiographic localization of nonunion is noted at surgery. (**C**) Iliac bone graft is seen across fracture line of reduced scaphoid fracture. Radiograph taken through a long arm plaster cast immobilization. (**D**) Scaphoid view taken 10 weeks after bone graft for scaphoid nonunion shows complete healing and incorporation of bone graft.

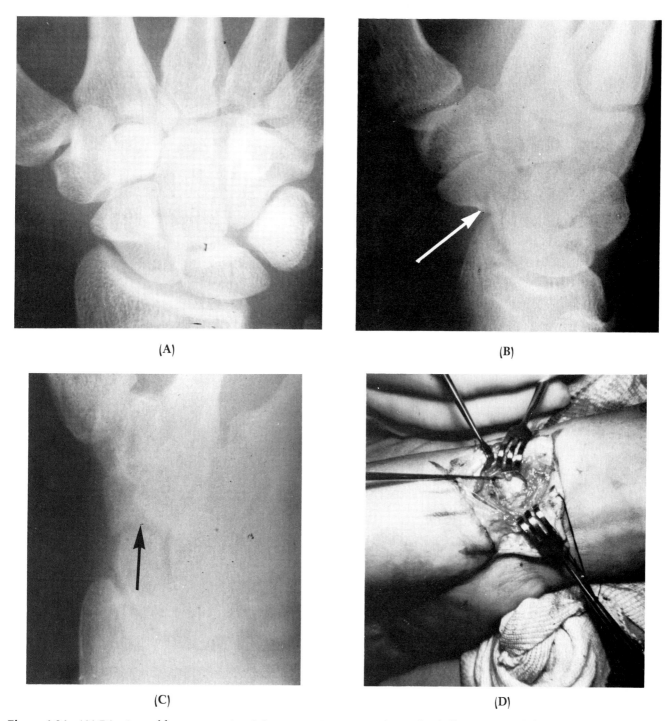

(A)

(B)

(C)

(D)

Figure 4-24 **(A)** PA view of hyperextension injury to wrist sustained in a football game. No definite fracture or dislocation can be seen. **(B)** Oblique radiograph shows fracture of scaphoid through its waist, but fracture was not diagnosed and no immobilization was provided. **(C)** After numerous visits to a chiropractor patient finally consulted an orthopedist 8 months after initial injury. Nonunion of the scaphoid fracture can be seen on scaphoid view taken at that time. **(D)** Long arm-thumb spica cast immobilization for 4 months did not unite fracture. About 1 year after initial injury, surgery was performed to insert an autogenous iliac graft across site of scaphoid nonunion. Surgical exposure shown here.

(continued)

Figure 4-24 *(continued)*
(E) Site of scaphoid nonunion exposed at surgery before insertion of iliac graft. **(F)** Scaphoid view postoperatively shows temporary Kirschner wire fixation of fracture necessary for stability after autogenous iliac bone graft across site of nonunion. **(G)** PA radiograph 3½ months after surgery shows union of scaphoid fracture and absence of internal fixation.

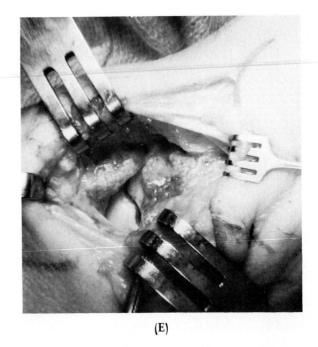

(E)

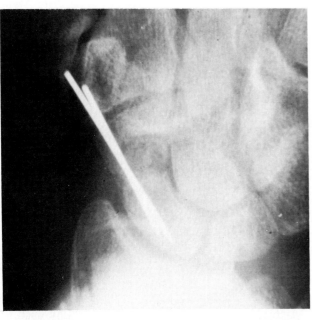
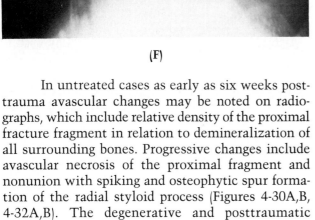

(F)

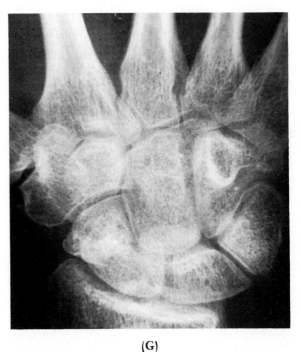

(G)

In untreated cases as early as six weeks posttrauma avascular changes may be noted on radiographs, which include relative density of the proximal fracture fragment in relation to demineralization of all surrounding bones. Progressive changes include avascular necrosis of the proximal fragment and nonunion with spiking and osteophytic spur formation of the radial styloid process (Figures 4-30A,B, 4-32A,B). The degenerative and posttraumatic changes of the radial styloid process are due both to the original trauma and to the repeated chronic impingement of the scaphoid tuberosity on that area, either because of flexion deformity at the site of scaphoid nonunion or because of scaphoid shortening due to advanced bone resorption at the nonunion (Figures 4-30A,B, 4-32A,B). This impingement is particularly evident in palmar flexion and radial deviation of the wrist.

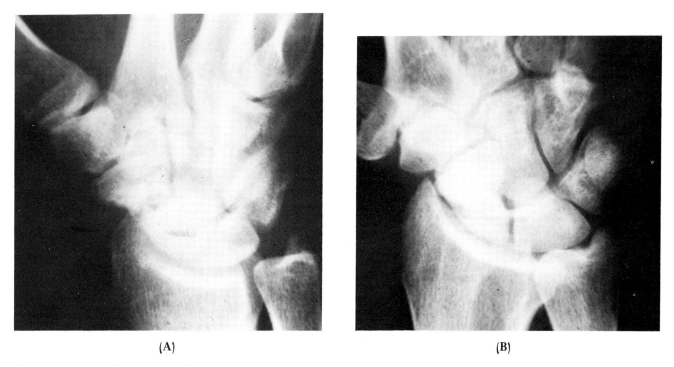

(A)   (B)

Figure 4-25 (A) Oblique view shows fracture of scaphoid 10 months prior to attempted autogenous iliac bone graft across site of nonunion. (B) PA view shows bone graft incorrectly placed across scapholunate joint rather than across site of scaphoid nonunion. There is narrowing of joint space between radial styloid process and scaphoid due to impingement of tuberosity of scaphoid on that process. Changes are also noted in the wrist joint area. *(Illustrations 4-25A,B courtesy of H.A. Yocum, M.D.)*

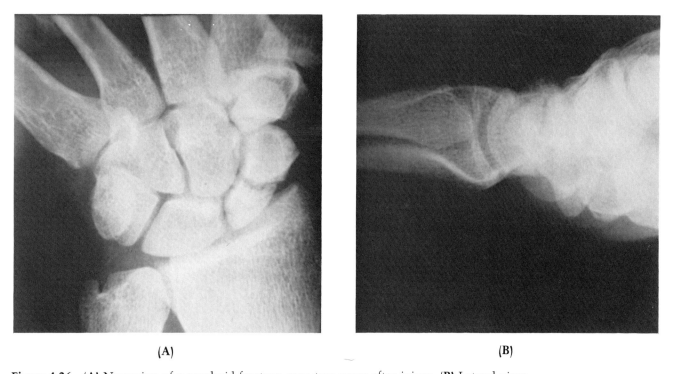

(A)   (B)

Figure 4-26 (A) Nonunion of a scaphoid fracture seen two years after injury. (B) Lateral view.

(continued)

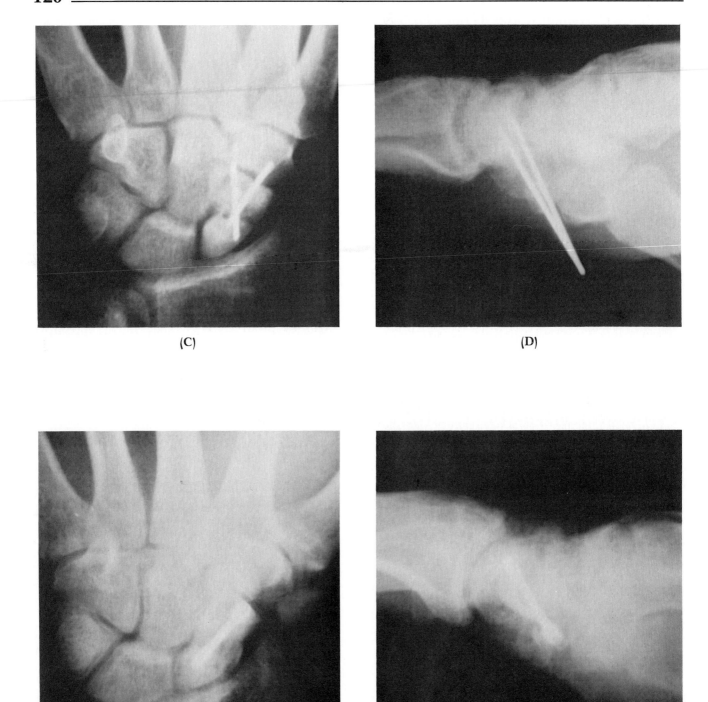

(C)

(D)

(E)

(F)

Figure 4-26 *(continued)*
(C) Open reduction, iliac bone graft, and Kirschner wire fixation did not achieve union at the fracture site, seen four months postoperatively with definite nonunion evident. **(D)** Same, lateral view. **(E)** Open reduction, insertion of a large corticocancellous iliac bone graft measuring 1.5 cm to restore scaphoid in length, combined with Herbert screw fixation. **(F)** Same, lateral view. *(Figures 4-26A–F courtesy of Marybeth Ezaki, M.D.)*

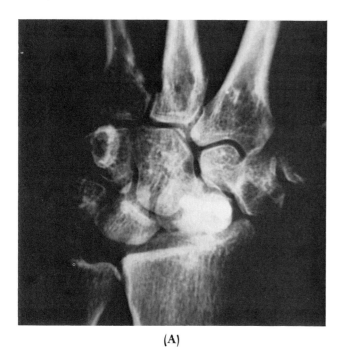

(A)

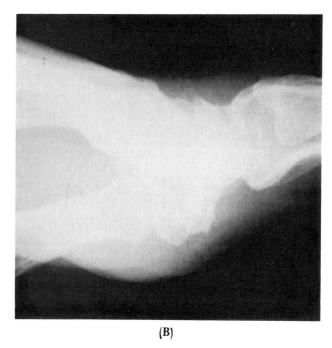

(B)

Figure 4-27 **(A)** Healed malunion of Herbert screw fixation of a scaphoid nonunion. Scaphoid length has not been restored and the distal scaphoid pole is angled palmarly. **(B)** Corresponding lateral view shows the palmar angulation of the distal scaphoid segment at the site of malunion and screw fixation. The solution was osteotomy and tri-scaphe arthrodesis. *(Figures 4-27A–B courtesy of Peter Carter, M.D.)*

Discovery of a nonunion in an old scaphoid fracture is not necessarily an indication for treatment (Figures 4-30A,B, 4-31, 4-32A,B). Sedentary workers, elderly people, and any adult with arthritic changes (whether posttraumatic, degenerative, or rheumatoid, involving multiple intercarpal joints or the wrist joint) usually should not undergo surgery specifically directed at the scaphoid. Bone graft of the scaphoid nonunion is contraindicated, particularly if arthritic changes involve the distal radial articular surface or the contiguous articular surfaces of the scaphoid, lunate, and capitate.

With or without union of the scaphoid fracture, pain caused by impingement of the radial styloid process on the scaphoid may be relieved by radial styloidectomy. However, solitary radial styloidectomy in the presence of radiocarpal posttraumatic or degenerative arthritic changes will be unsuccessful in relieving pain and increasing wrist motion. Osteoporosis and hypertrophic spur formation of the radial styloid may indicate trauma to the area of that process at the time of original injury, during which violent impingement against the scaphoid caused its fracture. Radial styloidectomy to remove this hypertrophic spur formation, either by itself or in combination with a bone graft for a scaphoid nonunion if articular surfaces are acceptable, may be an excellent procedure to diminish pain. The bone from the excised radial styloid should *not* be used as the bone graft for a scaphoid nonunion since this bone is much less suitable than that derived from either the iliac crest or a rib. If there is inattention to detail at the time of radial styloidectomy, arthritic changes with spicule formation may result at the site of styloid excision (Figures 4-28A,B).

Excision of the proximal portion of the scaphoid at the site of old nonunion may be considered but is generally contraindicated (Figures 4-29A,B). Excision of the entire scaphoid is definitely contraindicated. The entire carpal architecture eventually becomes distorted following either procedure. As seen in Figures 4-29A,B, the entire distal carpal row, not just the capitate, migrates proximally, which may result eventually in capitate articulation with the distal radius, ulnar migration of the lunate, and distortion of the hamate-triquetral joint due to proximal sliding of the hamate (Figures 4-29A,B).

Reconstruction of a wrist with an old scaphoid nonunion and diffuse changes of degenerative and posttraumatic arthritis includes arthroplasty or

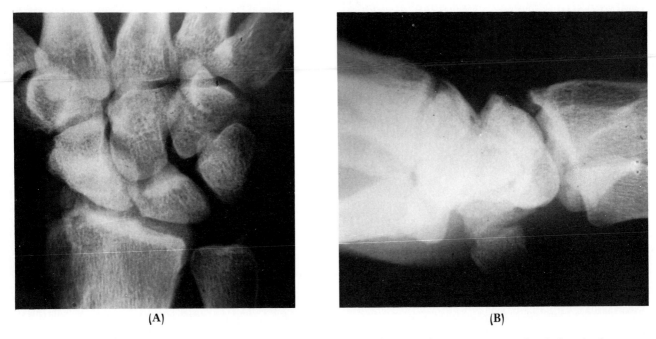

(A)   (B)

Figure 4-28 **(A)** PA radiograph shows healed scaphoid fracture after bone graft using section of radial styloid process. Arthritic changes are noted in radioscaphoid joint. **(B)** Oblique view demonstrates hypertrophic spur formation on distal radius in area from which bone graft was obtained. Debridement of hypertrophic osteophytic spurs from distal radius was performed and improved wrist motion.

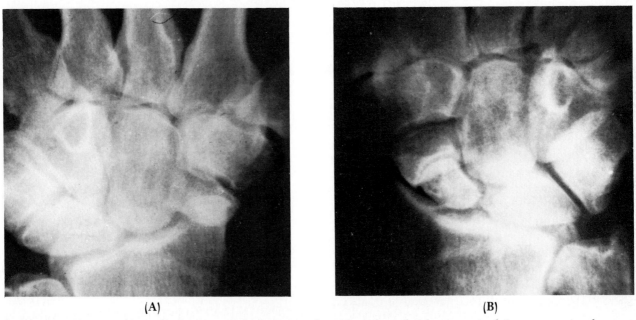

(A)   (B)

Figure 4-29 **(A)** PA radiograph of wrist in which proximal portion of scaphoid was excised 6 years previously for prolonged nonunion. Proximal migration of capitate and hamate area seen; capitate now articulates with distal radius. Distortion of carpus and arthritic changes in radiolunate articulation are noted, but patient was essentially asymptomatic and had excellent mobility. **(B)** Contralateral wrist shows nonunion of old scaphoid fracture with marked shortening of scaphoid and arthritic changes between distal radius and both scaphoid and lunate. Case does not demonstrate congenital bipartite or two-segmented scaphoid, despite bilateral findings. Radiographic evidence of arthritic changes in joints surrounding scaphoid supports diagnosis of old bilateral scaphoid fractures. *(Illustrations 4-29A,B courtesy of S.C. Santangelo, M.D.)*

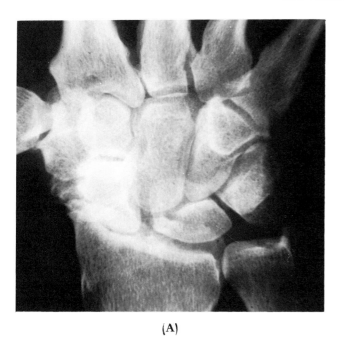

(A)

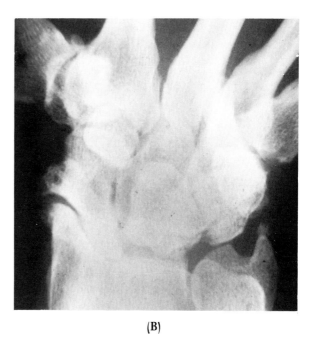

(B)

Figure 4-30 (A) PA radiograph of right wrist shows severe degenerative joint disease of radioscaphoid joint, diastasis of scapholunate joint, and marked distortion and shortening of scaphoid, with osteophytic spur formation of radial styloid process. (B) Scaphoid view demonstrates marked lipping and osteophytic formation of radial styloid process due to impingement of distorted scaphoid on this area, resulting in severe arthritic changes. (Radiographs of contralateral left wrist showed degenerative and arthritic changes of wrist joint, multiple intercarpal joints, and flattening of proximal scaphoid.) Case illustrates bilateral chronic severe trauma to both wrists, probably secondary to old healed bilateral scaphoid fractures.

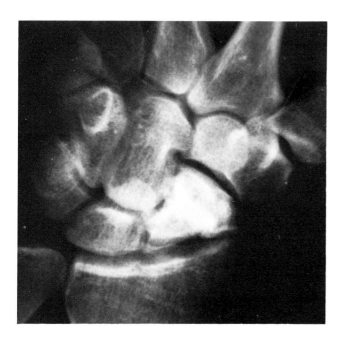

Figure 4-31 A 20-year scaphoid nonunion clearly shows marked shortening of scaphoid and sclerotic borders at site of scaphoid nonunion.

arthrodesis (Figures 4-30A,B, 4-31, 4-32A,B). Arthroplasty may include excision of the scaphoid and insertion of a silastic implant (Figures 4-33A–C). The wrist architecture at this late date is usually so destroyed that proper fit of a commercial implant is difficult unless it is handcarved and altered at surgery. However, this implant may act quite well as a buttress against the trapezium, capitate, and radius to maintain an acceptable position of the capitate and to retain minimally symptomatic wrist motion. Figures 4-33A–C illustrate the necessity of ligamentous reconstruction of the important radioscaphoidlunate portion of the deep palmar radiocarpal ligament at the time of implant arthroplasty, usually utilizing a section of the flexor carpi radialis tendon to restore the vital support of this ligament.

Silastic scaphoid implant arthroplasty is contraindicated if previously radial styloidectomy has been performed which removed its buttress effect necessary for implant stability.

If the implant arthroplasty fails, motion may be retained by a proximal row carpectomy, which includes excision of the lunate and the triquetrum in

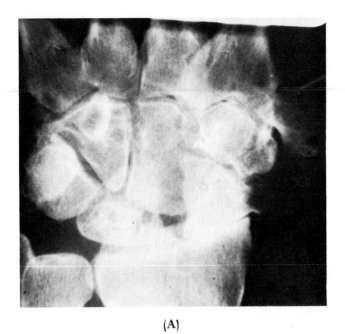
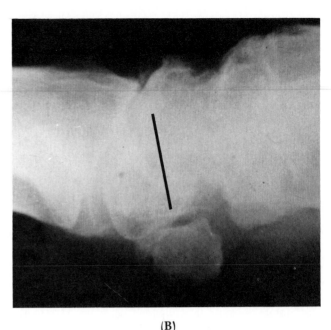

(A)   (B)

Figure 4-32 **(A)** PA radiograph of wrist illustrates marked distortion of scaphoid with secondary diastasis of scapholunate joint. Severe degenerative changes are noted in wrist joint area involving particularly radius and scaphoid. **(B)** Lateral view shows dorsal rotation of the lunate and severe degenerative joint disease secondary to old trauma and probably fracture of scaphoid. There is secondary distortion and diastasis of scapholunate articulation and scapholunate dissociation with dorsal rotation and subluxation of lunate.

addition to removal of the implant. If proximal row carpectomy is chosen initially, the lunate, triquetrum, and, usually, the entire scaphoid are excised (though if preferred the distal scaphoid pole can be retained) usually with simultaneous radial styloidectomy. Incorporation of a silastic hinge type implant (Swanson design manufactured by Dow Corning) is a refinement of the standard proximal row carpectomy. The proximal stem of the implant is inserted in a suitably prepared intramedullary hole in the shaft of the distal radius and the distal stem through a tunnel in the capitate, into an intramedullary hole in the long finger metacarpal shaft. A silastic cap is not necessary to cover the distal ulna if the distal radioulnar joint is reasonably normal. A relatively painless, stable wrist joint with acceptable motion results.

For a manual laborer who requires a painless, stable wrist, arthrodesis extending from the radius into the index and long metacarpals is the procedure of choice.

Other methods of treatment for old nonunion of the scaphoid have been attempted with variable results. These include localized fusion of the scaphoid, lunate, hamate, and capitate and fusion of the scaphoid to the capitate. Fusion of the scaphoid, lunate, and capitate are successful only if the sur-

rounding joints are essentially normal. Occasionally with nonunion of a scaphoid fracture in the proximal third, this small proximal fragment can be fused to the lunate rather than to the larger scaphoid fragment with acceptable results. There is little indication for these limited carpal fusions to treat old scaphoid nonunion with diffuse arthritic changes in adjacent joints. Wrist arthroplasty or arthrodesis is far more reliable.

Scaphoid Dislocation

Scaphoid dislocation almost invariably is associated with other simultaneous carpal trauma (Figures 4-34A,B). Isolated scaphoid dislocation is extremely rare and is a result of severe localized trauma (Figures 4-35A–D).

Transscaphoid Perilunate Fracture Dislocation and Perilunate Dislocation

General Discussion

Both transscaphoid perilunate fracture dislocation and perilunate dislocation occur dorsally in the vast majority of instances due to a forced hyperextension

Figure 4-33 **(A)** PA view shows nonunion 6 months after second attempt at iliac bone graft for chronic nonunion of a fractured scaphoid from a high-velocity missle injury. **(B)** PA radiograph shows displacement and rotation of scaphoid silastic implant inserted after excision of scaphoid noted in Figure 4-33(A). **(C)** PA radiograph illustrates excellent anatomic repositioning of carpus after removal of rotated scaphoid silastic implant and insertion of another, with accurate soft tissue reconstruction to maintain proper position of implant. *(Illustrations 4-33A–C courtesy of F.N. DeLuca, M.D.)*

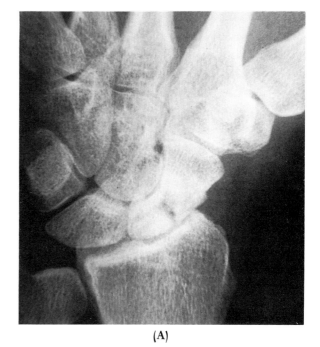

(A)

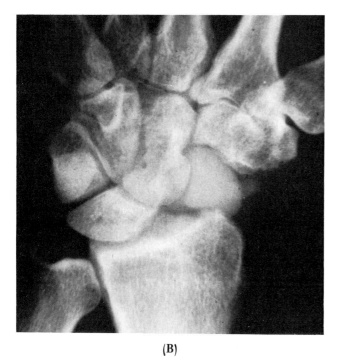

(B)

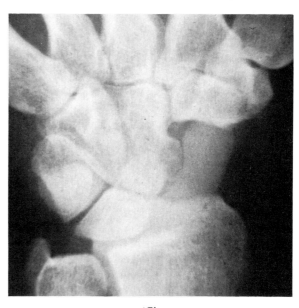

(C)

injury of the wrist. The rare palmar counterparts must necessarily be caused by severe hyperflexion injury to the wrist.

To achieve a dorsal displacement of the carpus from the lunate, which remains in its normal anatomic relationship to the distal radius, one of two injuries must occur: there must be complete scapholunate dissociation, resulting in a dorsal perilunate dislocation; or there must be a displaced fracture of the scaphoid, resulting in a dorsal transscaphoid perilunate fracture dislocation.

On physical examination in both injuries there is a dorsal displacement of the carpus just distal to the radiocarpal joint, which presents in the immediate posttraumatic period as a prominent ridge transversely across the carpus. Occasionally it may be possible to palpate the proximal pole of the capitate dorsally. The diffuse swelling will obscure these findings several hours after injury.

In both lesions all wrist motion is limited and painful. Pain is more severe if there is an associated scaphoid fracture, and there is discrete tenderness in

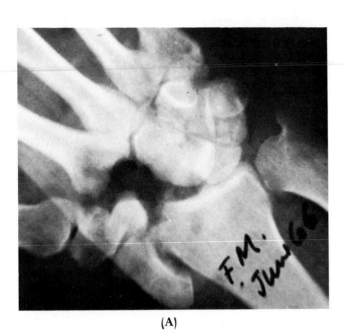
(A)

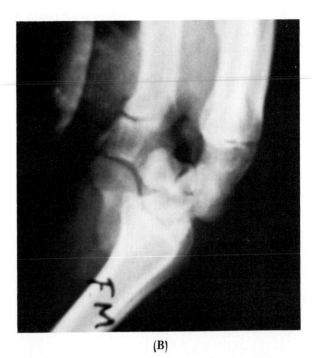
(B)

Figure 4-34 **(A)** PA radiograph shows complete distortion of carpal anatomy with total dislocation and displacement of scaphoid, trapezium, and trapezoid. Of interest is stability of index metacarpal base despite total avulsion of trapezoid. **(B)** Lateral radiograph shows dorsal dislocation of capitate, fracture of lunate with palmar tilt, and complete dislocation of scaphoid, trapezium, and trapezoid. Lesion was due to severe crushing injury to wrist which caused extreme distortion of carpus and avulsion of radial portion, including scaphoid, trapezium, and trapezoid and thumb metacarpal. Midcarpal dislocation (dorsal dislocation of capitate) also occurred. *(Reprinted, by permission, from G.W.D. Armstrong, M.D., Rotational subluxation of the scaphoid, Can J Surg 11:306–14, 1968.)*[10]

the area of the anatomic snuff box. In both lesions the lateral radiograph is vitally important for accurate diagnosis. The longitudinal axes of the capitate and the radius do not coincide, and the longitudinal axis of the capitate is noted to be dorsal to that of the radius. The lunate remains in its normal anatomic position in relation to the distal radius. Palmar tilt of the lunate, often found in dorsal perilunate dislocation, must not be confused with anterior subluxation or dislocation of the lunate.

After reduction and prior to cast immobilization, radiographic evaluation is most important to discover any rotational instability of the scaphoid, with or without scapholunate dissociation, and rotational instability of the lunate.

Following successful closed manipulation and reduction, immobilization should be continued for six to eight weeks if there is no fracture. A long arm cast is preferred, at least for the first three to four weeks. The elbow is flexed 90° and the wrist is held in neutral position, or 15° to 20° palmar flexion, with neutral pronation-supination. If the scaphoid is fractured and anatomic closed reduction is achieved, im-

mobilization usually must be continued for eight to ten weeks, at least.

Transscaphoid Perilunate Fracture Dislocation

The dorsal transscaphoid perilunate fracture dislocation is the most common of all fracture dislocations, fractures, and dislocations in the carpus except for dorsal avulsion fractures of the carpals and isolated fracture of the scaphoid.

The proximal portion of the scaphoid and the lunate are the most protected bones in the wrist in the position of wrist flexion and radial deviation. This security is afforded by various ligamentous attachments including the palmar radiocarpal ligament complex, the ulnocarpal ligament complex, the dorsal radiocarpal ligament, the dorsal capsule, and the scapholunate interosseous ligaments. The scaphoid itself, however, is very vulnerable to trauma in wrist extension since it is the only stable osseous link between the proximal and the distal carpal rows. In

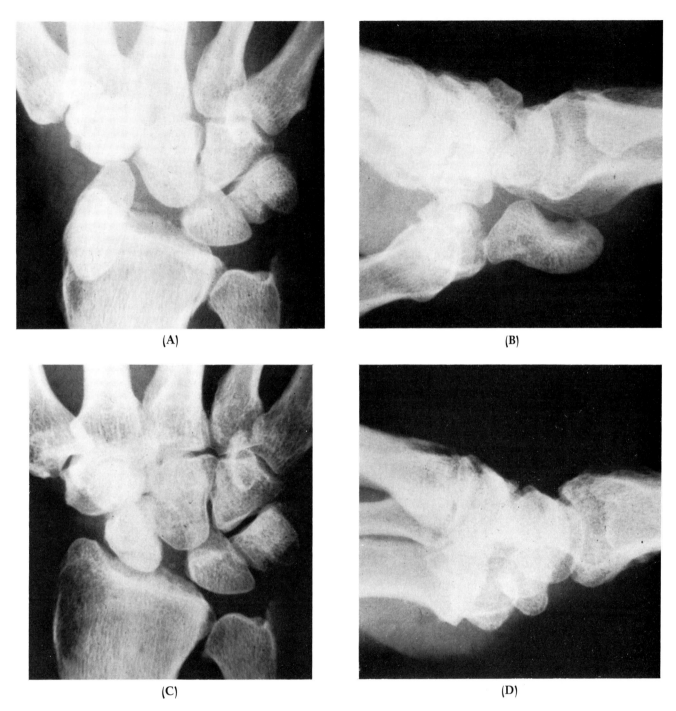

(A)

(B)

(C)

(D)

Figure 4-35 (A) PA view of wrist which sustained a severe blow from a crane wire. Complete scaphoid dislocation is noted with a few small bone fragments in space proximal to capitate head. Remainder of carpus appears normal. (B) Lateral view shows complete palmar dislocation of scaphoid, a rare lesion. Surgery was necessary for reduction, and all ligamentous attachments were found to be avulsed except that between radial aspect of scaphoid and trapezium. (C) PA view 3 weeks after surgery shows loss of scaphoid reduction with rather marked diastasis of scapholunate area and scapoid shortening. (D) Lateral radiograph shows palmar rotational deformity of scaphoid and slight dorsal rotational deformity of lunate. At this time open reduction and internal Kirschner wire fixation of scaphoid to lunate, to capitate, and probably to distal radius, perhaps combined with ligamentous reconstruction, is indicated. *(Reprinted, by permission, from Y. Murakami, Dislocation of the carpal scaphoid, Hand 9:79–81, 1977.)*[11]

scaphoid fracture the exact location is determined primarily by the position of the wrist at the time of injury and secondarily by the point of impact. Fracture usually occurs in the middle third or isthmus of the scaphoid. If the trauma is sufficiently violent, the entire carpus and distal scaphoid fragment are displaced dorsally, proximally, and radially, and the proximal portion of the scaphoid remains with the lunate, resulting in a dorsal transscaphoid perilunate fracture dislocation.

Occasionally one or more other carpals are fractured in addition to the scaphoid, most commonly the triquetrum (Figures 4-38A–C).

The physical findings of this lesion have been noted above and closely resemble those of the dorsal perilunate dislocation except that pain and tenderness are increased due to fracture of the scaphoid.

The lateral radiograph (Figures 4-36A, 4-37A, 4-38A, 4-39B) shows a normal relationship of the distal radius to the lunate. The distal concavity of the lunate which is normally filled by the proximal convexity of the capitate is vacant and looks like an "empty cup." The proximal pole of the scaphoid remains with the lunate, but the remainder of the car-

pus, including the distal pole of the scaphoid, is displaced dorsally and proximally. The longitudinal axis of the capitate is not in line with the longitudinal axis of the radius because of the dorsal displacement of the capitate which overrides the lunate. The lunate may also be tilted palmarly.

The PA radiograph (Figures 4-36B, 4-37B, 4-38B, 4-39C) shows an obvious displaced fracture of the scaphoid and complete disruption of the lunate-capitate relationship. No clear joint can be seen between these two carpals, and the proximal displacement of the capitate is evident. There is superimposition of the capitate on the lunate and the proximal portion of the scaphoid. All other radiographic views accentuate the vacant concavity of the distal lunate articular surface and the normal relationship of the lunate and the proximal pole of the scaphoid to the distal radius (Figure 4-38C).

Closed manipulation and reduction, if possible, is effected by longitudinal traction on the hand with an assistant exerting countertraction on the flexed elbow. The wrist is extended, and direct pressure applied dorsally over the capitate and palmarly on the lunate is accompanied by flexion of the wrist. The

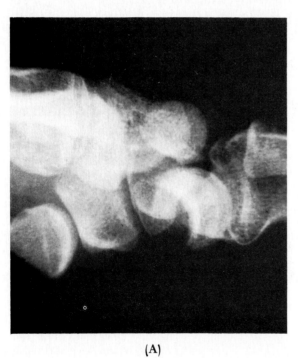

(A)

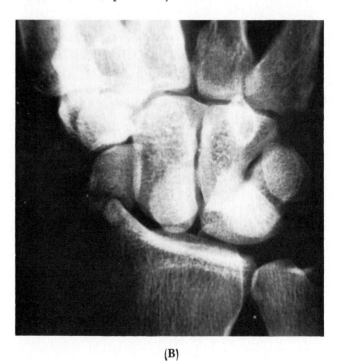

(B)

Figure 4-36 **(A)** Dorsal transscaphoid perilunate fracture dislocation seen on lateral view. Relationship of radius and lunate is normal with approximately 20° palmar tilt of lunate. Distal concave articular surface of lunate is vacant, and remainder of carpus is dorsally dislocated and displaced proximally. Longitudinal axes of capitate and distal radius do not coincide. **(B)** PA radiograph clearly illustrates fracture of scaphoid. Proximal portion of scaphoid and lunate are in normal relationship to each other and to distal radial articular surface, but both lunate-capitate and lunate-triquetral articulations are absent. Capitate proximally displaced.

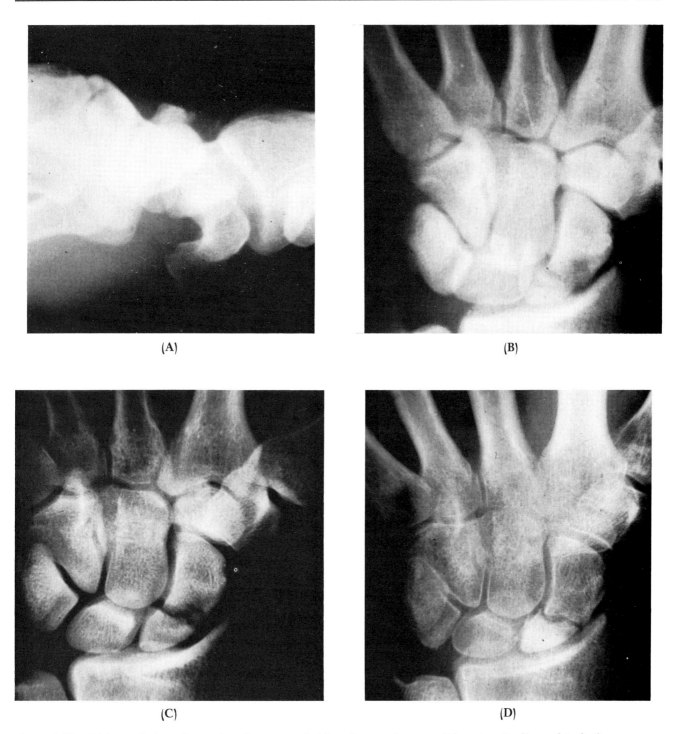

(A)

(B)

(C)

(D)

Figure 4-37 (A) Lateral view shows dorsal transscaphoid perilunate fracture dislocation. Radiographic findings similar to those in Figure 4-36A. (B) PA radiograph shows fracture of scaphoid, normal articulation of distal radius with proximal scaphoid segment and lunate, and abnormal relationship of lunate to triquetrum and capitate and of proximal scaphoid fragment to capitate. (C) PA radiograph shows normal anatomy of carpus with an obvious fracture through junction of proximal and middle thirds of scaphoid after successful closed manipulation and reduction and prior to cast immobilization. Lateral radiograph (not shown) showed normal carpal anatomy. (D) Delayed union of scaphoid fracture with avascular changes in proximal scaphoid segment 5 months after injury.

(continued)

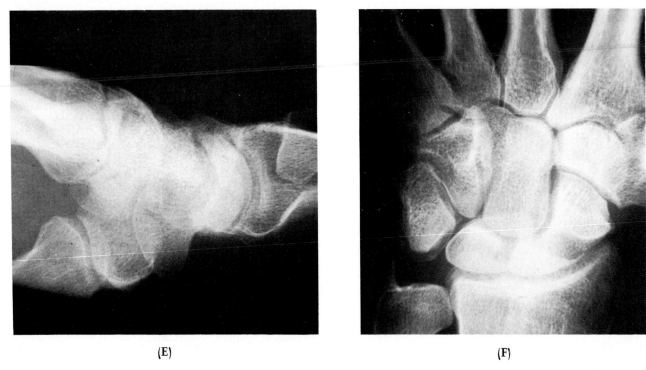

(E) (F)

Figure 4-37 *(continued)*
(E) All wrist motion was painful, and extension particularly was limited. Operative debridement of multiple small bone fragments from dorsal aspect of radioscaphoid articulation performed 11 months after injury. Lateral radiograph taken 1 year after original injury and 6 weeks after wrist debridement shows absence of bony fragments. Essentially normal carpal relationships are seen. **(F)** PA view shows complete healing of scaphoid fracture with no evidence of avascular necrotic changes.

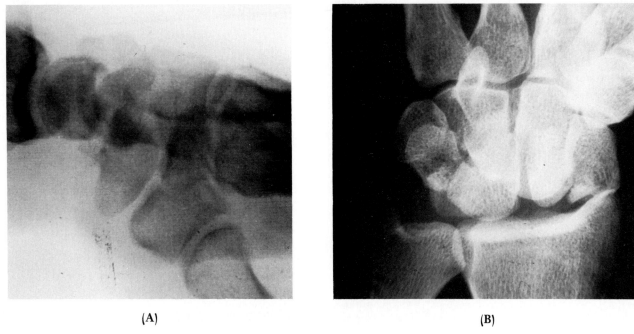

(A) (B)

Figure 4-38 **(A)** Lateral radiograph shows characteristic findings of dorsal transscaphoid perilunate fracture dislocation of wrist complicated by fracture of triquetrum. **(B)** PA radiograph shows dorsal transscaphoid perilunate fracture dislocation and fractured triquetrum.

Figure 4-38 *(continued)*
(C) Oblique view shows palmar tilt of lunate of approximately 45° and illustrates the fracture of triquetrum.
(D) PA radiograph 6 months after original injury and successful closed reduction and external immobilization shows healing of both scaphoid and triquetral fractures, with essentially normal architecture of wrist. **(E)** Lateral radiograph shows essentially normal carpal anatomy and correction of palmar tilt of lunate. *(Illustrations 4-38A–E courtesy of S.C. Santangelo, M.D.)*

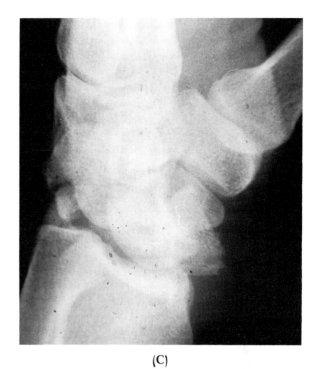

(C)

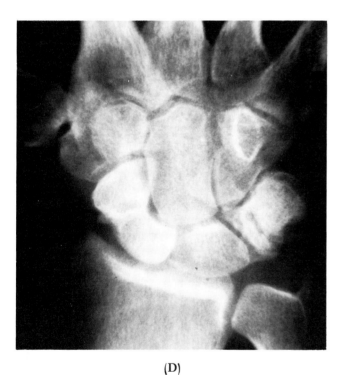

(D)

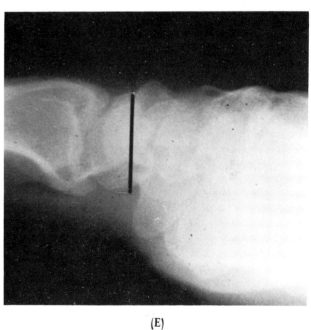

(E)

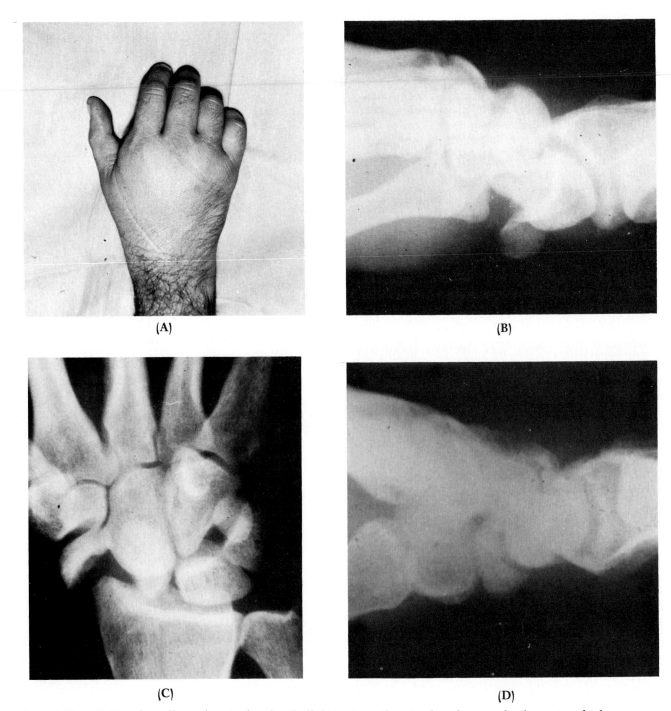

(A)

(B)

(C)

(D)

Figure 4-39 **(A)** Dorsal swelling of entire hand and all digits is evident in this photograph of a wrist which sustained a hyperextension injury 2 days previously. **(B)** Lateral radiograph illustrates dorsal transscaphoid perilunate fracture dislocation with characteristic findings. **(C)** PA view shows relatively small proximal and distal segments of scaphoid. **(D)** Lateral view after successful closed manipulation and reduction shows that essentially normal carpal anatomy was restored.

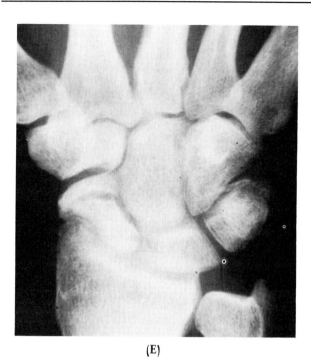

(E)

Figure 4-39 *(continued)*
(E) PA view after reduction discloses distinct incongruity between proximal and distal scaphoid segments, with blunting and rounding of contiguous bone edges at fracture site and marked loss of scaphoid length. Patient had sustained a scaphoid fracture some years previously which was not treated. Rounded bone edges at site of fracture and loss of scaphoid length are due to long-standing nonunion, with resorption of bone at fracture site. Patient's present injury was a dorsal transscaphoid perilunate fracture dislocation through area of old scaphoid fracture nonunion.

reduction is similar to that for Colles' fracture. Immobilization has been discussed previously and concerns healing of the scaphoid, which may be prolonged. If anatomic reduction of the fractured scaphoid or of the dislocation is impossible, open reduction from a dorsal approach and internal fixation is recommended. Sometimes reduction is hindered because of a rotation or displacement of the proximal scaphoid fragment. The fracture surface of the proximal fragment of the scaphoid may face directly palmarly and be irreducible.

If after successful reduction a diastasis persists between the lunate and the proximal scaphoid portion (indicating scapholunate dissociation and usually an associated rotational instability of the scaphoid), open reduction with Kirschner wire fixation is indicated when closed reduction and percutaneous Kirschner wire fixation does not achieve the desired anatomic result.

If discovered after two or more weeks posttrauma, ligamentous reconstruction of scapholunate dissociation with temporary Kirschner wire immobilization is recommended to reestablish a scapholunate articulation as anatomic as possible.

There is often a delay in healing (Figures 4-37C–F) and occasionally a nonunion (Figures 4-40A,B) of the scaphoid fracture. If no healing is seen after four months of immobilization, bone graft is indicated.

Avascular changes occur more commonly than in an isolated fracture of the scaphoid and involve the proximal portion (Figure 4-37D). Occasionally avascular necrosis of the lunate and/or the proximal pole of the scaphoid occur, but usually the avascular changes resolve spontaneously and do not progress to necrosis.

Additional complications include arthritis, if the scaphoid fracture results in malunion and, occasionally, delayed flexor tendon rupture and chronic carpal tunnel syndrome.

In the undiagnosed or untreated injury open reduction can be attempted up to three months posttrauma. It is essential to achieve anatomic reduction of a displaced or angulated scaphoid fracture or to reconstruct the normal relationship between the scaphoid and lunate.

After six months posttrauma reduction is usually impossible and reconstruction, if indicated, must be directed either to proximal row carpectomy, selected intercarpal fusions, or wrist arthrodesis (Figures 4-41A,B).

Proximal row carpectomy involves excision of the lunate, the triquetrum, and either the complete scaphoid or its proximal segment. (Refer to section on scaphoid fracture in this chapter for technique.) This procedure is a reasonable attempt to retain motion, but some power and stability is sacrificed, and some pain may remain.

For a successful proximal row carpectomy without use of a hinged implant, the distal radial articular surface and the proximal articular surface of the capitate should be essentially normal.

Selected intercarpal fusions include arthrodesis of the scapholunate-capitate joints and are occasionally recommended in an attempt to retain some radial carpal motion. This procedure is quite unpredictable, if any signs or symptoms of posttraumatic or degenerative arthritis in adjacent joints are present. The most predictable outcome follows radiocarpal fusion or wrist arthrodesis. The result is a painless stable wrist, but obviously motion is limited to pronation and supination, unless the bone

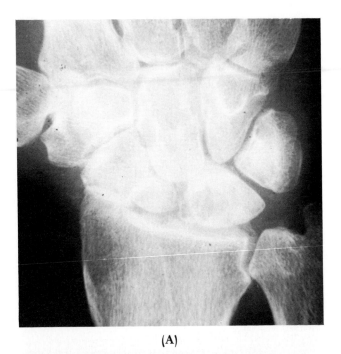

(A)

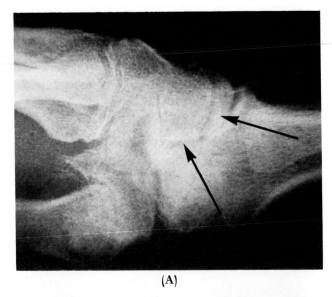

(A)

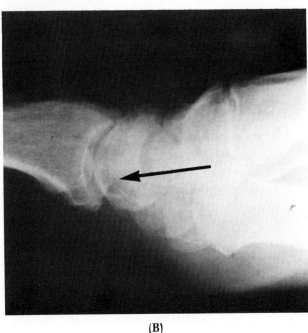

(B)

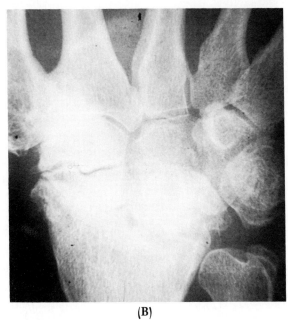

(B)

Figure 4-40 (A) PA radiograph of an untreated dorsal transscaphoid perilunate fracture dislocation sustained 8 years previously shows nonunion of scaphoid fracture, dissociation of scapholunate joint, and cystic changes in lunate. Arthritic changes noted between distal radius and distal scaphoid segment, with impingement of scaphoid tuberosity on radial styloid process. (B) Lateral radiograph shows diffuse arthritic changes of wrist joint and cystic changes in lunate.

Figure 4-41 (A) Lateral view shows findings of untreated dorsal transscaphoid perilunate fracture dislocation which had occurred 20 years previously. Spontaneous fusion of distal radius with scaphoid, marked irregularity of distal radial articulation with lunate, dorsal and proximal displacement of remaining carpus, and severe degenerative arthritis of trapezium-thumb metacarpal joint are seen. (B) PA radiograph accentuates shortening of carpus, with proximal displacement of capitate, fusion of radius and scaphoid, diffuse degenerative arthritic changes involving articulations of lunate with scaphoid and distal radius, and of scaphoid with triquetrum. Distal radius is not completely fused to lunate. *(Illustrations 4-41A,B courtesy of P.R. Sweterlitsch, M.D.)*

Figure 4-42 (A) Lateral view shows palmar radial transscaphoid perilunate fracture dislocation of wrist 3 weeks after injury. Note normal relationship of distal radius with lunate and proximal fragment of scaphoid. Remainder of carpus is dislocated anteriorly and proximally. (B) PA radiograph illustrates more clearly fracture of scaphoid and carpal shortening due to palmar dislocation, proximal displacement, and radial deviation. (C) Oblique view clearly shows scaphoid fracture and anterior subluxation of carpus in relation to normal position of lunate and proximal scaphoid segment at wrist joint. Attempt at open reduction was unsuccessful due to time lapse between injury and treatment. Therefore proximal carpal row, including the distal fragment of scaphoid, was excised. *(Reprinted, by permission, from A.H. Woodward, M.D., R.J. Neviaser, M.D., and F. Nisenfeld, M.D., Radial and volar perilunate transscaphoid fracture dislocation, S Med J 68:926–28, 1975.)*[12]

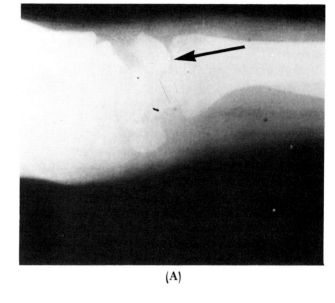

(A)

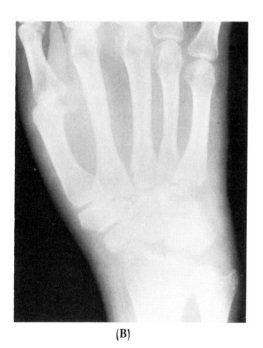

(B)

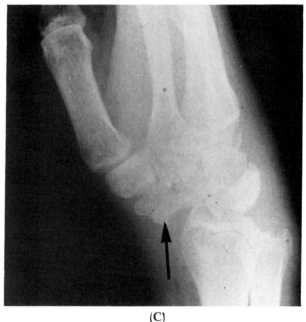

(C)

graft does not extend distally to include the index and long metacarpals and intervening carpometacarpal joints.

In dealing with fractures and fracture dislocations of the wrist it is important to differentiate between lesions incurred in a recent injury and those from old injuries. Often this differentiation may be difficult prior to reduction, but after anatomic repositioning of the carpus, accurate diagnosis should be less of a problem (Figures 4-39A–E). Again, radiographic evaluation after reduction and prior to cast immobilization is strongly recommended since some details such as rotational instability of the

scaphoid and scapholunate dissociation may be obscured by the overlying plaster cast.

Occasionally a patient is seen who sustained a dorsal transscaphoid perilunate fracture dislocation many years previously but received no treatment (Figures 4-40A,B, 4-41A,B). Variable limitation of motion and pain are noted on physical examination, and radiographs usually disclose rather marked degenerative and posttraumatic arthritic changes.

Palmar transscaphoid perilunate fracture dislocation often has associated radial displacement[12] (Figures 4-42A–C). A severe hyperflexion force causes the injury. Median nerve compression or occasionally ulnar nerve compression may be caused by this displaced mass, similar to the findings in the much more common palmar dislocation of the lunate. This displaced mass also may be palpated deep to the flexor tendons and creates a convexity on the palmar aspect of the wrist.

The lateral radiograph shows a palmar and proximal displacement of the carpus with an essentially normal relationship of the distal radius to the lunate and the proximal portion of the scaphoid. The PA radiograph discloses a fracture of the scaphoid with a distorted relationship between the lunate and the capitate and no discernible joint space. There is general foreshortening of the wrist, and the capitate is palmarly dislocated and proximally displaced. Other views aid in the diagnosis of the scaphoid fracture and any concomitant injury.

Closed reduction, if possible, is usually achieved by longitudinal traction with simultaneous dorsal pressure on the lunate and palmar pressure on the capitate with the wrist extended. After reduction the wrist is kept in neutral position or slight flexion and immobilized in the same manner as its dorsal counterpart. If anatomic reduction of the scaphoid has not been achieved by closed manipulation and reduction, open reduction and internal fixation is indicated.

Perilunate Dislocation

Perilunate dislocation signifies a normal relationship of the distal radial articular surface to the lunate with dorsal or palmar and proximal displacement of the entire remaining carpus from the lunate. Dorsal perilunate dislocation is rather common (Figures 4-43A–D, 4-44A–E, 4-62A), but palmar perilunate dislocation is rare.

Physical findings are essentially similar to those noted in transscaphoid perilunate fracture dislocations except that the pain and usually the edema and ecchymosis are not as severe because the scaphoid has not been fractured. The dorsal prominence noted transversely across the carpus just distal to the radiocarpal joint is similar to that seen in the dorsal transscaphoid perilunate fracture dislocation.

Differentiation between a dorsal perilunate dislocation and a palmar dislocation of the lunate is extremely important at initial diagnosis. The lateral radiograph is the key to the solution. In the neutral position the longitudinal axis of the capitate should normally coincide with the longitudinal axes of the radius and the lunate. In palmar dislocation of the lunate the longitudinal axes do not coincide since the lunate is palmar to the radius and the capitate. In dorsal perilunate dislocation, the longitudinal axis of the capitate is dorsal to those of the radius and the lunate because of the dorsal and proximal displacement of the capitate. The palmar tilt of the lunate, often associated with dorsal perilunate subluxation, must not be confused with palmar subluxation of the lunate.

Not infrequently, however, on lateral radiograph, the lunate may lie in a position transitionally between palmar lunate subluxation and dorsal perilunate subluxation.

Again, the lateral radiograph is the key to diagnosis and shows the normal relationship between the distal radius and the lunate (Figures 4-43A, 4-44A). The remainder of the carpus is dislocated proximally and dorsally to the lunate, and the capitate overrides the lunate. The longitudinal axis of the capitate is not in line with the longitudinal axis of the radius and is displaced dorsally. Palmar rotation of the scaphoid is often seen because of disruption of the scapholunate interosseous ligaments permitting rotational deformity of the scaphoid. The distal concave lunate articular surface usually occupied by the head of the capitate is vacant and looks like an "empty cup." The lunate is also often palmarly tilted at varying angles.

On the PA radiograph (Figures 4-43B, 4-44B) no joint can be seen between the lunate and the capitate, and a double density or bony superimposition is noted in this area, indicating overriding of the lunate by the capitate. The lunate does not have its normal quadrilateral appearance, and the scaphoid is foreshortened longitundinally. The scapholunate articulation is abnormal, and a wide diastasis is usually noted, as is a normal articulation between the distal radius and the lunate.

It should be remembered that a dorsal perilunate dislocation of the wrist may be produced during attempts to reduce a palmar lunate dislocation (discussed under Lunate Dislocation in this chapter). Reduction is achieved by techniques similar to those described for reduction of a dorsal transscaphoid perilunate fracture dislocation. Longitudinal traction is exerted on the hand with an assistant providing countertraction on the arm across the flexed elbow, followed by wrist extension with direct pressure exerted dorsally over the capitate and palmarly over the lunate. The wrist is then flexed, and reduction should be complete. Before plaster is applied, radiographic evaluation is extremely important. At this time a rotational deformity of the scaphoid with scapholunate dissociation may often be discovered since the

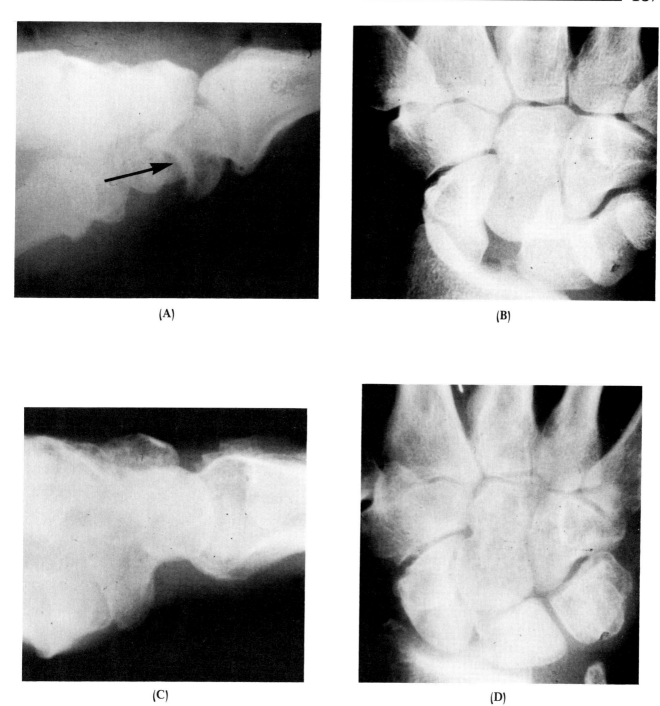

(A)

(B)

(C)

(D)

Figure 4-43 (A) Lateral radiograph shows dorsal perilunate dislocation of the wrist. There is normal relationship between distal radius and lunate, but distal lunate concave articular surface is vacant. Entire carpus is displaced dorsally and proximally in relation to lunate, which is palmarly angulated approximately 15°. Long axes of capitate and radius are not in the same plane. (B) PA view illustrates normal relationship of distal radius to lunate but abnormalities in lunate's relationship to scaphoid, capitate, and triquetrum. Scaphoid is shortened and does not articulate with distal radius. Wide diastasis between scaphoid and lunate. Following successful closed reduction of this type of injury it is mandatory to obtain radiographic reevaluation before plaster cast immobilization to assess accurately status of scapholunate joint (see text). (C) Lateral view 9 months after successful closed reduction and cast immobilization shows an essentially normal carpal configuration. (D) PA radiograph shows essentially normal carpal architecture with satisfactory scapholunate articulation.

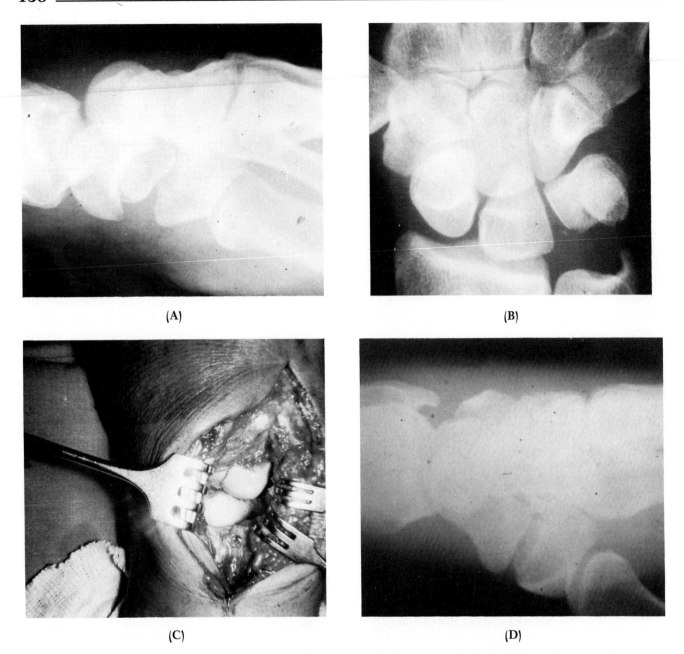

(A)

(B)

(C)

(D)

Figure 4-44 **(A)** Lateral radiograph shows dorsal perilunate dislocation of wrist and accentuates dorsal carpal dislocation with proximal displacement. **(B)** PA view shows shortening and cortical "ring" sign of scaphoid and abnormal articulations between lunate and scaphoid and capitate, with bony superimposition of capitate on lunate. **(C)** Lesion was irreducible by closed manipulation, and open reduction was necessary. Dorsal view of surgical exposure clearly shows dorsal position of capitate (superior to lunate) prior to reduction. **(D)** Lateral radiograph out of plaster 6 weeks after the original injury shows essentially normal carpal anatomy.

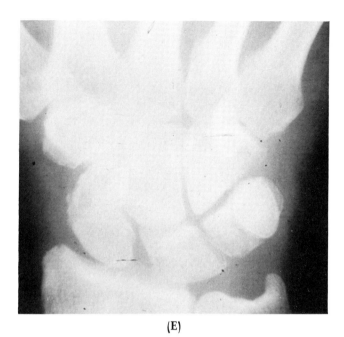

(E)

Figure 4-44 *(continued)*
(E) PA radiograph shows persistence of slight scapholunate diastasis and some scaphoid shortening indicating residual mild scapholunate dissociation. Wrist motion not impaired, and patient was asymptomatic. No further treatment indicated. *(Illustrations 4-44A–E courtesy of D.M. Junkin, M.D.)*

entire scapholunate articulation must be completely avulsed to permit dorsal dislocation of the scaphoid from the lunate. On occasions when closed reduction of a dorsal perilunate dislocation is impossible, open reduction from a dorsal approach (Figures 4-44A–E), usually with Kirschner wire immobilization, is necessary.

If scapholunate dissociation is not revealed, a long arm cast immobilization is provided with the elbow flexed 90° and the wrist flexed approximately 20°.

It is important to reevaluate the wrist radiographically at seven- to ten-day intervals for three to four weeks after the initial treatment since a scapholunate dissociation not present after initial reduction may become evident at a later date. This deformity must be discovered prior to two to three weeks posttrauma to enable reestablishment of the normal scapholunate anatomy without surgical intervention (Figures 4-62A,B). (Persistent scapholunate dissociation and/or rotational deformity of the scaphoid are discussed under Wrist and Carpal Instability in this chapter.)

If a residual scapholunate dissociation is noted and a closed reduction is unstable, percutaneous Kirschner wire fixation will be necessary to hold the scaphoid and the lunate properly reduced. If anatomic reduction is impossible by closed methods, open reduction from the palmar approach and primary ligamentous repair is advised.

If a residual scapholunate dissociation is discovered after three weeks posttrauma, closed reduction will usually be impossible and open reduction with ligamentous reconstruction and temporary Kirschner wire fixation will be necessary.

In the late unreduced perilunate dislocation open reduction may be achieved up to three to four months posttrauma. After this time reduction is usually impossible and the choice is either proximal row carpectomy, local intercarpal arthrodesis, or radiocarpal fusion (as previously discussed under dorsal transscaphoid perilunate fracture dislocation).

Physical and radiographic findings and treatment of the rare palmar perilunate dislocation are comparable to those of palmar transscaphoid perilunate fracture dislocation.

Lunate Dislocation

Lunate subluxation and dislocation is nearly always palmar (Figures 4-45A,B, 4-61A,B) and is caused by a hyperextension injury. Dorsal lunate dislocation is extremely rare and is caused by forced hyperflexion of the wrist.

Lunate displacement may be either complete dislocation or subluxation. In the former the lunate retains no articulation either with the radius or the carpus and may occasionally be found in the palmar aspect of the distal forearm. In the incomplete dislocation or subluxation the lunate still retains its articulation with the radius but not with the capitate, and is palmarly tilted. Palmar tilt of the lunate, often found in dorsal perilunate dislocation, must not be confused with anterior subluxation or dislocation of the lunate.

The mechanism of injury of palmar lunate dislocation is compared to the "squeezing out of a melon seed" by some authors. The hyperextension injury combines palmar distraction of the carpus with dorsal impaction, and the lunate is squeezed out palmarly by the remainder of the carpus as a result. Another opinion concerning the mechanism of injury is that the palmar dislocation of the lunate is the final result of what originally was a dorsal perilunate dislocation

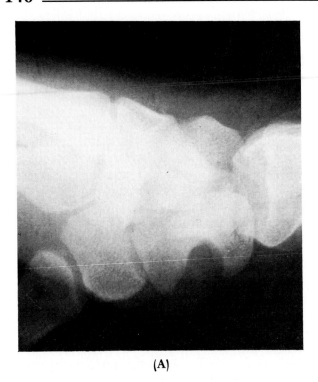

(A)

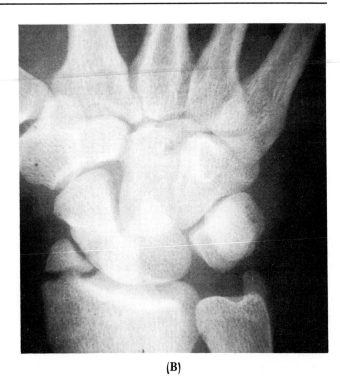

(B)

Figure 4-45 **(A)** Lateral radiograph illustrates anterior dislocation of lunate. Lunate is palmarly tilted approximately 60°, and longitudinal axis of capitate is in alignment with longitudinal axis of radius. **(B)** PA view clearly shows triangular or "pie shaped" configuration of lunate, characteristic of anterior dislocation of that bone; undisplaced fracture of scaphoid through middle third; and relatively undisplaced fracture of radial styloid process (chauffeur's fracture). Immobilization for 8 weeks after successful closed reduction provided normal carpal architecture, healing of scaphoid fracture, and healing of radial styloid fracture.

which proceeded to spontaneous relocation of the carpus, but in doing so, pushed the lunate anteriorly into subluxation or dislocation.

Actually, these injuries should be considered as interrelated segments of a spectrum of ligamentous damage ranging in severity from dynamic intercarpal instabilities with partial ligament tears through overt intercarpal instabilities (refer to section on carpal instabilities in this chapter) to complete dislocations (e.g., dorsal perilunate and palmar lunate dislocations).[13,14]

A very strong ligamentous attachment of the lunate to the distal radius by the radiolunate portion of the palmar radiocarpal ligament usually remains intact with palmar dislocation or subluxation of the lunate. Therefore, on the lateral radiograph 45° to 90° of anterior rotation of the subluxed lunate is usually seen. The lunate, however, may be rotated any extent up to 180° or may be completely displaced proximally from the carpus into the distal forearm. Usually the more severe rotation of complete displacement of the

lunate is due to complete avulsion of virtually all ligamentous restraints.

On examination of the recent injury the palmar displacement of the lunate often may be noted as a tender, palpable palmar prominence beneath the flexor tendons instead of the normal concavity in this region. The patient holds the fingers in flexion and any attempt to actively or passively extend or actively flex the digits is limited and painful, as is any attempt at wrist motion. If some time has passed since the injury, the palpable mass of the lunate may be obliterated by diffuse swelling on the palmar aspect of the wrist. Because of impingement of the displaced lunate on the median nerve there may be an acute carpal tunnel syndrome with hypesthesia and paresthesia in the median nerve distribution of the hand. Less commonly, an ulnar nerve compression syndrome may be noted.

The lateral radiograph (Figures 4-45A, 4-61A) is most important; it shows an essentially normal relationship between the distal radius and the entire carpus, except for the lunate which is anteriorly displaced. The lunate may be rotated from 45° to 180° or may be completely displaced proximally from the carpus. The vacant distal concave articular surface of the lunate resembles a cup which spills water palmarly. The key relation on the lateral radiograph is the longitudinal axis of the capitate directly in line with the longitudinal axis of the radius.

Anterior subluxation or incomplete dislocation of the lunate may be confused with a dorsal perilunate dislocation if attention is not paid to the details of the lateral radiograph (Figures 4-45A, 4-61A).

As mentioned above, not uncommonly on lateral radiograph, the lunate is in a transitional position making differentiation of a dorsal perilunate subluxation from a palmar lunate subluxation impossible.

The PA radiograph (Figures 4-45B, 4-61B) shows a triangular "pie shape" of the lunate rather than its normal quadrilateral configuration, due to its rotation. There is distortion of the scapholunate, the lunate-capitate, and the lunate-triquetral joints, with superimposition of the capitate and the triquetrum on the lunate.

Closed reduction under appropriate anesthesia may be successful up to one to two weeks after injury. Longitudinal traction on the hand with countertraction on the flexed elbow and extension of the wrist opens the space to receive the lunate. Direct pressure on the palmar aspect of the displaced lunate relocates the lunate into that space as the wrist is flexed. If the radiolunate portion of the palmar radiocarpal ligament remains attached to the proximal lip of the lunate, reduction is usually easily achieved using this ligament as a hinge. If reduction of the lunate is accomplished, the wrist remains flexed; if reduction has not been achieved, the wrist springs back into extension. As mentioned previously, during attempted reduction of a palmar lunate displacement a dorsal perilunate dislocation may be caused when the wrist is extended. Usually, however, after the lunate is properly seated, this dorsal perilunate dislocation can be adequately reduced.

If all ligamentous attachments are avulsed from the lunate, closed reduction may be more difficult or even impossible. Open reduction from the palmar approach is then necessary.

It is most important to evaluate the wrist radiographically after successful closed reduction to determine whether a rotatory deformity of the scaphoid and/or lunate, usually with a scapholunate dissociation, persists. If this finding is noted, the normal wrist

anatomy must be restored (treatment discussed in section Wrist and Carpal Instability in this chapter; Figure 4-61B).

If median nerve compression is present initially, early reduction of an anterior lunate dislocation or fracture dislocation usually relieves these symptoms rapidly. However, if reduction is some days following the trauma, surgical release of the transverse carpal ligament may be necessary to relieve persistent median nerve compression.

If satisfactory anatomic configuration of the wrist has been achieved after closed reduction, long arm cast immobilization for five to six weeks, with the wrist in slight palmar flexion, provides good treatment. However, at intervals of seven to ten days there should be radiographic reevaluation, since diastasis of the scapholunate joint may occur at a later date despite initial normal radiographs following closed reduction.

If closed reduction of a palmarly subluxed or dislocated lunate is unsuccessful, open reduction should be attempted up to six months posttrauma. Both palmar and dorsal approaches have been advocated, but the palmar approach permits median nerve decompression simultaneously with reduction of the lunate. Occasionally both palmar and dorsal incisions may be necessary.

Despite a bad reputation, actual avascular necrosis of the lunate is not common, although there is often a transient decrease in blood supply to that bone, noted radiographically by a relative sclerosis as compared to the surrounding carpal bones.

Reduction should usually not be attempted if treatment is instituted longer than six months posttrauma. Ideally, excision of the lunate with insertion of a silastic lunate implant is recommended if acceptable carpal anatomy can be restored. If implant insertion is not feasible, proximal migration of the capitate and distal carpal row into the space created is inevitable. If the proximal pole of the scaphoid is abnormal (e.g., concurrent aseptic necrosis, posttraumatic arthritis), proximal row carpectomy with silastic hinge implant arthroplasty should be considered.

An isolated palmar lunate-transscaphoid fracture dislocation is rare.[15] There is usually other associated skeletal trauma (Figures 4-46A,B). Early anatomic reduction and stable internal fixation, by as many Kirschner wires as necessary to restore stability, obtains the best results. In Figures 4-46A–D one wire proved to be insufficient.

Dorsal, radial, or ulnar (refer to Figures

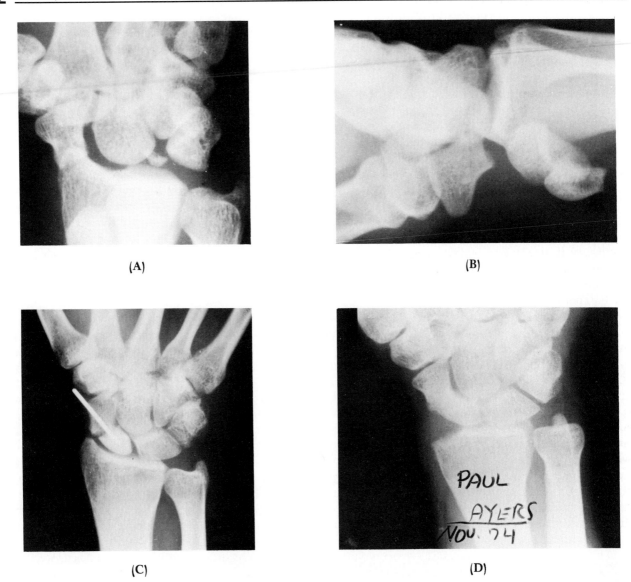

(A)

(B)

(C)

(D)

Figure 4-46 **(A)** On examination, wrist injured in motorcycle accident appeared swollen and showed signs of acute median nerve compression. PA view shows marked distortion of carpal architecture, with fracture of scaphoid at junction of proximal and middle thirds, proximal migration of capitate and distal portion of scaphoid, a small loose fracture fragment adjacent to ulnar aspect of capitate head, and complete displacement of lunate and proximal portion of scaphoid. "Pie shape" or triangular outline characteristic of anterior lunate dislocation is upside down, apex pointed proximally. **(B)** Lateral radiograph clearly shows complete anterior dislocation and proximal displacement of lunate with proximal portion of scaphoid. Severity of injury avulsed majority of soft tissue connections of lunate and proximal scaphoid fragment, which remained attached to radius by palmar capsule and palmar radiolunate ligament only. Distal concavity of lunate can be noted facing proximally due to 180° rotation. **(C)** PA radiograph 3 months after open reduction of dislocated lunate and displaced fracture of scaphoid with internal fixation by one Kirschner wire shows essentially normal carpal architecture, except for scaphoid. No avascular changes of the lunate, but some sclerosis of proximal scaphoid fragment can be seen, with nonunion and loss of position at fracture site. **(D)** PA radiograph 6 months later shows normal carpal architecture and complete healing of scaphoid fracture, with no evidence of avascular changes following an autogenous iliac bone graft to site of displaced nonunion of scaphoid. There is absence of radial styloid process, excised simultaneously due to its impingement on scaphoid. Wrist extension of 75° and flexion of 45° 18 months after injury enabled patient to return to full duty in U.S. Marine Corps. There is no indication for proximal row carpectomy as an initial procedure as this case demonstrates. Anatomic early reduction is the key to correct management. *(Illustrations 4-46A–D courtesy of S.F. Gunther, M.D.)*

3-27A–E in Chapter 3) dislocation of the lunate occurs only in massive wrist trauma.

Lunate Fractures

A dorsal avulsion fracture of the lunate resembles that of a similar avulsion type fracture of the triquetrum (Figure 4-75). Though a transverse undisplaced fracture of the lunate is rare, chip fractures are common. A palmar chip fracture may involve the proximal (Figure 4-47) or distal (Figure 4-48) articular lip, and it may be undisplaced (Figures 4-47, 4-48) or displaced (Figure 4-49). A small displaced articular fracture which does not result in joint instability and does not impinge on neurovascular structures (e.g., median nerve) does not have to be reduced surgically or excised (Figure 4-49).

The same characteristics and treatment apply to a dorsal chip fracture of the lunate (Figure 4-50).

Compression fracture of the lunate is probably the most common mechanism of injury and probably results from direct compression of that bone between the head of the capitate and the distal radial articular surface. Not infrequently an actual indentation or "step off" of the proximal articular surface can be seen where the distal radius caused an indented compression fracture (Figure 4-51). Special laminagraphic studies (polydirectional computerized tomography) may be particularly helpful in diagnosing fractures of the body of the lunate.

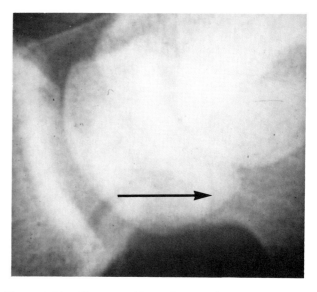

Figure 4-48 Close-up of lateral view shows comminuted palmarly displaced fracture of distal radius (Smith's fracture) associated with undisplaced fracture of palmar distal lip of lunate articular surface. *(Illustration courtesy of R.W. Godshall, M.D.)*

Avascular necrosis of the lunate (Kienböck's disease) (Figures 4-63A,B, 4-64A–D, 4-65A,B) may result following severe trauma to the lunate itself or its supporting structures. Though transient diminished blood supply to the lunate is not uncommon, actual necrosis of the bone is rather infrequent considering the total number of injuries involving this

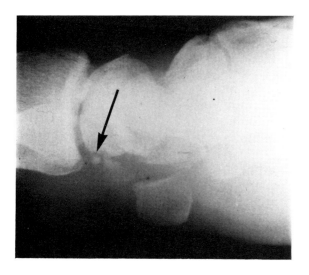

Figure 4-47 Lateral radiograph illustrates chip fracture on palmar aspect of proximal lip of lunate at its articulation with radius sustained 3 weeks previously.

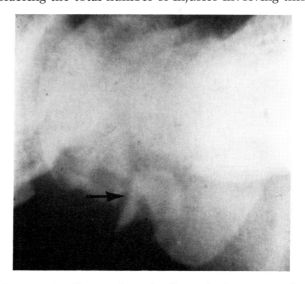

Figure 4-49 Close-up lateral radiograph shows rotated displaced palmar lip fracture of distal lunate articular surface. Patient sustained undisplaced fractures of scaphoid and distal radius. Immobilization for 8 weeks resulted in normal wrist function. No additional treatment necessary.

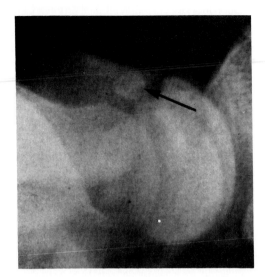

Figure 4-50 Close-up lateral radiograph shows minimally displaced fracture of dorsal lip of lunate distal articular surface. Immobilization for 5 weeks resulted in normal wrist function. *(Illustration courtesy of D.M. Junkin, M.D.)*

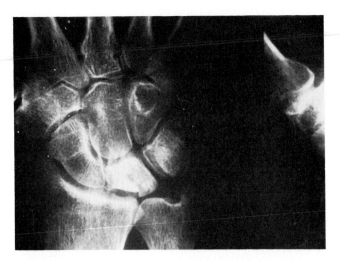

Figure 4-51 PA view of wrist shows flattening and sclerosis of lunate following severe longitudinal crush injury to carpus. There is flattening of proximal lunate articular surface caused by compression from direct contact with contiguous surface of distal radius at time of injury. Step-off appearance of proximal lunate articular surface is due to compression fracture, and sclerosis of lunate is secondary to avascular changes. *(Illustration courtesy of A.M. Larimer, M.D.)*

area of the wrist. Actual avascular necrosis of the lunate occurs following lunate fracture and also after severe soft tissue injury involving ligament and capsular avulsions. If marked flattening of the lunate and painful limited wrist motion result from severe avascular necrosis, excision of the lunate with insertion of a silastic implant is acceptable to restore the normal carpal architecture (Figures 4-64A–D). For this procedure to be successful the remaining intercarpal articulations and the distal radial articular surface should be essentially normal, with minimal, if any, posttraumatic or degenerative arthritic changes. Rotational instability of the scaphoid is frequently a sequela of this procedure because of the necessary sacrifice of the scapholunate interosseous ligaments (Figures 4-64C,D).

If the adjacent proximal pole of the scaphoid is also involved with aseptic necrosis and flattening, proximal row carpectomy combined with insertion of a silastic hinge implant should be considered if symptoms warrant.

Carpal and Wrist Instabilities

Carpal Instabilities[16,17,18]

Skeletal stability of the wrist area (e.g., wrist joint and carpus) is provided by the distal radius and the distal carpal row. The distal radial articular surface composed of the scaphoid and lunate fossae provides a stable fulcrum for wrist joint motion. The distal carpal row with the index and long metacarpals is anatomically and functionally a single stable osseoligamentous unit—the stable portion of the hand.

Ligamentous stability depends primarily on the integrity of the palmar radiocarpal ligament and the ulnocarpal ligament complex with their various components. (For details of anatomy, refer to Chapter 1 and Figure 1-6.) Motion of both the wrist joint and the midcarpal joint is focused on the proximal carpal row, primarily the scaphoid and lunate, the intercalated segment between the radius and the distal carpal row.

Proximally, the scaphoid and lunate articulate with the radius—the wrist joint. Distally the scaphoid, lunate, and to a lesser extent the triquetrum create the "socket" for the central point of intercarpal motion, the capitate head, which combined with the small proximal articular pole of the hamate forms the "ball" of the midcarpal ball-and-socket joint. (Refer to Figures 1-3 and 1-4 of Chapter 1.) The majority of carpal instability therefore, involves the intercalated segment—the proximal carpal row, primarily the scaphoid and lunate.

Any significant (and sometimes a seemingly insignificant) fracture, dislocation, subluxation or ligament avulsion (or fracture variant) can result in carpal instability if normal architecture is not restored early enough and maintained long enough for appropriate skeletal and ligamentous healing.

Carpal instability may:

1. occur as either a completely separate entity or in combination with other pathology,
2. be acute or chronic, and
3. be overt or dynamic.

Acute carpal instability most often occurs either as a separate condition or as the sequela of a dorsal perilunate dislocation, palmar lunate dislocation, a displaced or angulated scaphoid fracture, segmental articular fracture of the distal radius (particularly the radial variant—chauffeur's fracture), and after insertion of a lunate or scaphoid silastic implant. Less commonly, it occurs after dorsal or palmar trans-scaphoid perilunate fracture dislocation, scapho-capitate syndrome, displaced triquetral fracture with carpal distortion, or other types of segmental articular fractures of the distal radius.

Chronic instability, though often the result of the ravages of arthritis, particularly rheumatoid arthritis, occurs also in any of the above mentioned skeletal or ligamentous injuries which remain chronically unreduced. The chronic situation also may occur after malunion of a distal radial fracture which is either metaphyseal or segmental articular.

Carpal instability may be either overt or dynamic. Overt infers that the pathology is significant enough in most cases to permit accurate diagnosis by correlation of physical and routine radiographic findings.

The dynamic lesion, a partial ligament avulsion or tear or chronic attenuation is usually occult and is the prodromal stage of an overt instability.

Recognized types of carpal instability include:

1. Scaphoid rotational instability
2. Lunate rotational instability
   A. Dorsal intercalary segment instability (DISI)
   B. Palmar intercalary segment instability (PISI)
3. Scapholunate dissociation
4. Lunate-triquetral instability
5. Triquetral-hamate instability

Carpal instabilities should be considered a spectrum of injuries ranging from partial ligament tears (dynamic lesions) to complete ligament tears with joint diastasis and rotational instabilities (overt lesions). Each individual instability is usually an interrelated segment of a complex intercarpal liga-

ment disruption pattern. The most common is scaphoid rotational instability plus lunate rotational instability (DISI and less frequently PISI) plus scapho-lunate diastasis. *However, each instability may present as a separate distinct entity by itself, particularly the dynamic types.* The terms, therefore, are not "essentially synonymous."[20] The following discussion hopefully will clarify this interesting pathology.

Diagnosis

The patient's history, though negative in some cases, often is a fall on, blow to, or torsional strain of the wrist and hand and the mechanism of injury is usually hyperextension. Symptoms include variable pain and frequently a definite "pop" or "click" noted at the time of injury. Symptoms persist with generalized swelling correlating with tenderness on palpation of specific locations of the proximal carpal row. Sometimes a soft tissue mass is evident which is either a true ganglion or synovitis of either the wrist or intercarpal joints. All ranges of wrist (wrist joint and midcarpal joint) motion are limited and painful, particularly flexion and extension and grasp is painful and weak. Click can often be reproduced and may be associated with voluntary subluxation of either the lunate or scaphoid.

The key to diagnosis of the overt lesion rests with appropriate radiographs accurately interpreted. The views recommended include an AP of the wrist (hand supinated or palm up) in neutral, maximum radial deviation, maximum ulnar deviation and a clenched fist view. Lateral views in neutral, maximum flexion and maximum extension and two oblique views complete the series.

On a normal lateral radiograph in neutral position, as mentioned in the section on anatomy in Chapter 1, there is a longitudinal alignment of the long axes of the radius, lunate, capitate and long finger metacarpal (Figure 4-52). The capitolunate angle should be 0 and is estimated by determining the relation of the longitudinal axis of the lunate to the longitudinal axis of the capitate (Figure 4-52).

The radiolunate angle is determined by comparing the longitudinal axis of the radius to that of the lunate and also should be 0 (Figure 4-52). The scapholunate angle is that made by comparing the longitudinal axis of the scaphoid to that of the lunate with the normal range of 30° to 60° and an average of 47° (Figure 4-52).

The lunate triquetral angle is the angle formed between the longitudinal axis of the lunate and the

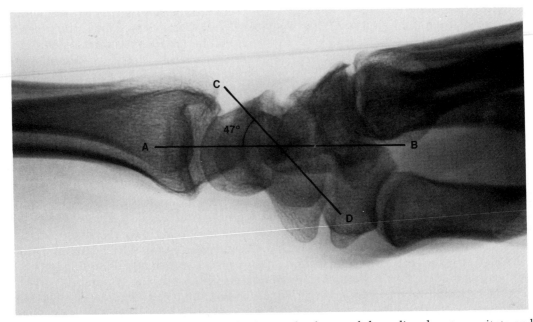

Figure 4-52 In the normal wrist, the alignment of the longitudinal axes of the radius, lunate, capitate and long finger metacarpal should coincide on the same horizontal line A–B. The capitolunate and radiolunate angles should be 0. The longitudinal axis of the scaphoid C–D should intersect the longitudinal axis of the lunate A–B at an average angle of 47° with a range of 30–60°.

longitudinal axis of the triquetrum which ranges from +31° to −3° and averages +14°. (Refer to Figure 4-59.)

Scaphoid Rotational Instability.[18] The scaphoid functions as the stabilizing skeletal connecting link between the proximal and distal carpal rows. It is bound firmly to the lunate by scapholunate interosseous ligaments and the radioscapholunate ligament, enabling the proximal scaphoid and the lunate to move synchronously.

Without the stability of the scapholunate articulation and normal anatomic configuration of the scaphoid bone itself (e.g., unstable angulated or displaced scaphoid fracture) the proximal carpal row acts as an unsupported, unrestricted middle link in a three link system of the radius, the proximal carpal row and the distal carpal row. This instability causes a zig-zag or accordian-like deformity with carpal collapse from axial compression.

Rotational instability of the scaphoid occurs only anteriorly with abnormal increase of the normal palmar tilt of the scaphoid which occasionally progresses until the scaphoid's longitudinal axis becomes parallel to the distal radial articular surface and perpendicular to the longitudinal axes of the radius and capitate.

Scaphoid rotational instability is usually accompanied by lunate rotational instability and scapholunate dissociation. Dorsal subluxation of the proximal pole of the scaphoid also may be present. Clinically, the scaphoid and scapholunate joint are tender to palpation and a dorsal subluxation of the proximal pole of the scaphoid may be either spontaneous or volitional.

The lateral radiograph shows increased angulation of the scaphoid and if the lunate does not show a palmar rotational instability, the scapholunate angle should be greater than 60° with a definite diagnosis of an angle greater than 80° (Figure 4-53A).

Taleisnik's V sign made by the intersection of the palmar outline of the scaphoid with the palmar margin of the radius creates a sharp V-shaped pattern (Figure 4-53A).

The PA radiograph in supination shows a truncated or shortened scaphoid with a cortical "ring" shadow representing overlap of the distal pole on the isthmus or proximal pole. Signs of scapholunate diastasis and lunate rotational instability also are often noted (Figure 4-53B). Dorsal or palmar lunate rotational instability is usually associated. However, scaphoid rotational instability may occur as an isolated entity without any lunate rotational instability or scapholunate diastasis. This is particularly true in the dynamic type of instability.

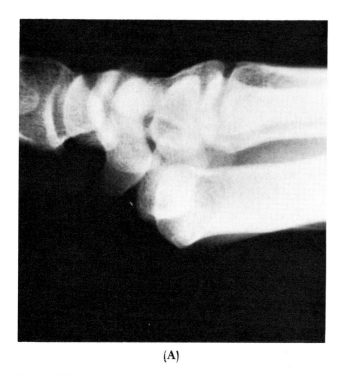

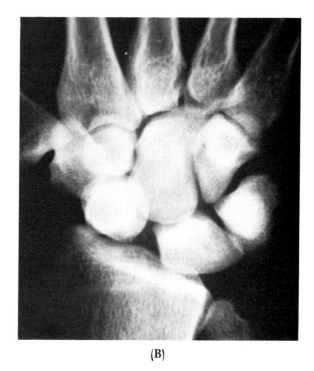

(A)   (B)

Figure 4-53 (A) Lateral view shows long axis of scaphoid perpendicular to longitudinal axes of capitate and lunate and parallel to distal radial articular surface. There is no associated lunate rotational instability. (B) PA view of rotational instability of scaphoid with scapholunate dissociation. Scaphoid is abnormally short, with cortical "ring" sign and there is abnormal space between scaphoid and lunate.

Lunate Rotational Instability. Ligaments on all borders of the lunate may be torn depending upon the severity of injury. Circumferentially these ligaments include: the scapholunate interosseous ligaments, the radioscapholunate ligament, the ulnolunate ligament portion of the ulnocarpal ligament complex, the lunate triquetral ligament and finally rupture of the radiolunate portion of the dorsal radiocarpal ligament (necessary for complete palmar lunate dislocation). (Refer to Figure 1-6 in Chapter 1.)

Lunate rotational instability may be either dorsal (DISI) or palmar (PISI) depending upon whether the point of impingement of the head of the capitate on axial load is either palmar to or dorsal to the lunate flexion-extension axis.

Scaphoid rotational instability and scapholunate diastasis are usually associated. Tenderness is noted on palpation of the scaphoid and lunate but is most pronounced at the scapholunate joint.

Dorsal intercalary segment instability (DISI) (Figure 4-54) — Dorsal rotational instability of the lunate is by far the more common and signifies that the distal concave lunate surface faces dorsally. The lateral radiograph demonstrates this angulation

which may be associated with a palmar subluxation of the lunate. The scapholunate angle is greater than 60° and both radiolunate and capitolunate angles should be greater than 15° (Figures 4-55, 4-56).

The AP view shows a notable elongation of the palmar lip of the lunate in a truncated "pie shape" instead of the normal quadrilateral shape (Figures 4-55A, 4-56A). Scaphoid rotational instability and scapholunate diastasis are almost always associated.

Palmar intercalary segment instability (PISI) (Figure 4-57) — Palmar rotational instability of the lunate (PISI) is much less common and is thought by some to be the result of a congenital ligamentous laxity in many cases. It may be associated with scaphoid rotational instability and scapholunate diastasis. However, it may also be associated with lunate-triquetral dissociation.

In addition to tenderness on palpation of the lunate, scaphoid, and scapholunate joint, dorsal subluxation of the lunate either spontaneous or volitional may be found.

The lateral radiograph shows palmar angulation of the distal lunate articular surface and in this instance the scapholunate angle may not be abnor-

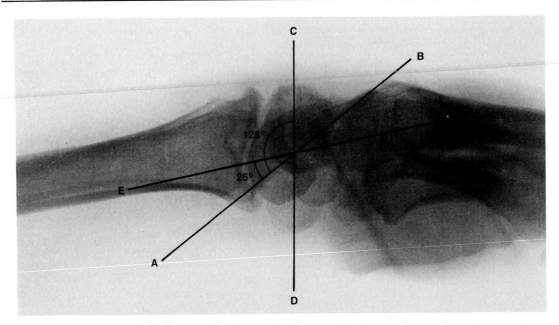

Figure 4-54 DISI instability of the lunate. The longitudinal axis of the lunate A–B is dorsally rotated. Longitudinal axis of the scaphoid C–D is palmarly rotated. The longitudinal axes of the radius and the capitate E–F coincide. The scapholunate angle is 180° in this case and the capitolunate and radiolunate angles are 25°.

mal since both the scaphoid and the lunate are abnormally palmarly rotated with associated scaphoid rotational instability (Figure 4-58). Radiolunate and capitolunate angles are usually greater than 15°.

Scapholunate Dissociation. The AP radiograph shows a widening of the scapholunate articulation (Figures 4-53B, 4-55A) which is emphasized by ulnar deviation (Figure 4-56C). A space greater than 2 mm is usually diagnostic but with any question, radiographs of the contralateral wrist should be taken in similar positions for comparison.

A marked diastasis of the scapholunate articulation has been nicknamed the "Terry Thomas" or the "Leon Spinks" sign (Figures 4-62B, 4-67A); often associated are scaphoid and lunate rotational instabilities.

Lunate—Triquetral Instability.[21] Symptoms of pain are centered on the ulnar aspect of the wrist. Tenderness is elicited on palpation of the lunate triquetral joint and a positive ballottement test is present in the overt lesion with complete tear or marked attenuation of the lunate-triquetral interosseous ligament. This test is performed by immobilizing the lunate between the thumb and index finger of one

hand while the triquetrum and pisiform are displaced dorsally and palmarly on the fixed lunate.

Radiographs of the overt lunate-triquetral dissociation are helpful. The normal angle made by intersecting the longitudinal axes of the lunate and triquetrum is +14° with a range of +31° to −3° on the lateral radiograph and the axis of the triquetrum is normally angled palmarly in relation to that of the lunate (Figure 4-59A).

In lunate-triquetral dissociation the average lunate triquetral angle is −16° with an average of −3° to −50° (Figure 4-59B). The AP radiograph usually shows a normal lunate-triquetral relationship in neutral and in radial deviation. In ulnar deviation (Figure 4-60), however, the lunate does not fully translate radially in the lunate fossa of the radius and the normal convex arc of the proximal carpal row is flattened and irregular because of disruption between the lunate and triquetrum. The triquetrum usually displaces proximally to the lunate and may overlap it (Figure 4-60). The lunate has a "truncated pie" configuration if a PISI deformity is associated, as often occurs.

Triquetral—Hamate Instability. This lesion may conceivably be a separate entity caused by injury to the ulnar aspect of the carpus.[22] However, the overt

Figure 4-55 (A) PA radiograph of wrist shows abnormal space between proximal scaphoid and lunate, with shortening of scaphoid. (B) Lateral view shows dorsal rotation of lunate and exaggerated palmar angulation of scaphoid, with dorsal protrusion and subluxation of proximal pole of scaphoid at wrist joint. Case represents dorsal rotational instability of wrist with scapholunate dissociation and dorsal subluxation of proximal pole of scaphoid following a severe wrist hyperextension injury. (C) Oblique view accentuates dorsal subluxation of proximal pole of scaphoid and diastasis of scapholunate joint. *(Illustrations 4-55A–C courtesy of F.N. DeLuca, M.D.)*

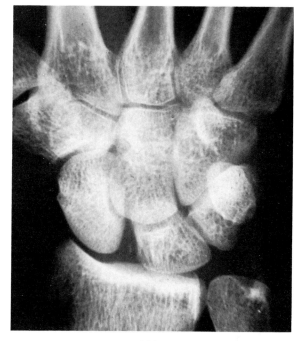

(A)

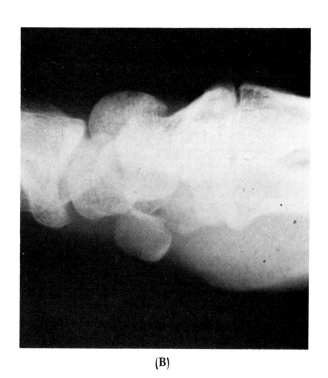

(B)

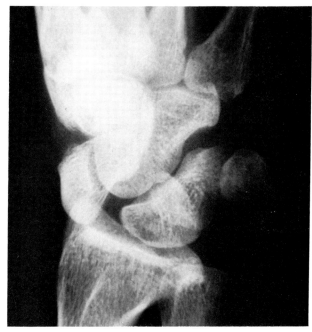

(C)

Figure 4-56 (A) PA radiograph of wrist which sustained a moderate hyperextension injury illustrates some diastasis of scapholunate articulation and some shortening of scaphoid. (B) Lateral radiograph shows a dorsal rotation of lunate. (C) AP radiograph in ulnar deviation accentuates scapholunate dissociation. Diagnosis: dorsal rotational instability with scapholunate dissociation of moderate degree. Patient declined any reconstruction of scapholunate articulation.

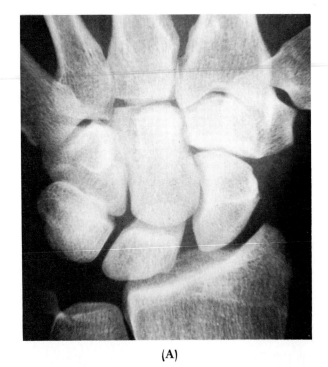

(A)

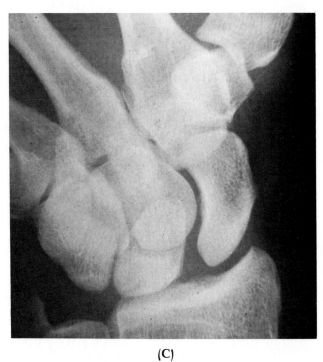

(B)

(C)

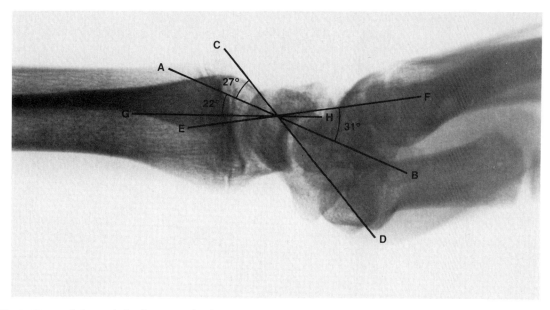

Figure 4-57 PISI instability of the lunate. The longitudinal axis of the lunate A–B is palmarly rotated. The axis of the scaphoid C–D is somewhat palmarly rotated. The axis of the capitate is slightly dorsally rotated E–F. The scapholunate angle is 27°, the radiolunate angle is 22° and the capitolunate angle is 31°.

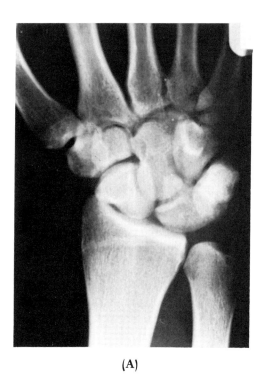

(A)

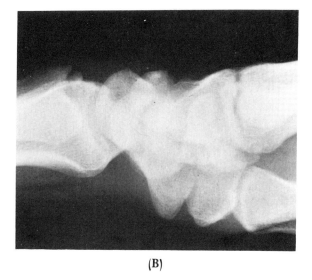

(B)

Figure 4-58 (A) PA view of wrist 6 weeks after a severe hyperextension injury. Abnormal space is seen between scaphoid and lunate; marked shortening of scaphoid with cortical "ring" sign is evident. (B) Lateral radiograph illustrates palmar rotational instability of wrist with palmar tilt of lunate and exaggerated palmar angulation of scaphoid. Diagnosis: palmar rotational instability of wrist with scapholunate dissociation. Physical examination disclosed a mild dorsal prominence in area of wrist and some "step off" or palmar displacement of metacarpus.

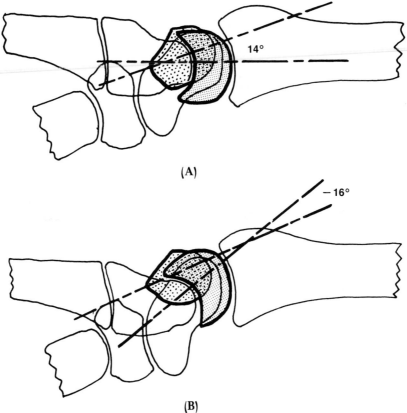

(A)

(B)

Figure 4-59 **(A)** Normal alignment of carpus, lateral view. LT angle averages +14°. **(B)** LT dissociation with average LT angle −16° *(Courtesy of R.L. Linscheid, M.D.)*[19]

lesion is most often found associated with proximal migration of the distal carpal row following significant lunate or scaphoid pathology (e.g., excision, traumatic loss (Figures 4-29A, 4-30A), or marked flattening) or marked diastasis of the scapholunate joint.

Dynamic Lesions. A dynamic carpal instability may occur as a prodromal lesion of any of the overt instabilities just discussed. Clinical findings may be minimal (e.g., wrist click and variable tenderness) and routine radiographs are essentially normal.

Diagnosis may depend on a reasonable suspicion verified by ancillary radiographic studies (e.g., fluoroscopy with stress evaluation, tomograms, and arthrograms which may show dye abnormally squirting through a partial ligament tear).

Treatment.

General theories — The specific treatment depends upon the time interval from the injury to the diagnosis. Since early diagnosis is of paramount im-

portance, one must be constantly aware of the very real possibility of a carpal instability pattern persisting after reduction of a dorsal perilunate dislocation or palmar lunate dislocation (Figure 4-61). Instability also commonly occurs with a displaced or angulated scaphoid fracture (whether a solitary lesion or part of a dorsal transscaphoid perilunate fracture/dislocation), a radial segmental articular fracture of the distal radius (chauffeur's fracture) (Figure 4-62) following malunion of any distal metaphyseal or segmental articular fracture of the distal radius[23] and with marked flattening (e.g., avascular necrosis) traumatic loss or surgical excision of the scaphoid or lunate (with or without silastic implant replacement) (Figures 4-63, 4-64, 4-65).

There are three time intervals which determine appropriate treatment:

1. Within the first three to four weeks after injury,
2. Eight–ten weeks or more after injury, and
3. Between four and 10 weeks after injury.

Within the first three to four weeks after injury, if stable closed anatomic reduction is possible, im-

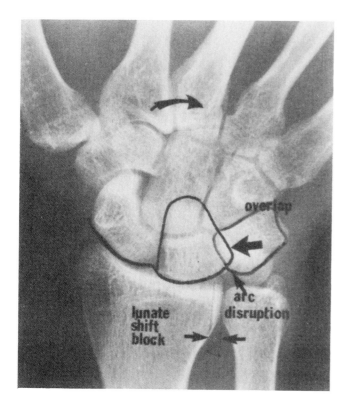

overlap

lunate
shift
block

arc
disruption

Figure 4-60 LT dissociation. In ulnar deviation the lunate is blocked and fails to fully translate radially in the lunate fossa of the radius. There is irregularity in the proximal convex arc and the lunate and triquetral image is overlapped with a "truncated pie" configuration of the lunate indicating a PISI lunate instability pattern. *(Courtesy of R.L. Linscheid, M.D.)*[19]

mobilization should continue for a minimum of six and preferably eight weeks, closely monitored by interval radiographs at seven to 10 day intervals.

If closed reduction is possible but unstable, percutaneous Kirschner wire fixations of the reduced carpals to each other and to adjacent stable carpals is indicated. If anatomic reduction is impossible, then open reduction and ligament repairs from the palmar approach or from both palmar and dorsal approaches are indicated.

Eight weeks or more after injury, generally indicates segmental carpal arthrodesis. Ligament reconstructions have been popular in the past and some still recommend attempting soft tissue reconstruction. However, generally the soft tissue procedures do not hold up in the long run and limited segmental arthrodesis becomes necessary later.[24]

Treatment in the time interval between three and eight weeks after injury is very controversial.

Many would recommend reduction and ligament repair or possibly ligament reconstruction using tendon grafts or transfer and others believe the die has been cast and the definitive procedure of limited carpal arthrodesis is indicated even at this early time. The answer to this problem is not definite and the surgeon should make his choice in each individual case according to age, occupation, patient's desire, etc.

Specific instability patterns — The DISI and PISI lunate rotational instabilities are usually accompanied by scaphoid rotational instability and scapholunate joint diastasis. Therefore, attention must be paid to restoring normal anatomy to each entity as soon as possible (Figure 4-66).

If normal anatomy can be restored by closed manipulation and reduction within the first three or four weeks after injury and percutaneous Kirschner wires are necessary to retain that reduction, the scaphoid should be pinned to the lunate and both pinned to the capitate (Figure 4-67).

Carpal instability caused by pathology of the distal radius necessitates restoration of distal radial anatomy to as near normal as possible before malunion (Figure 4-68).

For treatment eight to 10 weeks after injury, the author recommends one of two procedures:

1. Arthrodesis of the scaphoid, lunate and capitate, or
2. The "tri-schaphe" arthrodesis.[25–27]

Ideally, if the scaphoid and lunate could be arthrodesed at the scapholunate joint this would be most preferable.

Technically, however, this is very difficult though the Herbert screw or some modification may be the answer in the future. The success of arthrodesis of the scaphoid to the lunate and both to the capitate is virtually guaranteed resulting in a painless stable carpus with approximately 50% normal motion.

The tri-scaphe arthrodesis attacks the problem by reducing and holding the scaphoid proximal pole reduced by fusion of the scaphoid distal pole to the trapezium and trapezoid. Though this procedure is popular currently, it has not been performed for a sufficient period of time to evaluate long-term results.

Technically, each procedure is performed through dorsal approach. The scaphoid can be controlled for accurate reduction by driving a temporary Kirschner wire through the isthmus from dorsal to palmar direction which is used as a handle. An

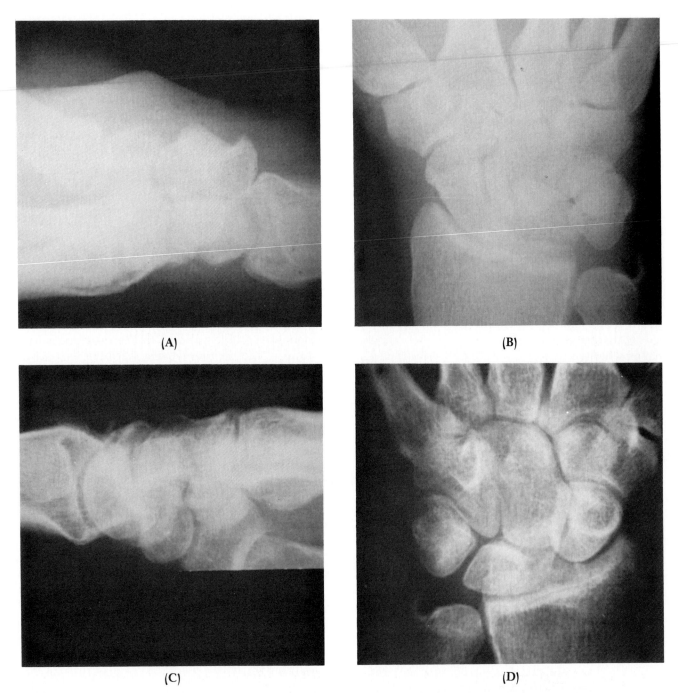

(A)

(B)

(C)

(D)

Figure 4-61 (A) Lateral radiograph of palmar dislocation of the lunate. The lunate is clearly seen palmar to the remainder of the carpus and the distal radius with its distal concave articular surface rotated 90° palmarly and the remainder of the carpus in direct line with the distal radial articular surface. (B) Corresponding PA radiograph illustrates the triangular or "pie-shaped" configuration of the lunate characteristic of this lesion and all borders of the lunate are indistinct with overlapping and no discernible normal joints. (C) Lateral radiograph made eight months after successful closed reduction of the lunate dislocation shows a DISI rotational instability of the lunate with rotational instability of the scaphoid. (D) Corresponding PA view shows an abnormally short scaphoid with the cortical "ring" sign, scapholunate diastasis, and a truncated "pie" shape of the lunate. This case illustrates the importance of early diagnosis of carpal instability to re-establish and maintain normal carpal anatomy after a successful closed reduction of a palmar lunate dislocation. *(Figures 4-61A–D courtesy of James G.T. Boyes, M.D.)*

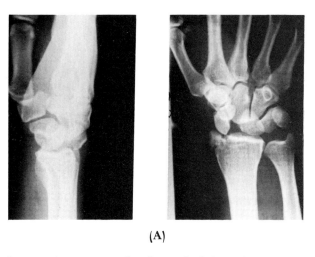
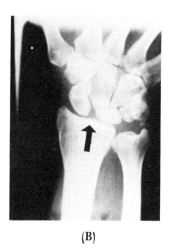

(A)   (B)

Figure 4-62 **(A)** Lateral radiograph, left, and PA view, right, show dorsal perilunate dislocation associated with somewhat proximally displaced chauffeur's fracture of distal radius (see section on dorsal perilunate disloca-tions). **(B)** Persistent deformities are seen 7 months postreduction and after unsuccessful open reduction and percutaneous Kirschner wire fixation of scapholunate dissociation and rotational instability of scaphoid. Severe rotational instability of scaphoid noted with marked palmar angulation, diastasis of scapholunate articulation and shortening of scaphoid. It is important to recognize rotational instability of wrist following initial reduction of dorsal perilunate dislocation. Chronic disability is prevented only by restoring normal carpal anatomy. *(Reprinted, by permission, from J.G.T. Boyes, Jr., M.D. Subluxation of the carpal navicular bone, S Med J 69:141–44, 1976.)*

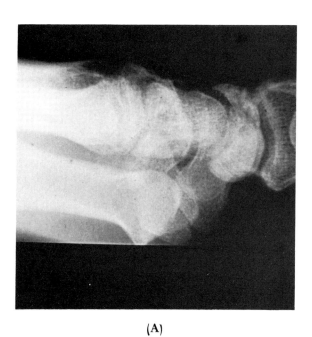
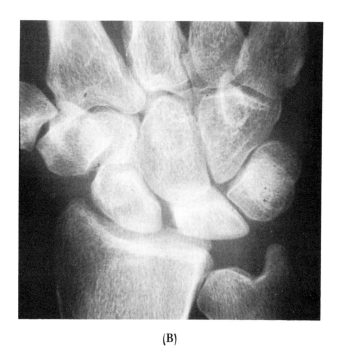

(A)   (B)

Figure 4-63 **(A)** Lateral radiograph of wrist which sustained a severe extension injury 8 months before shows increased palmar angulation of scaphoid and thinning and sclerosis of lunate, with minimal dorsal angulation. **(B)** PA radiograph shows definite thinning of lunate with avascular changes and shortening of scaphoid with diastasis of scapholunate articulation. Scapholunate dissociation is probably subsequent to abnormal wrist ar-chitecture following avascular necrotic changes and thinning of lunate. Original injury may have been palmar dislocation of lunate which reduced itself spontaneously.

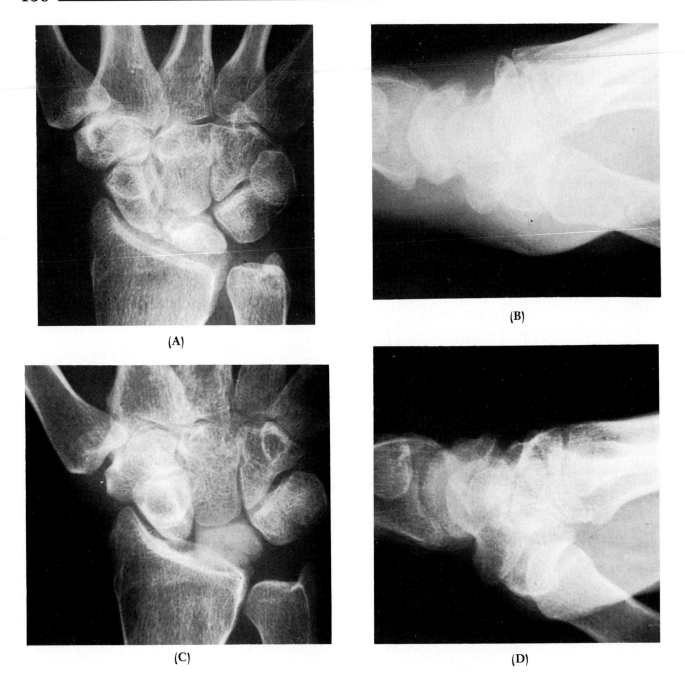

(A)

(B)

(C)

(D)

Figure 4-64 (A) PA view shows characteristic findings of aseptic necrosis of lunate with degenerative changes, including sclerosis and flattening, particularly on its radial aspect. Scapholunate joint is incongruous, and there is some shortening in length of scaphoid. Radioscaphoid and radiolunate joints also appear somewhat incongruous. No traumatic etiology was determined. (B) Lateral radiograph shows some distortion of lunate, particularly on its dorsal aspect, and rotational instability of scaphoid with increase of its palmar tilt. (C) PA view 6 months after insertion of silastic lunate implant shows good general position of carpus and its components, with a good joint space between distal radius and scaphoid and lunate. There is no abnormal space between scaphoid and silastic lunate implant, but scaphoid is foreshortened and cortical "ring" sign is evident. (D) Lateral radiograph shows good configuration of lunate silastic implant which is in good position and shows no rotational deformity. Scaphoid continues to show a palmar tilt and some continued rotational instability. Patient was completely asymptomatic and remained so at follow-up examination 5 years after surgery.

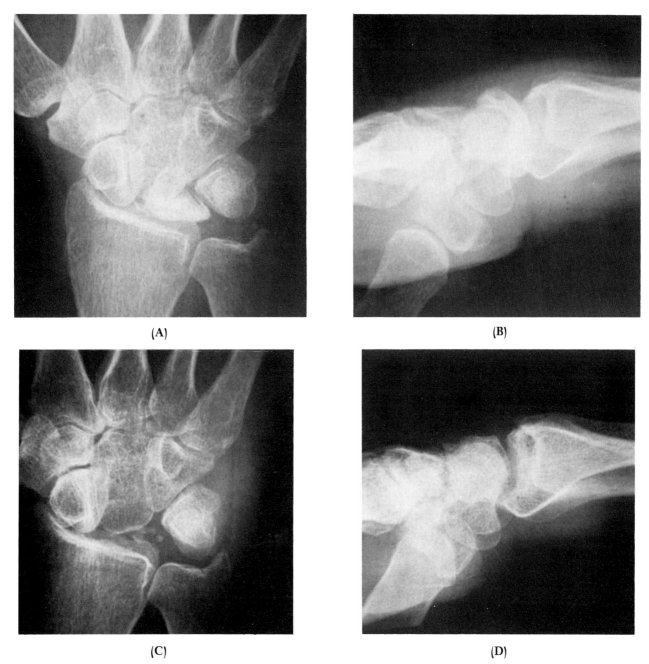

(A) (B)

(C) (D)

Figure 4-65 (A) PA view shows severe avascular necrosis of the lunate (Kienböck's disease) with irregularity and fragmentation, an abnormally short scaphoid with a cortical "ring" sign evident, and proximal migration of the entire distal carpal row, bringing the capitate head close to the distal radius. (B) Corresponding lateral view shows extreme flattening and spreading of the lunate with avascular changes and severe rotational instability of the scaphoid, which lies almost parallel to the distal radial articular surface. (C) This PA radiograph was made eight months after excision of the lunate and shows even more distortion of carpal anatomy. The scaphoid is seen on end with a prominent cortical "ring" sign, the capitate head is somewhat irregular and articulates with the distal radius, and the hamate-triquetral joint is somewhat irregular. (D) Corresponding lateral view shows complete rotational instability of the scaphoid which parallels the distal radial articular surface and an irregular joint between the distal radius and the capitate. Solitary excision of the lunate is contraindicated to treat aseptic necrosis of the lunate (Kienböck's disease). Consequently, the distal carpal row migrates proximally, eventually articulating the capitate head with the distal radius and severe scaphoid rotational instability occurs. *(Figures 4-65A–D courtesy of James G.T. Boyes, M.D.)*

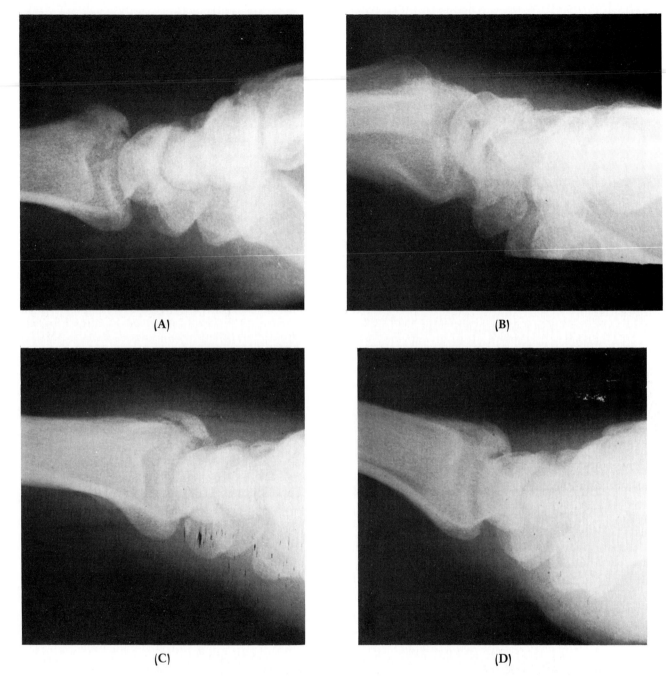

(A)

(B)

(C)

(D)

Figure 4-66 **(A)** Lateral radiograph of right wrist of patient who sustained bilateral wrist injuries shows normal configuration of carpus but flattening of distal radial articular surface, with loss of its palmar angulation and an essentially undisplaced dorsal segmental radial articular fracture (dorsal Barton's fracture). **(B)** Ten weeks later lateral view shows distinct palmar angulation of lunate and increase in palmar angulation of scaphoid. Some dorsal subluxation of lunate may be noted. **(C)** Initial lateral radiograph of left wrist which sustained an identical injury shows normal carpal architecture and a relatively undisplaced dorsal segmental articular fracture of distal radius (dorsal Barton's fracture). **(D)** Lateral view of left wrist 10 weeks after injury shows normal carpal architecture and good healing of dorsal articular fracture of distal radius. Case illustrates bilateral, apparently symmetrical wrist injuries of relatively undisplaced segmental articular fractures of dorsal distal radius (dorsal Barton's fractures). Right wrist developed palmar rotational instability with scapholunate dissociation. Minimal pain and somewhat diminished wrist motion did not warrant wrist arthroplasty or arthrodesis. Left wrist healed without complications. *(Illustrations 4-66A–D courtesy of R.W. Godshall, M.D.)*

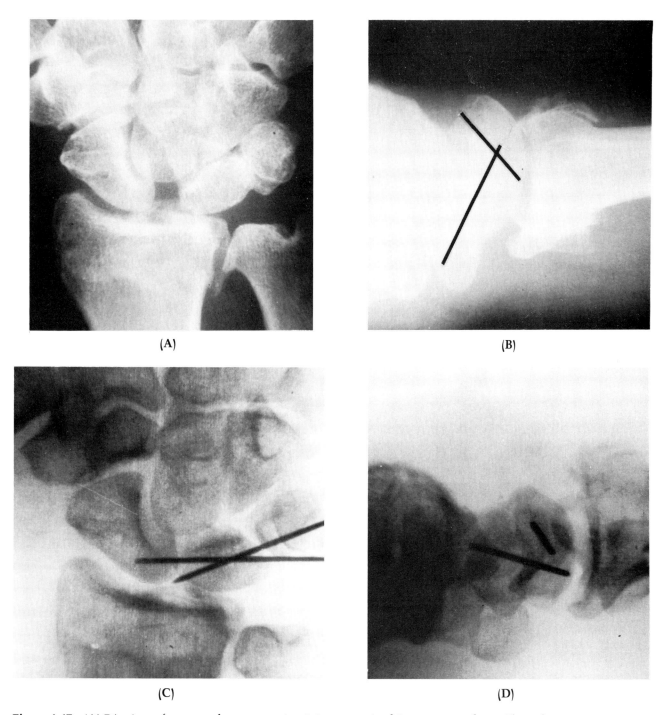

(A)

(B)

(C)

(D)

Figure 4-67 (A) PA view of a severe hyperextension injury sustained in a motorcycle accident shows comminuted fracture of distal radial articular surface, diastasis of scapholunate articulation, and some scaphoid shortening. (B) Lateral radiograph shows gross comminution of distal radial articular surface with dorsal subluxation and palmar angulation of lunate. Palmar angulation of scaphoid is accentuated. Case illustrates combination of comminuted distal radial articular fracture associated with scapholunate dissociation and dorsal subluxation of lunate. (C) PA radiograph following closed reduction and percutaneous pins-and-plaster treatment for fractured radius, with temporary Kirschner wire immobilization of scapholunate articulation following correction of scapholunate diastasis. (D) Lateral radiograph illustrates good correction of comminuted distal radial articular fracture and correction of palmar lunate and scaphoid angulations.

(continued)

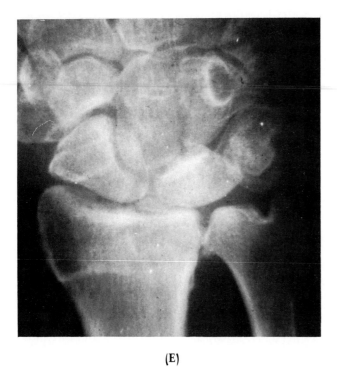

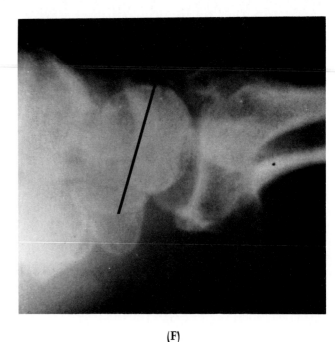

(E)   (F)

Figure 4-67 *(continued)*
(E) PA radiograph 6 months after injury shows some shortening of radius, posttraumatic changes of distal radioulnar articulation, some shortening of scaphoid, and avascular changes of lunate. **(F)** Lateral radiograph shows similar findings with broadening of distal radial articular surface and a somewhat vertical position of scaphoid. Patient's general wrist function was good, and he was essentially asymptomatic. *(Illustrations 4-67A–F courtesy of S.C. Santangelo, M.D.)*

autogenous bone graft should accompany multiple Kirschner wire fixations in both techniques.

In the time interval of four to 10 weeks, the choice is between soft tissue reconstructions or limited intercarpal arthrodeses. In the former, ligament repair from both dorsal and palmar approaches can be reinforced by tendon graft or transfer. One technique is use of a segment of the extensor carpi radialis brevis, tendon left attached at its insertion which is threaded through the scaphoid and lunate and back into the dorsal radius. This procedure attempts reconstruction of the scapholunate interosseous ligaments and the radioscapholunate ligament. Temporary Kirschner wire fixation of the reduced carpals protects healing ligament repairs and tendon transfers.

If a limited intercarpal arthrodesis is preferred for a more predictable definitive procedure, either arthrodesis of the scaphoid, lunate and capitate or the tri-scaphe arthrodesis is available. Reconstruction of lunate triquetral diastasis and triquetral hamate instability is similar.

Likewise, at the same time intervals after injury, similar procedures are recommended for lunate triquetral and triquetral hamate lesions: 1) Anatomic reduction with or without percutaneous Kirschner wire fixations for the first three or four weeks post-injury, 2) Ligament reconstruction combined with appropriate tendon transfer or limited arthrodesis between four and 10 weeks post-injury, and 3) Limited carpal arthrodesis (triquetrum to lunate or triquetrum to hamate 10 weeks or longer).

Corrective osteotomy of the distal radius for malunion of distal radial metaphyseal fractures with secondary carpal instability may restore the carpal architecture (Figures 4-68A,B). However, carpal anatomy must be restored before arthritic changes develop.

The symptomatic chronic instability with diffuse arthritic changes of intercarpal joints and the wrist joint is best treated by either proximal row carpectomy[28] with or without incorporation of silastic hinge implant or wrist arthrodesis extending to the distal carpal row.

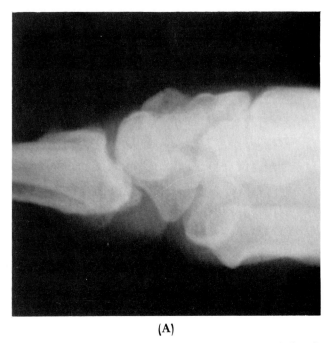

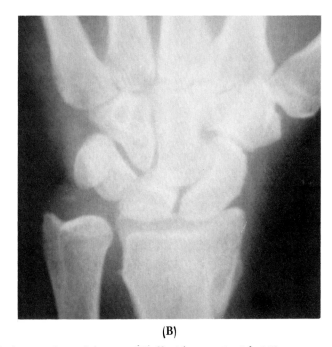

(A)   (B)

Figure 4-68 **(A)** Lateral view of malunited dorsal distal radial metaphyseal fracture (Colles' fracture) with 25° dorsal angulation of the distal articular surface. Secondary carpal instabilities include palmar rotational instability of the scaphoid and dorsal rotational instability of the lunate. **(B)** Corresponding PA view shows shortening of the distal radius but no apparent scapholunate dissociation.

Dynamic instabilities are usually diagnosed longer after injury because of two factors:

1. The disability is not severe and the patient, thinking the injury is "just a sprain which will heal by itself" does not seek medical consultation early, and
2. The diagnosis as noted above may be very difficult to determine. Early diagnosis of an acute dynamic lesion facilitates conservative cast immobilization for a minimum of six and preferably eight weeks.

Late diagnosis with verification of a partial ligament tear by arthrography[1] indicates ligament repair with temporary Kirschner wire fixation. An undiagnosed and untreated dynamic lesion probably will progress to an overt carpal instability.

An untreated or inadequately treated, overt carpal instability results in degenerative joint disease from a collapse deformity of the carpus. Rotation of the scaphoid or flexion of the distal segment of a displaced scaphoid fracture impinges the scaphoid tuberosity on the radial styloid process particularly in radial deviation. Degenerative and posttraumatic changes of the radial styloid process include erosion of the articular surface, a "spiking" deformity and

often exuberant hypertrophic spur formation. All wrist motion becomes diminished and painful particularly radial deviation and extension. Dorsal subluxation of the proximal scaphoid pole and/or lunate associated with chronic scapholunate dissociation induces degenerative joint changes both at the radial scaphoid articulation and often at the scaphoid, trapezium-trapezoid articulations. With marked scapholunate diastasis, proximal migration of the entire distal carpal row occurs with attenuation of the triquetrum-hamate interosseous ligaments (Figure 4-69A,B).

Chronic lunate-triquetral instability also naturally progresses to arthritic changes of that joint (Figure 4-70). The chronic instability with arthritic changes in a patient who is relatively sedentary in both occupation and avocation and who is essentially asymptomatic should not be reconstructed. However, those patients with significant painful disability and arthritic changes of both the wrist and intercarpal joints are best treated by one of two procedures: 1) proximal row carpectomy with or without incorporation of a silastic hinged implant, or 2) wrist arthrodesis including the distal carpal row.

An alternative to treat the SLAC wrist (scapholunate advanced collapsed pattern of degenerative ar-

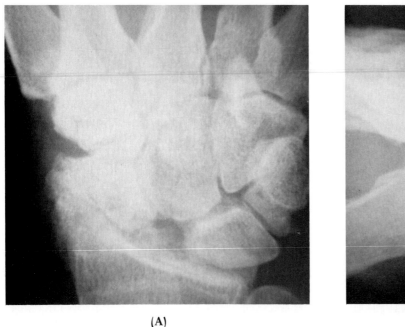

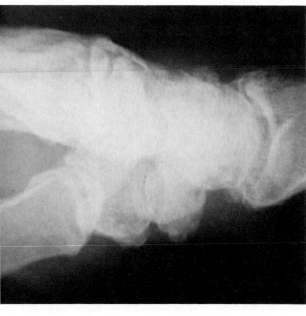

(A)

(B)

Figure 4-69 **(A)** PA view shows marked diastasis of the scapholunate joint, proximal migration of the distal carpal row with changes of lunate-triquetral and hamate-triquetral joints and marked arthritic changes of the radial styloid process and radioscaphoid joint. The proximal scaphoid pole was excised many years previously with this result of progressive symptomatic wrist and intercarpal arthritis. **(B)** Corresponding lateral radiograph shows palmar position of the remaining distal scaphoid segment but surprisingly no apparent rotational instability of the lunate.

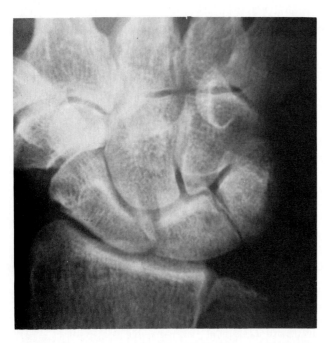

Figure 4-70 PA view shows virtual absence of cartilage space between the lunate and triquetrum resulting from chronic lunate-triquetral instability.

thritis) was recently proposed by Watson.[29] The purpose is to stabilize the wrist so the lunate will transmit the functioning load through the preserved radiolunate joint. The procedure combines capitate-lunate arthrodesis with or without inclusion of the hamate and triquetrum with excision of the scaphoid and replacement by a silastic scaphoid implant.

Wrist Joint Instabilities

Dorsal Subluxation and Dislocation. Marked dorsal subluxation of the scaphoid (Figure 4-55B) and/or the lunate (Figures 4-66, 4-67B) and dorsal subluxation and dislocation of the entire carpus on the radius (refer to Figure 4-10A) follow severe ligamentous injuries.

On the lateral radiograph there is dorsal displacement, subluxation, or dislocation of the scaphoid, lunate, or the entire proximal carpal row on the distal radial articular surface.

A dorsally and proximally displaced segmental articular fracture of the distal radius, accompanied by subluxation of the carpus, is found in a displaced dorsal segmental articular fracture of the distal radius (dorsal Barton's fracture) (refer to Articular Fractures of the Distal Radius in Chapter 3).

Palmar Subluxation and Dislocation. Palmar subluxation or dislocation of the carpus noted in acute injury usually occurs secondarily to a palmar articular fracture displacement of the distal radial articular surface (palmar Barton's fracture) (Figures 4-89A–C). In the chronic state it is associated almost exclusively with rheumatoid arthritis (Figure 4-71).

The lateral radiograph shows palmar and proximal displacement of the proximal carpal row of any extent (Figure 4-71), from mild subluxation to complete dislocation from the distal radial articular surface or in association with a palmarly displaced segmental articular fracture of the distal radius (palmar Barton's fracture—Figure 4-89C).

Ulnar Subluxation. Rheumatoid arthritis is the most common cause of this deformity (Figures 4-72, 4-73), particularly if resection of the distal ulna (Darrach procedure) has been performed previously (Figure 4-74). Ulnar subluxation of the carpus may be second-

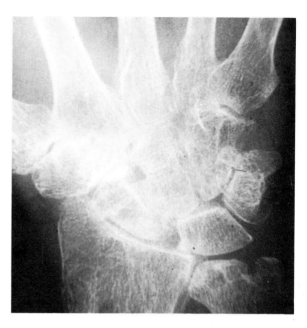

Figure 4-72 PA radiograph illustrates ulnar slide of entire carpus on distal radius and ulna due to rheumatoid arthritis. Lunate is seen distal to ulna; intercarpal arthritic changes are seen throughout carpus as well as in distal ulna and radius.

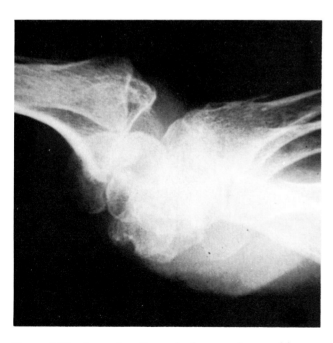

Figure 4-71 Lateral radiograph shows palmar subluxation and proximal displacement of entire carpus on distal radius due to rheumatoid arthritis. Multiple carpal irregularities with some palmar flexion of lunate are seen.

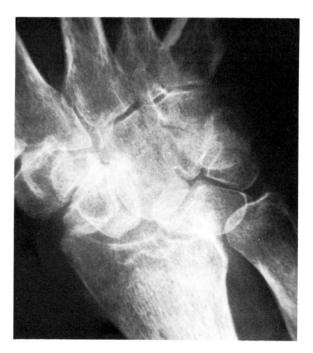

Figure 4-73 PA radiograph shows ulnar slide due to rheumatoid arthritis with increased angulation of distal radius towards ulna; also, rather marked scapholunate dissociation and rotational deformity of scaphoid with proximal migration of distal carpal row into space between scaphoid and lunate. Arthritic changes are evident in the intercarpal joints.

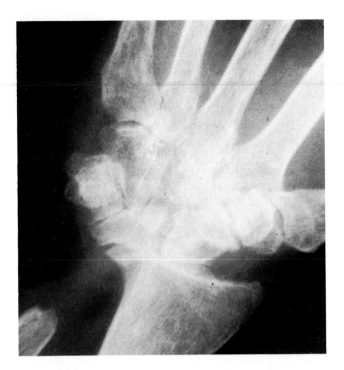

Figure 4-74   PA view shows result of Darrach procedure performed 7 years previously. Marked ulnar slide of carpus on distal radius with changes on ulnar aspect of distal radial articular surface. Case demonstrates inadvisability of Darrach procedure in patient with rheumatoid arthritis. In addition, too large a segment of distal ulna was excised.

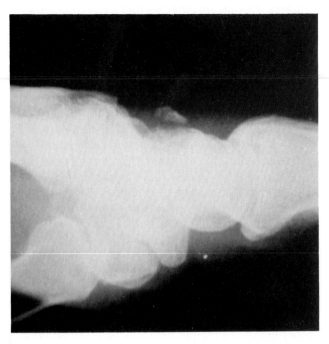

Figure 4-75   Lateral view illustrates dorsal chip avulsion fracture on dorsal aspect of triquetrum. Treated by plaster splint immobilization for 3 weeks until patient was asymptomatic.

ary to malunion of a distal radial metaphyseal fracture which may or may not involve multiple articular fragments of the distal radial articular surface, resulting in an exaggerated ulnar angulation and causing a progressive "ulnar slide" of the carpus due to chronic ligament attenuation and laxity.

On the PA radiograph there is an increased ulnar angulation of the distal radial articular surface. There should be an abnormal space between the radial styloid and the scaphoid, as a result of which the lunate becomes located distal to the ulnar articular surface. For ulnar slide of the carpus to occur, the radioscaphoid lunate ligament must be markedly attenuated or ruptured.

Radial Subluxation.   Radial and proximal displacement of a segmental articular fracture of the radial styloid or radial aspect of the distal articular surface (chauffeur's fracture) accompanied by subluxation of the carpus. The PA radiograph is diagnostic (Figure 4-62A).

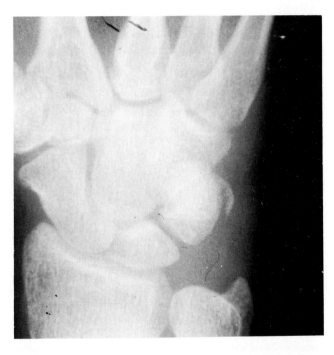

Figure 4-76   PA radiograph of wrist shows minimally displaced avulsion fracture of ulnar nonarticular surface of triquetrum. Immobilization for 3½ weeks provided asymptomatic wrist function.

Less Common Carpal Fractures, Dislocations, and Fracture Dislocations

Fracture of the triquetrum may involve an avulsion fracture on the dorsal aspect (Figure 4-75), a fracture through its body (Figure 4-38), or a fracture on the ulnar aspect (Figure 4-76) due to either avulsion or direct trauma. A significant fracture of the triquetrum

should be treated by cast or splint immobilization for about six weeks or until fracture healing is diagnosed by physical examination and radiographs. The dorsal and palmar avulsion fractures are rather inconsequential and are treated by immobilization for two and one-half to three weeks as noted above.

Dorsal transtriquetral perilunate fracture dislocation is an uncommon solitary wrist injury (Figure 4-77) and usually other carpal and/or distal

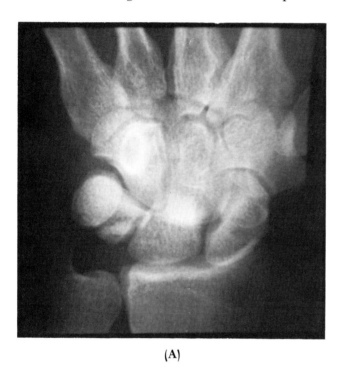

(A)

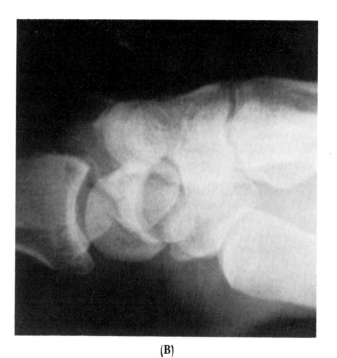

(B)

Figure 4-77 (A) PA view of a dorsal transtriquetral perilunate fracture dislocation of the wrist. The changes include generalized distortion of the proximal carpal row with transverse fracture of the triquetrum, "truncated pie" shape of the lunate, absent radioscaphoid cartilage space, and distortion of the scapholunate, lunate-triquetral and triquetral-hamate joints. (B) Corresponding lateral radiograph shows anatomic position of the lunate with dorsal displacement of the majority of the remaining carpus except for a segment of the triquetrum with obvious dorsal protrusion of the proximal pole of the scaphoid. (C) PA radiograph after open reductions and Kirschner wire fixations shows acceptable carpal, intercarpal and wrist joint anatomy restored. *(Figures 4-77A–C courtesy of Michael Doyle, M.D.)*

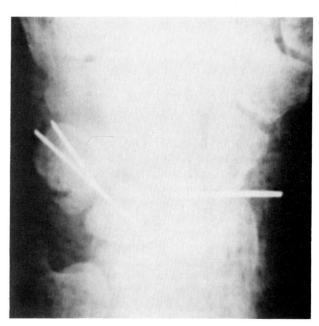

(C)

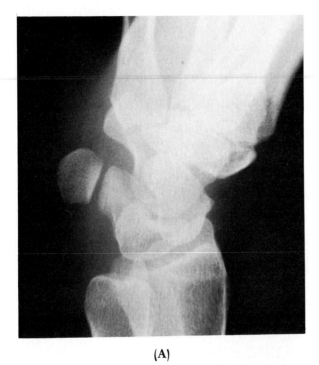

(A)

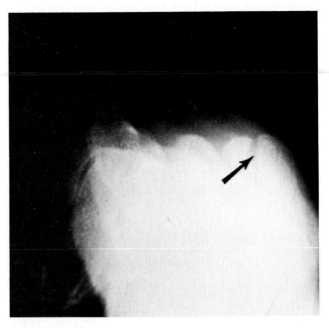

Figure 4-79 Modified carpal tunnel view of another patient shows a definite fracture of the pisiform. Case illustrates necessity of obtaining special views when indicated to enable positive diagnosis of skeletal lesions if fracture is suspected by physical examination and history. *(Illustration courtesy of R.G. Eaton, M.D.)*

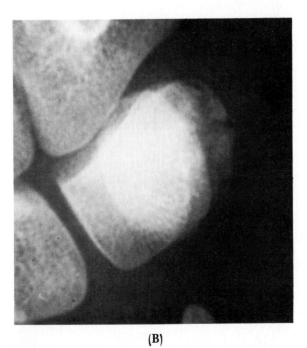

(B)

Figure 4-78 (A) Oblique view of wrist accentuates lateral profile of pisiform. Patient had point tenderness upon palpation of pisiform following a fall on ulnar aspect of wrist. No fracture is seen on this view. (B) Close-up of corresponding PA view of wrist clearly illustrates comminution of undisplaced fracture of pisiform. *(Illustrations 4-78A,B courtesy of D.M. Junkin, M.D.)*

radial pathology is concomitant (refer to Figure 16-8 of Chapter 16). Closed reduction in the closed injury is usually impossible and open reduction from either the dorsal or dorsal and palmar approaches is necessary.

Fracture of the pisiform is uncommon (Figures 4-78A,B, 4-79); it is diagnosed by point tenderness of the pisiform which may be associated with symptoms of ulnar nerve compression (neurapraxia). This is verified by radiographic localization which often requires multiple views (Figure 4-79). A ragged appearance of the pisiform in a skeletally immature patient is most often due to the irregularity of ossification of this bone (Figure 4-80). Examination and palpation of the pisiform discloses no tenderness in the area and a fracture may be ruled out.

Discrete fracture or fracture dislocation of the trapezium is uncommon. Fracture dislocation requires a very severe injury to avulse the trapezium from its extremely strong connection to both the trapezoid and scaphoid (Figures 4-81A,B).

Injuries to the capitate are not common due to its central protected position in the carpus. Dorsal

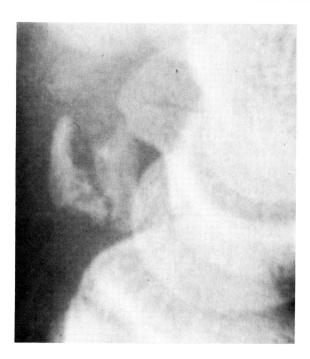

Figure 4-80 Oblique view of pisiform shows gross irregularity of normal pisiform ossification in a skeletally immature person (10-year-old male), not a fracture. If patient had discrete tenderness in area of pisiform, it would be extremely difficult to differentiate between fracture and normal ossification process.

dislocation of the capitate is rare (Figures 4-82A–D) and is best diagnosed on a lateral radiograph. Normal configuration of the carpus is seen except at the distal concavity of the lunate, which does not contain the head of the capitate. The capitate is dorsal to the remainder of the carpus and somewhat displaced proximally (Figure 4-82A). The PA radiograph shows distortion of the scaphoid-capitate and lunate-capitate joints, with some bony superimposition of the capitate on these other two bones (Figure 4-82B). Reduction is achieved as with most other fracture dislocations. Dislocations of the capitate are treated by traction distally with dorsal pressure on the dislocated capitate. If closed reduction is impossible or if there is an associated unstable scapholunate dissociation, surgical intervention and restoration of normal joint and soft tissue anatomy by appropriate ligamentous repairs and temporary internal fixation is advised.

Fracture of the capitate results from a severe direct blow to the central portion of the carpus directly on the capitate. Cast immobilization for six to eight weeks is sufficient.

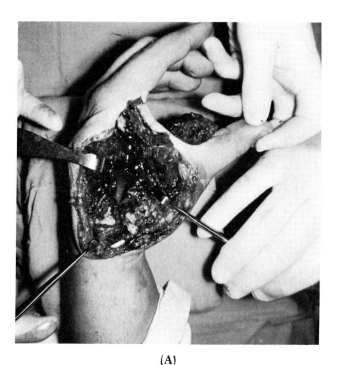

(A)

(B)

Figure 4-81 (A) Photograph illustrates severe dorsal avulsion crush injury to radial aspect of hand, producing open fracture dislocation of trapezium from trapezoid and scaphoid. (B) Oblique radiograph of hand prior to surgery does not reveal unstable fracture dislocation of trapezium.

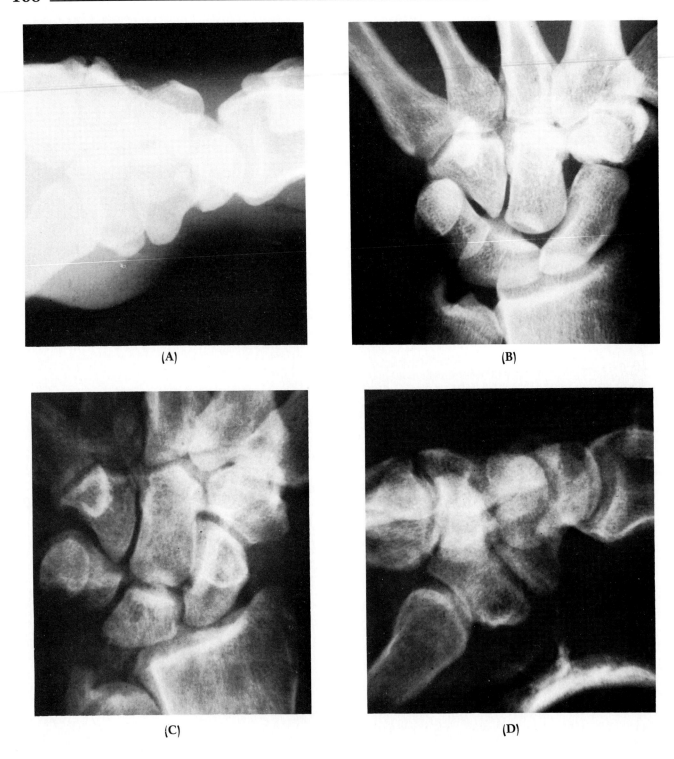

(A)

(B)

(C)

(D)

Figure 4-82 **(A)** Lateral radiograph of wrist illustrates dorsal dislocation of capitate. Capitate is seen dorsal to lunate and is proximally displaced. A vacant distal lunate concave articular surface can be visualized. **(B)** PA view is not diagnostic but does show incongruous articulations of both scaphoid and lunate with capitate. **(C)** PA radiograph after successful closed manipulation and reduction illustrates restoration of normal carpal anatomy. **(D)** Lateral radiograph also shows restoration of normal carpal anatomy. *(Illustrations 4-82A–D courtesy of A.M. Larimer, M.D.)*

A very interesting lesion, usually due to severe trauma, is transverse fracture of the capitate through its center, resulting in 180° rotation of the proximal fragment. Usually this rotated fracture of the capitate head occurs in association with fracture of the scaphoid, the so-called scapho-capitate syndrome (Figures 4-83A–E). The majority of these syndromes occur in association with dorsal transscaphoid perilunate fracture dislocations. Since closed reduction of the capitate fracture is usually impossible, open reduction and internal fixation is necessary to reestablish normal carpal anatomy (Figures 4-83B,C). Avascular necrosis of the proximal fragment (head of the capitate) is not uncommon.

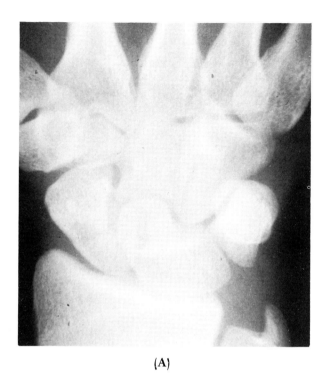

(A)

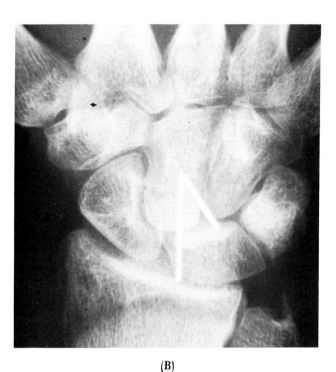

(B)

Figure 4-83 (A) PA view of wrist shows undisplaced transverse fracture of scaphoid through junction of proximal and middle thirds and transverse fracture through center of capitate, with rotation of head of capitate 180° and fractured surface facing proximally. (B) PA view shows normal carpal anatomy after open reduction and temporary Kirschner wire fixation of capitate fracture, irreducible closed. (C) Similar findings noted in lateral view. Normal relationship of scaphoid with lunate is seen in both Figures 4-83B and C.

(C)   *(continued)*

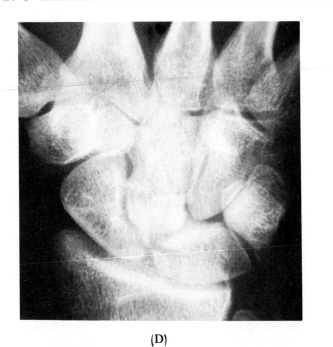

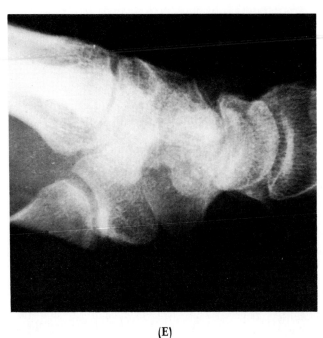

(D)

(E)

Figure 4-83 *(continued)*
(D) PA view 7 months after surgery shows normal architecture of carpus with absence of temporary Kirschner wire fixation. **(E)** Lateral view also shows essentially normal carpal anatomy. *(Illustrations 4-83A–E courtesy of D.M. Junkin, M.D.)*

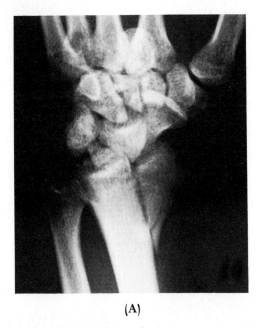

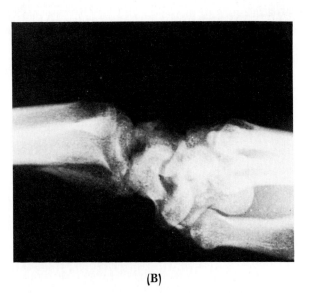

(A)

(B)

Figure 4-84 **(A)** PA radiograph shows complete distortion of carpal anatomy with a large proximally displaced radial segmental articular (chauffeur's) fracture of distal radius. Hazy outline seen between bases of index and long metacarpals is head of capitate, which is rotated 180° and completely displaced in this abnormal position. There also can be seen displaced scaphoid fracture, fractures of lunate and triquetrum, and distortion of ring and little finger metacarpal bases. **(B)** Lateral view shows capitate head completely displaced palmarly to index and long metacarpal bases and rotated 180° with its articular surface facing distally. Lunate is palmarly subluxed, and its distal articular surface is vacant. Multiple intercarpal fractures and dorsal fracture dislocation, with displacement of ring finger metacarpal, are also noted.

Distal displacement of the capitate head associated with complete 180° rotation is rarely encountered and then only in massive injuries to the carpus (Figures 4-84A,B). Similar treatment of open reduction and internal fixation as necessary is indicated.

A much less common lesion is fracture of the capitate with rotation of the head not associated with scaphoid fracture. Open reduction and fixation solves this problem (Figures 4-85A–C).

Fracture of the hamate is often associated with fracture subluxation of the fifth metacarpal (see Figure 5-2). Closed reduction of the fifth metacarpal fracture subluxation is often augmented by percutaneous Kirschner wire fixation to secure the metacarpal to the carpus, thus preventing recurrent subluxa-

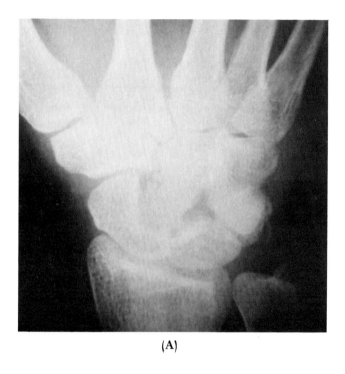

(A)

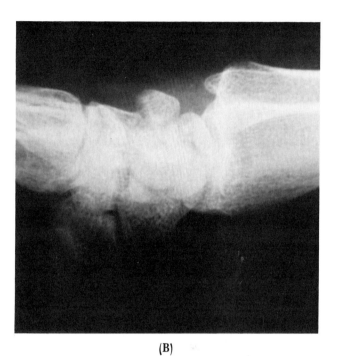

(B)

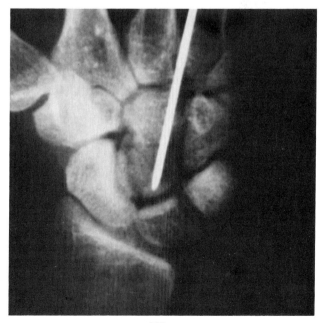

(C)

Figure 4-85 **(A)** PA radiograph shows distortion of the mid-carpal joint with irregularity of the head of the capitate and small fracture fragment of the triquetrum. At open reduction this injury proved to be a displaced fracture through the capitate with 180° rotation of the capitate head. This isolated capitate lesion is much less common than the scaphocapitate syndrome. **(B)** Lateral view shows fracture comminution and distortion in the area of the lunate-capitate articulation with no joint discernable. **(C)** Following open reduction and internal fixation, anatomy of the capitate and the mid-carpal joint have been restored. *(Figures 4-85A–C courtesy of Marybeth Ezaki, M.D.)*

tion. The fracture of the hamate is incidental. Solitary fracture of the body of the hamate is uncommon (Figure 4-86).

Isolated fracture of the hook of the hamate is rare (Figures 4-87, 4-88) and usually due to direct blunt

trauma. In addition to point tenderness, symptoms and findings of ulnar nerve compression (neurapraxia) may be associated. This fracture may be a solitary lesion or it may be associated with multiple trauma to the wrist (Figures 4-89A–C), as any of these unusual

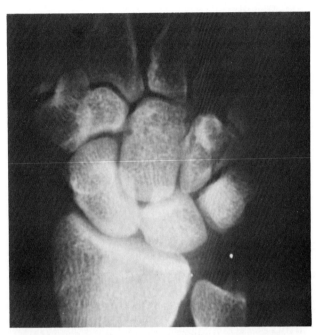

Figure 4-86 Unusual solitary longitudinal fracture through the body of the hamate.

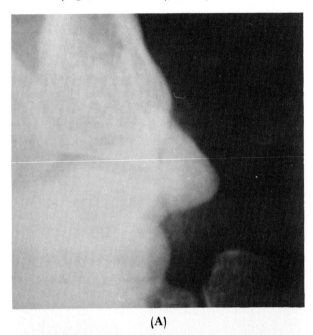

(A)

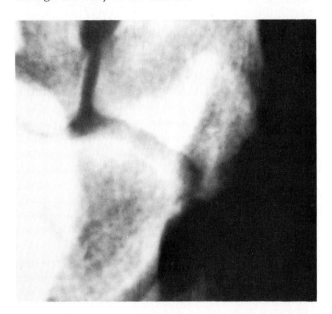

Figure 4-87 Close-up of oblique view of wrist shows minimally displaced fracture of hook of hamate. This discrete lesion is rare and is sustained by blunt trauma directly to this structure *(Illustration courtesy of R.G. Eaton, M.D.)*

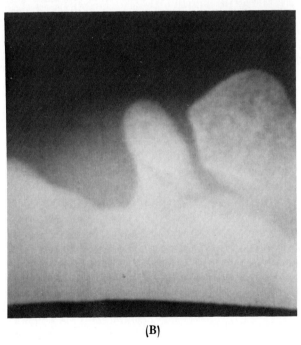

(B)

Figure 4-88 **(A)** Fracture through the hook of the hamate, seen on oblique view. **(B)** Same fracture seen through a profile view with the fractured hook of the hamate on the left and pisiform on the right. *(Courtesy of Michael Doyle, M.D.)*

fractures may be. Multiple radiographs are often necessary to visualize this fracture adequately.[1,30]

Trapezoid dislocation is very rare[31] and also is usually associated with multiple skeletal trauma (Figure 4-90). The index metacarpal remains attached to the trapezoid because of the intimate skeletal relationship (refer to section on anatomy in Chapter 1).

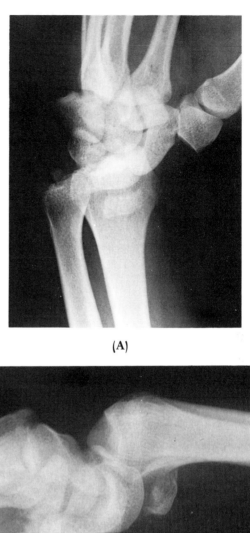

(A)

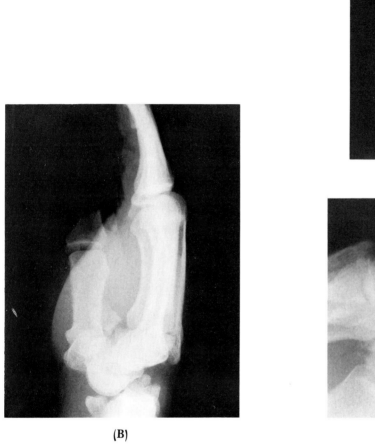

(B)

(C)

Figure 4-89 **(A)** PA radiograph illustrates distortion of entire wrist joint, fracture of distal radius, dislocation of scaphoid-trapezium joint, rotational deformities of ring and little finger metacarpals, and distortion of index and long finger carpometacarpal joints. Injuries were sustained when hand was pinned between motorcycle and police van as rider was thrown over handlebars. **(B)** Lateral view shows dorsal subluxation of index and long metacarpal bases, anterior subluxation of ring and little finger metacarpal bases, abnormality in area of scaphoid-trapezium joint noted previously as a dislocation, palmar and proximal displacement of entire carpus associated with displaced segmental articular fracture of palmar aspect of distal radius (palmar Barton's fracture), and fracture of hook of hamate. **(C)** Close-up of lateral view of wrist clearly illustrates palmar proximal displacement of the entire carpus and displaced segmental articular fracture of anterior articular surface of distal radius (palmar Barton's fracture subluxation). Other lesions are seen as noted in Figure 4-89B. Two weeks after severe wrist injury noted here open reduction and internal fixation, with capsular repair of carpometacarpal subluxations (index through little finger), open reduction and capsular repair of scaphoid-trapezium dislocation, and closed reduction of palmar Barton's fracture subluxation were carried out. Temporary Kirschner wire immobilization removed 15 weeks postoperatively; 6 months after that patient had full ranges of digital motion. Wrist motion of 45° extension and 60° flexion allowed return to full duty as a police officer. *(Illustrations 4-89A–C courtesy of S.F. Gunther, M.D.)*

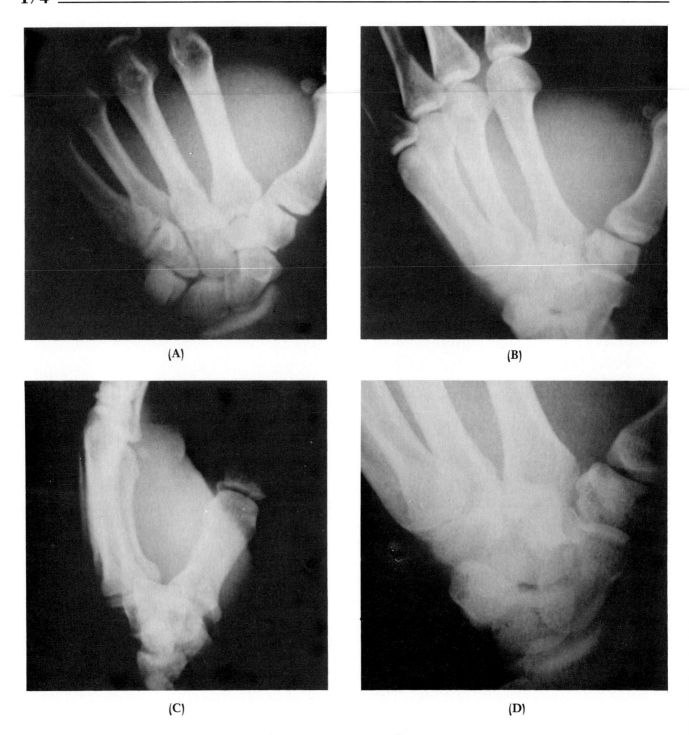

(A)

(B)

(C)

(D)

Figure 4-90 **(A)** PA view of the wrist and the hand shows distortion of the carpometacarpal joints, index through long fingers, with indefinite outline of the trapezoid. **(B)** The oblique view shows an abnormal linear parallel configuration of the metacarpus indicative of carpometacarpal pathology. The trapezoid, again, cannot be accurately defined. **(C)** Lateral view illustrates complete dorsal dislocation of the trapezoid with the base of the index metacarpal. **(D)** Closeup of the oblique view shows better the complete dorsal trapezoid dislocation with the contiguous index metacarpal base. This lesion is complete dislocation of index, long, and ring carpometacarpal joints with associated complete dislocation of the trapezoid.

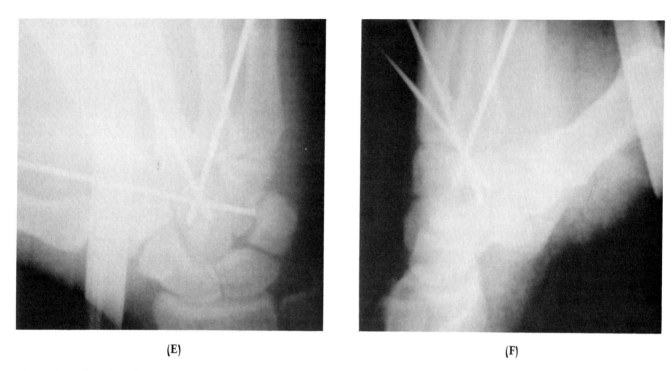

(E)   (F)

Figure 4-90 *(continued)*
(E) Anatomic closed reduction preceded Kirschner wire percutaneous fixations, PA view. **(F)** Corresponding lateral view.

General References

Dobyns JH, Linscheid RL: Fractures and dislocations of the wrist, in Rockwood CA Jr, Green DP: *Fractures in Adults*. Philadelphia, J.B. Lippincott Co., 1984, vol 1, pp 411–509.
Taleisnik J: Fractures of the carpal bones, in Green DP (ed): *Operative Hand Surgery*. New York, Churchill Livingstone, 1982, vol 1, pp 669–702.

References

1. Egawa, M, Asai T: Fracture of the hook of the hamate: Report of six cases and the suitability of computerized tomography. *J Hand Surg* 1983;8(4):393.
2. Palmer AK, Levinsohn EM, Kuzma GR: Arthrography of the wrist. *J Hand Surg* 1983; 8:15–23.
3. Cope JR: Carpal coalition. *Clin Radiol* 1974;25:261–266.
4. O'Rahilly R: A survey of carpal and tarsal anomalies. *J Bone Joint Surg (Am)* 1953;35-A: 626–642.
5. Watson HK, Maglana W: Complications of fracture management of the hand and wrist, in Gossling, HR, Pillsbury SL (eds): *Complications of Fracture Management*. Philadelphia, J.B. Lippincott Co., 1984, pp 389–398.
6. Cooney WP, Dobyns JH, Linscheid RL: Nonunion of the scaphoid: Analysis of the results from bone grafting. *J Hand Surg* 1980;5(4):343–354.
7. Mezet R Jr: Fractured scaphoid. *Am Acad Orthop Surgeons*, sound slide no. 367, 1972.
8. Faithfull DK, Herbert TJ: Small joint fusions of the hand using the Herbert bone screw. *J Hand Surg* 1984; 9-B:167–168.

9. Herbert TJ: Management of the fractured scaphoid bone using a new surgical technique. Proc Rep Universities Colleges Councils Associations Soc. *J Bone Joint Surg* 1982; 64-B:633.

10. Armstrong GWD: Rotational subluxation of the scaphoid. *Can J Surg* 1968;11:306–314.

11. Murakami Y: Dislocation of the carpal scaphoid. *Hand* 1977;9:79–81.

12. Woodward AH, Neviaser RJ, Nisenfeld F: Radial and volar perilunate transscaphoid fracture dislocation. *S Med J* 1975;68:926–928.

13. Mayfield JK, Johnson RP, Kilcoyne RK: Carpal dislocations: Pathomechanics and progressive perilunar instability. *J Hand Surg* 1980;5(3):226–241.

14. O'Brien ET: Lunate and perilunar dislocations. *Am Acad Orthop Surgeons*, sound slide no. 392, 1973.

15. Stern PJ: Transscaphoid-lunate dislocation: A report of two cases. *J Hand Surg* 1984; 9A:370–373.

16. Boyes JGT Jr: Subluxation of the carpal navicular bone. *S Med J* 1976;69:141–144.

17. Dobyns JH, Linscheid RL, Chao EYS, et al: Traumatic instability of the wrist, in *Instructional Course Lectures, Am Acad of Orthop Surgeons* XXIV. St. Louis, C.V. Mosby Co., 1975, pp 182–199.

18. Howard FM, Fahey T, Wojcik E: Rotary subluxation of the navicular. *Clin Orthop* 1974; 104:34–39.

19. Linscheid RL, Dobyns JH, Beabout JW, et al: Traumatic instability of the wrist: Diagnosis, classification, and pathomechanics. *J Bone Joint Surg (Am)* 1972;54-A:1612–1632.

20. Green DP: Carpal dislocations, in Green DP (ed): *Operative Hand Surgery*. New York, Churchill Livingstone, 1982, vol 1, pp 703–742.

21. Reagan DS, Linscheid RL, Dobyns JH: Lunotriquetral sprains. *J Hand Surg* 1984;9A: 502–514.

22. Lichtman DM, Schneider JR, Swafford AR, et al: Ulnar midcarpal instability—Clinical and laboratory analysis. *J Hand Surg* 1981;6(5):515–523.

23. Taleisnik J, Watson HK: Midcarpal instability caused by malunited fractures of the distal radius. *J Hand Surg* 1984;9A:350–357.

24. Glickel SZ, Millender LH: Ligamentous reconstruction for chronic intercarpal instability. *J Hand Surg* 1984;9A:514–527.

25. Kleinman WB, Steichen JB, Strickland JW: Management of chronic rotary subluxation of the scaphoid by scapho-trapezio-trapezoid arthrodesis. *J Hand Surg* 1982;7(2):125–136.

26. Watson HK: Limited wrist arthrodesis. *Clin Orthop* 1980;149:126–136.

27. Watson HK, Hempton RF: Limited wrist arthrodesis I: The triscaphoid joint. *J Hand Surg* 1980;5:320–327.

28. Neviaser RJ: Proximal row carpectomy for posttraumatic disorders of the carpus. *J Hand Surg* 1983;8:301–305.

29. Watson HK, Ballet FL: The SLAC wrist: Scapholunate advanced collapse pattern of degenerative arthritis. *J Hand Surg* 1984;9A:358–365.

30. Carter PR, Eaton RG, et al: Ununited fracture of the hook of the hamate. *J Bone Joint Surg (Am)* 1977; 59:583–588.

31. Goodman ML, Shankman GB: Update: Palmar dislocation of the trapezoid—A case report. *J Hand Surg* 1984;9A:127–131.

Carpometacarpal Joints: Fractures, Dislocations, and Fracture Dislocations

The distal carpal row (trapezium-trapezoid-capitate-hamate) is firmly bound together by multiple ligaments, including dorsal, palmar, and interosseous ligaments; these make the distal carpal row plus the index and long metacarpals the stable portion of the hand. The central metacarpal (long finger) is the central pillar of the longitudinal and transverse arches of the hand (see section Functional Arches of the Hand in Chapter 1, Anatomy). Therefore any fracture, dislocation, or fracture dislocation which interrupts normal anatomic configuration adversely influences the functional longitudinal and transverse arches.

Motion at the carpometacarpal joints is extremely variable, ranging from the trapezium-thumb metacarpal joint, one of the most highly mobile joints of the hand, to the carpometacarpal joints of the index and long fingers (trapezoid-index metacarpal joint and capitate-long finger metacarpal joint), two of the most stable joints of the hand. The carpometacarpal joint of the little finger (hamate-fifth metacarpal) resembles the anatomic configuration of the thumb carpometacarpal joint, but its mobility, though good, is not as great. The third most mobile carpometacar-

pal joint is that of the ring finger (hamate-ring finger metacarpal joint).

Injury to the thumb carpometacarpal joint is most common due to its vulnerable position. Next in frequency of injury is the carpometacarpal joint of the little finger (Figures 5-1A–C–5-5A–E), also because of its less protected position as a marginal ray. Carpometacarpal injury is more common in the mobile area of the hand (ring and little finger area) than in the stable portion (index and long). Though the little finger metacarpal base may suffer solitary dislocation or fracture dislocation, injury to the ring finger carpometacarpal joint or metacarpal shaft (dislocation, fracture dislocation, or shaft fracture) often occurs simultaneously. Therefore if trauma to the little finger carpometacarpal joint is diagnosed, the ring finger carpometacarpal joint and metacarpal shaft also should be closely examined for possible concomitant injury (Figures 5-3A–C–5-5A–E).

Dislocation or fracture dislocation of the metacarpal base of the index or long finger, or both combined, is less common because they are stably tethered to their respective carpals (trapezoid and

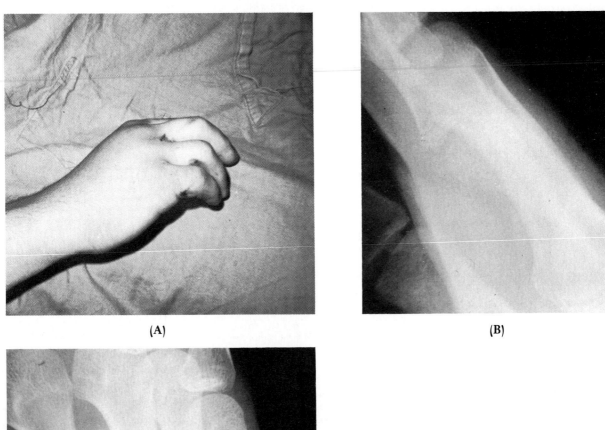

(A)

(B)

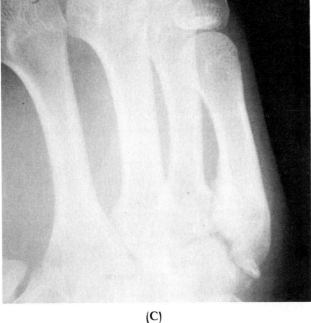

(C)

Figure 5-1 **(A)** Moderately severe edema accompanying carpometacarpal injury to ulnar aspect of hand.
(B) Lateral radiograph shows palmar angulation of little finger metacarpal shaft, protrusion of metacarpal head palmarly, and protrusion of metacarpal base dorsally with chip fracture of hamate. Diagnosis: dorsal fracture subluxation of little finger carpometacarpal joint.
(C) Oblique view shows palmar angulation of metacarpal, loss of alignment of fifth metacarpal to adjacent metacarpals, and displaced fracture of hamate.

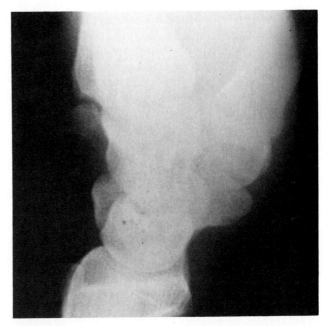

Figure 5-2 Lateral radiograph shows large avulsion fracture of hamate dorsally displaced with fifth metacarpal base. Diagnosis: dorsal fracture subluxation of fifth metacarpal base at carpometacarpal joint.

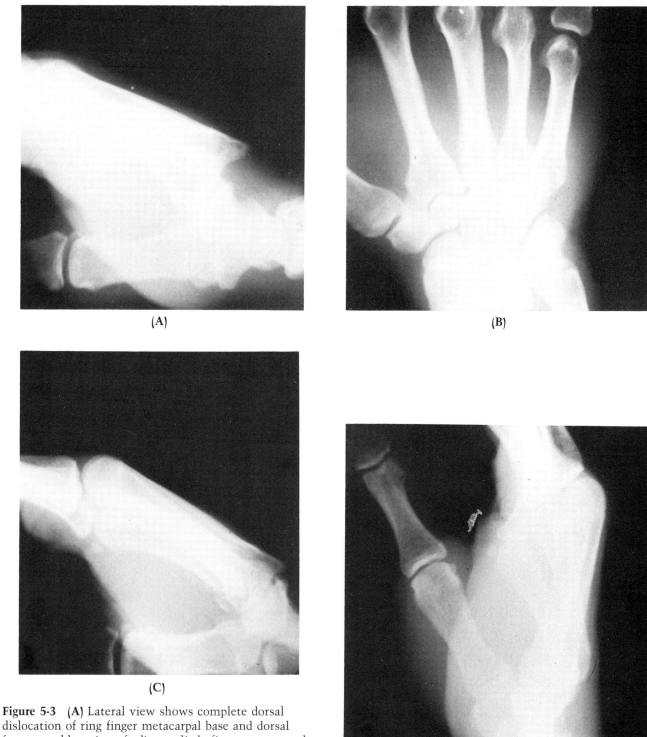

(A)

(B)

(C)

Figure 5-3 (A) Lateral view shows complete dorsal dislocation of ring finger metacarpal base and dorsal fracture subluxation of adjacent little finger metacarpal base at carpometacarpal joint, with palmar angulation of shaft and prominence of metacarpal head palmarly. (B) PA radiograph illustrates difficulty in diagnosing injury from this single view. (C) Lateral radiograph following satisfactory stable closed reduction not requiring Kirschner wire fixation.

Figure 5-4 Lateral radiograph shows dorsal dislocation of little finger metacarpal base with palmar angulation of shaft and palmar protrusion of metacarpal head. Also associated was comminuted fracture of ring finger metacarpal base seen on PA view (not included).

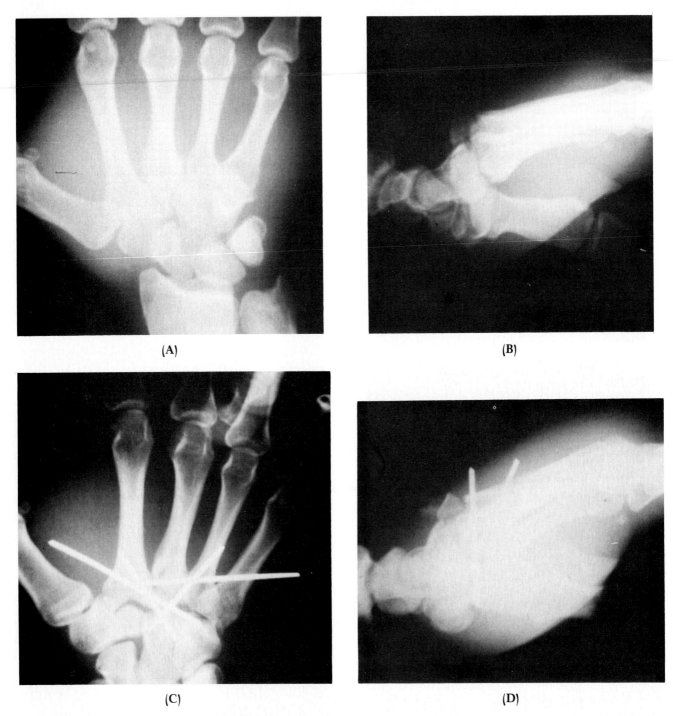

(A)

(B)

(C)

(D)

Figure 5-5 (A) PA radiograph illustrates multiple injuries in carpometacarpal joint area, including dorsal dislocation of index metacarpal base and dorsal fracture subluxations of long, ring, and little finger metacarpal bases. Displaced avulsion fracture of hamate also noted. (B) Lateral radiograph shows dorsal fracture subluxations of long, ring, and little finger metacarpal bases but not dorsal dislocation of index finger metacarpal base. (C) PA radiograph after closed manipulation and percutaneous Kirschner wire stabilizations. (D) Lateral radiograph after closed manipulation shows reductions achieved and maintained following percutaneous wire stabilizations.

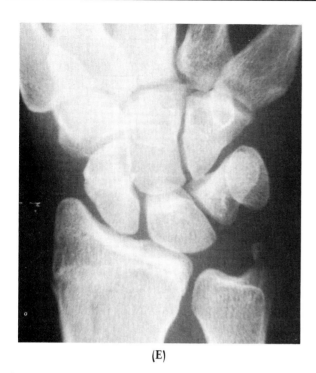

(E)

Figure 5-5 *(continued)*
(E) PA radiograph of contralateral wrist shows fractures of distal radius, ulnar styloid process, and scaphoid. Case illustrates importance of examining both extremities, particularly after massive injury is diagnosed in one hand. *(Illustrations 5-5A–E courtesy of A.M. Larimer, M.D.)*

capitate) (Figures 5-6A,B, 5-7A–E). Their central position in the hand also makes them less vulnerable to injury. The base of the index metacarpal is concave to accept the adjacent trapezoid which is anatomically "keyed" in position for additional security. (See Chapter 1, Anatomy, Carpometacarpal Joints.)

Dislocation or fracture dislocation of any carpometacarpal joint may be associated with a shaft, proximal metaphyseal, or distal metaphyseal (neck) fracture of an adjacent metacarpal or metacarpals.

The vast majority of carpometacarpal dislocations occur dorsally from a blow to or fall on the palmar aspect of the hand, but in massive injuries dislocations of multiple metacarpal bases may occur either dorsally (Figures 5-5B, 5-6A, 5-7B), palmarly, or both (Figure 4-89B in Chapter 4, Wrist Injuries), depending on the direction and severity of the injuring force.

Physical examination usually discloses rather marked swelling on the dorsum of the hand and wrist (Figure 5-1A), particularly if the hand has been held dependently. There is diffuse tenderness upon gentle

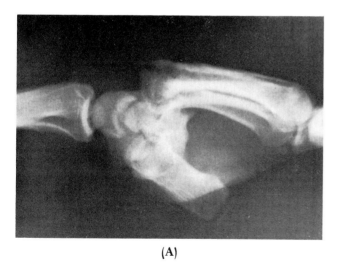

(A)

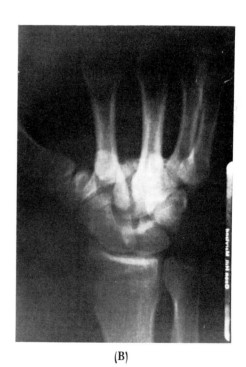

(B)

Figure 5-6 **(A)** Complete dorsal fracture dislocations of index, long, ring, and little finger metacarpal bases at carpometacarpal joints are seen in lateral radiograph. Injury was sustained in motorcycle accident. Severe skeletal trauma indicates massive soft tissue trauma, with edema and ecchymosis. **(B)** PA view illustrates, in addition to complete dorsal fracture dislocation of entire metacarpus except for thumb, a sagittal fracture of trapezoid and large dorsal avulsion fracture of capitate. *(Illustrations 5-6A,B courtesy of S.F. Gunther, M.D.)*

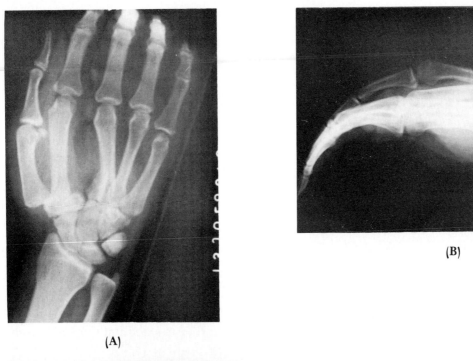

(A)

(B)

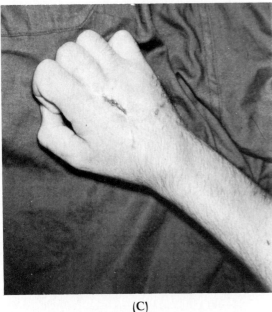

(C)

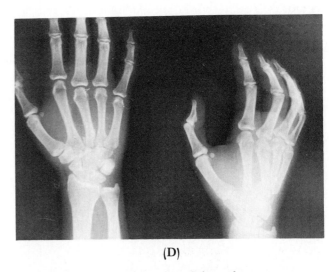

(D)

Figure 5-7 (A) PA radiograph illustrates massive carpometacarpal trauma due to through-and-through injury from high-velocity projectile (A-K-47 round). Injuries included dorsal dislocation of thumb metacarpal base and dorsally displaced fracture subluxations of index and long finger metacarpal bases. (B) Lateral radiograph illustrates well dorsal dislocation of thumb metacarpal base and dorsal fracture subluxations of index and long metacarpal bases. (C) Dorsal photograph approximately 2 months after initial injury. Wounds are nearly healed, but MP joints maintained in extension are improperly positioned and transverse arch of hand is flattened. (D) PA and oblique radiographs show partial reduction of index and long finger metacarpal bases, reduction of thumb metacarpal base, and incorrect complete extension of MP joints. Loss of long finger metacarpal length is due to comminution and bone loss and to angulation at site of fracture of base.

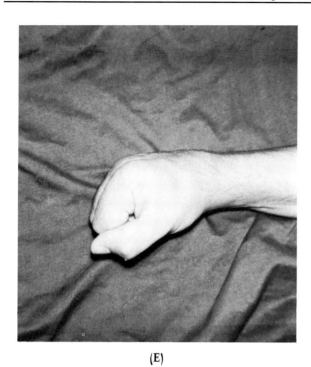

(E)

Figure 5-7 *(continued)*
(E) Following aggressive therapy of active and passive MP joint ranges of motion, flexion of 65° to 70°, extension to neutral, and strong grasp were obtained 3 months after initial injury.

palpation, but maximal tenderness may usually be elicited at the area of carpometacarpal subluxation, dislocation, or fracture dislocation.

The PA radiograph may not be diagnostic for carpometacarpal pathology. Most often the lateral radiograph or one or both oblique views are necessary for accurate diagnosis (Figures 5-1B,C). On the lateral radiograph palmar angulation of the involved metacarpal shaft is often found with palmar protrusion of the involved metacarpal head in addition to dorsal displacement of the metacarpal base.

The oblique views clearly show pathology of the ring and little finger metacarpals.

Though reduction of a carpometacarpal joint dislocation or fracture dislocation is rarely difficult, maintenance of reduction may be virtually impossible without fixation. Though some authorities advocate initial percutaneous Kirschner wire immobilization of the reduced metacarpal, one attempt at closed reduction with external immobilization is justified if stability has been achieved. If redislocation occurs, a repeat closed reduction is combined with percutaneous Kirschner wire fixation of the reduced metacarpal into the adjacent carpus or metacarpals, according

to preference. Rarely is open reduction of a carpometacarpal joint dislocation or fracture dislocation necessary. (Exceptions are the thumb and little finger carpometacarpal joints discussed in Chapter 6, The Thumb, section on Articular Fractures.)

Multiple carpometacarpal joint dislocations and/or fracture dislocations indicate a very severe injury, usually with marked soft tissue trauma and massive edema. Therefore in such multiple injuries, constant elevation often should be provided for a few days until edema and congestion subside sufficiently to allow satisfactory closed reduction and immobilization or fixation as necessary. For multiple injuries Kirschner wire fixation is usually recommended (Figures 5-5A–D, 5-6A,B) (also refer to Figure 4-90 of Chapter 4). The case in Figures 5-6A,B, for example, was treated by closed manipulation and reduction of the complete dorsal dislocation of the metacarpus (except for the thumb), with percutaneous Kirschner wire fixation and open reduction and internal fixation of the trapezoid fracture. The patient regained full digital motion, 40° wrist flexion and extension, and grip strength 75% of the normal contralateral hand.

A through-and-through injury, particularly one caused by a high-velocity missile, can cause massive damage to the carpometacarpal area (Figures 5-7A–E, 5-8). Initial treatment is that designated for a large

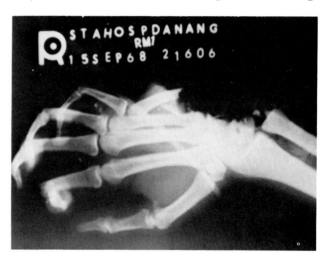

Figure 5-8 Massive injury to ulnar aspect of carpus and little finger metacarpal includes bone loss of that metacarpal, triquetrum, and hamate sustained in a through-and-through injury by a high-velocity projectile (A-K-47 round). Massive destruction of carpometacarpal area may cause irreparable vascular damage, necessitating primary amputation distal to injury. However, all viable structures should be retained at initial treatment for possible use in later reconstructive procedures.

open contaminated wound, most often with delayed primary closure or coverage. Reduction of the carpometacarpal dislocations or fracture dislocations should be performed as soon as possible to provide as near normal anatomy as possible. The case in Figures 5-7A–E illustrates the importance of functional immobilization with the MP joints flexed to prevent needless joint contractures. Immobilization with the MP joints completely extended is definitely contraindicated in any situation. Only aggressive therapy in a very cooperative patient can rectify longstanding MP joint extension contractures.

Occasionally injury to the carpometacarpal area is so massive that either primary or secondary deletion is necessary (Figure 5-8). Primary deletion is advocated only for the digit or digits sustaining irreparable vascular trauma with obvious digital non-viability. Otherwise all viable structures should be preserved at the time of initial treatment, particularly in the severely injured hand, to provide available sources of material for secondary reconstruction. Then at the time of secondary deletion of a completely functionless digit, some components—skin utilized as a free skin graft or as a neurovascular island pedicle transfer or rotational pedicle with its subcutaneous tissue, tendon for transfer or free tendon graft, bone for bone graft, and nerve for nerve graft—can be effectively used for reconstruction.

Isolated fractures, fracture dislocations, and dislocations of the thumb carpometacarpal joint (trapezium-thumb metacarpal joint) are found in the section on Articular Fractures in Chapter 6, The Thumb.

General References

Green DP, Rowland SA: Fractures and dislocations in the hand, in Rockwood CA Jr, Green DP (eds): *Fractures in Adults*, ed 2. Philadelphia, J.B. Lippincott Co., 1984, vol 1, pp 313–409.

O'Brien ET: Fractures of the metacarpals and phalanges, in Green DP (ed): *Operative Hand Surgery*. New York, Churchill Livingstone, 1982, vol 1, pp 583–635.

O'Brien ET: Fractures of the hand and wrist region, in Rockwood CA Jr, Wilkins KE, King RE (eds): *Fractures in Children*, ed 2. Philadelphia, J.B. Lippincott Co., 1984, vol 3, pp 229–272.

Sandzén SC Jr: Complex injuries of the wrist and hand, in Meyers MH (ed): *The Multiply Injured Patient with Complex Fractures*. Philadelphia, Lea & Febiger, 1984, pp 365–400.

CHAPTER
6

The Thumb: Dislocations, Ligamentous Injuries, and Fractures

Dislocations and Ligamentous Injuries

Carpometacarpal Joint

Acute subluxation or dislocation of the thumb metacarpal base (Figures 6-1A,B to 6-3A,B), the result of a longitudinal impact on the flexed thumb metacarpal, is not a common injury.

All the ligamentous structures surrounding and reinforcing the thumb carpometacarpal joint (trapezium-thumb metacarpal joint), including the most important deep ulnar or anterior oblique carpometacarpal ligament which connects the palmar beak of the thumb metacarpal base to the deep intercarpal ligaments and to the tuberosity of the trapezium, must be avulsed to completely dislocate the metacarpal base. Although the posterior oblique carpometacarpal ligament is reinforced by the diffuse, often multiple insertions of the abductor pollicis longus into the thumb metacarpal base on its dorsoradial aspect, it is weak and incapable of resisting forceful dorsal displacement of the metacarpal base.

If subluxation rather than dislocation occurs, the associated ligamentous injuries are not as severe, but treatment may be equally perplexing.

Physical examination discloses a dorsal protuberance at the base of the thumb metacarpal which is discretely tender upon palpation and which often may be anatomically reduced without difficulty (Figure 6-3A). Although closed reduction of the metacarpal base subluxation or dislocation is usually achieved initially, it is often unstable. If reduction can be maintained satisfactorily by external immobilization using a thumb spica cast or molded plaster splint for a period of four to five weeks, and if recurrent subluxation does not occur, healing usually progresses without later recurrent dislocation (Figure 6-1A,B). Some surgeons prefer initial percutaneous Kirschner wire fixation of the thumb metacarpal to the trapezium or to the adjacent metacarpals (index and/or long finger) to insure maintenance of anatomic reduction during the healing phase. If closed reduction is impossible because of soft tissue interposition (Figure 6-3C), or if resubluxation or redislocation occur after initial conservative treatment, ligamentous reconstruction may be necessary. Some surgeons favor repair or reconstruction of the dorsal ligaments only (Figure 6-3D), using a segment of the palmaris longus or extensor pollicis longus tendon; others favor a palmar approach to allow repair of the important

185

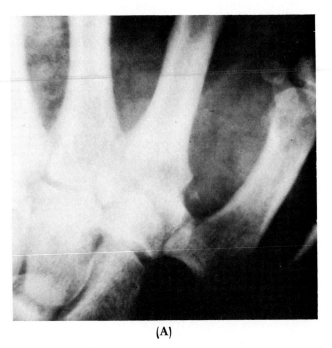

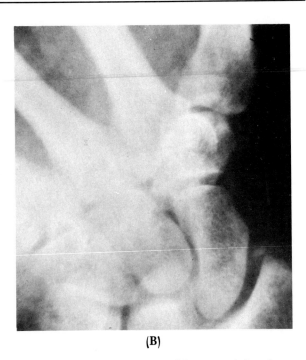

(A)

(B)

Figure 6-1 **(A)** Lateral view of complete dorsal dislocation of thumb metacarpal base. Note adduction of thumb metacarpal toward index metacarpal and proximal displacement. **(B)** Lateral radiograph after successful closed manipulation, reduction, and 4½ weeks in plaster immobilization. Satisfactory functional stability resulted.

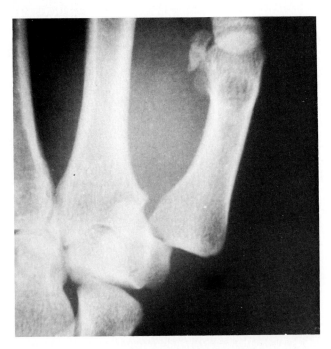

Figure 6-2 Dorsal subluxation with near dislocation of thumb carpometacarpal joint. Conservative treatment of closed reduction and 4½ weeks plaster splint immobilization resulted in acceptable functional stability.

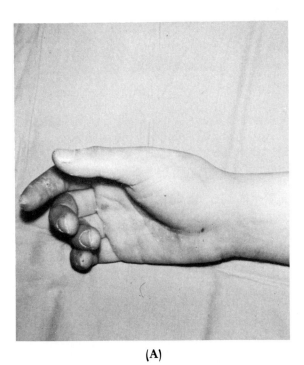

(A)

Figure 6-3 **(A)** Palmar radial view of hand accentuates an abnormal dorsal protuberance at base of thumb metacarpal. Patient sustained blunt trauma to tip of partially flexed thumb in a football game 1 week previously.

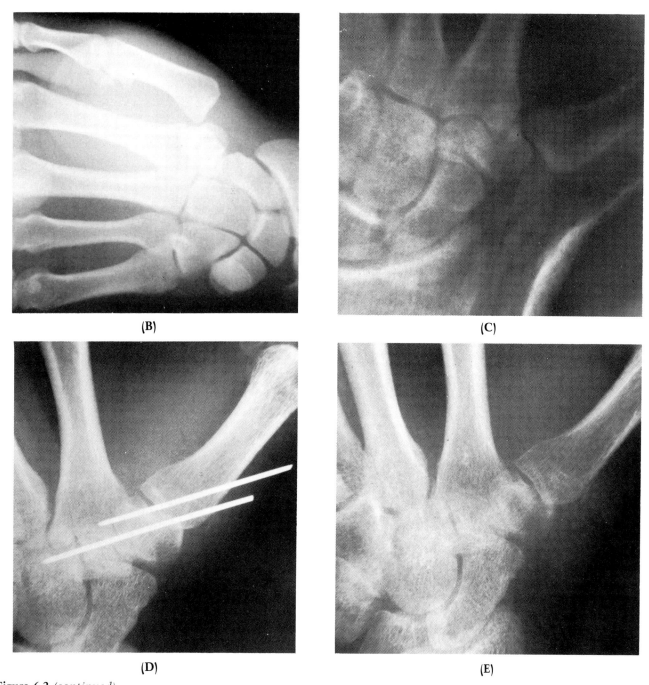

(B)

(C)

(D)

(E)

Figure 6-3 *(continued)*
(B) Radiograph shows marked dorsal subluxation and near dislocation of thumb metacarpal base at car-pometacarpal joint. **(C)** Attempted closed manipulation and reduction was unsuccessful; in lateral view persistent subluxation noted of thumb carpometacarpal joint in plaster immobilization. Operative intervention necessary to release dorsal capsule of carpometacarpal joint trapped beneath thumb metacarpal base, which prevented closed reduction. **(D)** Lateral view shows complete reduction of carpometacarpal joint subluxation after open reduction and internal temporary Kirschner wire fixation. Reconstruction of posterior oblique carpo-metacarpal ligament and dorsal capsule accomplished utilizing segment of extensor pollicis longus tendon routed through remnants of dorsal ligamentous and capsular structures on trapezium and thumb metacarpal base. **(E)** Radiograph shows maintenance of stable carpometacarpal joint after removal of temporary Kirschner wire fixation 5 weeks after open reduction and ligament reconstruction. Strong pinch and normal motion resulted.

deep ulnar carpometacarpal ligament, if technically feasible. If this ligament is irreparable, a longitudinal segment of the flexor carpi radialis tendon of insertion may be used to provide stability (Eaton procedure).[1]

If posttraumatic arthritic changes incapacitate normal function, arthrodesis of the carpometacarpal joint is indicated.

Much more common than dislocation or subluxation of the metacarpal base is extraarticular fracture of the thumb metacarpal base (proximal metaphysis) or articular displaced fracture avulsion of the thumb metacarpal palmar beak (Bennett's fracture), or a variation thereof.

Metacarpophalangeal Joint

Hyperextension Injury. This injury of the thumb MP joint may be divided into three relatively distinct categories depending on the specific ligaments damaged, which in turn is determined by the severity of injury:[2]

1. Avulsion of the palmar plate, usually proximal to the sesamoids, allowing 20° to 30° hyperextension (Figures 6-4A,B)

2. Rupture of the palmar plate and the accessory collateral ligaments of the MP joint, allowing hyperextension of 60° to 90°

3. Complete rupture of the palmar plate, the accessory collateral ligaments, and at least the greater portion of one lateral collateral ligament allowing 90° or more hyperextension

Physical examination discloses ecchymosis, hematoma, and discrete tenderness at the site of palmar plate and ligament avulsion. Pain and deformity at the site of avulsion is demonstrated on stress-testing of the joint, performed if necessary under appropriate anesthesia.

Closed reduction and immobilization for four to five weeks with the MP joint flexed 15° to 20° is recommended for the majority of hyperextension injuries.

Though more unusual, the palmar plate may rupture distal to the sesamoids, or may be accompanied by transverse fracture through the sesamoids. Avulsion of the palmar plate in these areas is generally a more severe injury since proximal migration of the sesamoids, or the proximal portions of the fractured sesamoids in that case, results due to muscle action of the oblique head of the adductor pollicis,

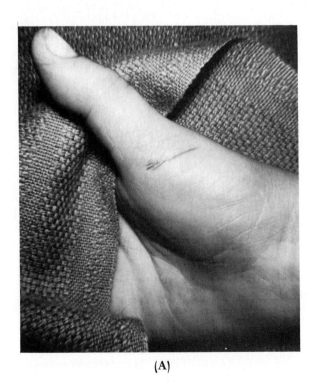

(A)

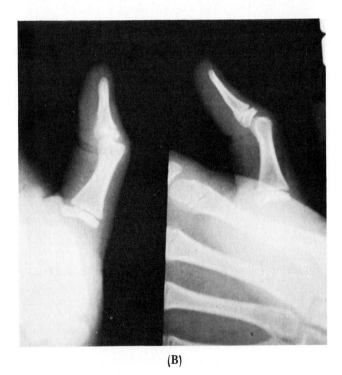

(B)

Figure 6-4 **(A)** Mild hyperextension deformity of thumb MP joint of approximately 20° to 25°. Approximately 15° of IP joint flexion is associated. **(B)** Radiograph shows a hyperextension injury with dorsal subluxation and recurvatum deformity of thumb MP joint without dislocation.

which inserts partially on the ulnar sesamoid, and of the flexor pollicis brevis, which inserts on the radial sesamoid and the base of the proximal phalanx. Careful scrutiny of the radiograph is necessary to determine whether the sesamoids are in proper anatomic relation to the base of the proximal phalanx or if they have migrated proximally. If proximal migration is marked and proximal phalangeal stability is impaired, serious consideration should be given to surgical reattachment of the palmar plate and repositioning of the proximally migrated tendons of the thenar muscles, or to reduction and fixation of the fracture fragments of the sesamoids with their appropriate attached tendons of thenar muscle insertion. If chronic instability results after conservative treatment, ligamentous reconstruction is indicated for the palmar plate and ligamentous avulsions.

Subluxation and Dislocation. Varying degrees of dorsal subluxation or complete dorsal dislocation occur as a direct result and exaggeration of a hyperextension type injury.

Complete MP joint dislocation is actually the same injury as complete dorsal subluxation, but in addition there is the exaggerated deformity of complete loss of continuity of the joint's articulation (Figures 6-5A,B). Dislocation occurs most commonly either dorsally or laterally, and it is, in fact, the most common dislocation occurring in the hand. (See section on Gamekeeper's Thumb in this chapter.) Very rarely it occurs palmarly, and then usually in an open injury.

For complete dislocation, the palmar plate must be completely ruptured transversely. This occurs most commonly at or near the proximal attachment to the metacarpal. More rarely the avulsion occurs distal to the sesamoids, and occasionally fracture avulsion occurs through the sesamoids.

Proximal palmar plate avulsion is easily documented in the skeletally mature adult on the lateral radiograph since the sesamoids retain their normal anatomic position in relation to the proximal phalanx and therefore dislocate dorsally with it (Figure 6-5B). Usually the thenar intrinsic muscles remain attached by their appropriate tendons to the

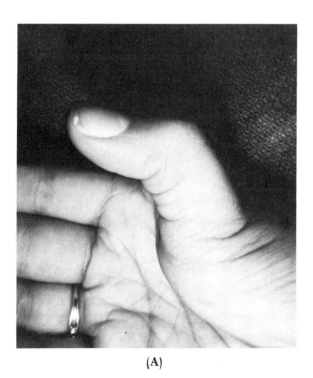
(A)

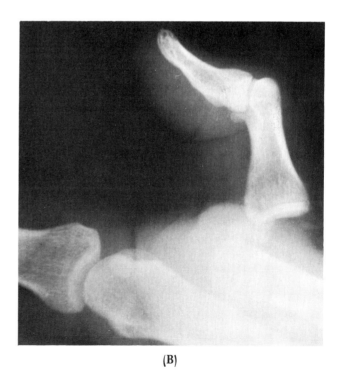
(B)

Figure 6-5 (A) Marked MP joint hyperextension of approximately 60° to 70° with a bayonet type deformity and transverse dorsal skin dimpling associated with 50° to 60° of IP joint flexion. (B) Lateral radiograph clearly shows bayonet configuration of complete dorsal dislocation of thumb proximal phalanx on metacarpal head and neck. Sesamoids are in normal anatomic relationship to proximal phalanx, which indicates rupture of MP joint palmar plate from its proximal attachment.

sesamoids (oblique head of the adductor pollicis to the ulnar sesamoid and the flexor pollicis brevis to the radial sesamoid. As the dislocation is reduced, the intrinsics help to guide the palmar plate around the metacarpal head back into its normal position and prevent its impingement within the joint. If either or both of these intrinsic muscles are avulsed from their appropriate sesamoid, or if the segments of the fractured sesamoids have displaced, or if the palmar plate has been avulsed from its distal attachment to the proximal phalangeal base, reduction will be more difficult. Surgical intervention may then be necessary to achieve reduction, to reattach an avulsed tendon or tendons, to reattach the palmar plate distal insertion, or to reduce and fix fractured sesamoids to provide satisfactory MP joint stability.

Dorsal dislocation is easily diagnosed by the characteristic deformity of dorsal and proximal displacement of the proximal phalanx on the thumb metacarpal head (Figures 6-5A,B). This bayonet type deformity is due to palmar protrusion of the thumb metacarpal condyle or condyles through a palmar plate tear or through the thenar muscles. This deformity actually results from malposition of the thumb metacarpal in its flexed adducted position; the apparent dorsal dislocation of the proximal phalanx is a secondary occurrence. As noted, the degree of proximal phalangeal hyperextension or dorsal displacement depends on the specific damage to specific ligaments (palmar plate and lateral collateral and accessory collateral ligaments). Hyperextension at the MP joint is maintained by pull of the extensor pollicis longus augmented by the thenar intrinsics which are displaced dorsally and exert traction both at their insertions on the proximal phalanx base and into the extensor aponeurosis. Interphalangeal joint flexion is primarily due to pressure of the palmarly protruding metacarpal head onto the flexor pollicis longus tendon and also to relative laxity of the extensor pollicis longus tendon across that joint.

Closed reduction is usually easily accomplished by attempting gently to reposition the metacarpal head by exerting pressure on the dorsal aspect of the base of the proximal phalanx, minimal longitudinal traction, and palmar pressure on the metacarpal head, maintaining the hyperextended deformity until reduction is achieved. After successful closed manipulation and reduction, joint ligamentous stability should be tested. Of particular importance is the integrity of both the lateral and medial collateral ligaments.

Occasionally reduction is difficult or impossible because of metacarpal head entrapment in a tear in the palmar capsule or in the thenar muscles

(oblique head of the adductor pollicis or flexor pollicis brevis). By gentle manipulation the metacarpal head may be maneuvered through the tear in the palmar plate or the muscle, but excessive longitudinal traction is contraindicated; it does nothing more than tighten the soft tissue constriction and produce a "button hole" effect about the metacarpal head, thus preventing reduction. Occasionally the palmar plate avulses distal to the sesamoids, and more rarely the flexor pollicis longus tendon becomes impinged in the dislocated joint and prevents closed reduction.

Satisfactory closed reduction is followed by immobilization of the MP joint in about 10° flexion for a period of five to six weeks to guarantee good healing of the avulsed extensor pollicis brevis insertion and the palmar plate insertion.

Surgical intervention initially or for reconstruction is indicated for:

1. Irreducible dislocation or incomplete MP joint reduction
2. Marked MP joint instability usually associated with tendon avulsion of either the oblique head of the adductor pollicis or the flexor pollicis brevis, or both
3. Displaced fractures of the sesamoids
4. Complete avulsion of a collateral ligament, usually the ulnar collateral ligament (see section on Gamekeeper's Thumb)

Surgical reconstruction through a palmar approach is advised for all the above conditions except a collateral ligament avulsion. Great care must be taken to avoid damage to either of the palmar proper digital nerves of the thumb which are protruding palmarly in their stretched position over the protruding metacarpal head in the irreducible dorsal dislocation and which are directly in the operative site. Any soft tissue impingement within the joint, such as the palmar plate or sesamoids (Figures 6-8A,B) or, rarely, the flexor pollicis longus tendon which is irreducible by closed manipulation, must be surgically exposed and extracted, with repair of the palmar plate combined with reattachment of avulsed tendons of thenar muscles as indicated. In Figures 6-8A,B, the patient sustained dorsal subluxation of the MP joint with entrapment of a sesamoid. Closed manipulation and reduction successfully released the entrapped sesamoid and reduced the MP joint subluxation (Figure 6-8B). Five years later the same lesion recurred, and closed manipulation and reduction was again successful (Figure 6-8A). It is interesting to note that the sesamoid was not visible on the radiograph of the initial injury since the cartilage anlage had not yet ossified. Stability was achieved after five weeks of conservative immobilization of the recent injury and no recurrent chronic subluxation persisted. If sesamoid subluxation should become chronic, palmar plate reconstruction, using either local tissue or a fascial or tendon graft, is necessary to prevent arthritic damage and to provide stability. (Lateral dislocations of the thumb MP joint are discussed under the next section in this chapter, Gamekeeper's Thumb.)

Acute palmar dislocation of the thumb MP joint in the acute injury has not been encountered by this author but must necessarily involve avulsion or attenuation of the extensor pollicis brevis tendon of insertion on the proximal phalanx, both lateral collateral and accessory collateral ligaments, the dorsal capsule, and possibly the palmar plate insertion. Arthrodesis is recommended for an old chronic undiagnosed or untreated MP joint dislocation (Figures 6-6A–C).

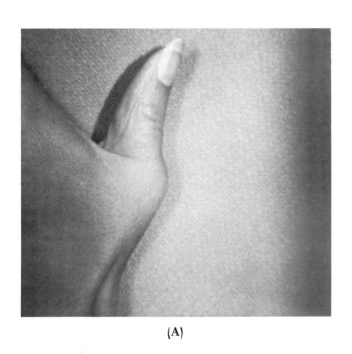

(A)

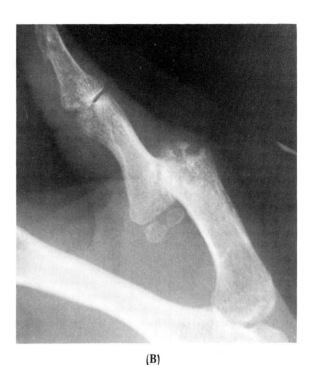

(B)

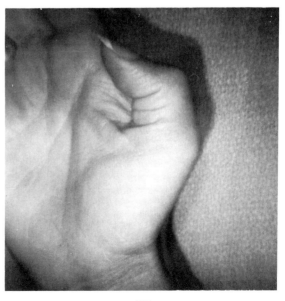

(C)

Figure 6-6 (A) Dorsal view of hand shows an abnormally short thumb, dorsal protuberance at MP joint, and hyperextension of IP joint. Injury to MP joint occurred 25 years previously but was not treated. (B) Lateral view of thumb shows an old, chronic palmar dislocation of MP joint with severe posttraumatic and degenerative arthritic changes. Protruding metacarpal head accounts for dorsal protuberance. (C) Maximum flexion of joints shows good IP flexion but no motion in MP joint area. Arthrodesis of MP joint in 30° flexion provided a stable, painless MP joint (patient's main symptoms were pain and tenderness in MP joint area). Painless strong pinch resulted.

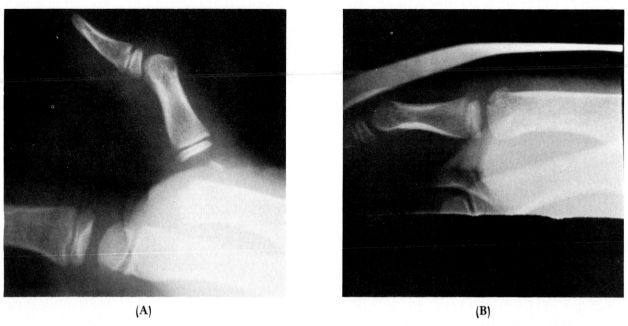

(A)   (B)

Figure 6-7 **(A)** Lateral view illustrating severe hyperextension deformity and bayonet type configuration of thumb MP joint associated with IP joint flexion. Fracture fragment dorsal to thumb metacarpal neck avulsed from defect on dorsal aspect of metacarpal head. Diagnosis: dorsal fracture subluxation of thumb MP joint. **(B)** Lateral view following closed manipulation and successful reduction of fracture subluxation shows acceptable position of both reduced articular fragment and joint.

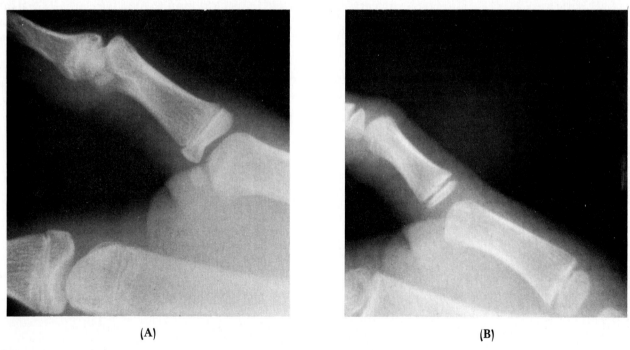

(A)   (B)

Figure 6-8 **(A)** Close-up view shows dorsal subluxation of thumb MP joint with interposition and entrapment of sesamoid. Lesion is caused by avulsion or partial avulsion of palmar plate from its metacarpal attachment. Closed manipulation successfully released trapped sesamoid and reduced MP joint subluxation. **(B)** Lateral radiograph of same patient 5 years earlier. Dorsal subluxation at MP joint is seen in this recurvatum injury, but entrapment of sesamoid and palmar plate is not visualized because sesamoid ossification was not present at that time.

Fracture dislocation of the thumb metacarpophalangeal joint is treated as fracture dislocations elsewhere (Figures 6-7A,B). If the fragment is small and irreducible, it should be excised and the ligament reconstructed. However, if the articular fragment is large and irreducible by closed means, open reduction and internal fixation should replace and fix it anatomically.

Gamekeeper's Thumb. The term *Gamekeeper's thumb* was originally associated with chronic laxity of the ulnar collateral ligament of the thumb MP joint caused by recurrent chronic pressure on the ulnar aspect of the thumb proximal phalanx in a maneuver used by British gamekeepers to kill a wild hare. Currently the term designates an acute or chronic partial or complete tear of the ulnar collateral ligament of the thumb MP joint or fracture avulsion, usually of the insertion of the ulnar collateral ligament from the base of the thumb proximal phalanx (Figures 6-12A,B).[3]

Diagnosis of this injury is made by physical findings of swelling and usually ecchymosis on the ulnar aspect of the thumb MP joint, associated with tenderness. Radiographic examination may be negative or show an avulsion fracture of the ulnar collateral ligament insertion or, more rarely, origin. If this fracture is undisplaced (Figure 6-9), conservative

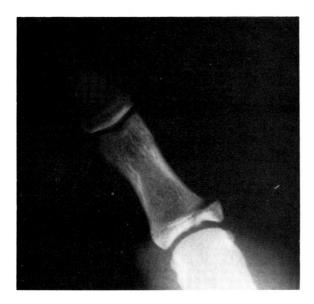

Figure 6-9 PA radiograph shows a relatively undisplaced Salter type III physeal injury extending through articular epiphysis of proximal phalanx base; ulnar collateral ligament of MP joint is attached to this relatively undisplaced fracture fragment.

immobilization for four weeks in plaster is indicated. If the fracture is displaced and irreducible, allowing marked abduction of the ulnar collateral ligament (Figures 6-10A,B), surgical exposure with anatomic repositioning and temporary internal fixation should be effected to provide good stability and the best functional result (Figures 6-10A–D). If a small avulsion fracture is noted on radiographs (Figure 6-11) or if the radiograph is negative but physical examination (under appropriate anesthesia, if necessary) discloses marked abduction of the ulnar aspect of the MP joint upon stress, surgical exploration with reattachment of the avulsed ulnar collateral ligament is strongly recommended (Figures 6-11, 6-12A,B). Only by operative intervention can the best prognosis be offered. A certain percentage of these lesions of complete ligament avulsion will heal with stability restored, but many will heal with ligament attenuation and result in some chronic joint instability. However, in many cases the ruptured distal end of the ulnar collateral ligament folds back upon itself beneath the adductor aponeurosis. Obviously healing will not be satisfactory under these conditions; at best, there will be ligamentous laxity with variable MP joint instability resulting.

Again, it is strongly advised that the completely avulsed ulnar collateral ligament be reattached into its anatomic insertion at the ulnar aspect of the proximal phalangeal base and secured by means of a pullout wire, which can be removed approximately four weeks after surgery (Figures 6-11, 6-12A,B).

If only minimal laxity is discerned on stress abduction, conservative immobilization for four to five weeks in plaster is recommended in place of surgery.

Chronic instability following chronic attenuation (laxity) or avulsion of the ulnar collateral ligament predisposes the MP joint to unnecessary posttraumatic and degenerative arthritic changes. If ligamentous reconstruction (either utilizing available tissues, if possible, or fabricating an ulnar collateral ligament from the palmaris longus or other suitable tendon) (Figures 6-13A,B), or if adductor advancement by the method of Neviaser[4] does not provide the desired asymptomatic stability, fusion of the MP joint will be necessary (Figures 6-14A,B). Primary repair of the acute rupture will prevent these difficulties and thus obviate the more sophisticated and less satisfactory reconstructions.

Rupture of the radial collateral ligament of the thumb is not as common and is caused by an adduction injury of the radial collateral ligament of the thumb MP joint (Figures 6-15A–E). Findings are the mirror image of those described for Gamekeeper's

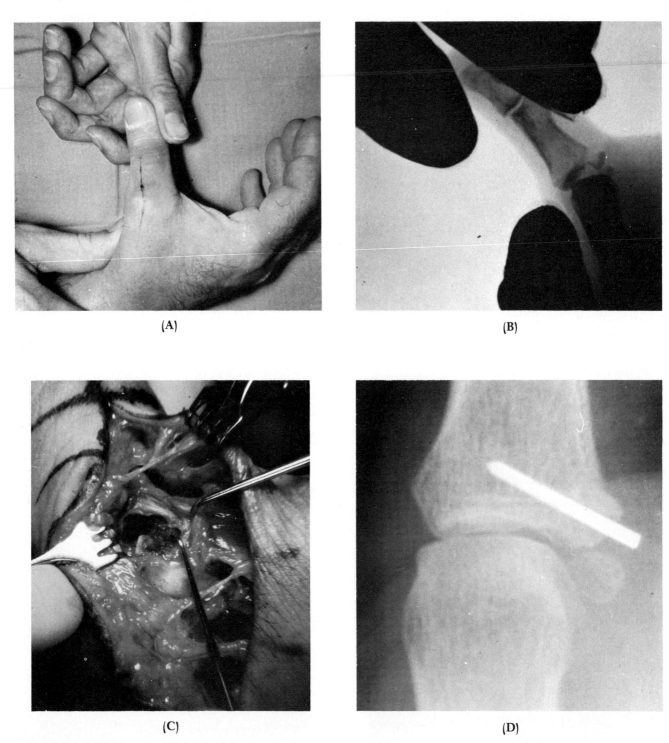

(A)

(B)

(C)

(D)

Figure 6-10 (A) Photograph shows abduction of ulnar aspect of thumb joint upon stress, indicating complete tear of ulnar collateral ligament or displaced articular fracture of proximal phalanx base at insertion of that ligament. (B) PA view shows on stressed abduction, displacement of articular fracture fragment from ulnar aspect of proximal phalanx base. Stress test of an undisplaced articular fracture, therefore, is contraindicated. (C) MP joint was exposed by dorsal chevron-type incision to anatomically replace avulsed articular fracture fragment. Close-up view at surgery shows fracture fragment pulled back inferiorly by small hook retractor. (D) PA radiograph after healing of anatomically replaced articular fracture fragment avulsion to reestablish stability of ulnar collateral ligament insertion and normal articular congruity.

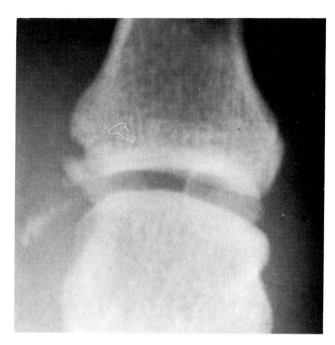

Figure 6-11 Close-up of PA radiograph of thumb MP joint illustrating small flake fracture avulsion of ulnar collateral ligament insertion. Instability necessitated surgical exposure and reinsertion of avulsed ulnar collateral ligament insertion into base of proximal phalanx by temporary pullout wire fixation, after debridement of small fracture fragment.

thumb, and treatment is the same—primary repair of the complete ligament avulsion, anatomic replacement of the fracture avulsion (Figure 6-16), and conservative immobilization for the partial ligament tear.

Partial tear of the palmar plate and occasionally of the extensor mechanism is often associated with rupture of either the ulnar or radial collateral ligament. At the time of surgical exploration and ligament repair, reconstruction of associated ligament or tendon damage should be performed.

Interphalangeal Joint

Thumb interphalangeal joint subluxation and dislocation are rather uncommon and usually occur dorsally (Figure 6-17). Lateral and palmar dislocation most often accompany open wounds. Palmar dislocation or subluxation also may occur with a drop finger of the thumb distal phalanx secondary to a large displaced articular fracture in association with the insertion of the extensor pollicis longus tendon. (See section on Drop Finger Injuries in Chapter 8, Phalangeal Fractures.)

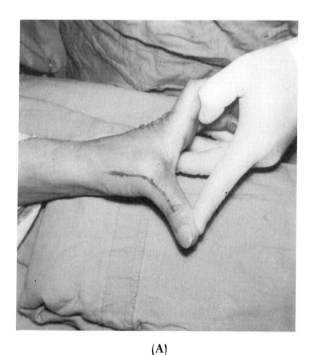

(A)

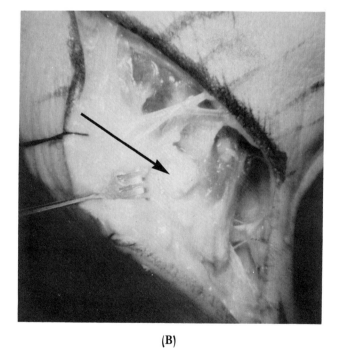

(B)

Figure 6-12 (A) Marked abduction of thumb MP joint upon stress under anesthesia. (B) Close-up of surgical exposure shows completely avulsed ulnar collateral ligament insertion. Ligament was reinserted and fixed into proximal phalanx base by temporary pullout wire fixation.

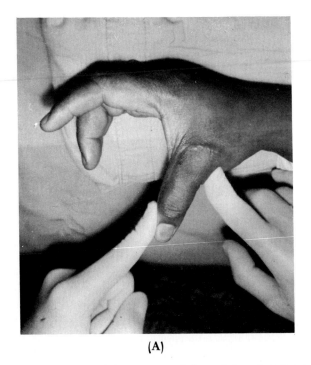
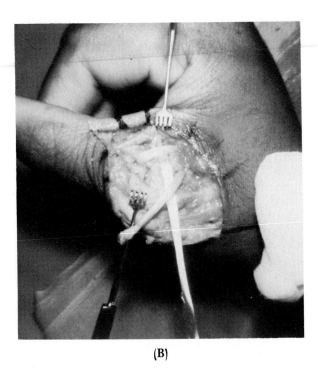

(A)   (B)

Figure 6-13 **(A)** Abduction instability of thumb MP joint on stress evaluation under anesthesia. Note dorsal scar at site of unsuccessful previous attempt at surgical reconstruction of chronic ulnar collateral ligament avulsion utilizing local tissues. **(B)** Close-up dorsal view showing reconstruction of ulnar collateral ligament by threading of palmaris longus tendon in a figure-of-eight fashion through transverse drill holes in proximal phalanx base and ulnar aspect of thumb metacarpal metaphysis.

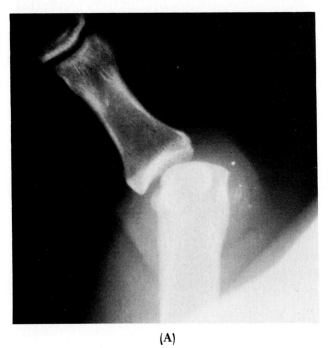
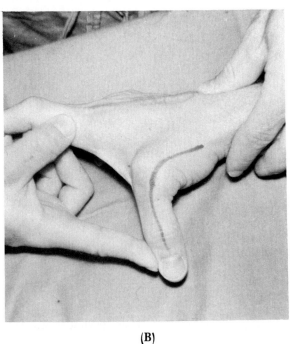

(A)   (B)

Figure 6-14 **(A)** Radiograph of chronic Gamekeeper's thumb with chronic ulnar collateral ligament laxity. Note degenerative arthritic changes of metacarpal head and calcifications in soft tissue on ulnar aspect at area of ligament trauma. **(B)** Photograph shows severe chronic abduction laxity on stress under anesthesia. After failure of an adductor advancement procedure due to persistent pain, thumb MP joint was fused.

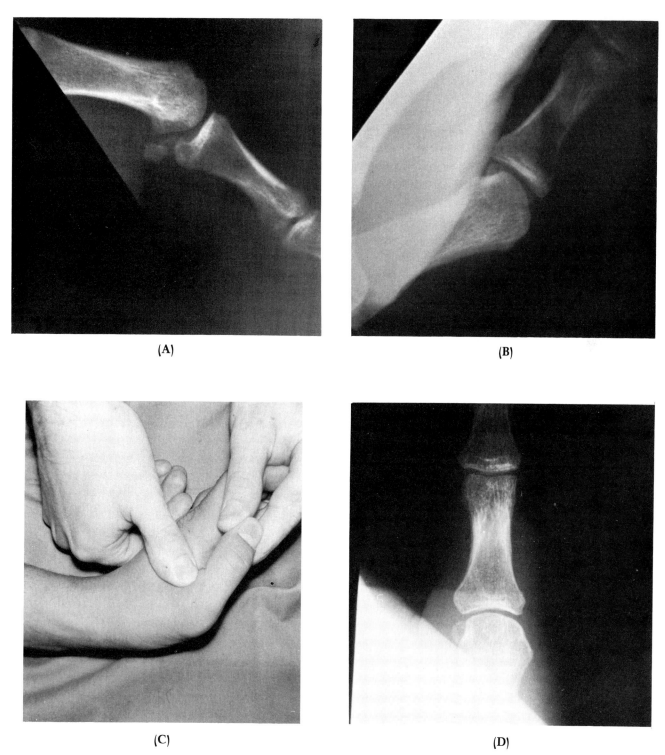

Figure 6-15 **(A)** Lateral radiograph of thumb MP joint area in 18-year-old football player who sustained adduction injury. Some palmar subluxation of proximal phalanx and incomplete active extension is evident. **(B)** PA view with stressed adduction of thumb MP joint shows significant ligamentous laxity. **(C)** Marked radial instability of thumb MP joint on stressed adduction. **(D)** PA radiograph after surgical reinsertion of radial collateral ligament into radial aspect of thumb proximal phalanx base and reconstruction of extensor pollicis brevis insertion and dorsal MP joint capsule.

(continued)

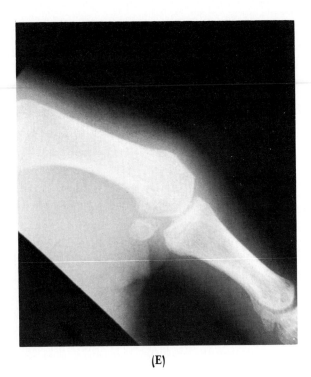

(E)

Figure 6-15 *(continued)*
(E) Lateral radiograph shows normal anatomy of thumb MP joint with correction of previous palmar subluxation. Excellent stability and nearly normal MP joint flexion and extension resulted.

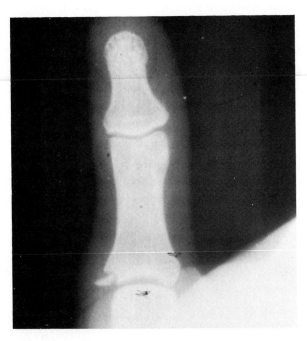

Figure 6-16 Radiograph of thumb MP joint showing 3-week-old fracture avulsion of radial collateral ligament insertion into thumb proximal phalanx base. Not treated because of long interval since injury. If seen shortly after injury, surgical reconstruction would have prevented ligamentous laxity due to the 90° rotation and proximal displacement of fracture fragment.

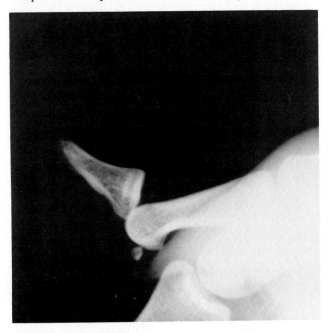

Figure 6-17 Lateral view of closed, complete dorsal dislocation of thumb IP joint. Note sesamoid position indicating rupture of palmar plate from insertion on base of distal phalanx. Note sesamoid remains with the palmar plate.

Thumb interphalangeal joint subluxation or dislocation results from severe trauma which often may cause an open wound either by direct or torsional injury. In the dorsal hyperextension injury the palmar plate may rupture either at its attachment to the base of the distal phalanx or from its proximal phalangeal attachment. The extensor pollicis longus tendon is rarely avulsed from its insertion. Reduction by simple manipulation and traction is not difficult, but occasionally subluxation persists because of entrapment of a proximally avulsed palmar plate which remains in the joint at the time of reduction. The flexor pollicis longus rarely becomes entrapped. If palmar plate interposition is diagnosed, a palmar surgical approach allows extraction of the structure with repair.

Dorsal fracture subluxation or dislocation of the thumb interphalangeal joint may be treated in a fashion similar to the dorsal fracture subluxation of the PIP joint of other digits (Figures 6-18A–C). In the palmar approach, the palmar plate is exposed after partial removal of the flexor sheath and retraction of the flexor pollicis longus tendon. The palmar plate is detached at its distal insertion and on each side to permit proximal retraction, like a trap door, to enable

Figure 6-18 (A) Lateral radiograph of diffusely swollen thumb, which could be actively flexed 15° to 20° at IP joint, shows dorsal subluxation of that joint due to an unstable comminuted fracture of palmar aspect of distal phalangeal articular surface. (B) Lateral view after removal of comminuted fracture fragments, reduction of dorsal fracture subluxation, palmar plate advancement, and temporary Kirschner wire fixation of IP joint in 20° flexion. (C) Lateral view 7 weeks after surgery and removal of pullout wire and temporary Kirschner wire fixation shows maintenance of IP joint reduction by palmar plate advancement, which is securely fixed into palmar indentation of distal phalangeal base from which comminuted fracture fragments had been removed. Asymptomatic stable, active flexion of 45° IP joint range of motion was achieved.

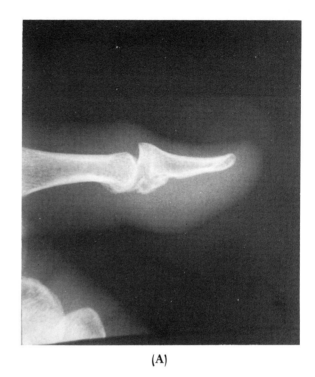

(A)

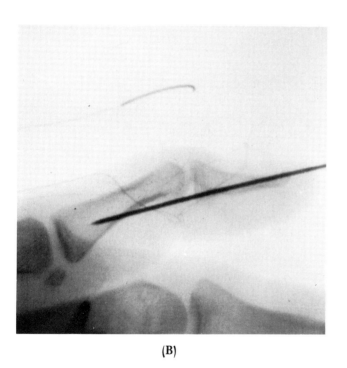

(B)

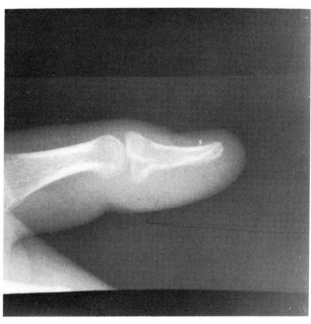

(C)

joint irrigation, fracture reduction, or removal of small fracture fragments accompanied by palmar plate advancement. (See description of this procedure under the section on fracture subluxation of the PIP joint in Chapter 9.)

Open dislocation of the thumb IP joint is treated like any open dislocation by meticulous wound toilet prior to definitive reduction, often along with temporary Kirschner wire fixation. In Figures 6-19A–C, an open IP joint dislocation, initial treatment included meticulous cleansing, irrigation, debridement, and loose skin approximation, with no attempt at any primary deep repairs. Viability was maintained solely by a segment of dorsoradial skin

Figure 6-19 (A) A massive saw avulsion injury to thumb IP joint area caused this open IP joint dislocation. (B) Corresponding radiograph shows complete interphalangeal joint dislocation. Findings at surgery included avulsive loss of flexor pollicis longus and extensor pollicis longus tendons, proper neurovascular bundle on ulnar aspect of the thumb, ulnar collateral ligament and capsule of IP joint. (C) Complete extension is shown here 3 months after injury.

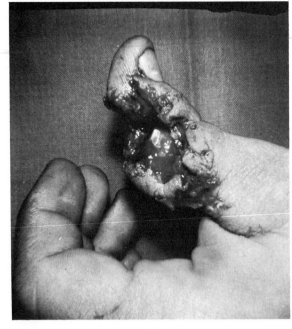

(A)

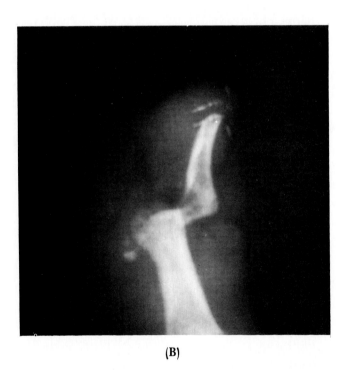

(B)

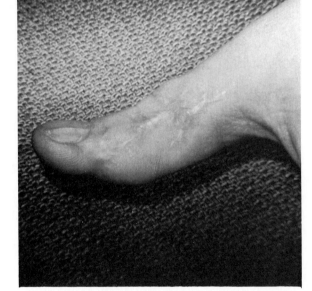

(C)

and a severely contused proper neurovascular bundle on the radial aspect. Complete functional thumb length was maintained and, remarkably, protective sensation was sufficient to obviate a reconstructive nerve graft. Active, stable flexion of 20° to 25° resulted from scarring of the flexor pollicis longus tendon. No secondary graft of either the long thumb flexor or extensor or ligament was necessary.

If it is possible to do so without either additional vascular compromise or surgical exposure, a collateral ligament avulsion may be repaired. If the flexor pollicis longus tendon has been avulsed, it may be repaired at this time. However, if there is any danger of additional vascular compromise (either through prolonged surgery, additional dissection, or a vascularly compromising postoperative immobilization), tendon or ligament reconstruction should be carried out as a delayed primary or secondary procedure, depending upon the status of the injured digit's vascularity and the presence or absence of any complications of wound healing.

Fractures

Metacarpal Fractures

Fractures of the thumb metacarpal usually occur at the base, either in the metaphysis or articularly. Frac-

tures of the metaphysis are either transverse or oblique, and in the skeletally immature person physeal separation occurs. Articular fractures include the palmar beak alone (Bennett's fracture, the palmar beak and the dorsal aspect in a "Y" or "T" fashion (Rolando fracture), or a markedly comminuted articular fracture of the metacarpal base. The classification proposed by Green[5] is excellent (Figure 6-20).

Proximal Metaphyseal Fractures, Including Physeal Separation. Transverse fractures of the thumb metacarpal proximal metaphysis which are minimally

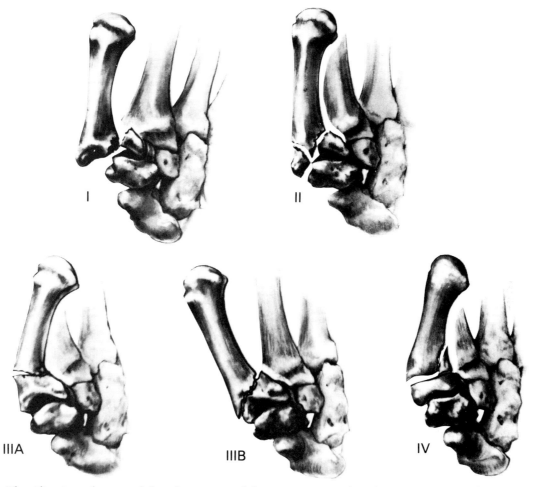

Figure 6-20 Classification of types of thumb metacarpal fractures (Green classification): **I**—Typical Bennett's fracture subluxation of the thumb metacarpal base. The fragment of the palmar beak of the thumb metacarpal remains in its normal anatomic position, and the thumb metacarpal is proximally displaced and adducted, primarily because of action of the abductor pollicis longus. **II**—A comminuted, essentially undisplaced fracture of Rolando consists of fracture of the palmar beak and dorsal lip of the thumb metacarpal base. **III-A**—A transverse fracture of the proximal thumb metacarpal metaphysis with characteristic palmar angulation. **III-B**—An oblique fracture of the thumb metacarpal proximal phalanx with some proximal displacement. **IV**—The characteristic traumatic physeal separation of the thumb metacarpal in a skeletally immature patient, which usually is a Salter type II configuration associated with palmar angulation, ulnar displacement, or both. *(Reprinted, by permission, from David P. Green, M.D., Fractures of the thumb metacarpal, S Med J, 65:807, 1972.)*[5]

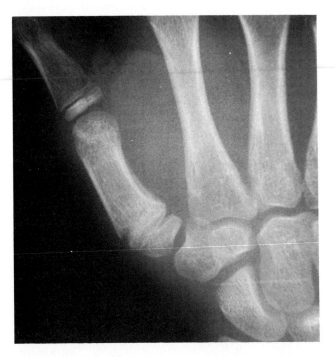

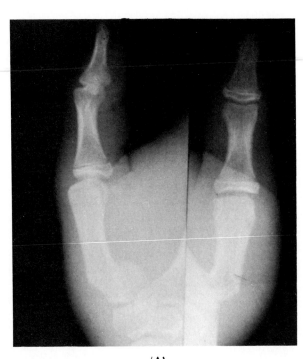

(A)

Figure 6-21 Transverse proximal metaphyseal fracture of thumb metacarpal with 20° to 30° palmar angulation at fracture site.

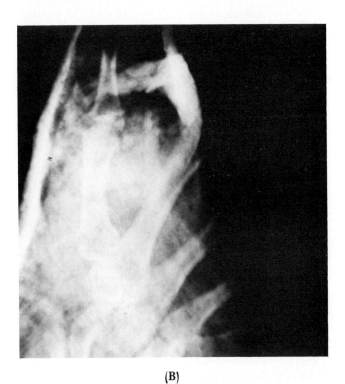

(B)

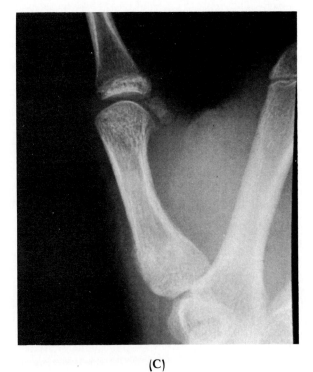

(C)

Figure 6-22 (A) More severe manifestation of transverse proximal metaphyseal fracture showing 50° palmar angulation deformity. (B) Lateral view following closed manipulation and reduction with immobilization of thumb metacarpal in physiologic position of extension, abduction, and opposition. (C) After complete healing. Immobilization was maintained for 5 weeks to prevent recurrence of angulation deformity.

angulated or minimally displaced need no reduction but if stable, should be immobilized for four weeks in a short arm-thumb spica cast or plaster splint which includes the wrist and forearm (Figure 6-21).

Angulation characteristically occurs palmarly (Figure 6-22A) due to the stong pull of the thenar intrinsic muscles augmented by the flexor pollicis longus. If displacement occurs, the adductor pollicis causes ulnar or medial displacement of the proximal metacarpal shaft distal to the fracture site. Closed manipulation and reduction is generally successful if angulation is unaccompanied by displacement (Figure 6-22B), but immobilization should be continued for a minimum of four weeks to insure that

angulation does not recur due to the excessive deforming factors (Figure 6-22C).

Though reduction of the angulated fracture is recommended, persistent moderate palmar angulation, either recurring after reduction (Figures 6-23A–C) or appearing in cases diagnosed late, does not usually cause functional disability. Likewise, some medial angulation or displacement of the proximal metacarpal shaft (adduction) will not limit physiologic thumb metacarpal functioning if allowed to persist (Figures 6-24A–C).

If stable reduction is not maintained by closed methods, marked unstable medial displacement and/or palmar angulation of the metacarpal metaphysis is best treated by closed reduction and

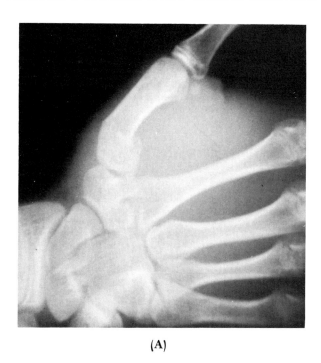

(A)

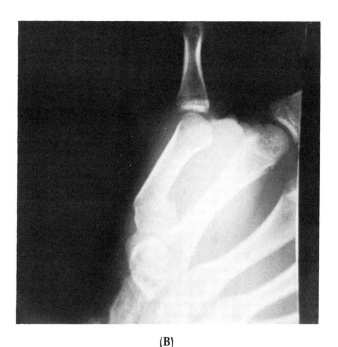

(B)

Figure 6-23 (A) A 35° flexion angulation of transverse proximal metaphyseal fracture of thumb metacarpal. (B) A 45° angulation recurred because of premature discontinuation of immobilization after successful closed fracture manipulation and reduction. (C) Normal thumb-index web (injured hand, left) with normal thumb opposition despite healing of fracture in palmar angulation.

(C)

Figure 6-24 **(A)** Lateral view of transverse fracture of thumb metacarpal proximal metaphysis. **(B)** PA view following closed manipulation and partial reduction of adduction displacement and palmar angulation. Some residual ulnar displacement persists at fracture site. **(C)** Comparable abduction of both thumb metacarpals noted 10 weeks after original injury (injured thumb, left).

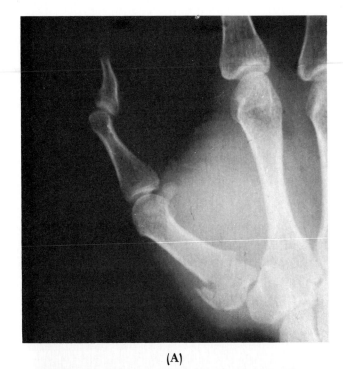

(A)

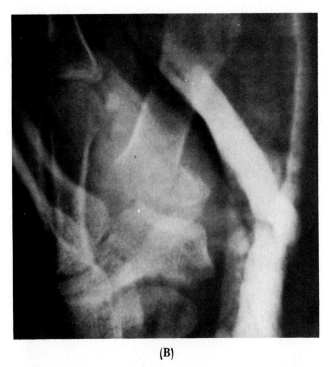

(B)

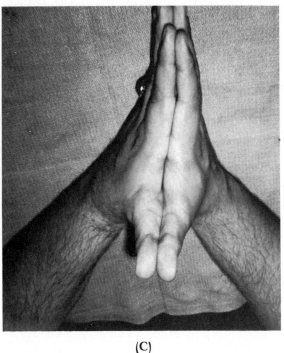

(C)

percutaneous Kirschner wire fixation of the thumb metacarpal to adjacent index and/or long metacarpals or the carpus (Figures 6-25A–D). An unstable physeal separation should be treated in a similar manner for the best result (Figures 6-26A–D).

Oblique fracture of the thumb metacarpal proximal metaphysis may be relatively stable (Figures 6-27A,B) or may be complicated by unacceptable proximal displacement or slipping of the metacarpal on this small proximal fragment, with impingement on the carpometacarpal joint (Figure 6-28A).

If proximal migration or displacement of the thumb metacarpal is excessive, there will be impingement upon the carpometacarpal joint, causing

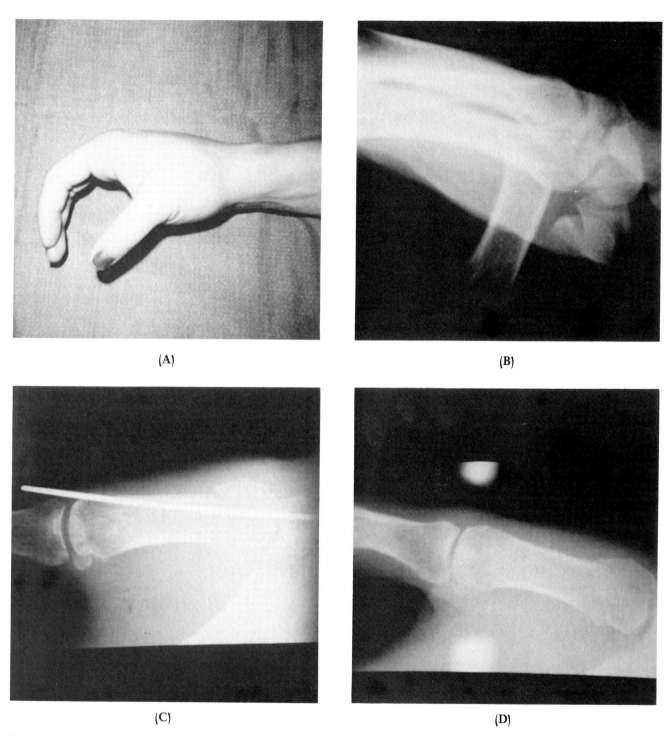

(A)

(B)

(C)

(D)

Figure 6-25 **(A)** Marked swelling of the radial aspect of the hand with adduction of the thumb metacarpal base, seen two days after severe closed crush injury of the hand with no evidence, however, of a closed compartment syndrome. **(B)** Corresponding PA radiograph of the thumb shows extreme displacement and adduction at the transverse fracture of the thumb metacarpal base. **(C)** Closed reduction and single percutaneous longitudinal Kirschner wire fixation provided stability. **(D)** Excellent healing occurred, as noted, three months after injury.

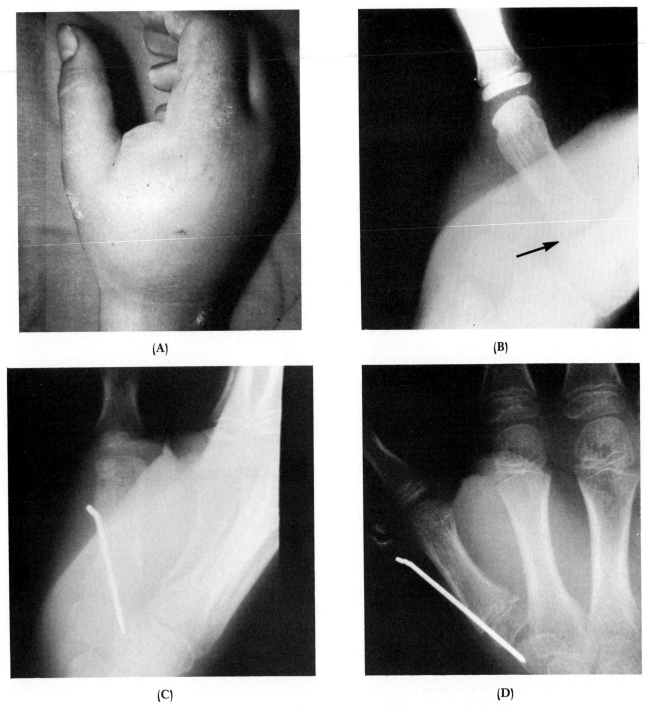

(A)

(B)

(C)

(D)

Figure 6-26 **(A)** Marked edema of entire hand centered about thumb-index web space. **(B)** PA view of a complete ulnar displacement with adduction deformity of metacarpal shaft through a Salter II physeal separation of the thumb metacarpal. **(C)** PA view following closed manipulation and reduction of physeal separation with percutaneous Kirschner wire fixation. Initial successful closed manipulation and reduction redisplaced while in plaster immobilization. **(D)** Lateral radiograph.

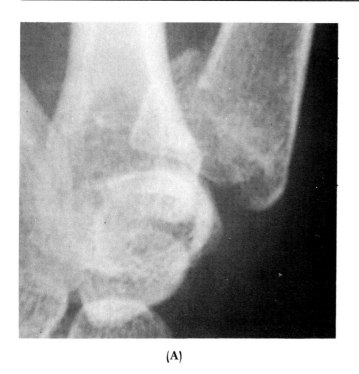

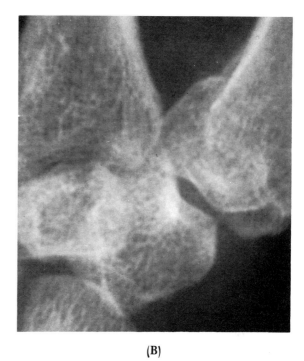

(A)   (B)

Figure 6-27 **(A)** Oblique, somewhat proximally displaced fracture of thumb metacarpal base noted on close-up lateral view of thumb metacarpal. Diagnosis: oblique extraarticular fracture of the thumb metacarpal base. Compare to Figure 6-30, a displaced articular fracture of thumb metacarpal base (Bennett's fracture). **(B)** Lateral radiograph 4½ weeks after injury illustrates maintenance of position at fracture site with no further proximal displacement of thumb metacarpal shaft and an essentially normal trapezium-thumb metacarpal joint. Treated by thumb spica cast immobilization.

restricted motion and secondary arthritic changes. If reduction is unstable, percutaneous Kirschner wire fixation is a quite acceptable method to maintain the closed reduction (Figures 6-28A–C).

In the elderly, particularly the senile, some carpometacarpal overriding by the proximally displaced metacarpal shaft after closed manipulation and reduction may be preferable to surgery (Figures 6-29A,B).

Proper positioning of the thumb metacarpal in wide abduction and opposition during immobilization after closed manipulation and reduction, or after closed manipulation and percutaneous Kirschner wire fixation, *is of the utmost importance.*

It is also most important to differentiate an oblique proximal metaphyseal fracture which is extraarticular (Figure 6-27A) from a Bennett's fracture with a large palmar fragment (Figure 6-30). The former may usually be treated adequately by closed manipulation, reduction, and immobilization for four weeks (Figures 6-27A, B), but the latter often requires fixation of some type (Figures 6-32A–C), such as percutaneous Kirschner wire stabilization, after closed manipulation and reduction. (Refer to section on Articular Fractures in this chapter.)

Articular Fractures

Bennett's Fracture. This is an articular fracture through the palmar lip of the thumb metacarpal base. The undisplaced or minimally displaced fracture (Figures 6-31A,B) is treated by immobilization in the physiologic position in a thumb spica cast or suitable plaster splint for four weeks. Emphasis is placed on taking serial radiographs (Figures 6-31A,B) at seven- to ten-day intervals to be certain that the position at the fracture site is not lost.

Displacement of a Bennett's fracture includes proximal displacement or retraction of the entire thumb metacarpal away from the small palmar beak, which remains in normal anatomic position owing to the integrity of its stong, deep ulnar ligament firmly attached to the deep intercarpal ligaments and to the crest of the trapezium (Figures 6-30, 6-32B). (Refer to section on Carpometacarpal Joint in this chapter.) The strong pull of the abductor pollicis longus muscle proximally displaces the metacarpal shaft, and displacement is augmented by the transverse pull exerted by the transverse head of the adductor pollicis on the distal metacarpal. To achieve

Figure 6-28 **(A)** Proximally displaced oblique fracture of thumb metacarpal base is seen on lateral radiograph of thumb metacarpal. Impingement of dorsal aspect of thumb metacarpal shaft on trapezium required reduction. However, original closed manipulation and reduction redisplaced during external immobilization. **(B)** Lateral radiograph after closed manipulation, reduction, and percutaneous Kirschner wire fixation of reduced metacarpal shaft to adjacent index metacarpal shaft. **(C)** Lateral radiograph 6 weeks after injury shows healed fracture following removal of Kirschner wire.

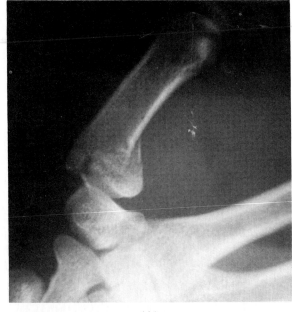

(A)

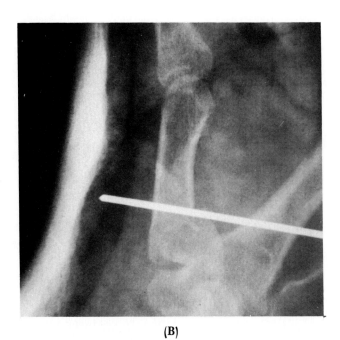

(B)

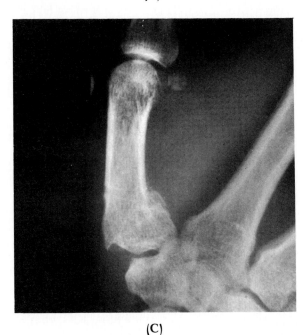

(C)

reduction, the thumb metacarpal must be replaced by longitudinal traction into its proper anatomic position in relation to the small undisplaced palmar beak fragment.

If closed reduction of the displaced fracture is satisfactory, some surgeons advocate thumb spica cast immobilization in the physiologic position, with particular emphasis on molding the cast at the metacarpal base to maintain proper position. Radiographs at seven- to ten-day intervals are essential to diagnose any redisplacement (Figures 6-33A,B).

For an unstable Bennett's fracture, percutaneous Kirschner wire fixation of the metacarpal base to the adjacent carpus or stable metacarpals (index and/or long finger metacarpals) is advocated after acceptable closed reduction has been achieved (Figures 6-32A–C).

If acceptable reduction is impossible by closed manipulation, then open reduction and either percutaneous Kirschner wire fixation or internal Kirschner wire fixation is recommended. Usually, however, open reduction is not necessary to restore

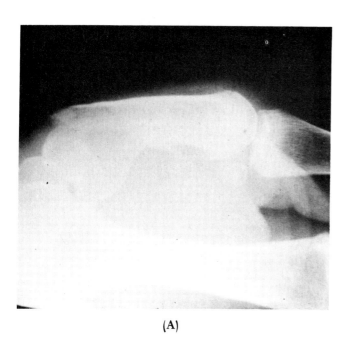

(A)

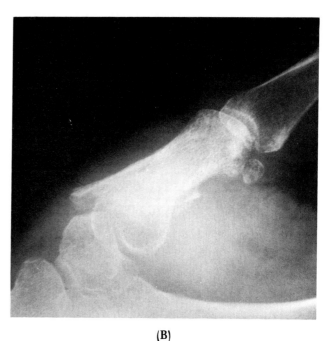

(B)

Figure 6-29 **(A)** Lateral radiograph of thumb metacarpal shows flexion deformity and slight proximal displacement of oblique fracture of thumb metacarpal base in 80-year-old man. **(B)** Lateral radiograph after healing 6 weeks following injury shows some impingement of dorsal metacarpal shaft on trapezium. Malunion was preferable to subjecting this elderly patient to surgery.

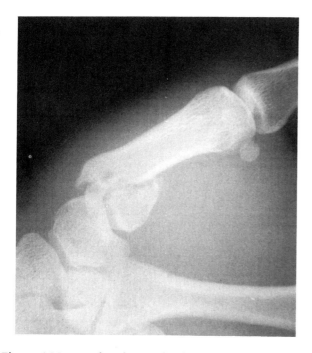

Figure 6-30 Displaced articular fracture of thumb metacarpal base with large palmar fragment (Bennett's fracture). This case should be compared to the extraarticular fracture noted in Figures 6-27A,B.

acceptable congruity to the proximal metacarpal articular surface.

For the symptomatic undiagnosed or untreated Bennett's fracture with posttraumatic changes, arthrodesis of the carpometacarpal joint is advised in the young, physically active person (Figure 6-34). In the middle-aged person, or if the scaphotrapezial joint is involved with degenerative or posttraumatic changes, excision of the trapezium and silastic implant arthroplasty is preferred.

It is unusual to encounter an old undiagnosed Bennett's fracture dislocation which is essentially asymptomatic (Figure 6-35). Even with marked proximal metacarpal displacement and metacarpal adduction, reconstruction is usually not advised at that late date.

Bennett's Fracture of the Little Finger Metacarpal. A mirror image of the Bennett's type fracture of the thumb may occur at the little finger metacarpal base (Figures 6-36, 6-37A,C). Proximal displacement of the entire little finger metacarpal results by proximal pull of the extensor carpi ulnaris insertion augmented by

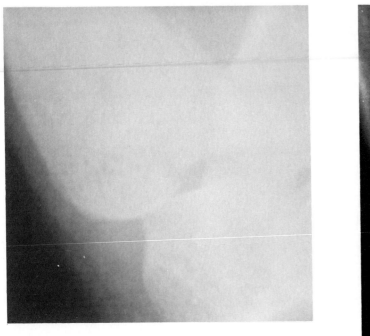

(A)

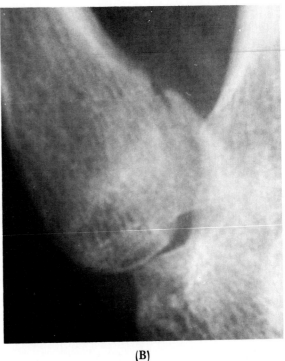

(B)

Figure 6-31 (A) Lateral radiograph of thumb metacarpal shows a minimally displaced Bennett's fracture of thumb metacarpal palmar beak 1 week after injury. Original satisfactory position is seen to be maintained at this most important radiographic reevaluation. (B) Healed fracture is noted on similar radiograph 5 weeks after initial injury, with good position maintained.

the deforming pull of distal prolongations of fibers of the flexor carpi ulnaris insertion (Figure 6-37C).[6]

Conservative immobilization for four weeks is all that is necessary in the undisplaced or relatively undisplaced fracture, but it should involve both the little and ring fingers out to the tips with MP joints flexed and the wrist slightly extended (Figure 6-36).

Successful closed manipulation and reduction of a displaced similar type fracture can be treated in the same manner, but if the fracture is unstable, percutaneous Kirschner wire fixation of the little finger metacarpal transversely to adjacent metacarpals is most effective (Figures 6-37A–D). Open reduction and percutaneous Kirschner wire or internal fixation is advisable if satisfactory closed reduction is impossible.

In undiagnosed or inadequately treated fractures in this area, posttraumatic arthritic changes are inevitable (Figure 6-38), as in Bennett's fracture of the thumb. Carpometacarpal arthrodesis of the little finger metacarpal base to the hamate is indicated if symptoms are severe enough.

Rolando's Fracture. Fracture of Rolando of the thumb metacarpal base involves fracture both of the palmar beak and of the dorsal aspect of the metacarpal base in a "T" or "Y" fashion (Figures 6-39A,B, 6-40A, 6-41A). If this fracture is undisplaced, conservative immobilization in the physiologic position suffices (Figures 6-39A,B). If, however, distortion of the carpometacarpal joint occurs, any method which reasonably restores the articulation is acceptable. Methods include open reduction and Kirschner wire fixation if the fragments are large enough, open or closed reduction with percutaneous Kirschner wire fixation of the thumb metacarpal in the physiologic position (Figures 6-40A–C), or dynamic skeletal traction to retain reduction by means of a transverse Kirschner wire through the proximal phalanx (Figures 6-41A–C).

The discriminating study of radiographs of any fracture of the thumb metacarpal base prior to treatment is most important to determine if the fracture is articular or extraarticular and how much comminution is present. Only after these conditions have been

Figure 6-32 (A) Lateral radiograph of displaced Bennett's fracture after closed reduction and percutaneous Kirschner wire fixation shows thumb metacarpal shaft reduced to palmar beak fragment and immobilized to adjacent carpus. (B) Close-up of unstable displaced fracture prior to treatment shows proximal displacement of thumb metacarpal shaft from normal anatomically situated articular fragment of palmar beak. (C) Note congruous articular surfaces of trapezium and of thumb metacarpal base 4½ weeks after initiation of treatment.

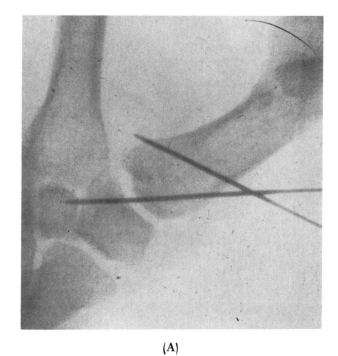

(A)

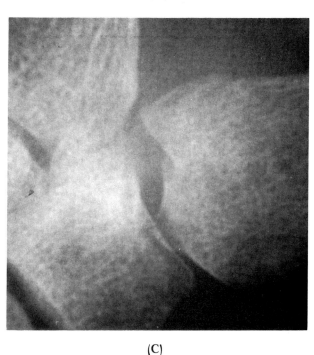

(B)   (C)

determined can effective treatment and immobilization be provided, incorporating either:

1. Closed manipulation and reduction with or without percutaneous Kirschner wire fixation

2. Open reduction with percutaneous or internal Kirschner wire fixation
3. Closed reduction with dynamic skeletal traction immobilization
4. Open reduction and skeletal fixation

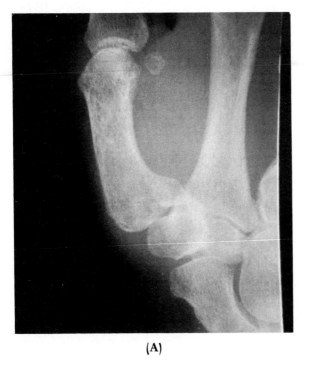
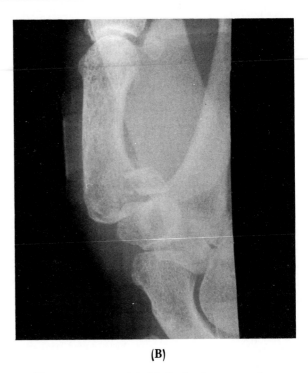

(A)   (B)

Figure 6-33 (A) Minimally displaced Bennett's fracture in 45-year-old woman treated initially by improper, inadequate aluminum splint immobilization. (B) Displacement of fracture is evident 4½ weeks later. Inadequate initial treatment compounded by lack of proper serial radiographic evaluations at 7- to 10-day intervals to document maintenance of reduction or to facilitate diagnosis and appropriate treatment of instability and displacement of the fracture which developed.

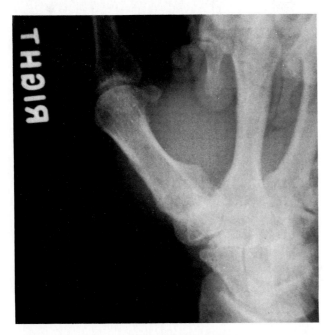
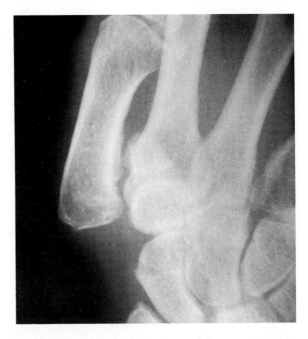

Figure 6-34 The alternative to painful traumatic arthritis of thumb carpometacarpal joint at the stage seen in Figure 6-33(B) is arthrodesis, shown here in lateral radiograph of thumb carpometacarpal area.

Figure 6-35 Marked adduction and proximal displacement of thumb metacarpal in untreated Bennett's fracture dislocation sustained 20 years earlier. Although this patient had a marked thumb-index web contracture, he was relatively asymptomatic.

Figure 6-36 Undisplaced articular fracture of little finger metacarpal base which may be designated a Bennett's type fracture of little finger metacarpal base. Fracture is mirror image of Bennett's fracture of thumb metacarpal base.

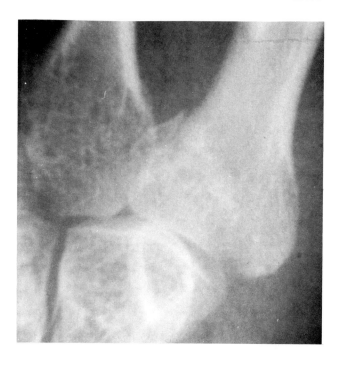

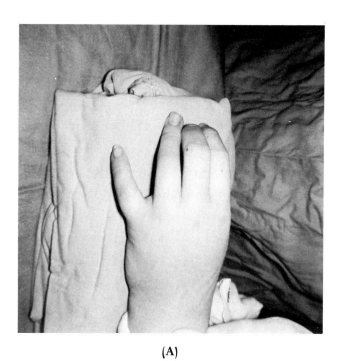

(A)

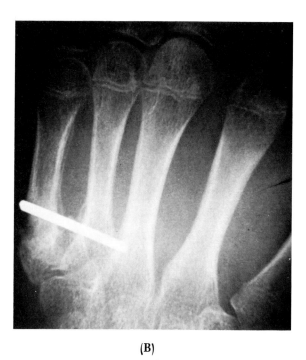

(B)

Figure 6-37 **(A)** Generalized swelling of hand with abduction of little finger in area of proximal phalanx base in 12-year-old girl. Gross appearance of injury would suggest traumatic physeal separation of little finger proximal phalanx. **(B)** PA view following manipulation, reduction, and percutaneous Kirschner wire fixation of reduced little finger metacarpal shaft to adjacent ring and long finger metacarpals.

(continued)

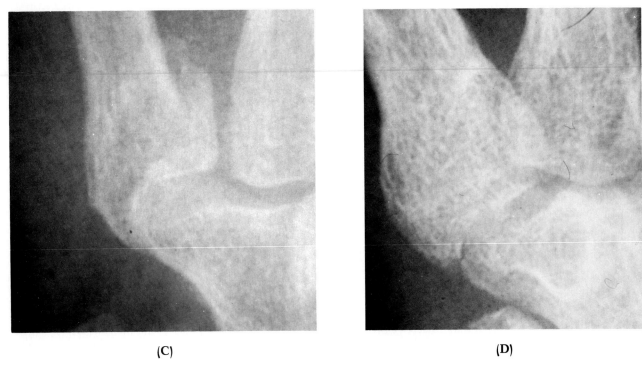

(C)   (D)

Figure 6-37 *(continued)*
(C) Close-up of displaced articular fracture of little finger metacarpal base prior to treatment illustrates proximal displacement of little finger metacarpal shaft away from normal position of radial beak of metacarpal by extensor carpi ulnaris. **(D)** Close-up of fracture after healing, about 5 weeks following reduction and percutaneous Kirschner wire immobilization. Note essentially normal hamate–little finger metacarpal articulation. Normal anatomy of little finger in relation to other digits and normal flexion and extension of all joints restored.

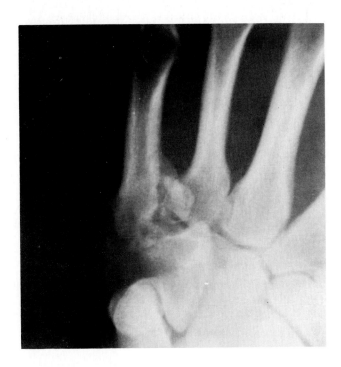

Figure 6-38 PA view of untreated proximally displaced Bennett's type fracture dislocation of fifth metacarpal base sustained 10 weeks previously, with secondary posttraumatic and degenerative arthritic changes of hamate–fifth metacarpal joint. Carpometacarpal fusion is indicated if symptoms warrant.

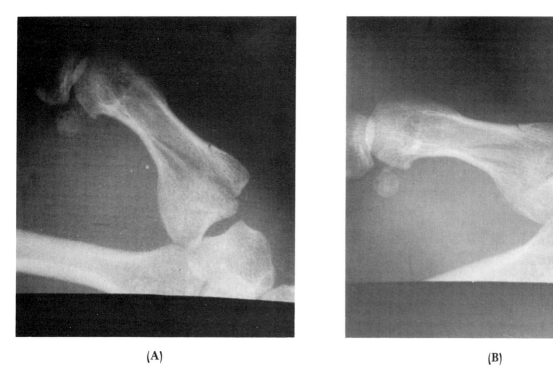

(A) (B)

Figure 6-39 (A) Lateral radiograph of comminuted fracture of Rolando of thumb metacarpal base shows fracture of palmar beak and dorsal aspect of thumb metacarpal base, both undisplaced. (B) A different view of same case shows extensive fracture comminution.

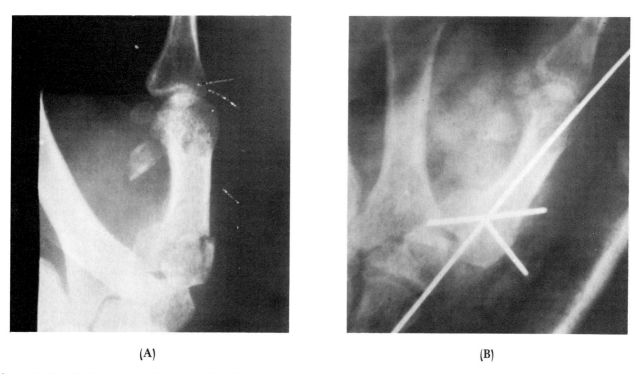

(A) (B)

Figure 6-40 (A) Comminuted, proximally displaced fracture of Rolando of thumb metacarpal base. (B) Same case after open reduction and Kirschner wire fixation of larger fragment and temporary percutaneous longitudinal Kirschner wire fixation of reduced thumb metacarpal to carpus.

(continued)

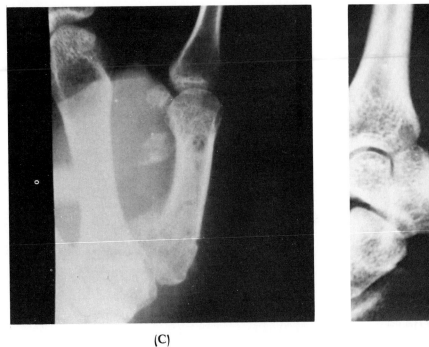

(C)

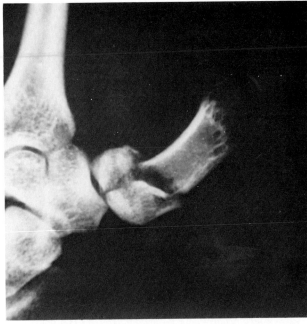

(A)

Figure 6-40 *(continued)*
(C) Lateral radiograph 6 weeks following surgery and removal of Kirschner wires. *(Illustrations 6-40(A–C) courtesy of R.G. Eaton, M.D.)*

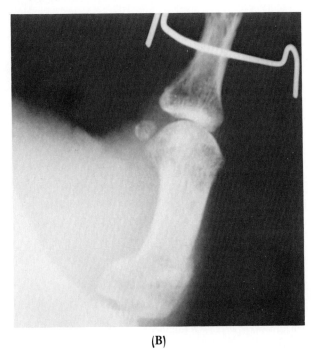

(B)

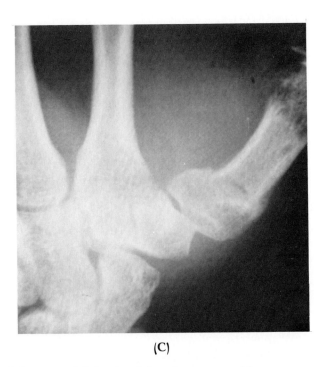

(C)

Figure 6-41 **(A)** Extensively comminuted proximally displaced fracture of Rolando of thumb metacarpal base. **(B)** PA radiograph following closed manipulation and transverse dynamic skeletal wire traction exerted through proximal phalanx. Note good joint space between trapezium and thumb metacarpal base. **(C)** Same case after healing of fractures 5 weeks following application of dynamic skeletal traction. Good joint space maintained between the trapezium and the thumb metacarpal base.

Fractures in the Vicinity of the Thumb MP Joint

Fractures of the distal thumb metacarpal are rare. Exceptions are an uncommon fracture avulsion of a metacarpophalangeal joint collateral ligament origin or an articular fracture of the metacarpal head usually associated with MP joint subluxation or dislocation. The stress of trauma to the metacarpophalangeal joint area usually causes fracture of the base of the proximal phalanx, avulses the ulnar collateral ligament insertion (or fracture avulsion), or causes traumatic separation through the physis of the proximal phalanx. A displaced intraarticular osteocartilaginous fracture of the metacarpal head which is impossible to reduce either by open or closed methods should be removed from the joint to prevent posttraumatic arthritic changes (Figure 6-42). Rarely is fracture of a sesamoid encountered (Figure 6-43).

The most common injury to the metacarpophalangeal joint area of the thumb is dorsal subluxation or dislocation, followed in frequency by ulnar collateral ligament avulsion with or without an associated articular fracture of the proximal phalangeal base.

Proximal Phalangeal Fractures

Undisplaced or minimally displaced or angulated (Figure 6-46) fractures of the proximal phalangeal base involving the articular surface should be treated by conservative immobilization for three to four weeks (Figures 6-44A,B). Follow-up radiographs are important to determine if any loss of position has occurred (Figures 6-45A,B). Manipulation of a comminuted fracture involving a large, essentially undisplaced articular fragment, as in Figures 6-47A–D, may be gently attempted. If moderate angulation persists, it is usually advisable to permit healing rather than perform more strenuous manipulation, possibly displacing the articular fragment and necessitating open reduction and internal fixation. If angulation causes functional impairment after healing, corrective osteotomy can be performed to realign the phalanx, but the initial conservative treatment to preserve a good articular surface is the most important aspect. Initial open reduction and internal fixation of both the articular and the shaft fractures is technically quite difficult, but may be preferred.

Shaft fractures may be either oblique or transverse. The characteristic deformity is dorsal angulation at the fracture site due to the distorting pull of the extensor aponeurosis, resembling the configuration

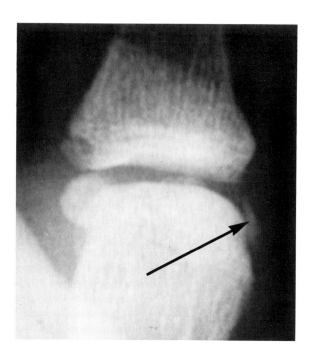

Figure 6-42 PA view of articularly displaced articular fracture of thumb metacarpal head. Treatment involved surgical removal of fragment to prevent posttraumatic and degenerative arthritic changes secondary to joint erosion from this free osteocartilaginous fragment which acted as a loose body.

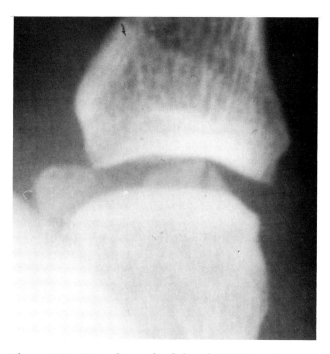

Figure 6-43 PA radiograph of thumb MP joint shows fracture of radial sesamoid seen in "cartilage space" of joint.

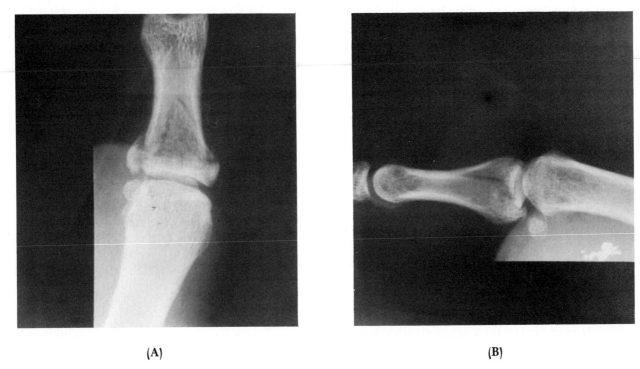

(A)   (B)

Figure 6-44 **(A)** Undisplaced fractures of both radial and ulnar aspects of thumb proximal phalanx base associated with an undisplaced articular shaft and metaphysis fracture of proximal phalanx. Conservative treatment of 3 to 4 weeks immobilization achieved satisfactory function. **(B)** Lateral view of the same injury.

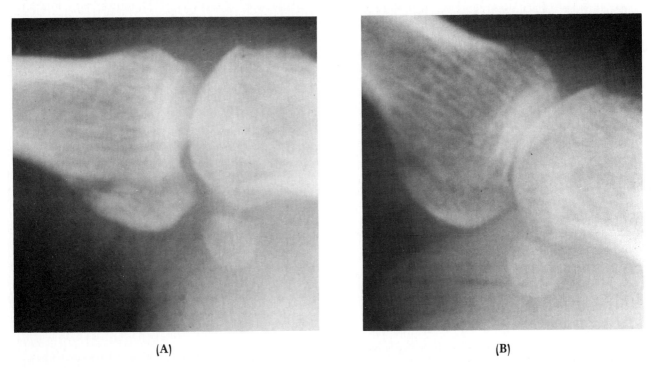

(A)   (B)

Figure 6-45 **(A)** Undisplaced fracture of palmar beak of thumb proximal phalanx treated by conservative immobilization for 3 weeks. **(B)** Lateral radiograph taken 10 weeks later shows healing of fracture with minimal callus and no loss of position. Serial radiographs had been made at 10- to 12-day intervals during first 4 weeks of immobilization to be sure that no fracture displacement occurred.

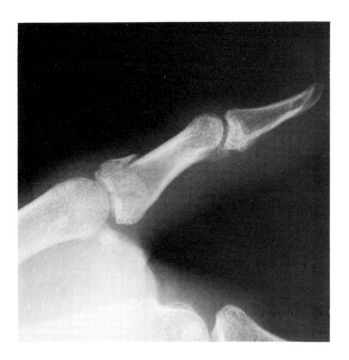

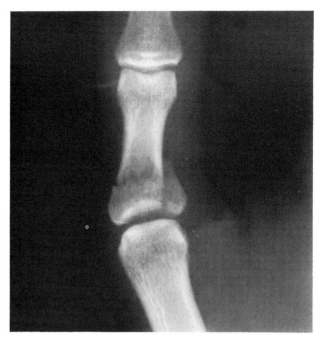

(A)

Figure 6-46 Lateral radiograph showing comminuted articular fracture of thumb proximal phalanx base and metaphysis with minimal dorsal angulation. Good MP and IP joint flexion and extension resulted after 3 to 4 weeks of conservative immobilization.

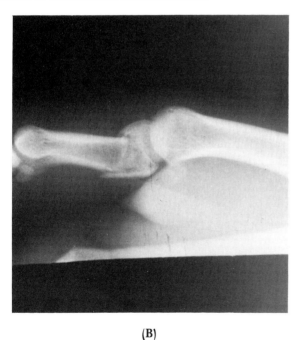

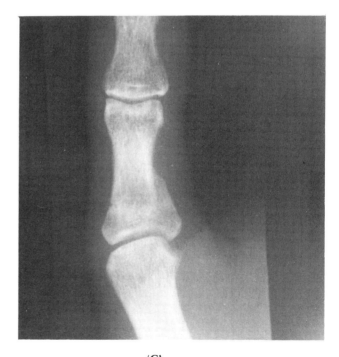

(B)

(C)

Figure 6-47 (A) PA radiograph of longitudinal, minimally displaced fracture of ulnar condyle of thumb proximal phalangeal base with some ulnar angulation of proximal phalanx. (B) Lateral view shows dorsal angulation of 20° at a comminuted proximal metaphyseal fracture of proximal phalangeal base. (C) Ten weeks after injury longitudinal alignment of thumb is acceptable although there is some ulnar angulation at MP joint.

(continued)

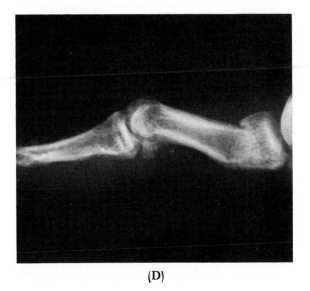

(D)

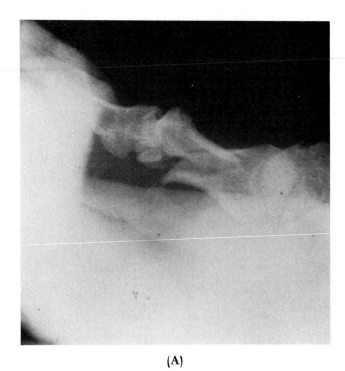

Figure 6-47 *(continued)*
(D) Lateral view shows persistent hyperextension or recurvatum deformity of proximal phalangeal base fracture. Strong stable pinch and acceptable MP and IP joint ranges of motion resulted. Corrective osteotomy was not necessary.

(A)

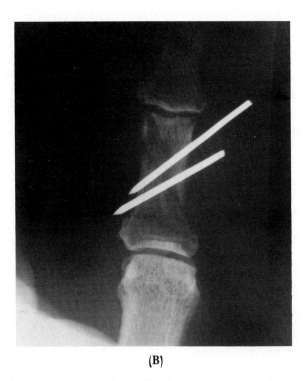

(B)

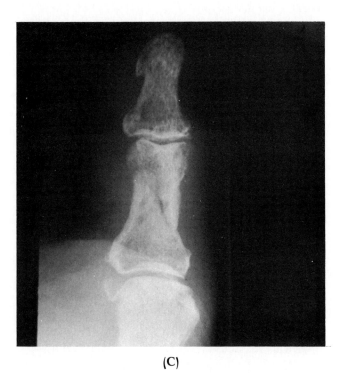

(C)

Figure 6-48 **(A)** Radiograph of open comminuted saw injury of thumb proximal phalanx shows dorsally angulated oblique fracture of thumb proximal phalanx. Initial treatment included meticulous wound toilet and delayed primary skin closure for this potentially contaminated wound. **(B)** PA view 10 days postinjury following open reduction and internal Kirschner wire fixation. **(C)** PA view after fracture healing and removal of temporary Kirschner wire fixation 3 weeks after surgery, at which time light range of motion exercises were commenced.

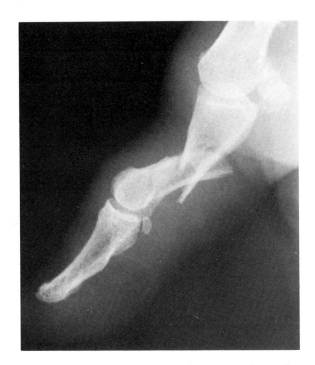

Figure 6-49 Lateral radiograph shows dorsal angulation of severely comminuted oblique proximal phalangeal crush fracture.

(recurvatum) of the proximal phalangeal fracture of the other digits (Figures 6-48A–C, 6-49).

The palmar protrusion of the apex of angulation impinges upon the flexor pollicis longus tendon and causes flexion of the IP joint. If closed manipulation does not result in satisfactory reduction, open reduction and internal or percutaneous Kirschner wire fixation is recommended to establish the proper balance between extensors and flexors (Figure 6-48B).

Uncorrected proximal phalangeal angulation results in persistence of the proximal phalangeal recurvatum deformity and IP joint flexion (Figures 6-50A,B). Corrective osteotomy can at least partially restore proper balance.

Occasionally a transverse fracture of the proximal phalanx is completely unstable and requires fixation (Figures 6-51A,B). Longitudinal percutaneous Kirschner wire fixation across the IP joint provides the necessary stability without impingement on the MP joint. (Refer to Chapter 13, Crush Injuries, for additional information on thumb proximal phalangeal fractures [Figures 13-4A–E]).

Undisplaced articular fractures of the distal end of the proximal phalanx are treated conservatively

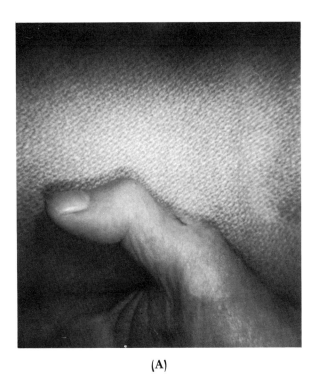

(A)

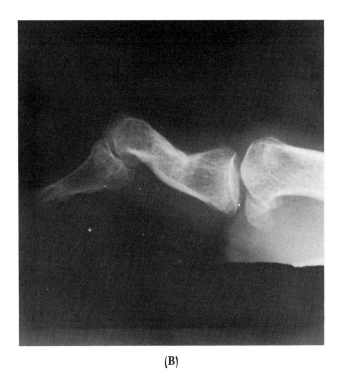

(B)

Figure 6-50 **(A)** Old, healed fracture of thumb proximal phalanx illustrates chronic recurvatum deformity of proximal phalanx and flexion contracture of IP joint. **(B)** Lateral view shows a healed old proximal phalangeal fracture with persistent recurvatum of proximal phalanx at healed fracture site and flexion contracture of IP joint.

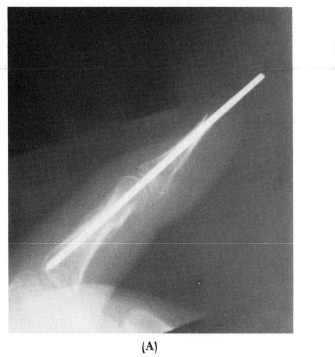

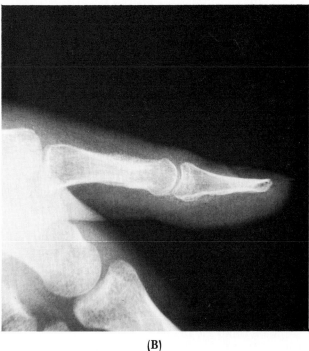

(A) (B)

Figure 6-51 **(A)** Lateral view of thumb following longitudinal Kirschner wire fixation to stabilize completely unstable transverse proximal phalangeal fracture. **(B)** Lateral radiograph after removal of Kirschner wire fixation 4 weeks postoperatively illustrates anatomic position of proximal phalanx.

(Figure 6-52), with emphasis on serial radiographic evaluation to be certain the proper position is maintained. Displaced condylar fractures often associated with IP joint subluxation or dislocation should be anatomically reduced and immobilized by Kirschner wire fixation (Figures 6-53A,B).

Distal Phalangeal Fractures

The majority of thumb distal phalangeal fractures are sustained in crush injuries which cause comminuted open or closed fractures of the distal tuft but may also involve the diaphysis and base. Occasionally fracture sustained by blunt trauma or torsional forces occurs through the diaphysis and may be transverse, longitudinal, or oblique, or may occur at the base of the distal phalanx. Torsional forces usually cause injury proximally at some location in the thumb ray (metacarpal, proximal phalanx or MP joint) because of the great inherent strength in the short, broad configuration of the distal phalanx.

If the distal phalangeal fracture is undisplaced or relatively undisplaced, three weeks of immobiliza-

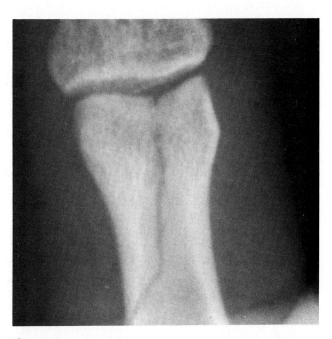

Figure 6-52 PA radiograph of thumb proximal and distal phalanges and IP joint shows a large undisplaced articular fracture of radial condyle of proximal phalanx and both radial and ulnar condyles of distal phalanx, treated by conservative immobilization for 3 weeks.

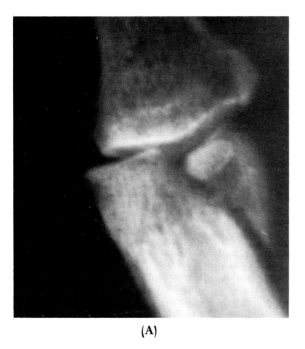

(A)

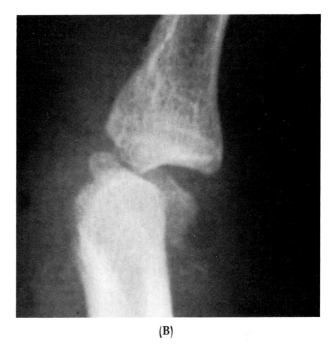

(B)

Figure 6-53 (A) PA radiograph of open palmar injury of thumb proximal phalanx illustrates a displaced radial condylar fracture and lateral subluxation of the IP joint. (B) Lateral radiograph shows prominent dorsal subluxation of the IP joint. Case demonstrates importance of multiple views to determine accurate diagnosis of skeletal injury or injuries. Treatment recommended was open reduction and internal fixation of open articular fracture subluxation, but patient refused any treatment other than wound toilet and primary skin closure.

tion are sufficient (Figures 6-52, 6-54). Manipulation of a displaced shaft fracture usually results in a satisfactory, stable reduction in both closed and open injuries (Figures 6-55A–D); occasionally, however, longitudinal Kirschner wire fixation must be included to maintain adequate reduction, particularly in a transverse fracture. Fracture avulsion of the flexor pollicis longus insertion is rare and is treated by immediate reinsertion. (See section DIP Joint Injuries in Chapter 9, Injuries to Digital Soft Tissue Structures for similar treatment of flexor digitorum profundus fracture avulsion and also section DIP Joint in Chapter 10, Articular Fractures.)

Malunion of either a thumb metacarpal or proximal phalangeal fracture can be treated by osteotomy and realignment with internal fixation to achieve a more stable physiologic thumb-index pinch. The most important goal is gross alignment of the MP and IP joints. The physiologic alignment of these joint axes determined in extension and flexion is much more important than attempting to produce a pleasing radiographic picture.

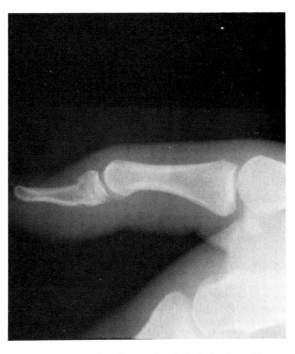

Figure 6-54 Lateral radiograph of slightly dorsally angulated fracture of distal phalanx proximal metaphysis or base, treated by external immobilization for 2½ weeks before commencing light activity.

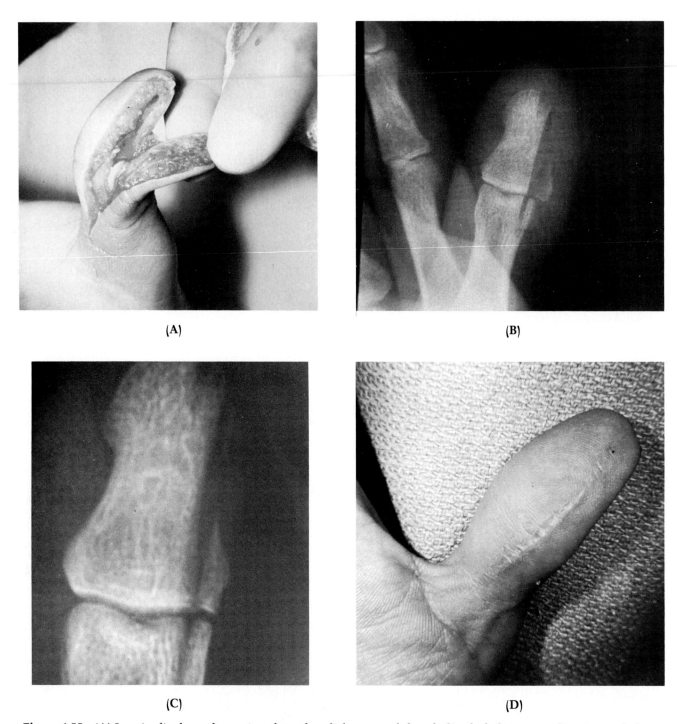

(A) (B)

(C) (D)

Figure 6-55 **(A)** Longitudinal saw laceration through radial aspect of thumb distal phalanx extending into radial condyle of proximal phalanx. View shows longitudinally split distal phalanx and radial condyle of proximal phalanx. **(B)** PA view shows longitudinal fractures of distal and proximal phalanges crossing IP joint. **(C)** PA radiograph after meticulous wound toilet and anatomic replacement of soft tissues with no internal fixation of distal phalangeal fracture shows maintenance of a good joint space. **(D)** Palmar view 10 weeks after injury shows good healing of pulp soft tissue. Good sensation resulted since this longitudinal injury did not lacerate any important sensory nerves.

References

1. Eaton RG: *Joint Injuries of the Hand.* Springfield, Ill, Charles C Thomas, 1971.
2. Stener B: Hyperextension injuries to the metacarpophalangeal joint of the thumb—rupture of ligaments, fracture of sesamoid bones, rupture of flexor pollicis brevis: An anatomical and clinical study. *Acta Chir Scand* 1963;125:275–293.
3. Smith RJ: Posttraumatic instability of the metacarpophalangeal joint of the thumb. *J Bone Joint Surg (Am)* 1977;59-A:14–21.
4. Neviaser RJ, Wilson JN, Lievano A: Rupture of the ulnar collateral ligament of the thumb (gamekeeper's thumb); correction by dynamic repair. *J Bone Joint Surg (Am)* 1971; 53-A:1357–1364.
5. Green DP, O'Brien ET: Fractures of the thumb metacarpal. *S Med J* 1972;65:807–814.
6. Sandzén SC Jr: Fracture of the fifth metacarpal resembling Bennett's fracture. *Hand* 1973;5:49–51.

CHAPTER
7

Metacarpal Fractures

Metacarpal fractures can be divided into four categories depending on their anatomic location: metacarpal base, metacarpal neck or distal metaphysis, metacarpal shaft, and chip avulsion fracture of the base.

Regardless of the site of metacarpal fracture, immobilization must be in the functional position of wrist extension, MP joint flexion approaching 90°, PIP and DIP joints in complete or nearly complete extension, and with wide thumb metacarpal abduction and opposition.

(Articular fractures of the metacarpal head are discussed in Chapter 10, Articular Fractures.)

Metacarpal Base Fractures

Fracture of a single metacarpal base, particularly of either the long or ring finger, is usually stable because of the tethering effect of the deep transverse metacarpal ligaments, the intervening interosseous musculature, and the secure fixation provided by ligaments binding the carpometacarpal articulations. The index and little finger metacarpals, together comprising the marginal or border rays (digits), are firmly secured only on their ulnar and radial borders, respectively (Figure 7-1). The majority of metacarpal base fractures are suffered on the ulnar border of the hand, most commonly the little finger, and are usually due to a direct blow. The little finger metacarpal is particularly mobile because of its carpometacarpal joint and is second in mobility only to the thumb. Some displacement of the metacarpal base fracture is acceptable (Figure 7-1), but reduction should be achieved if displacement is significant. Closed manipulation and reduction often suffices (Figures 7-2A,B), but if necessary, closed or open reduction and percutaneous Kirschner wire fixation should be utilized. Immobilization should include the entire digit with the adjacent ray on either side or the single adjacent ray of a border digit (index or little finger) distally to include the fingertips and proximally extending across the wrist to prevent malrotation. This immobilization in the functional position should be continued for three to three and one-half weeks after injury.

It is most important to recognize that a metacarpal base fracture is often associated with

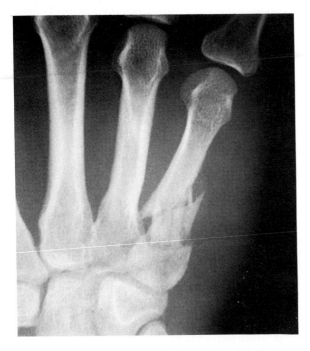

Figure 7-1 PA radiograph of relatively undisplaced oblique fracture of fifth finger metacarpal base. Treatment was conservative immobilization for 3 weeks.

dislocation of an adjacent metacarpal base or bases. The two oblique radiographs may be particularly helpful for accurate diagnosis. If reduction of the dislocation is unstable, percutaneous Kirschner wire fixation of the reduced metacarpal base to the adjacent carpus is necessary. Often skeletal fixation of the reduced metacarpal base dislocation provides the necessary stability for maintaining stable reduction of an adjacent fracture of a metacarpal base. If the fracture remains unstable, reduction may be held by similar percutaneous Kirschner wire fixation from the metaphysis distal to the fracture site into the metacarpal base or the carpus.

Single or multiple fractures of metacarpal bases must be accurately reduced to prevent malrotation and malalignment and angulation deformities of involved digits which would seriously impair functional anatomic synergistic digital flexion. (Refer to Figures 15-9A–G, Chapter 15, Multiple Fractures.)

(Dislocations and fracture dislocations of the metacarpal base are discussed in Chapter 5, Carpometacarpal Joints.)

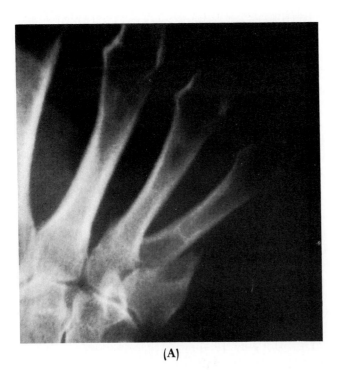

(A)

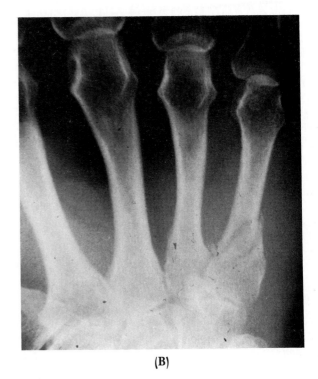

(B)

Figure 7-2 **(A)** PA view of oblique proximally and radially displaced fracture of fifth finger metacarpal base. **(B)** After closed manipulation and reduction. Treatment was conservative immobilization for 3½ weeks.

Avulsion Fracture of a Metacarpal Base

A small chip fracture avulsion of a tendon insertion of a wrist extensor or flexor, usually caused by a direct blow or torsional injury, is inconsequential but may often be quite symptomatic initially. These small fracture avulsions may involve the insertion of the extensor carpi radialis longus at the dorsal aspect of the index metacarpal base, the extensor carpi radialis brevis from a similar location on the long finger metacarpal base, the extensor carpi ulnaris from the little finger metacarpal base, the flexor carpi radialis from the palmar aspect of the index (and long) metacarpal bases, and, rarely, the flexor carpi ulnaris from the pisiform. Immobilization should be provided for roughly two to three weeks after the injury or until it is asymptomatic.

Metacarpal Neck (Distal Metaphyseal) Fractures

The distal metaphysis is the weakest portion of the metacarpal because it is composed primarily of cancellous bone (Figures 7-3A,B). It cannot withstand direct or torsional trauma as well as the adjacent metacarpal diaphysis which is primarily thick cortical bone. Longitudinal compression (e.g., direct blow on the metacarpal head of the clenched fist) comminutes the palmar cortex of the metaphysis and results in the common "boxer's fracture" with palmar angulation of the metacarpal head. Malunion in this angled position usually causes minimal disability in the little finger but becomes of increasing consequence toward the radial border of the hand (Figures 7-5A,B, 7-6A,B). The mobility of the ring finger metacarpal and especially of the little finger metacarpal at their carpometacarpal joints allows sufficient motion to compensate for malunion with palmar angulation at the distal metaphysis, causing some protrusion of the metacarpal head into the palm. However, the stability of the index and long metacarpal bases due to their secure carpometacarpal articulations (stable portion of the hand) does not permit such compensatory motion. Therefore any angulation with palmar protrusion of the index and long metacarpal head may become a distinct disability upon grasp. The metacarpal head protrudes palmarly similarly to its protrusion in an MP joint dislocation (see section on MP joint dislocations in Chapter 9, Injuries to Digital Soft Tissue Structures, and Figures 9-32A–E). In the skeletally immature person physeal separation occurs instead of fracture (see Chapter 12, Posttraumatic

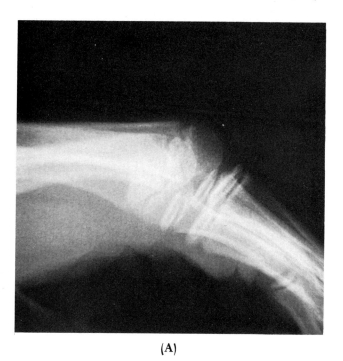

(A)

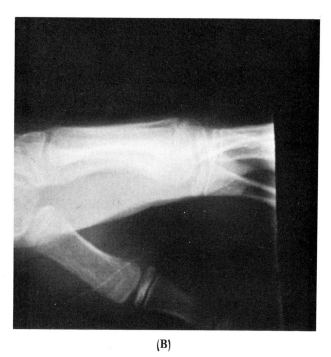

(B)

Figure 7-3 (A) Lateral view shows 80° palmar angulation of closed distal metaphyseal fracture of index metacarpal (boxer's fracture). Note index metacarpal shortening. (B) Lateral view, after closed reduction. Note persistence of minimal metacarpal shortening.

Figure 7-4 (**A**) Oblique view of angulated fracture of fifth metacarpal shaft with displaced fracture of distal metaphysis of ring finger and undisplaced fracture of index metacarpal distal metaphysis (Boxer's fracture). (**B**) PA view after open reduction and longitudinal intramedullary fixation of ring finger distal metaphyseal fracture. Note reduced healed fracture of little finger metacarpal shaft and healed oblique fracture of long finger proximal metaphysis. Surgery performed 8 weeks after original injury because of severity of soft tissue trauma. (**C**) Healed result 10 weeks after surgery.

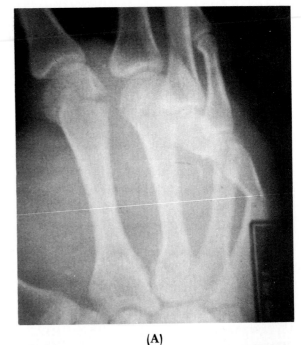

(A)

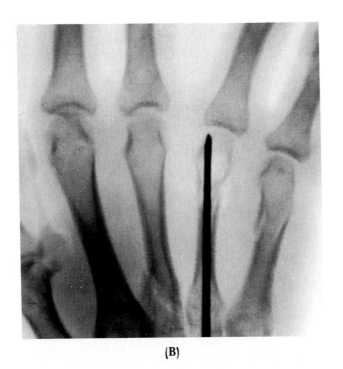

(B)

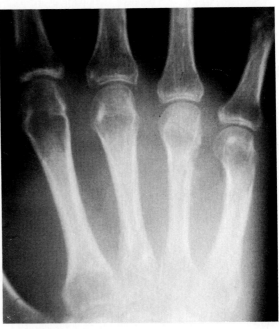

(C)

Skeletal Remodeling, Figures 12-5A–E). Therefore, there should be manipulation and reduction of any angulated distal metaphyseal fracture (boxer's fracture) in the index and long fingers (Figures 7-3A, 7-6A), and in the ring and little fingers usually, if angulation is greater than 25° to 30° (Figures 7-4A, 7-5A, 7-9A,B). *Most importantly any malrotation must be corrected* (Figures 7-7A,B).

Reduction of this angulation deformity is performed after adequate anesthesia by maximal MP flexion, followed by longitudinal pressure on the condyles of the proximal phalanx. Occasionally in an

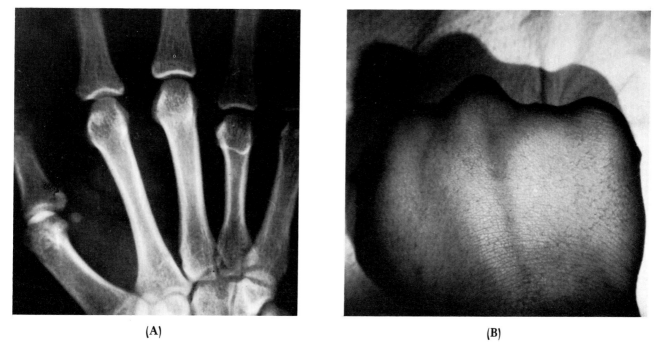

(A)   (B)

Figure 7-5 **(A)** PA view of old healed shortened ring finger distal metaphyseal fracture. **(B)** Note recession of ring finger metacarpal head.

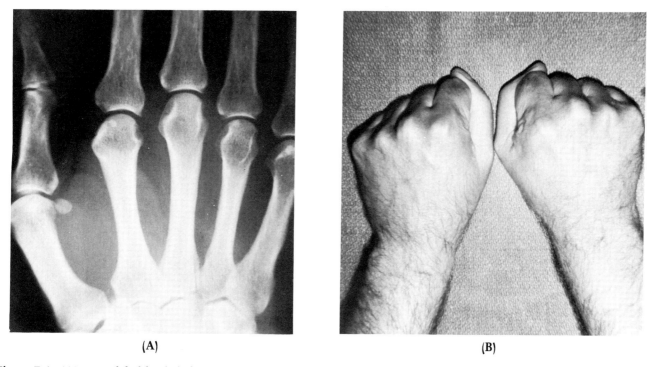

(A)   (B)

Figure 7-6 **(A)** Remodeled healed shortened distal index metacarpal metaphyseal fracture sustained 40 years previously. **(B)** Comparison to normal left hand of same patient. Note marked shortening of index metacarpal with recession of index metacarpal head.

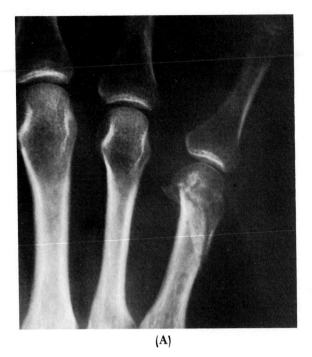

(A)

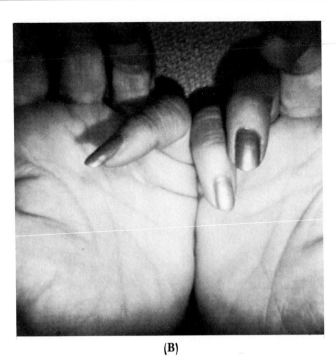

(B)

Figure 7-7 **(A)** Malrotation of healed distal metaphyseal fracture of little finger metacarpal. Note PA view of long and ring finger metacarpals and oblique view of distal metacarpal metaphysis and phalanges of little finger. **(B)** Malrotation of little finger compared to contralateral normal little finger in semiflexion.

impacted fracture, traction and manipulation are required to disimpact the fracture prior to reduction. Length is thereby restored, and the palmar metacarpal head protrusion is relieved. Constant immobilization is provided for three weeks and protective for an additional two weeks with maximal MP flexion. *Pressure is applied only to achieve the reduction and not to maintain the reduction.* Unrelieved pressure to maintain reduction will cause soft tissue slough due to pressure ischemia. After proper reduction the majority of distal metaphyseal fractures are stable in MP flexion and pose no problem (Figures 7-3A,B).

If the fracture is unstable and deformity recurs, percutaneous Kirschner wire fixation should be considered. Following closed reduction with maximum MP joint flexion, a percutaneous Kirschner wire or wires are drilled from the head in the area just proximal to the articular cartilage, proximally across the reduced fracture into the shaft. The wires should not penetrate the articular cartilage, nor should they impinge on or penetrate the extensor tendon or impinge on the MP joint (Figure 7-8). Plaster immobilization with MP flexion of the involved digit and adjacent digits should augment the Kirschner wire fixation, with pin removal approximately three weeks later.

At that time, light range of motion exercises are commenced and protective immobilization afforded at night and with strenuous activity for an additional two weeks.

Occasionally complete displacement or severe angulation of a distal metaphyseal fracture which is irreducible or grossly unstable upon reduction necessitates open reduction and internal fixation. Different methods may be utilized including transverse fixation of the reduced metacarpal head to adjacent metacarpal(s), crossed Kirschner wire anatomic fixation at the fracture site at open reduction, or longitudinal intramedullary Kirschner wire fixation. For maintaining reduction, the author prefers longitudinal Kirschner wire internal fixation discussed in the section following, Metacarpal Shaft Fractures (see Figures 7-15A–G). By this method MP joint motion can begin immediately, and wrist motion can be commenced in approximately three to four weeks (after removal of the Kirschner wire) (Figures 7-4A–C).

An old malunion of a ring finger distal metaphyseal fracture sustained in an altercation is shown in Figures 7-5A,B. Note the distinct metacarpal shortening both on radiograph and corresponding photograph. Complete remodeling of an index finger

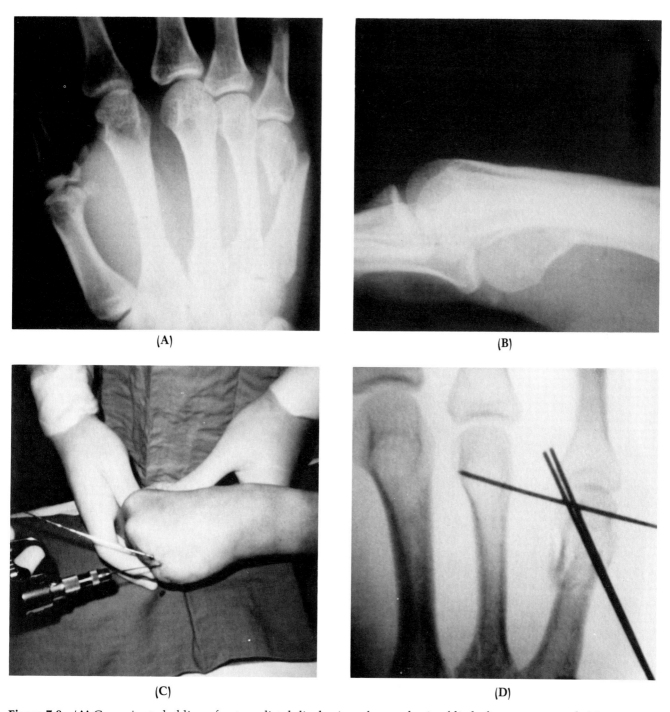

(A)

(B)

(C)

(D)

Figure 7-8 **(A)** Comminuted oblique fracture distal diaphysis and metaphysis of little finger metacarpal. **(B)** Lateral view illustrates 50° palmar angulation. **(C)** Method of percutaneous Kirschner wire fixation using a cannulated power drill after anatomic reduction. The articular cartilage must not be damaged. **(D)** PA radiograph shows secure fixation by one Kirschner wire extending transversely from the little finger metacarpal head into the adjacent ring finger metacarpal distal metaphysis and two oblique Kirschner wires extending across the fracture site.

(continued)

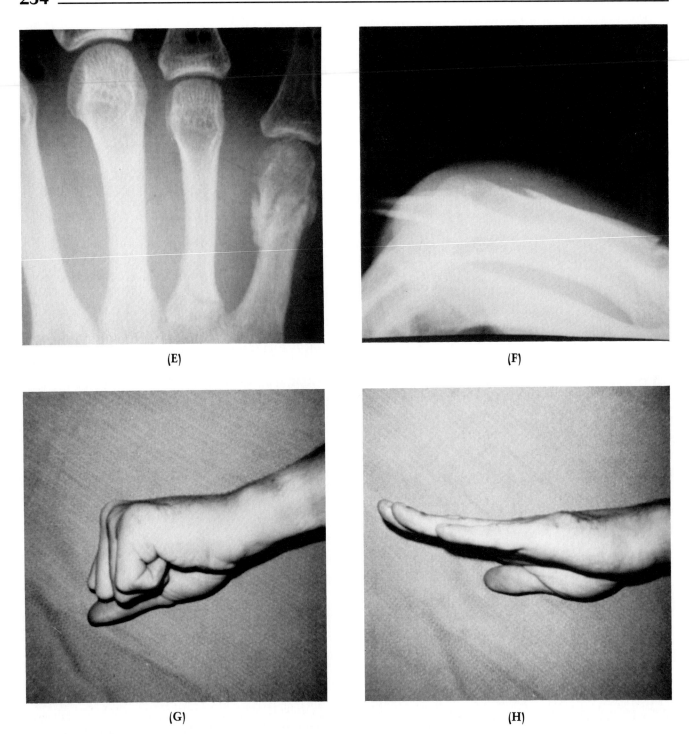

(E)

(F)

(G)

(H)

Figure 7-8 *(continued)*
(E) Healed result six weeks after fracture and after Kirschner wire removals. **(F)** Lateral view shows correction of palmar angulation. **(G)** Normal MP joint flexion. **(H)** Normal MP joint extension.

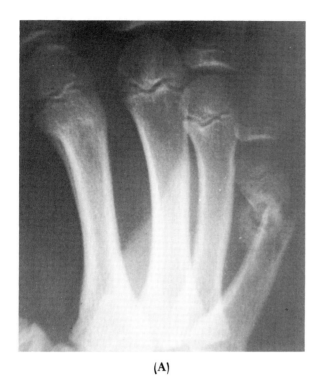

(A)

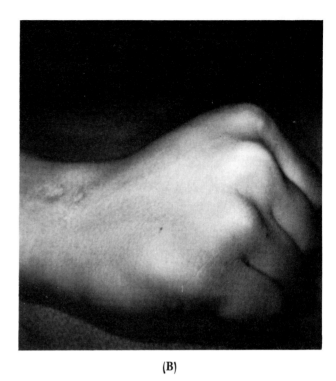

(B)

Figure 7-9 **(A)** Oblique radiograph shows abundant callus formation with palmar and radial angulation at fracture site of malunited little finger metacarpal fracture (boxer's fracture), first seen 3½ weeks after injury. Note metacarpal shortening. **(B)** Flexion illustrates shortening of little finger metacarpal and incomplete MP flexion. Minimal extensor lag at PIP joint (not shown) was noted on extension.

metacarpal is seen in the radiograph taken 40 years after injury (Figures 7-6A,B). The patient complained of his short index finger, particularly when use of this dominant right hand required coordination and maximal digital spread, as when playing the piano. Only if malunion occurs with angulation severe enough to interfere with the normal use of the hand (e.g., gripping) should osteotomy be considered (Figures 7-9A,B).

Proper alignment and rotation of the distal metaphyseal fracture is achieved and assured by correct anatomic relation of the injured digit to adjacent digits in flexion and extension and by comparing with the corresponding digits of the opposite hand (Figures 7-7A,B). Immobilization for three weeks, as noted, should involve the digit adjacent on each side, unless the injured digit is a bordering digit (index or little finger).

Metacarpal Shaft Fractures

Metacarpal shaft fractures may be divided into comminuted, transverse, and oblique types.

Comminuted impacted stable shaft fractures require protection for approximately two and one-half to three weeks, with guarded motion begun after 14 to 16 days (Figures 7-10A,B). Prior to activity, radiographic evaluation and examination should certify maintenance of position and inherent fracture stability. Unstable comminuted shaft fractures are best treated by transverse Kirschner wire fixation to adjacent stable metacarpals.

Transverse metacarpal shaft fractures, if stable, are treated conservatively by protective immobilization for three weeks. Minimal angulation can be accepted and the ultimate functional result will not be impaired, though there is some slight residual cosmetic abnormality due to depression of the distal metacarpal shaft and metacarpal head and protrusion dorsally at the apex of the angulation (Figures 7-11A,B). Transverse metacarpal shaft fractures tend to angulate with the apex of angulation dorsally, and the shaft distal to the fracture angulated palmarly. This characteristic deformity (Figures 7-12–7-15) is due to the pull of the interosseous muscles which insert partially on the base of the proximal phalanx and, to a lesser extent, the lumbrical muscles, all of which pass palmar to the MP joint, augmented by the powerful long flexors (flexor digitorum superficialis and flexor digitorum profundus). If closed manipulation

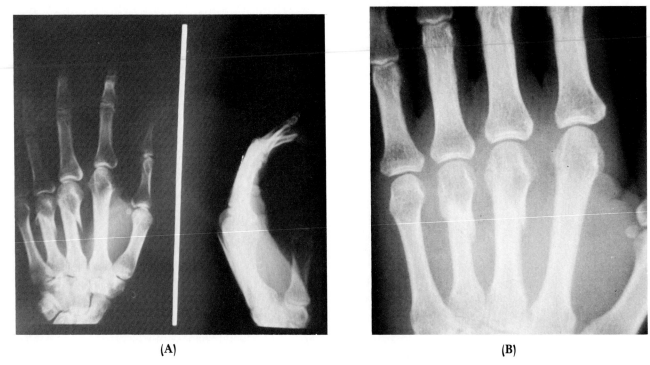

(A)   (B)

Figure 7-10 **(A)** A comminuted, impacted stable oblique metacarpal shaft fractures of long and ring fingers, PA and lateral views. **(B)** PA view after 2½ weeks of conservative immobilization.

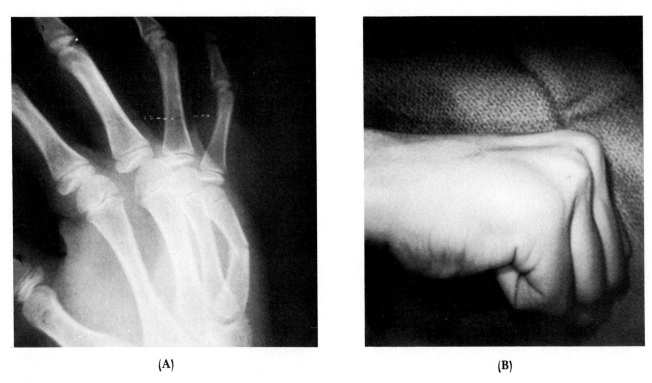

(A)   (B)

Figure 7-11 **(A)** Healing transverse metacarpal shaft fracture of little finger with 20° palmar angulation 3 weeks posttrauma. **(B)** Complete MP joint flexion resulted with some recession and palmar angulation of little finger metacarpal head but with no functional impairment of extension or flexion.

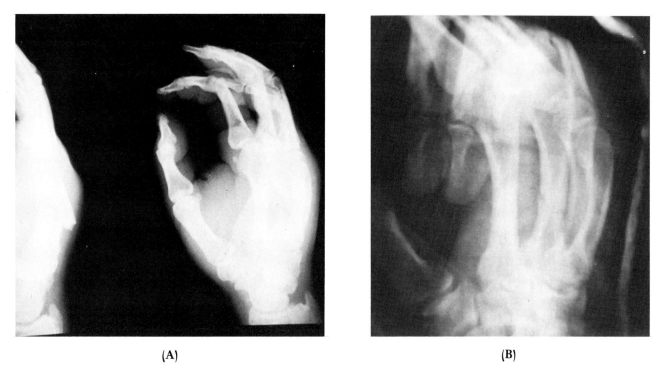

(A)   (B)

Figure 7-12 (A) Displaced angulated transverse metacarpal shaft fracture of long finger. (B) After stable closed reduction.

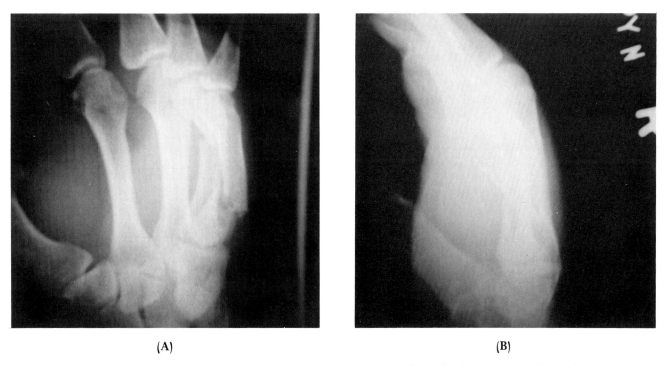

(A)   (B)

Figure 7-13 (A) Transverse fracture through the ring finger metacarpal distal diaphysis and the little finger metacarpal at the junction of the proximal metaphysis and diaphysis with displacement and palmar angulation at both fracture sites. (B) Lateral view accentuates palmar angulation.

(continued)

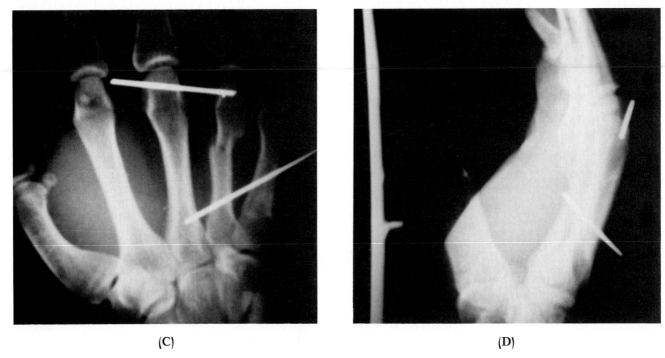

(C)   (D)

Figure 7-13 *(continued)*
(C) Ten days following percutaneous transverse Kirschner wire fixation of the reduced ring finger distal metaphysis into the long finger distal metaphysis and of the little finger metacarpal diaphysis into both the ring finger diaphysis and base of the long finger proximal metaphysis. **(D)** Lateral view shows correction of palmar angulation after reduction and percutaneous Kirschner wire fixations.

and reduction of an angulated or displaced transverse shaft fracture is successful (Figures 7-12A,B), immobilization should be continued for three and one-half to four weeks, including the wrist and extending out to include the distal phalanges of the involved digit (and the adjacent digits on either side) for the first 12 to 14 days with MP joints flexed and IP joints extended. Immobilization of the marginal ray metacarpals (index and little fingers) may be more difficult to maintain because of protection by an adjacent ray on only one side. After three weeks light motion of MP and IP joints may be commenced.

If a transverse shaft fracture is unstable, various alternatives are available. If closed reduction is satisfactory, percutaneous transverse Kirschner wire immobilization of the injured metacarpal to adjacent stable metacarpals may be used (Figures 7-13, 7-14). *However, great care should be taken to restore anatomic rotation of the transversely fixed fractured metacarpal*, particularly of the index and long fingers, to prevent rotational deformity.

A good method for unstable or irreducible metacarpal shaft fractures is open reduction and

longitudinal intramedullary Kirschner wire fixation (Figures 7-15A–G). The fracture site is exposed, followed by retrograde drilling of a double-ended Kirschner wire through the proximal metacarpal shaft emerging at the wrist which is maximally flexed (Figure 7-15C). The fracture is then reduced under direct vision, and the Kirschner wire is drilled anterograde across the reduced fracture site into the medullary canal of the distal shaft into the metaphysis without violating the MP joint. In this way the MP joints of all digits may be actively and passively moved during the entire treatment of the metacarpal shaft fracture. The Kirschner wire may be removed from the wrist area approximately four weeks after surgery to permit gradual wrist extension, but immobilization should be continued for the involved metacarpal for two weeks more since surgery and longitudinal intramedullary fixation will delay healing. The rationale for this immobilization is that restoration of wrist motion is much easier than restoration of MP motion would be if that latter joint were violated by entrance of the Kirschner wire, which also would make that joint more susceptible

Figure 7-14 (**A**) Displaced transverse fracture of ring finger metacarpal mid-diaphysis and displaced fracture of little finger metacapal proximal diaphysis. (**B**) After reductions secure percutaneous Kirschner wire fixation using two Kirschner wires to immobilize the ring finger distal metacarpal fragment to the long finger and little finger metacarpal to the ring finger proximal diaphysis and metaphysis. (**C**) Healed result six weeks later after removal of transverse Kirschner wires.

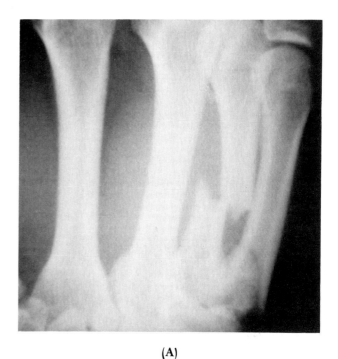

(A)

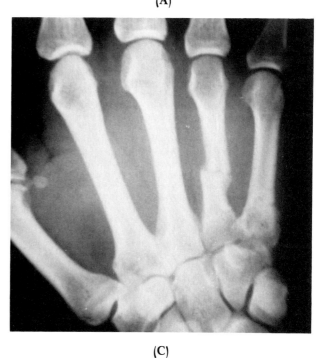

(B)   (C)

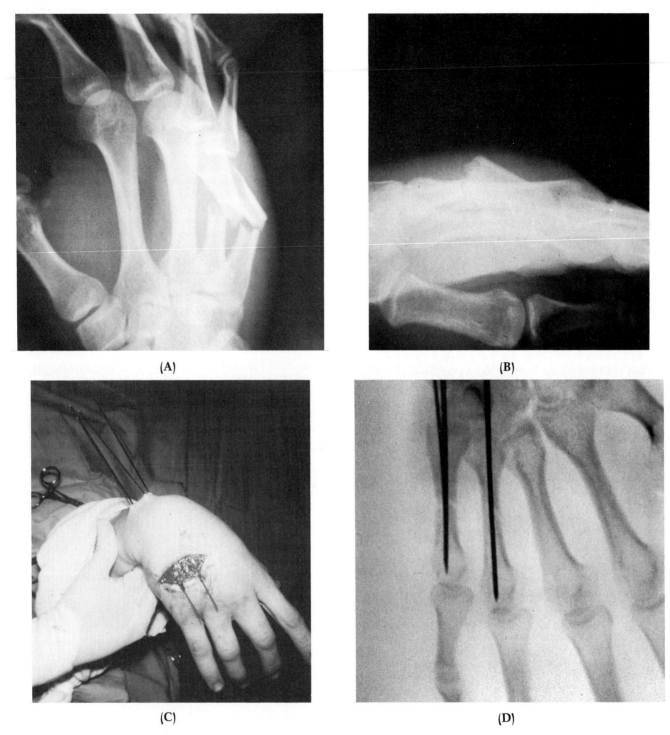

(A)

(B)

(C)

(D)

Figure 7-15 **(A)** Displaced angulated transverse unstable midshaft metacarpal fractures of ring and little fingers, oblique view. **(B)** Lateral view shows pronounced angulation at fracture sites with dorsal protuberance of proximal ends of distal fragments. **(C)** Open reduction and longitudinal intramedullary fixation with Kirschner wires. Each wire is introduced into proximal metacarpal shaft from exposed fracture site. Wire is driven proximally, far enough to allow fracture reduction, and then distally into distal metacarpal shaft, but should not impinge on MP joint. **(D)** Postoperative PA view shows normal anatomic restoration of ring and little finger metacarpals.

Figure 7-15 *(continued)*
(E) Lateral view 10 weeks after surgery. (F) PA view.
(G) Normal flexion and normal extension (not shown) resulted.

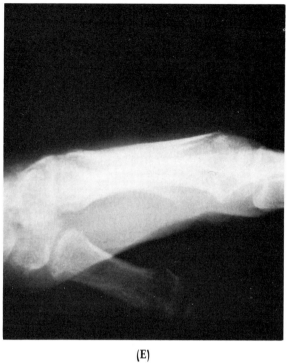

(E)

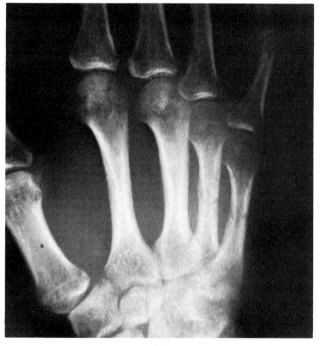

(F)

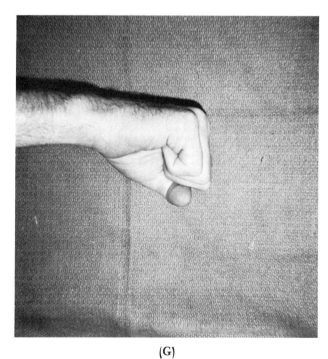

(G)

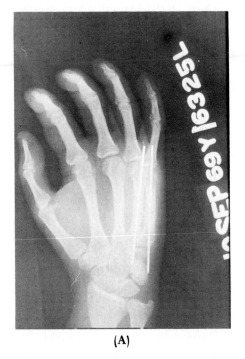
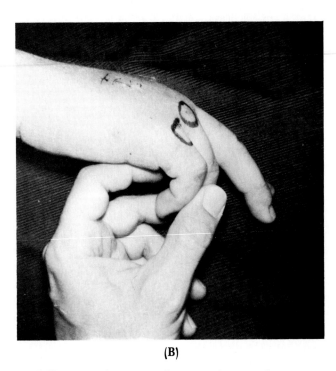

(A)   (B)

Figure 7-16 **(A)** PA view showing improper longitudinal intramedullary Kirschner wire fixation of ring and little finger transverse metacarpal shaft fractures. Note impingement of Kirschner wires across ring and little finger MP joints maintained in extension. **(B)** Lateral view showing approximately 45° flexion of ring finger MP joint and 35° flexion of little finger MP joint due to tight collateral ligaments after improper prolonged immobilization in extension.

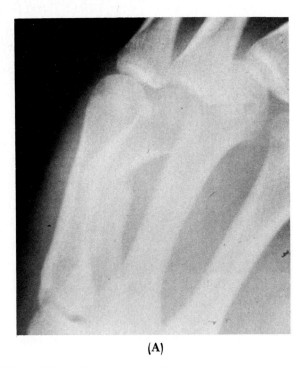
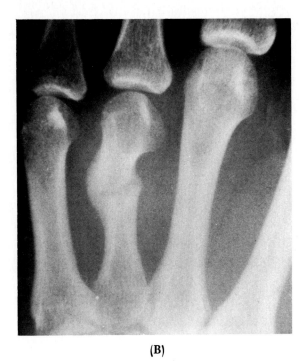

(A)   (B)

Figure 7-17 **(A)** Four-week old malunion of transverse midshaft ring finger metacarpal fracture with dorsal displacement of proximal end of distal fragment at fracture site and 45° to 50° palmar angulation of distal fragment. **(B)** PA view shows excessive shortening of ring finger metacarpal shaft and callus at site of malunion.

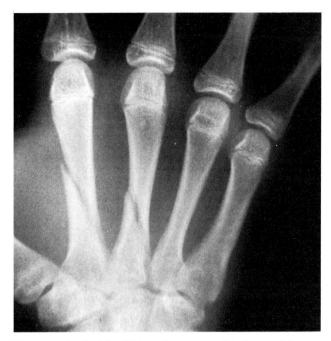

Figure 7-18 Stable oblique fractures of index and long metacarpal shafts, PA view.

to posttraumatic arthritic complications (Figures 7-16A,B).

Small compression plates particularly suited for metacarpal shaft fractures are occasionally used. If malunion with significant shortening and angulation occurs, reconstructive osteotomy should be seriously considered (Figures 7-17A,B).

Stable oblique metacarpal shaft fractures are treated similarly to the stable transverse shaft fractures by conservative immobilization (Figure 7-18).

Proximal displacement is a common deformity associated with unstable oblique shaft fractures, combined with some angulation, but not the marked angulation associated with transverse shaft fractures. If the proximal displacement of the oblique shaft fracture is minimal, there will be no functional impairment since some metacarpal shortening can be accepted with no hindrance to the complicated extensor-flexor interrelated synergistic mechanisms of action (Figures 7-19A–C). However, if displacement is more marked, closed or open reduction and percutaneous fixation if feasible, or open reduction and fixation, is recommended. The injury in Figures 7-20A–C,

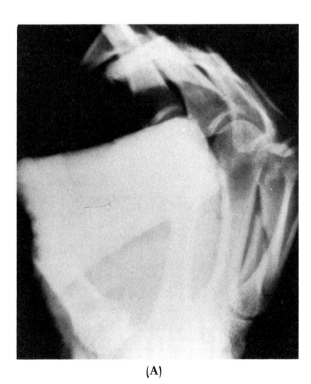

(A)

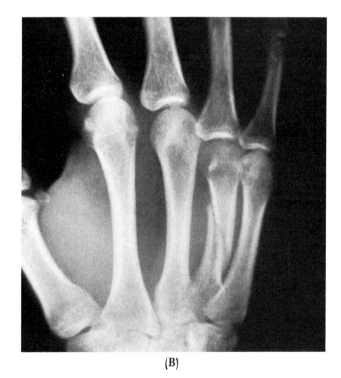

(B)

Figure 7-19 (A) Oblique view of minimally displaced ring finger oblique metacarpal shaft fracture accentuating displacement and angulation at fracture site with dorsal protuberance of spicule of distal shaft. (B) Oblique view 10 weeks after injury showing slight displacement and angulation at fracture site but essentially no change of position and relative absence of callus formation.

(continued)

Figure 7-19 *(continued)*
(C) Comparison of flexion of healed oblique metacarpal shaft fracture on left (X) with minimal loss of length compared to normal right ring finger metacarpal head. Flexion and extension are normal.

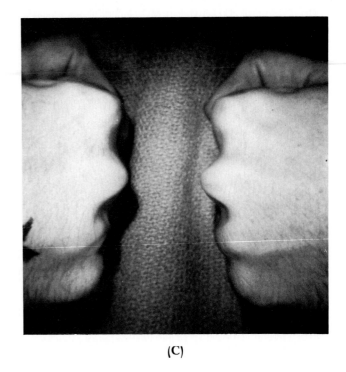

(C)

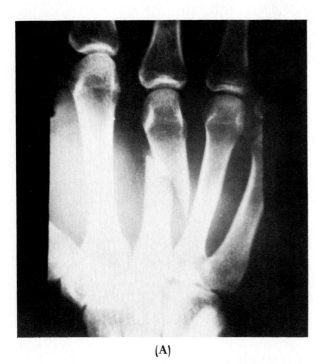

(A)

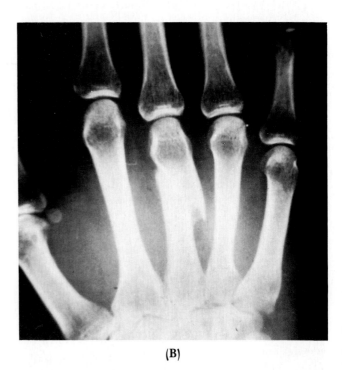

(B)

Figure 7-20   **(A)** PA view of moderately displaced and palmarly and radially angulated oblique metacarpal shaft fracture of long finger 5 weeks after injury. **(B)** PA view shows good healing 9 weeks after injury. Note blunting of spicule of proximal end of distal fragment.

Figure 7-20 *(continued)*
(C) Comparison of flexion of both hands. There was no functional impairment except for recessed left long finger metacarpal head, ulnar angulation of proximal phalanx, 0.75 cm of metacarpal shortening, and dorsal protuberance of bone spicule at proximal end of distal fragment.

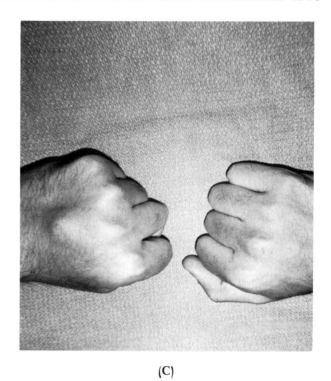

(C)

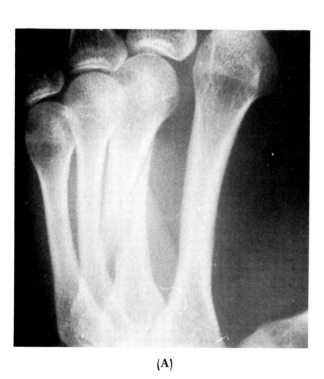

(A)

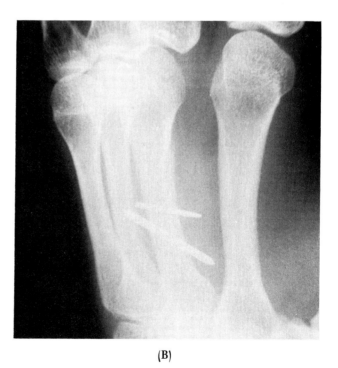

(B)

Figure 7-21 **(A)** Oblique view of oblique, slightly displaced long finger metacarpal shaft fracture. **(B)** Oblique film 2 weeks after open reduction and transverse Kirschner wire fixation.

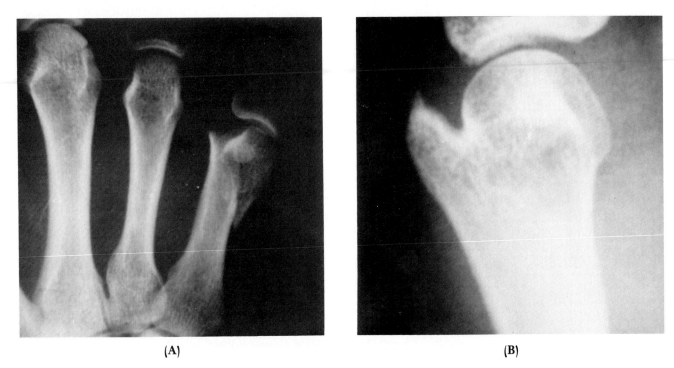

(A)   (B)

Figure 7-22 **(A)** Comminuted oblique displaced fracture of little finger metacarpal distal metaphysis with impingement on the MP joint and ulnar angulation of approximately 30°. Reduction was advised to relieve the MP joint impingement and to correct the angulation. **(B)** Surgery was declined and malunion occurred. Interestingly, the impingement of the spicule on the MP joint did not hinder motion since it was not in the flexion-extension axis and the persistent ulnar angulation and shortening were of minimal disability.

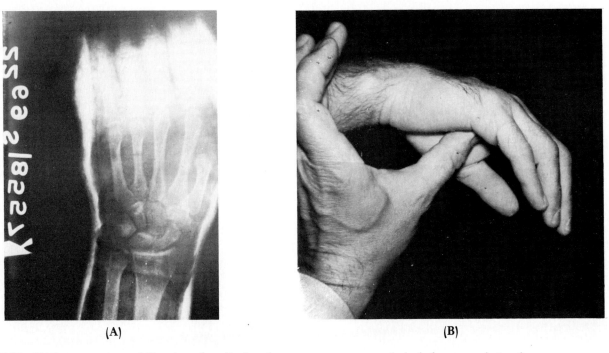

(A)   (B)

Figure 7-23 **(A)** Improper immobilization of undisplaced transverse metacarpal shaft fracture of ring finger. Note PA view of both metacarpals and proximal phalanges, indicating improper extension at all MP joints. **(B)** Minimal flexion of all MP joints, index through little finger, at discontinuation of immobilization 5 weeks posttrauma. Position was improper and period of immobilization too long.

for example, would have been better treated by either operative method. If shortening remains, the metacarpal head will remain indented and dorsal protuberance by the distal fragment spicule will persist. In this case, the functional result, however, was acceptable. This dorsal spicule might be expected to impinge upon the extensor tendons as seen on lateral radiographs (Figures 7-19A and 7-21A), but this is rarely a problem.

Exposure of the oblique fracture site with open reduction and Kirschner wire or screw fixation across the fracture site restores normal anatomy if a single attempt at closed reduction and percutaneous pin fixation is unsuccessful (Figures 7-21A,B). An oblique fracture may also be treated by longitudinal Kirschner wire fixation similar to the technique described for transverse metacarpal shaft fractures (Figure 7-15C).

Generally, an oblique fracture through a metacarpal distal metaphysis should be reduced and fixed to prevent impingement on the MP joint (Figure 7-22).

Severe metacarpal shaft fractures with significant bone loss[1] are discussed in Chapter 14, Retained Foreign Bodies and Through-and-Through Injuries (Figures 14-7A–L, 14-8A,B).

Proper immobilization for metacarpal fractures must include MP joint flexion as a prerequisite (Figures 7-23A,B).

General References

Green DP, Rowland SA: Fractures and dislocations in the hand, in Rockwood CA Jr, Green DP (eds): *Fractures in Adults*, ed 2. Philadelphia, J.B. Lippincott Co., 1984, vol 1, pp 313–409.

O'Brien ET: Fractures of the metacarpals and phalanges, in Green DP (ed): *Operative Hand Surgery*. New York, Churchill Livingstone, 1982, vol 1, pp 583–635.

O'Brien ET: Fractures of the hand and wrist region, in Rockwood CA Jr, Wilkins KE, King RE (eds): *Fractures in Children*, ed 2. Philadelphia, J.B. Lippincott Co., 1984, vol 3, pp 229–272.

Sandzén SC Jr: Complex injuries of the wrist and hand, in Meyers MH (ed): *The Multiply Injured Patient with Complex Fractures*. Philadelphia, Lea & Febiger, 1984, pp 365–400.

References

1. Littler JW: Metacarpal reconstruction. *J Bone Joint Surg (Am)* 1947;29:723–737.

CHAPTER
8

Phalangeal Fractures

Proximal Phalangeal Fractures

Proximal phalangeal fractures resemble metacarpal fractures in their mechanism of injury, usually either torsional stress or direct trauma. Fractures of the proximal phalanx primarily involve the shaft, but the distal metaphysis and proximal metaphysis also may be involved. (Articular fractures of the base and condyles are discussed in Chapter 10, Articular Fractures.) Restoration of proper alignment, rotation, and length is extremely important in the treatment of proximal phalangeal fractures to avoid malunion and to restore the physiologic synergistic function of the extensor and flexor mechanisms.

Any fracture of the proximal phalanx is apt to involve the tendon of the flexor digitorum superficialis in the healing callus since that tendon is deep to the profundus at this level. The profundus tendon has already passed through the decussation of the superficialis and lies superficial to the latter as it travels through to its insertion on the distal phalanx. Particularly prone to binding down the superficialis tendon in callus are crush fractures or even severe soft tissue crush injuries. Therefore motion should be

commenced as soon as possible to restore superficialis gliding function.

Fractures of the Distal Metaphysis

Anatomic reduction of distal metaphyseal fractures should be strived for to prevent angulation and rotational deformities (Figures 8-1A–C) and to restore full proximal phalangeal length. (Condylar fractures of the proximal phalanx are discussed in Chapter 10, Articular Fractures.)

Fractures of the Proximal Metaphysis or Base

Slight rotational or angulation deformities at the base of the proximal phalanx are greatly magnified at the tip of the digit (Figures 8-2A,B, 8-3). In this location anatomic fracture reduction should be strived for to prevent these complications. (Refer to Figures 10-2A,B in Chapter 10, Articular Fractures and compare this case to Figures 10-1A–D in the same chapter.)

249

Figure 8-1 (A) Ulnar angulation, rotational deformity, and shortening at site of malunion of little finger proximal phalangeal distal metaphyseal fracture. PA view of distal metacarpals and proximal phalanges (of index-little fingers) associated with oblique view of little finger proximal phalangeal distal metaphysis, distal to site of malunion, and little finger middle and distal phalanges is clue to rotational deformity at fracture site. (B) Palmar view shows malrotation of little finger due to previously noted malunion. Little finger markedly crosses over long and ring fingers upon attempted complete flexion. (C) Correction of alignment after osteotomy through site of malunion to correct rotational deformity.

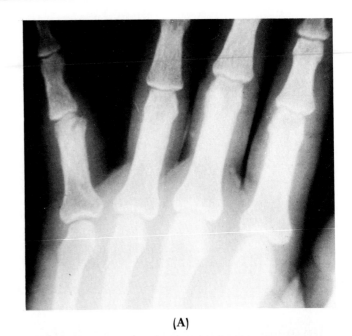

(A)

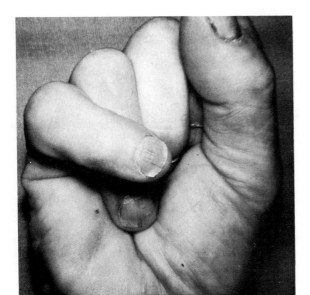

(B)

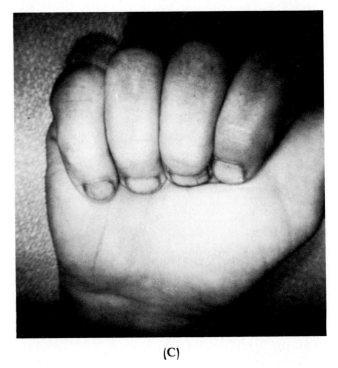

(C)

Shaft Fractures

Stable fractures (Figure 8-4) are protected by immobilization for 12 to 14 days with proximal and distal interphalangeal joints in complete or nearly complete extension and the metacarpophalangeal joint flexed. Light activity may begin at the end of that time, but protection during strenuous activity should be continued for an additional 10 days to two weeks.

Shaft fractures may be divided into three categories: transverse, oblique, and comminuted.

The typical configuration of an angulated transverse proximal phalangeal fracture is dorsal angulation of the shaft distal to the fracture with apex of the angulation deformity palmar (Figures 8-5A–C,

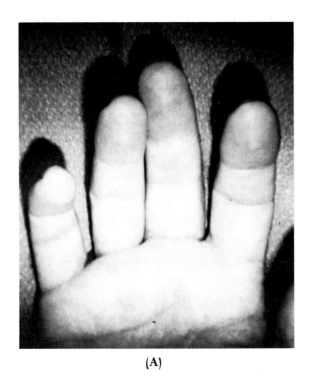

(A)

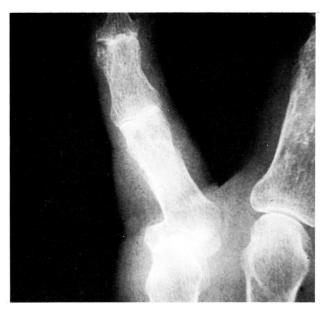

Figure 8-3 PA radiograph shows marked displacement and ulnar angulation at site of proximal metaphyseal fracture malunion of proximal phalanx.

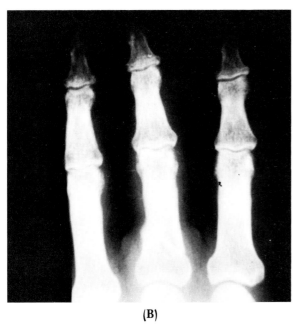

(B)

Figure 8-2 (A) Slight rotational and angulational deformity of long finger, palmar view in semiflexed attitude. (B) Radiograph shows malunion of proximal metaphyseal fracture of long finger proximal phalanx with persistence of some rotational and ulnar angulational deformity.

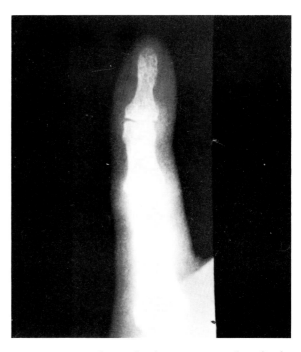

Figure 8-4 PA radiograph of a comminuted undisplaced proximal phalangeal fracture treated conservatively with immobilization for 2½ weeks, after which light range of motion was commenced.

Figure 8-5 (A) Lateral radiograph of dorsal angulation at site of comminuted fracture at junction of proximal metaphysis and diaphysis of proximal phalanx extending into MP joint. (B) PA radiograph. (C) Lateral radiograph after successful initial closed manipulation and reduction. Immobilization was continued for 3 weeks with MP joint flexed and PIP joint extended. Aggressive, active therapy lysed adhesions of superficialis tendon, and ranges of motion returned to normal.

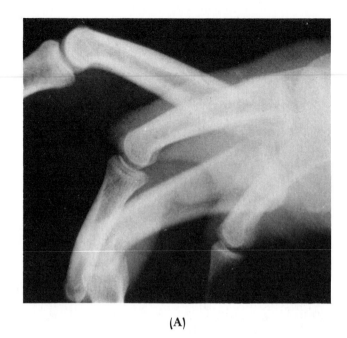

(A)

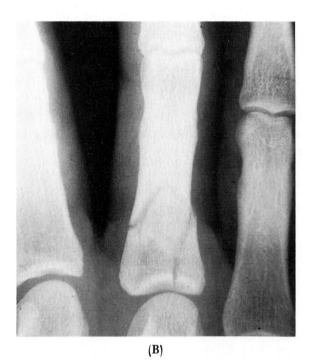

(B)

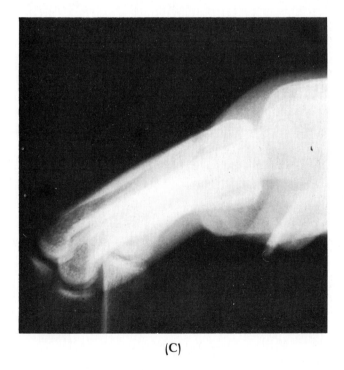

(C)

8-6A–E). Angulation may also occur laterally (radially or ulnarly) (Figure 8-6C). This characteristic deformity is a result of flexion of the proximal fragment by the interosseous muscles inserting into the base of the proximal phalanx and hyperextension of the shaft distal to the fracture site by extensor elements crossing that fracture site dorsally. The angulated proximal phalanx fracture therefore resembles a recurvatum configuration, often with flexion of the PIP and DIP joints due to impingement of the apex of the palmar

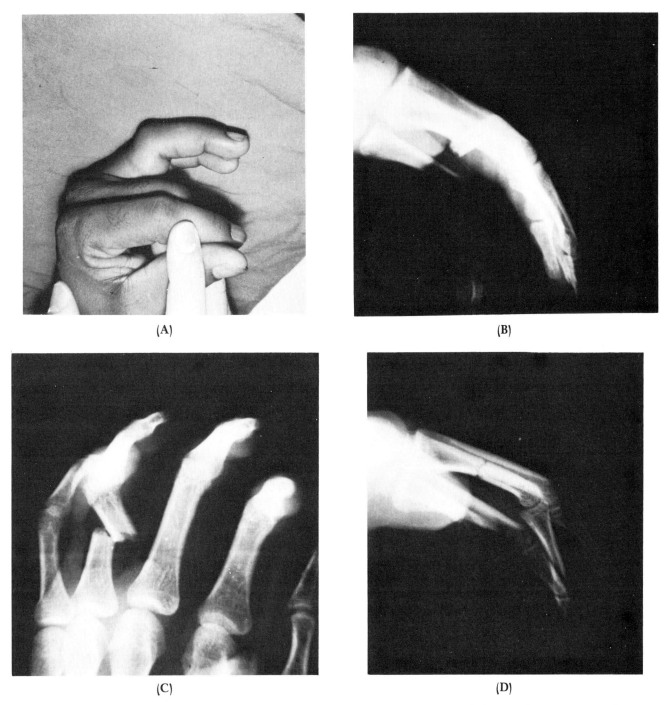

(A) (B)

(C) (D)

Figure 8-6 **(A)** Typical configuration of angulated transverse fracture of proximal phalanx with recurvatum of proximal phalanx and flexion of PIP and DIP joints. **(B)** Lateral radiograph shows dorsal angulation of distal fragment with apex of angulation palmarly and PIP and DIP flexion. **(C)** PA view shows shortening of proximal phalanx and angulation. **(D)** Lateral radiograph after closed manipulation and reduction shows anatomic reconstitution of proximal phalanx.

(continued)

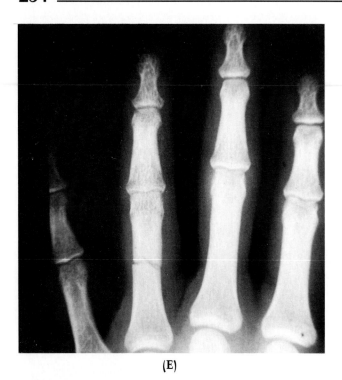

(E)

Figure 8-6 *(continued)*
(E) PA radiograph shows anatomic position. Immobilization was continued for 3 weeks after manipulation and reduction.

angulation upon the flexor digitorum superficialis and profundus tendons. (This recurvatum configuration is exactly opposite to that noted for angulated metacarpal fractures.)

If reduction is stable after closed manipulation, immobilization should be continued for about three weeks (Figures 8-5A–C, 8-6A–E).

Unstable proximal phalangeal shaft fractures should be anatomically reduced and skeletally fixed to maintain that reduction. Closed manipulation and percutaneous pin fixation is preferred, although often it is very difficult to achieve. If one attempt fails, open reduction and internal fixation should be carried out. Longitudinal intramedullary fixation, particularly for extremely comminuted fractures, may be helpful. Rarely is dynamic skeletal traction used.

An unstable fracture, either through the diaphysis or at the junction of the proximal metaphysis and diaphysis of the proximal phalanx, is best treated by open reduction and fixation of the fracture site (Figures 8-7A–C, 8-8A–C, 8-9A,B). Fracture site fixation should not impinge upon any adjacent joint, if

possible, to permit joint motion during healing. Early motion of the superficialis tendon is desired to prevent binding down of that tendon at the site of fracture and reduction, particularly after open reduction and internal fixation. If Kirschner wire fixation at the fracture site cannot be satisfactorily obtained—since this technique may be quite difficult to perform (Figure 8-7B)—longitudinal Kirschner wire fixation may align the proximal phalanx well, but unfortunately it impinges on the metacarpophalangeal joint (Figure 8-8B).

Oblique proximal phalangeal fractures often result in both shortening and rotational or angulation deformities. Closed anatomic reduction must be strived for (Figures 8-10A,B, 8-11A–E); if this is inadequate or impossible, fixation must be provided after closed or open anatomic reduction.

An unstable oblique proximal phalangeal fracture should be anatomically reduced closed and fixed by percutaneous Kirschner wire fixation, if possible. However, open reduction and internal fixation often is necessary, as with a transverse shaft fracture (refer to Figures 8-7B and 8-13A–C).

An obliquely placed Kirschneer wire which avoids impingement on either the MP or PIP joints may be used to maintain reduction (Figures 8-9A,B).

Occasionally surgical exposure of an irreducible shaft fracture allows removal of soft tissue interposition and anatomic reduction with no necessity for skeletal fixation (Figures 8-12A–C). Exposure of the fracture site allows anatomic reduction and fixation at the fracture site under direct vision if necessary (Figures 8-13A–C).

Aluminum splint immobilization of a displaced, somewhat angulated or rotated proximal phalangeal fracture which is partially reduced is obviously contraindicated. Malalignment angulation and malrotation are certain to result with corresponding functional disability. A fracture of this type, either transverse or oblique, when irreducible closed, should be opened and internally fixed if satisfactory percutaneous fixation is impossible (Figures 8-14A–C).

Anatomic reduction of a proximally displaced oblique shaft fracture which impinges on the PIP joint is mandatory. Otherwise, corrective reconstructive surgery to eliminate the impinging spicule will be necessary to regain acceptable PIP joint motion (Figures 8-15A–E, 8-16).

Comminuted shaft fractures should be held in as anatomic reduction as possible by any means available. Occasionally a longitudinal Kirschner wire fixation affords satisfactory positioning and stability

Figure 8-7 (**A**) Oblique view of displaced, rotated, angulated fracture of proximal phalanx at junction of proximal metaphysis with diaphysis. (**B**) Radiograph after open reduction and internal fixation with crossed Kirschner wires. (**C**) PA radiograph 6 weeks after open reduction and internal fixation shows maintenance of anatomic reduction after removal of Kirschner wires.

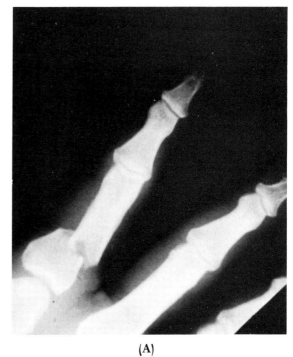

(A)

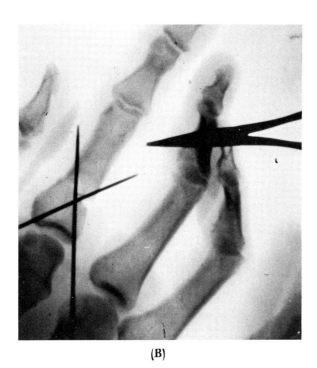

(B)

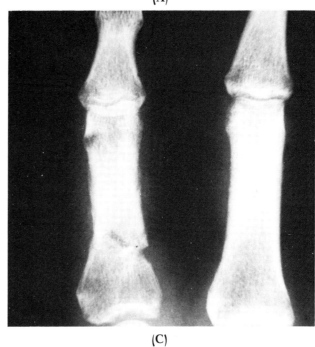

(C)

Figure 8-8 (A) Lateral view shows typical configuration of transverse proximal phalangeal fracture dorsally angulated with excess callus 2½ weeks after injury with no treatment. (B) Lateral radiograph after open reduction and longitudinal intramedullary Kirschner wire fixation. (C) Lateral radiograph 3 weeks after surgery showing anatomic position after removal of Kirschner wire.

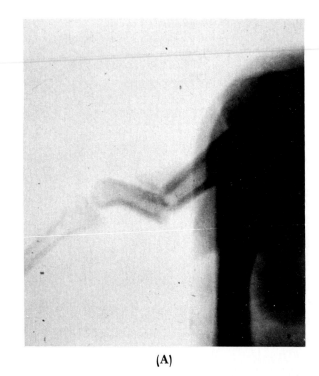

(A)

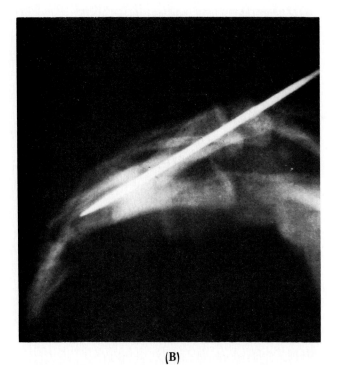

(B)

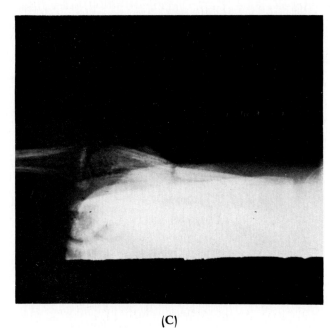

(C)

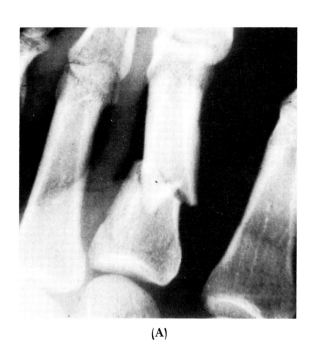
(A)

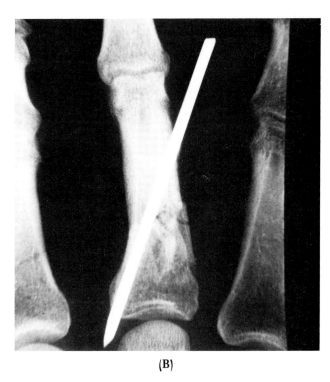
(B)

Figure 8-9 (A) Lateral radiograph of comminuted proximal phalangeal fracture with characteristic recurvatum deformity due to dorsal angulation of distal fragment. (B) PA view after open manipulation, reduction, and oblique large Kirschner wire fixation of this extremely unstable fracture. Note attempt to avoid impingement of Kirschner wire on MP and PIP joints to allow early postoperative motion. Good healing with acceptable alignment and almost normal MP and PIP joint motion resulted.

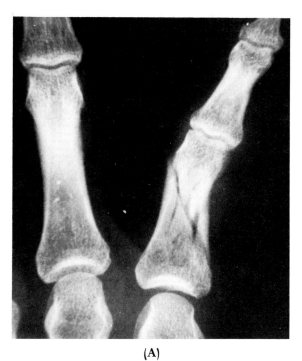
(A)

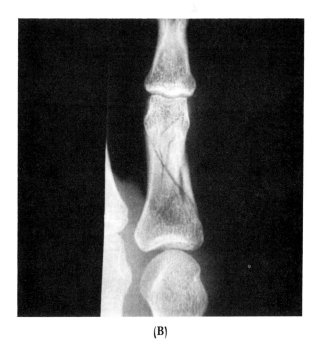
(B)

Figure 8-10 (A) PA view shows angulated comminuted proximal phalangeal fracture. (B) PA view shows maintenance of reduced position 10 days posttrauma and after closed reduction.

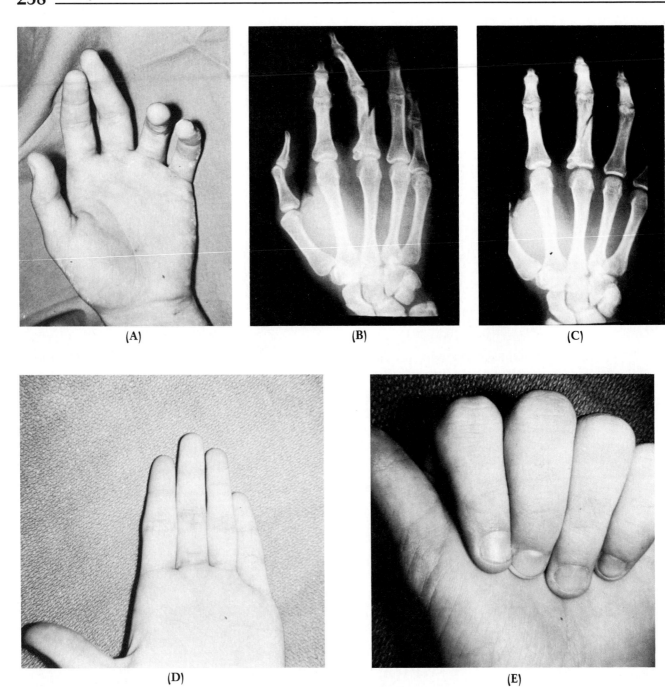

Figure 8-11 **(A)** Palmar view showing obvious rotational deformity of long finger. At first glance this would appear to be a physeal separation of proximal phalanx in a youth. **(B)** PA radiograph shows oblique fracture of proximal phalanx with rotational deformity. Upon close study, condylar fracture of radial condyle of long finger proximal phalanx also may be seen. It is important to scrutinize other areas closely to check for less overt simultaneous injuries when evaluating an obvious deformity. **(C)** PA radiograph 2 weeks after closed manipulation and reduction shows maintenance of anatomic position. **(D)** Palmar view 8 weeks after injury shows proper alignment of long finger to adjacent index and ring fingers. **(E)** Anatomic physiologic flexion of long finger in alignment with adjacent digits was achieved.

Figure 8-12 **(A)** Abduction of little finger in a youth, indicating probable physeal separation of proximal phalanx (dorsal view). **(B)** PA radiograph shows ulnar angulation of oblique fracture of proximal phalanx. Dorsal angulation of distal fragment of proximal phalanx was associated. **(C)** PA view after open reduction and no internal fixation shows excellent position. Open reduction was necessary because soft tissue interposition prevented closed reduction, but no internal fixation was necessary since reduced fracture was stable.

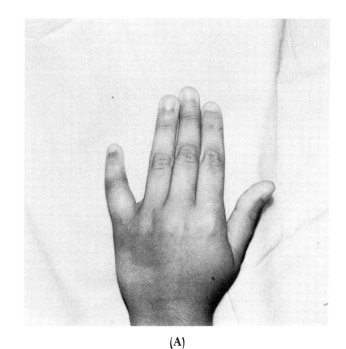

(A)

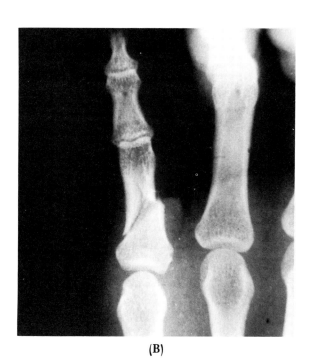

(B)

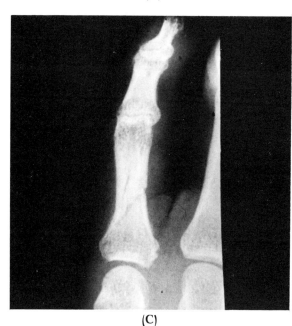

(C)

Figure 8-13 (A) PA radiograph of crushing injury shows oblique displaced fractues of both long and ring finger proximal phalanges and rotation at long finger fracture site. (B) Radiograph after open reduction and internal fixation of both fractures. Long finger fracture involved a separate butterfly fragment, necessitating reduction of fragment to base of proximal phalanx, followed by reduction of distal aspect of proximal phalanx to butterfly fragment. (C) PA radiograph 5 weeks after open reduction and internal fixation of both fractures following removal of internal fixation shows anatomic position restored.

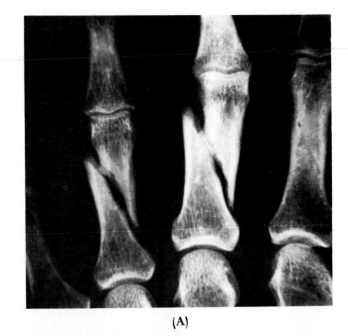

(A)

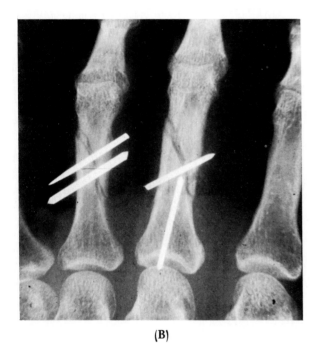

(B)

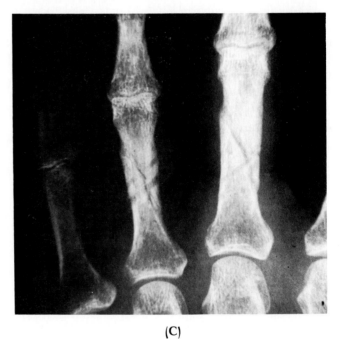

(C)

Figure 8-14 (A) PA radiograph after inadequate reduction and attempt at fixation with longitudinal Kirschner wire of oblique unstable proximally displaced shaft fracture of ring finger proximal phalanx. (B) Functional result after malunion shows significant rotational deformity of ring finger proximal phalanx impinging across dorsal aspect of little finger on attempted flexion.
(C) Good flexion after corrective osteotomy at site of malunion of ring finger proximal phalanx.

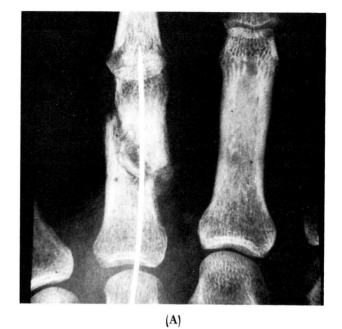

(A)

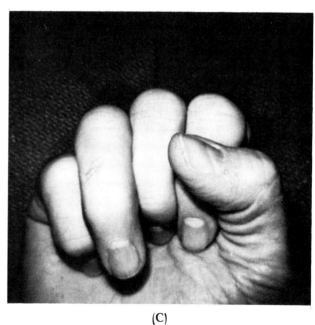

(B)

(C)

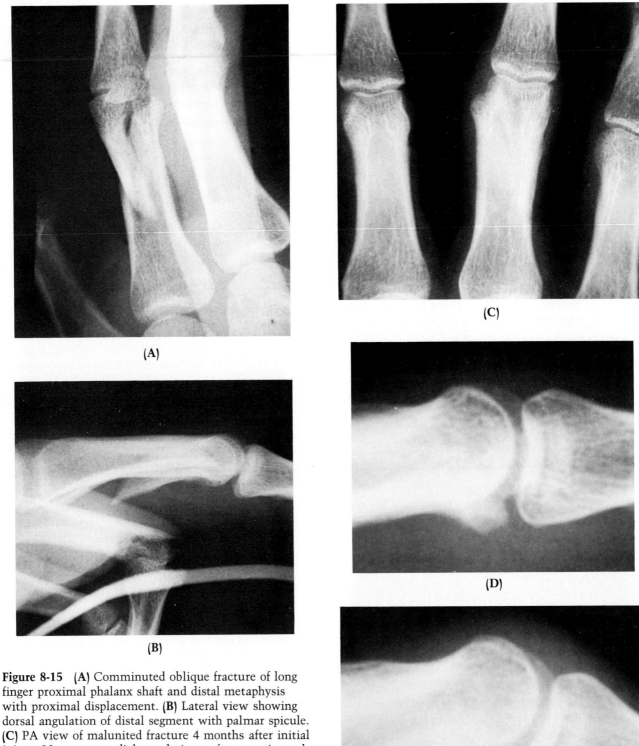

Figure 8-15 (**A**) Comminuted oblique fracture of long finger proximal phalanx shaft and distal metaphysis with proximal displacement. (**B**) Lateral view showing dorsal angulation of distal segment with palmar spicule. (**C**) PA view of malunited fracture 4 months after initial injury. Note some radial angulation at fracture site and ulnar protuberance of spicule of proximal fragment. (**D**) Close-up showing malunion, with impingement of spicule of proximal phalanx on PIP joint preventing adequate flexion. (**E**) Lateral radiograph after surgical excision of protruding fragment. Greatly improved PIP flexion resulted.

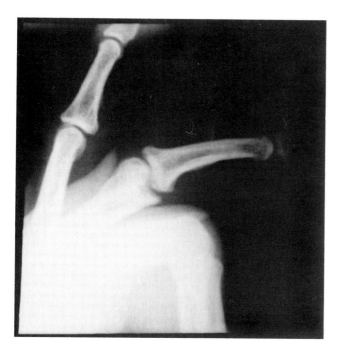

Figure 8-16 More severe malunited oblique proximal phalangeal fracture with virtually no PIP joint flexion because of impingement.

(refer to Chapter 15, Multiple Fractures, Figures 15-11A–E).

Skeletal traction to maintain reduction of a comminuted unstable fracture must be used with extreme discretion (Figures 8-17A–H). This traction should never be applied to the pulp but should always be through the skeleton, preferably transversely through the middle phalanx (Figure 8-17D). This dynamic skeletal traction requires meticulous attention to detail to avoid rotational deformities, malalignment, and angulation deformities. There should be no distraction at the fracture site since this will cause delay in union and, occasionally, nonunion. Skeletal traction, properly employed, is time-consuming and requires application of a short arm cast, followed by a palmar plaster splint incorporating the injured digit and the adjacent digit on either side to control proper rotation (Figures 8-17G,H). There is no place in the current treatment of digital fractures for the banjo splint which necessitates complete MP and IP joint extension.

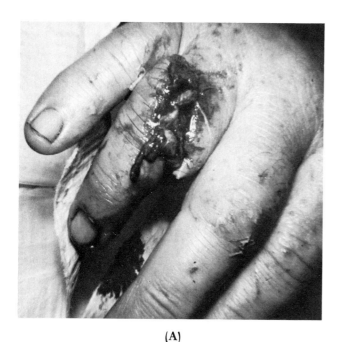

(A)

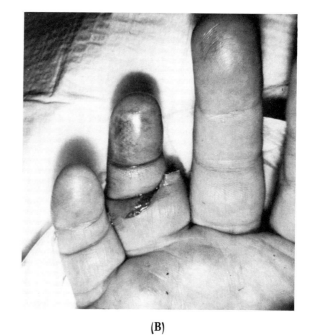

(B)

Figure 8-17 **(A)** Severe crush injury of proximal phalanx with marked comminution and shortening due to massive compression injury. **(B)** Palmar view shows nearly circumferential crush laceration of proximal phalangeal skin.

(continued)

Figure 8-17 *(continued)*
(C) PA view shows extensive comminution of proximal phalangeal crush fracture. **(D)** Close-up PA view after open manipulation and reduction followed by dynamic skeletal traction to maintain proper alignment and rotation of this extremely unstable comminuted proximal phalangeal fracture. After satisfactory healing flexor digitorum superficialis tendon was excised from fracture callus and almost normal digital function of digit resulted. **(E)** Healed fracture in good alignment 7 weeks after injury.

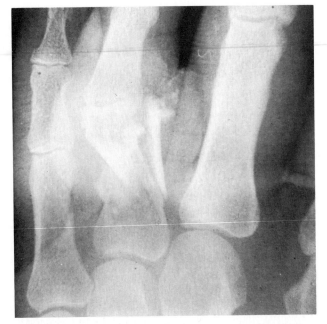

(C)

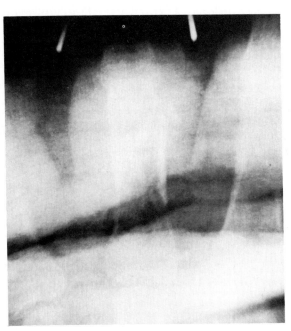

(D)

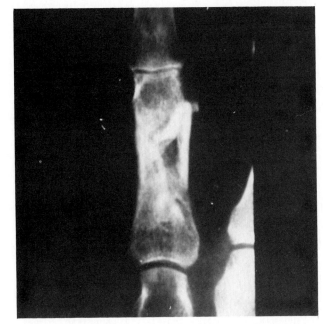

(E)

Figure 8-17 *(continued)*
(F) Lateral view. **(G)** Dynamic skeletal traction without compressive immobilization. Short arm cast immobilization augmented by palmar plaster splint supporting involved digit with adjacent digit on each side to allow uniform traction upon palmar surface of entire digit and to align injured digit properly both in rotation and alignment to adjacent digits. **(H)** Dorsal view shows traction as described. Traction should be sufficient to maintain reduction without distracting fragments at site of comminuted fracture.

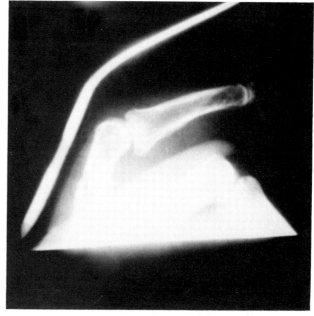

(F)

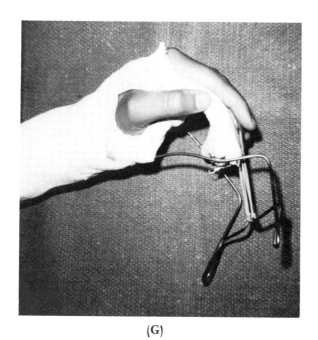

(G)

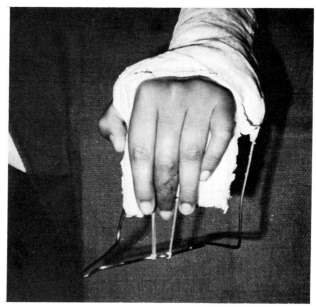

(H)

Figure 8-18 (A) Open comminuted displaced fracture of proximal phalanx. (B) PA radiograph shows displaced oblique comminuted proximal phalangeal fracture of little finger. (C) PA radiograph after open manipulation and stable reduction of fracture with no internal fixation necessary.

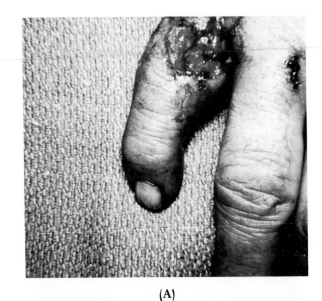

(A)

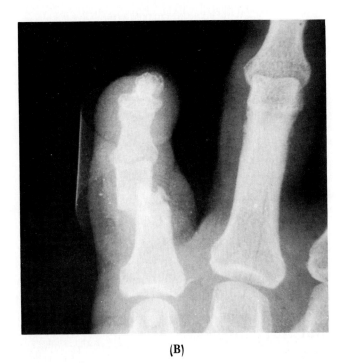

(B)

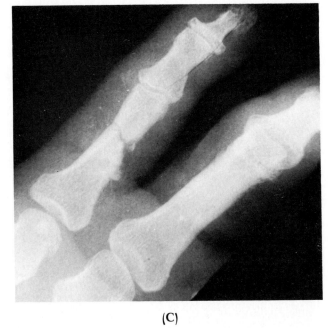

(C)

Initial meticulous cleansing, irrigation, and wound debridement (Figures 8-17A–D, 8-18A–C) are of primary importance in open fracture reduction. If open reduction is stable, the problem is solved. If advisable, internal fixation may be provided at primary care, at delayed primary treatment, or at secondary treatment after primary wound healing has occurred with no evidence of infection.

If malunion of a proximal phalangeal fracture has occurred (Figures 8-1A–C, 8-2A,B) correction of rotational, angulational, or alignment deformities is possible in the majority of instances by reconstructive osteotomy and digital realignment (Figures 8-1A–C). This rotational osteotomy may be performed occasionally in the metacarpal shaft or base to correct deformities in the proximal phalanx.

Arthroplasty and excision of a bone fragment impinging on a joint resulting from malunion may be carried out to restore better joint motion (Figures 8-15A–E).

Middle Phalangeal Fractures

Fracture of the middle phalanx is far less common than that of either the metacarpal or proximal phalanx. Crushing injuries or open wounds such as those from a saw or lawn mower typically cause this trauma. Torsional forces do not involve the middle phalanx to any extent since this bone is short and broad and thus much stronger than the adjacent proximal phalanx, metacarpal, and PIP joint.

Fractures may be divided according to their sites: distal metaphyseal, shaft, and basilar or proximal metaphyseal. Stable fractures should be immobilized with the PIP and DIP joints in extension for approximately 14 to 17 days, with light motion beginning at that time.

At reduction of displaced or angulated fractures, malrotation and angulation deformities must be prevented and length restored. It is important to strive for anatomic reduction in order to avoid complications involving the extensor mechanism (insertion of the central slip at the dorsal base of the middle phalanx and continuation of the lateral bands distally to insert in the base of the distal phalanx) in its synergistic action with the flexor digitorum superficialis (which inserts on the proximal two-thirds of the palmar aspect of this phalanx). Of great importance is accurate MP and PIP joint alignments at reduction.

Crush injuries involving the proximal two-thirds of the middle phalangeal shaft characteristically involve the superficialis tendon in cicatrix and callus, whereas in the distal third the profundus tendon may be similarly entrapped in callus.

Distal Metaphyseal Fractures

Undisplaced distal metaphyseal fractures are usually caused by blunt trauma and are treated by conservative immobilization for 12 to 14 days as noted above. Malunion with angulation, shortening, and rotational deformities causes severe functional impairment. Impingement of a bone spicule at a site of oblique fracture malunion may restrict PIP or DIP (Figure 8-19) joint motion.

Malrotation and malalignment deformities of the involved digit cause impingment on an adjacent digit or digits (Figures 8-20A,B). Some displacement may be accepted if proper alignment and rotation are achieved.

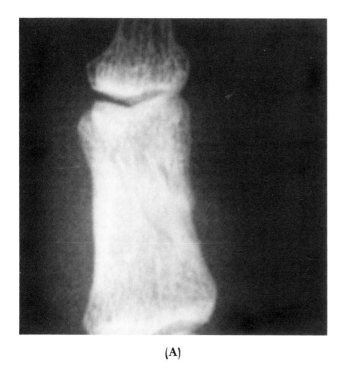

(A)

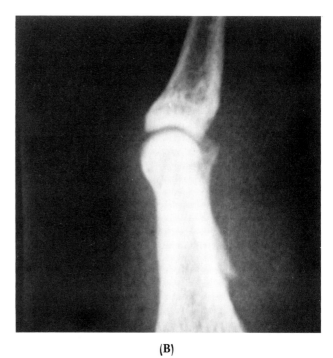

(B)

Figure 8-19 **(A)** Oblique fracture through distal metaphysis of middle phalanx. **(B)** Impingement of fracture spicule on palmar aspect of distal phalanx base limiting DIP joint flexion.

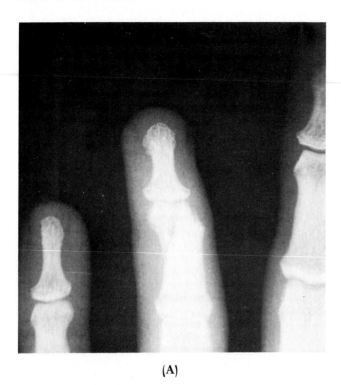

(A)

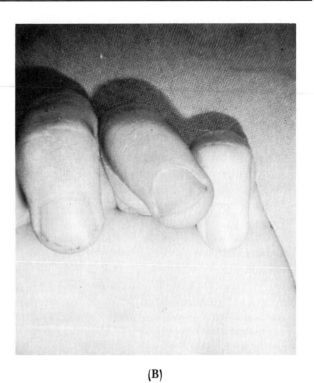

(B)

Figure 8-20 **(A)** PA view 3 weeks postinjury shows ulnar angulation with some rotational deformity at fracture site through distal metaphysis of ring finger middle phalanx. **(B)** Angulation and crossover of ring finger upon attempted complete digital flexion due to malunion shown in Figure 8-20A.

Shaft Fractures

The configuration of a middle phalangeal shaft fracture, if angulated, depends on the relation of the flexor digitorum superficialis tendon insertion to the fracture site. If the superficialis insertion is proximal to the fracture site, the phalanx proximal to the fracture will be flexed palmarly due to pull of that muscle. The shaft distal to the fracture site therefore will be angled dorsally, with the apex of that angulation palmarly. This protruding palmar angulation at the fracture site impinges on the flexor digitorum profundus and, combined with laxity of the extensor mechanism (lateral bands), causes DIP flexion (Figures 8-21A,B). If the superficialis tendon inserts distal to the fracture site, the shaft distal to the fracture angulates palmarly and the proximal shaft angulates dorsally, with the apex of angulation dorsally. The superficialis tendon causes flexion of the distal fragment, and the central slip of insertion of the extensor tendon extends the proximal fragment. This concept is best seen in palmar fracture dislocation of the PIP joint with avulsion of a portion of the dorsal cortex of the base in continuity with the central slip of insertion. Refer to Figures 9-53A, 9-54A, and

9-55A in Chapter 9, Injuries to Digital Soft Tissue Structures.

If the fracture is unstable, closed reduction (open, if necessary) with percutaneous Kirschner wire fixation or internal fixation will be necessary.

If closed reduction is impossible, open anatomic reduction and percutaneous Kirschner wire or internal fixation are suggested as the best treatment (Figures 8-21C,D).

A typical angulated transverse shaft fracture shows deformities described above most often with the apex of angulation palmarly causing a recurvatum deformity of the middle phalanx similar to the deformity of an angulated proximal phalangeal shaft fracture (Figures 8-21A,B). Fixation may be provided by longitudinal (Figures 8-21C,D) or oblique Kirschner wire fixation. Direct Kirschner wire fixation at the site of the fracture may be technically very difficult due to the small size of this bone. If longitudinal fixation is utilized, the DIP joint should be maintained in extension. Displacement with or without separation at the fracture site may result from a severe crush injury, which is often open (Figures 8-22A,B).

Stable undisplaced oblique fractures of the shaft, whether extending intraarticularly or not, are

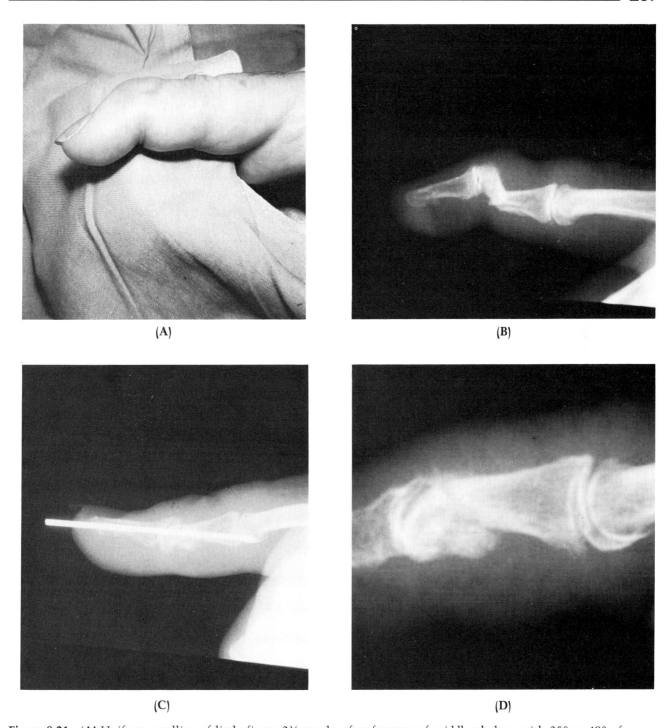

(A)

(B)

(C)

(D)

Figure 8-21 **(A)** Uniform swelling of little finger 2½ weeks after fracture of middle phalanx with 35° to 40° of incomplete extension at DIP joint. **(B)** Characteristic deformity with dorsal angulation of middle phalangeal segment distal to comminuted transverse middle phalangeal shaft fracture. **(C)** Lateral view of longitudinal Kirschner wire fixation after open reduction. **(D)** Lateral radiograph 10 weeks after open reduction and longitudinal Kirschner wire fixation (removed 3½ weeks after insertion). Nearly complete extension of PIP and DIP joints were noted at this time.

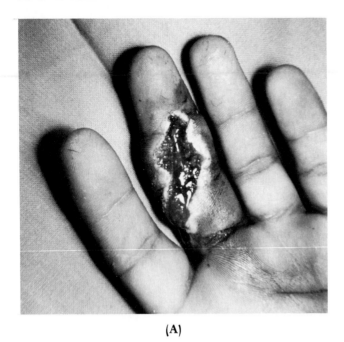

(A)

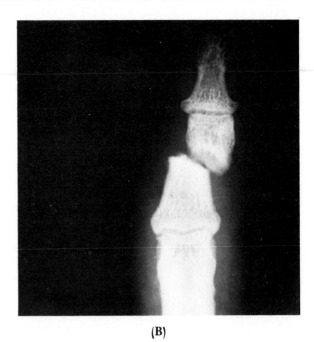

(B)

Figure 8-22 **(A)** Severe open crush fracture of middle phalanx 5 days after initial trauma. Severity of vascular impairment and marked swelling still prevented delayed primary closure and fracture reduction. **(B)** PA view shows significant distraction at middle phalangeal fracture site due to severity of injury. Treatment should include reduction and Kirschner wire fixation after circulation has improved to allow definitive treatment. Fracture may be treated simultaneously with delayed primary wound closure or as a secondary procedure, if necessary.

treated conservatively as noted above (Figure 8-23). If unstable, these fractures tend to displace and also angulate somewhat. If the fracture extends into the vicinity of either the PIP or DIP joint, proximal displacement may cause either a fracture fragment or callus to impinge upon that adjacent joint, with resulting decrease in motion (Figures 8-24A,B). It is strongly advised, therefore, that unstable oblique fractures be reduced and fixed either by closed reduction and percutaneous Kirschner wire fixation, if feasible, or by open reduction and internal fixation.

If a middle phalangeal fracture is extremely comminuted and unstable, fixaton should be provided by whatever means will establish the closest approximation to normal anatomy. Kirschner wire longitudinal fixation or dynamic skeletal traction through the distal phalanx (either transversely through the base or in a PA direction through the nail plate and tuft) may be attempted if vascular impairment is not caused by the latter.

Fractures of the Proximal Metaphysis or Base

If fracture at the proximal metaphysis or base of the middle phalanx involves angulation or rotational

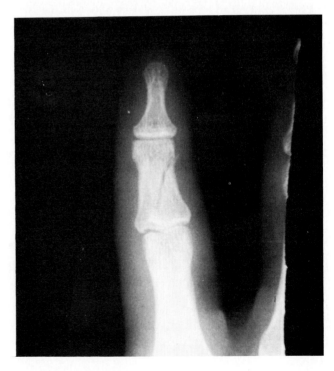

Figure 8-23 Oblique undisplaced shaft fracture of middle phalanx extending into PIP joint.

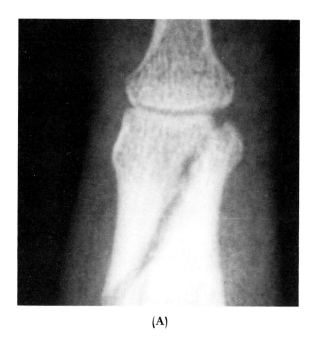

(A)

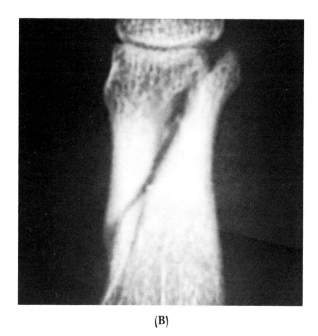

(B)

Figure 8-24 (A) PA view of oblique fracture of middle phalanx shows impingement of proximal bone spicule into DIP joint. A rotational element of deformity can be suspected because of incongruity of opposing surfaces at fracture site. (B) Close-up showing increased displacement with further impingement upon DIP joint 4 weeks later. Preferred initial treatment would include open reduction and Kirschner wire fixation to restore proper rotational alignment and to relieve impingement on DIP joint.

deformity, the anatomy should be restored to normal (Figures 8-25 and 8-26A–C).

Growth and remodeling often will provide acceptable correction of palmar or dorsal angulation in children, according to Wolff's law. (See Chapter 12, Posttraumatic Skeletal Remodeling, Figures 12-4A–E.)

Lateral, palmar, or dorsal angulation, rotational deformity, and shortening, particularly in adults, causes functional disability if uncorrected at initial treatment of the fracture (Figures 8-25, 8-26A–C). Later realignment may be achieved by corrective osteotomy.

Open fractures are treated by meticulous wound toilet and appropriate treatment for the specific fracture.

Distal Phalangeal Fractures

The vast majority of distal phalangeal fractures are caused by crushing injuries from heavy objects or by avulsive crushing injuries from saws, lawn mowers, snow blowers, etc. Therefore care of the soft tissue is the most important aspect of primary treatment (Figures 8-27A–D, 8-28A–D).

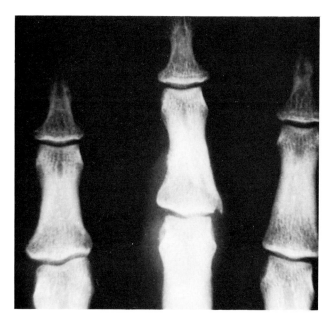

Figure 8-25 Angulation at site of comminuted impacted fracture through proximal metaphysis or base of middle phalanx.

Figure 8-26 (A) Grossly comminuted middle phalangeal fracture involving shaft and base of proximal metaphysis. (B) Lateral view shows complete fracture displacement through metaphysis. (C) Lateral radiograph 6 months after original injury shows gross malunion of completely displaced middle phalanx base and essentially no PIP flexion.

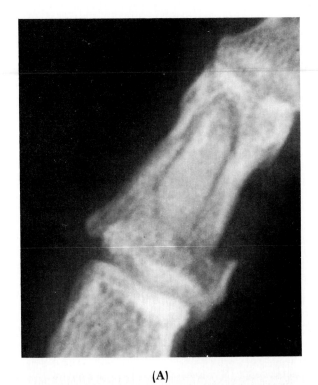

(A)

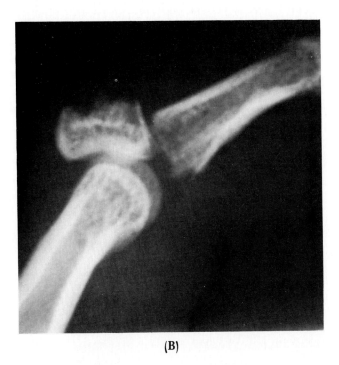

(B)

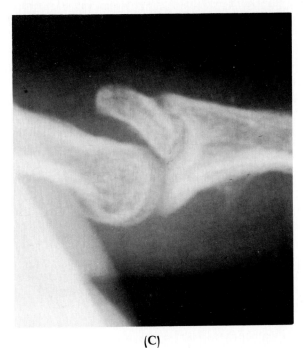

(C)

Many distal phalangeal fractures are open injuries and must be meticulously cleaned, irrigated, and debrided prior to any primary fracture care[1] (Figures 8-27A–D, 8-28A–D). If there is marked swelling, the wound should remain open or be closed very loosely to allow escape of edema and hemorrhage.

Any viable germinal epithelium which is not badly damaged should be retained (Figures 8-27A–D, 8-28A–D). If a painful or cosmetically unacceptable nail plate results, the aberrant germinal epithelium remnant may be excised under magnificaton as a secondary reconstructive procedure.

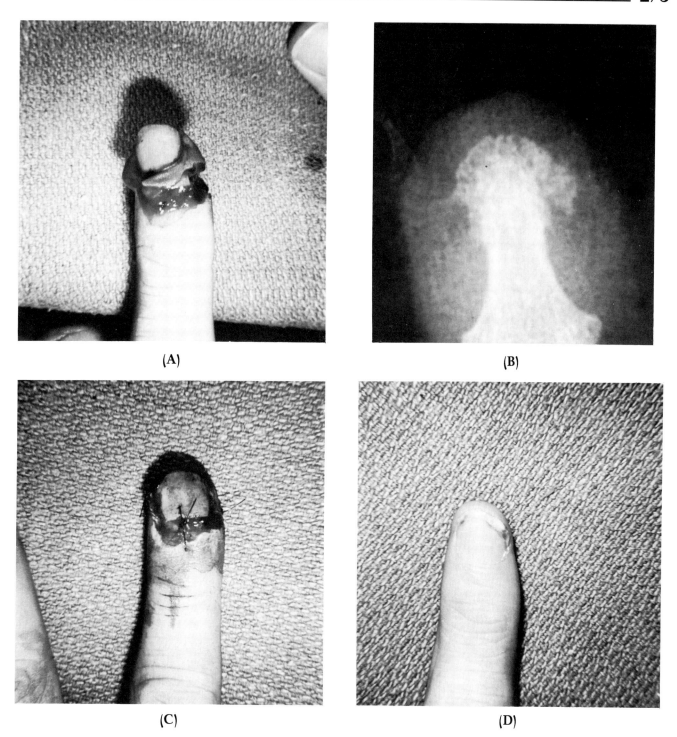

(A)

(B)

(C)

(D)

Figure 8-27 **(A)** Dorsal view of near amputation by saw through middle of distal phalanx. **(B)** Radiograph shows comminuted, essentially undisplaced tuft fracture of distal phalanx. **(C)** Dorsal photograph after meticulous wound toilet, debridement of proximal 40% of nail plate to prevent sequestration of any possible contaminated material in nail plate cul-de-sac, and primary soft tissue suture. **(D)** Dorsal view 5 months after injury showing nail plate regrowth, indicating germinal epithelium was minimally damaged.[2]

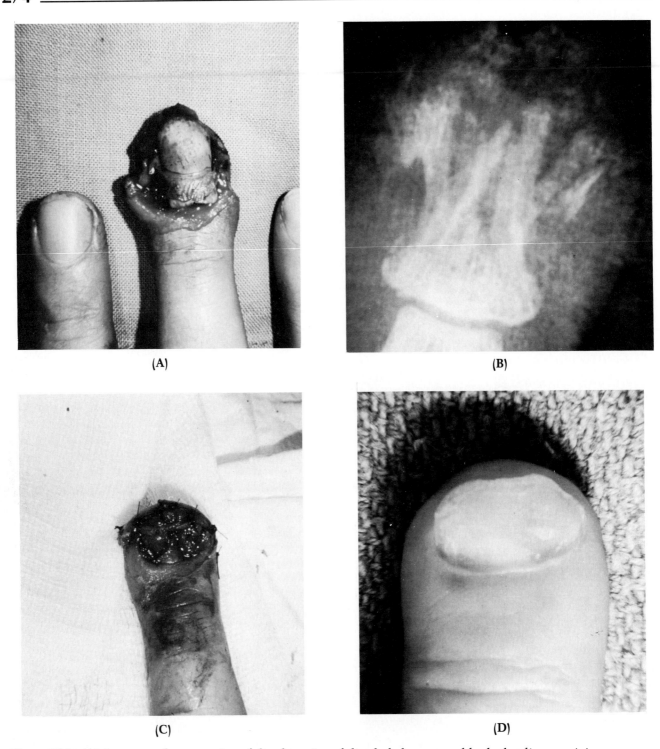

(A)

(B)

(C)

(D)

Figure 8-28 **(A)** Severe crush amputation of distal portion of distal phalanx caused by hydraulic press injury. Note complete avulsion of proximal nail plate and severe soft tissue damage. **(B)** Radiograph shows "blast" or "bursting" type injury with extensively comminuted fractures of tuft and shaft of distal phalanx. **(C)** Dorsal photograph after meticulous wound toilet, complete removal of nail, and use of palmar skin for primary closure. Nail bed itself was not treated other than to cleanse and restore it as anatomically as possible. **(D)** Dorsal view 6 months after injury shows surprisingly good nail plate regrowth and good digital contour despite some shortening.

Fractures of the Tuft

The most common lesion is a fracture of the tuft of the distal phalanx which is usually due to a crushing injury[2] (Figures 8-27B, 8-28B). The various degrees of fracture which occur include:

1. Undisplaced chip fracture of tuft
2. Slightly comminuted undisplaced fracture of tuft (Figure 8-27B)
3. An explosive or bursting variety in which both tuft and shaft are completely comminuted (Figure 8-28B)
4. Completely displaced transverse fracture at base of tuft and shaft (Figure 8-36A)
5. Undisplaced transverse fracture through distal portion of tuft (Figure 8-29), central portion of tuft (Figure 8-30), or base of tuft at its junction with the diaphysis or shaft (Figure 8-31)

No attempt should be made to remove any bone fragments unless they are completely devoid of soft tissue attachment and are literally washed out when the open injury is irrigated. In the extremely comminuted bursting type injury (Figures 8-28A–D) gross molding is acceptable after proper wound toilet, debridement, and loose closure. In general, however, manipulation of distal phalangeal tuft fractures is unnecessary unless the tuft is completely displaced.

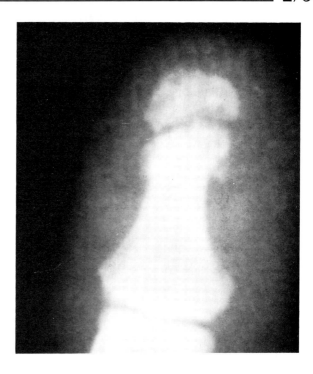

Figure 8-30 Transverse fracture through middle of distal phalangeal tuft.

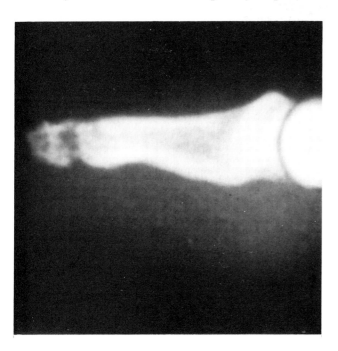

Figure 8-29 Transverse fracture through distal end of tuft of distal phalanx.

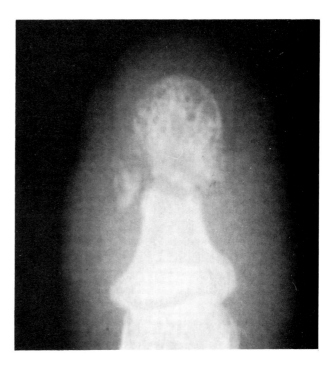

Figure 8-31 Transverse, somewhat comminuted fracture at base of distal phalangeal tuft at its junction with diaphysis.

Immobilization for fractures of the tuft (whether comminuted, transverse, or the occasional longitudinal type) should continue for at least three to three and one-half weeks to protect both the soft tissue and bone. Healing progresses much better and more rapidly with fewer complications of tenderness and aggravated cicatrix if the digit is properly immobilized and guarded. Initial immobilization by an aluminum splint extending across both PIP and DIP joints combined with compressive soft tissue dressing for the first week is changed to aluminum splint immobilization across the DIP joint only for an additonal two to three weeks. A retained subungual hematoma should be evacuated after appropriate cleansing. This can be done by penetration of the nail plate with a large hot paper clip, a No. 18 sterile hypodermic needle, or a No. 11 scalpel blade.

Shaft Fractures

Shaft fractures are usually transverse but occasionally may be longitudinal (Figure 8-32) or oblique. Transverse shaft fractures may occur at the distal end of the diaphysis at its junction with the tuft (Figure 8-31), through the middle of the diaphysis (Figure 8-32), or at the junction of the base with the diaphysis (Figures 8-33, 8-34A, 8-35A,B). Angulation is occasionally dorsal (Figure 8-34A), but is usually palmar (Figures 8-35A,B) with avulsion of the nail plate base. Since the extensor inserts on the dorsal aspect of the proximal epiphysis or base of the distal phalanx and the profundus tendon inserts on the palmar aspect of the proximal metaphysis, the extensor maintains the base in extension and the profundus flexes the shaft palmarly distal to the fracture site. Fracture of the distal phalanx with palmar angulation may mimic a drop finger, emphasizing the importance of radiographic studies (Figures 8-35A,B). A stable reduction after closed manipulation (Figures 8-35A–C) is treated by splint immobilization for three weeks. Occasionally, however, such a shaft fracture is grossly unstable, and longitudinal Kirschner wire fixation must be used to maintain satisfactory position (Figures 8-36A–E). Dorsal angulation (Figure 8-34A) may occur and is managed similarly (Figures 8-34A,B).

It is important to achieve proper reduction of an angulated shaft fracture, particularly if the nail plate has been avulsed. If incomplete reduction is discovered after initial treatment, remanipulation and adequate reduction should be followed by proper immobilization (Figures 8-35A–C). Often with such an injury permanent nail plate damage results from ini-

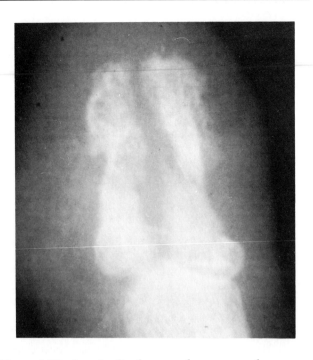

Figure 8-32 Longitudinal, somewhat separated comminuted crush fracture of distal phalanx extending into DIP joint. (Note also undisplaced transverse fracture through midshaft.)

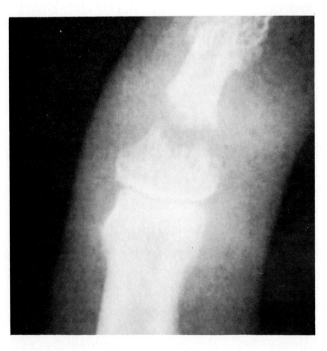

Figure 8-33 Undisplaced transverse fracture with some bone loss at junction of base and diaphysis of distal phalanx.

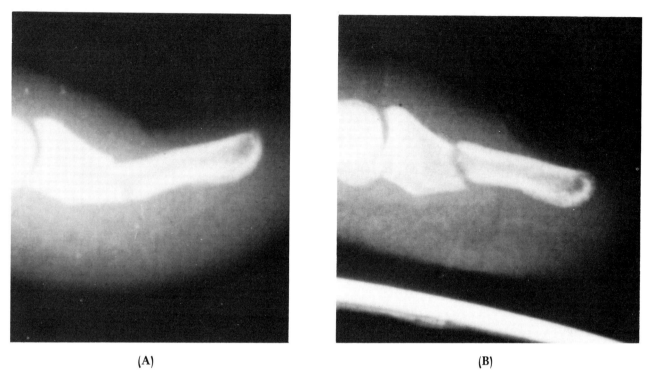

(A)   (B)

Figure 8-34 (A) Fracture at junction of base and shaft of distal phalanx with dorsal angulation of shaft distal to fracture site. (B) Satisfactory alignment after closed manipulation, reduction, and immobilization.

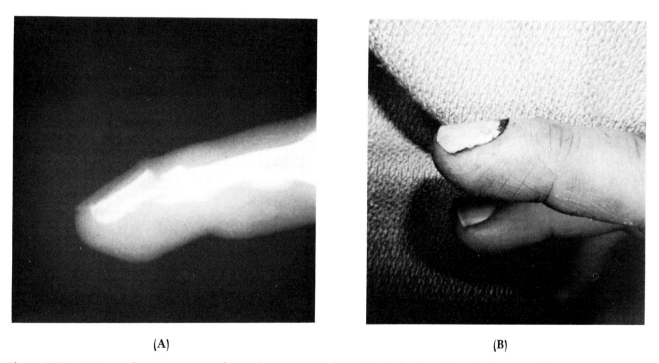

(A)   (B)

Figure 8-35 (A) Lateral view at time of initial treatment of angulated displaced distal phalangeal fracture at junction of diaphysis and base. (B) One day after injury and primary care there is persistent palmar angulation of distal phalanx. Radiograph shows no change of position after initial manipulation and attempted fracture reduction.

(continued)

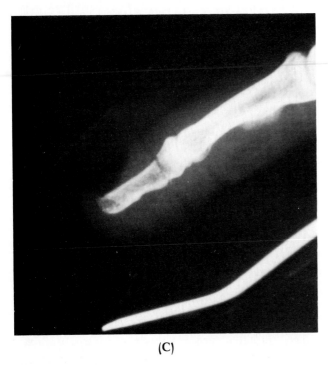

(C)

Figure 8-35 *(continued)*
(C) Lateral radiograph after successful second manipulation and reduction.

tial irreparable trauma to the germinal epithelium of the nail plate. If the proximal portion of the nail plate is avulsed from its cul-de-sac, it is desirable to debride the proximal 40% to 50% of the nail plate base (proximal portion) to prevent sequestration of a possibly contaminated hematoma and debris in the cul-de-sac at the time of fracture reduction.

Complex injuries of the distal phalanx must be treated by whatever method is appropriate, and often surgical intervention is necessary to achieve satisfactory results (Figures 8-36A–E). A rare occurrence is transverse fracture of the distal phalangeal shaft with protrusion of the distal fragment through the pulp palmarly. The tuft of the distal phalanx lies subcutaneously and must be reduced anatomically beneath and adjacent to the nailbed to prevent a chronic tender distal phalangeal tip and to protect it by sufficient subcutaneous tissue (Figure 8-37A–D).

Since the majority of proximal metaphyseal fractures involve the articular surface, they are discussed under Drop Finger in this chapter.

Closed Space Compression Injuries of the Distal Phalanx Pulp

Severe crush injury to the distal phalanx produces an open injury in the majority of instances (Figures

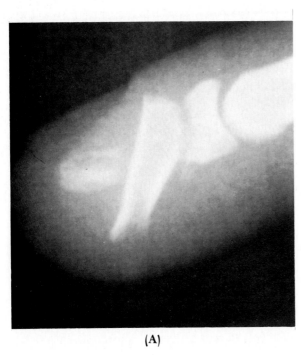

(A)

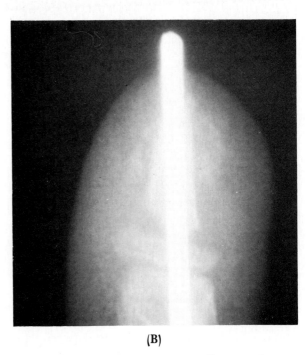

(B)

Figure 8-36 (A) Gross displacement of entire shaft of distal phalanx with tuft and base in essentially normal position. (B) Open reduction and longitudinal Kirschner wire fixation through DIP joint was necessary for stability.

Figure 8-36 *(continued)*
(C) PA radiograph 4 months after injury shows delayed union of diaphysis to base and telescoping of diaphysis into extremely comminuted tuft. **(D)** Lateral radiograph 2 years after injury shows nearly normal contour of distal phalanx and good DIP joint cartilage space. **(E)** PA view shows a short but normally contoured distal phalanx and good cartilage space of DIP joint.

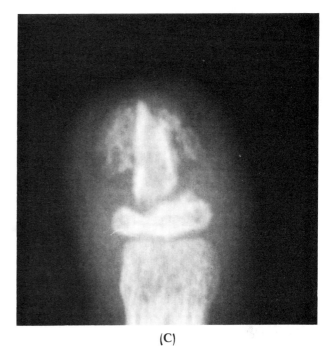

(C)

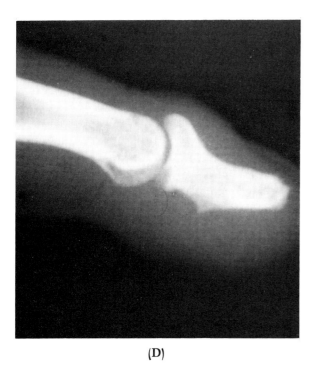

(D)

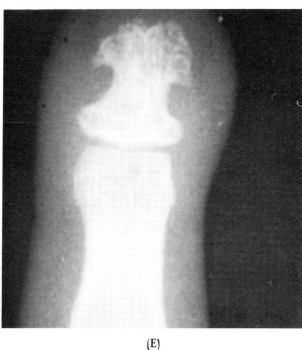

(E)

8-27A–D, 8-28A–D). If such trauma is sustained and the injury remains closed, compression within the loculated pulp may occur and result in ischemic changes to the skin and subcutaneous tissue (Figures 8-38A,B). Compression dressing, ice, and elevation with immobilization generally resolve the majority of these cases. Occasionally, however, pressure within this closed space is great enough to cause gangrenous changes if it is not relieved (Figures 8-39A–D). Wide incision just beneath the distal end of the nail plate from the midline extending proximally as far as necessary toward the nondominant midaxial line is necessary to sharply incise the fibrous septae at their origin from the periosteum and allow

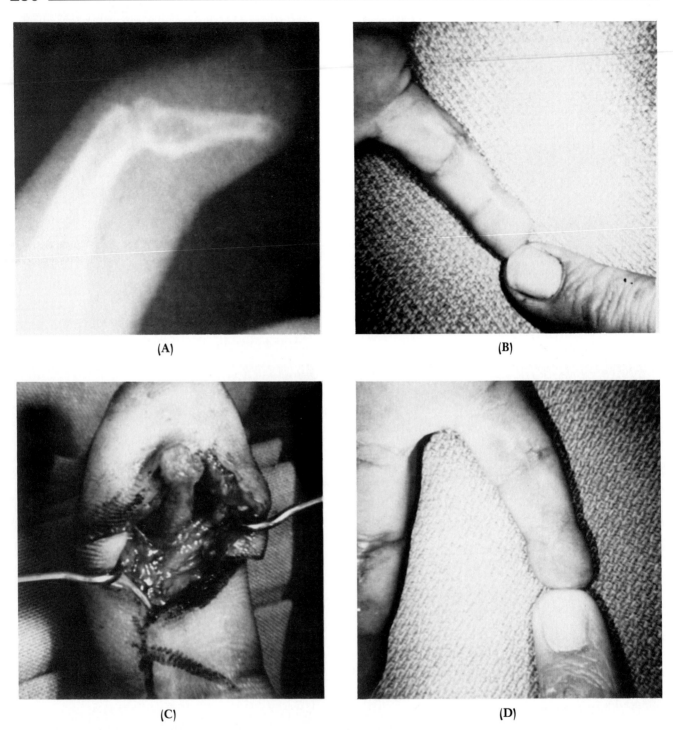

(A)

(B)

(C)

(D)

Figure 8-37 (A) Unusual injury in which the fractured distal phalanx has separated from the nailbed and protrudes deeply into the palmar pulp. (B) Pressure on the tip of the distal phalangeal segment shows protrusion of the distal phalanx tip subcutaneously. (C) Surgical exposure demonstrates palmar angulation of the distal phalanx with protrusion of the distal end. (D) Postoperatively after removal of the distal 40% of the distal phalanx and Z-plasty revision of the longitudinal scar, good protective pulp resurfaces the remainder of the phalanx.

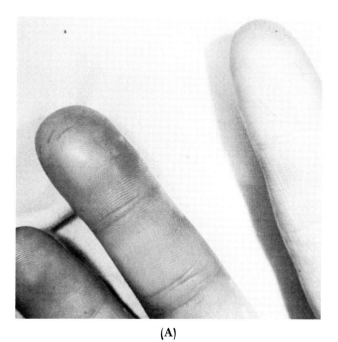

(A)

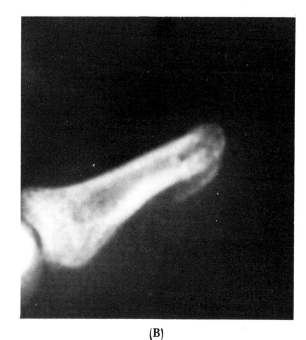

(B)

Figure 8-38 **(A)** Distended skin of distal phalanx from retained hematoma in closed space of distal phalangeal pulp. **(B)** Lateral radiograph of undisplaced chip fracture of distal phalangeal tuft. Injury was treated by compressive dressing, constant elevation, ice, and immobilization for 24 hours. Edema and congestion subsided considerably.

release of the hematoma. Healing occurs promptly, and minimal, if any, soft tissue necrosis ensues if the pressure is relieved prior to irreversible soft tissue changes. Similar ischemic changes occasionally occur after primary surgical closure of an open pulp injury of the distal phalanx. Treatment consists of removal of the sutures and wide opening of the wound.

Drop (Mallet) Finger

Drop finger—also known as mallet or baseball finger—consists of the inability to extend completely either the thumb at its IP joint or any of the other digits at its DIP joint due to laceration, avulsion or fracture avulsion of the extensor insertion. The usual mechanism of injury is a blow, often caused by a thrown object such as a baseball, to the tip or dorsum of the distal phalanx during vigorous active extension of the DIP joint. Forced extension of the DIP joint can cause fracture of the dorsal aspect of the base of the distal phalanx by direct abutment against the condyles of the middle phalanx. Proximal migration of the extensor insertion occurs after avulsion of its distal attachment from the base of the distal phalanx. Increased tension on the central slip of the extensor tendon,

which inserts into the epiphysis or base of the middle phalanx, results in a secondary recurvatum or hyperextension deformity of the PIP joint. The overall configuration is inability to extend the DIP joint and recurvatum or hyperextension of the PIP joint (Figure 8-40). This lesion may be caused by any of the following:

1. Avulsion of the extensor tendon insertion from the base of the distal phalanx or laceration of that tendon just proximal to its insertion (Figures 8-41A,B)
2. Chronic attrition and attenuation of the extensor tendon in the area of insertion by external pressure (e.g., arthritic spur) (Figure 8-42)
3. Small chip avulsion or small comminuted fracture of the dorsal aspect of the base of the distal phalanx associated with extensor tendon avulsion (Figure 8-43)
4. Large displaced articular fracture of the dorsal aspect of the base of the distal phalanx (usually 25% or more of the articular surface) in association with extensor tendon insertion (Figures 8-44, 8-46A,B, 8-47A,B)
5. Large displaced articular fracture (25% or more of the articular surface) with attached extensor insertion with palmar subluxation of the distal phalanx at the DIP joint (Figures 8-45A, 8-48A, 8-49A,B)

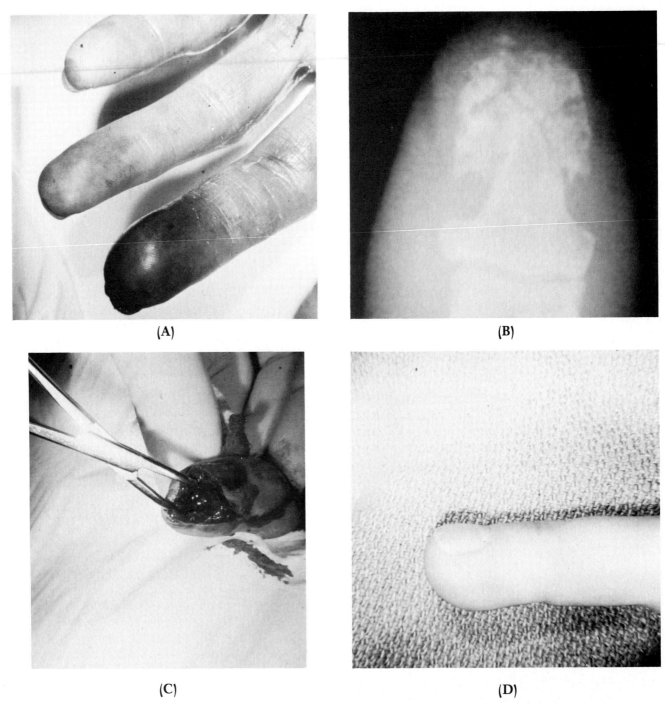

(A)

(B)

(C)

(D)

Figure 8-39 **(A)** Pregangrenous changes of distal phalangeal skin and pulp due to more severe closed crushing injury of distal phalanx with hematoma retained in closed space of pulp. **(B)** Radiograph shows gross comminution of distal phalangeal tuft fracture responsible for the hematoma. **(C)** Wide incision of pulp releases hematoma by incising septal fibers with care to protect digital nerves. **(D)** Healed incision 4 months after surgery. General function, including durability and sensation of pulp skin, was essentially normal.[2]

Figure 8-40 Lateral radiograph of acute drop finger due to avulsion of extensor tendon insertion. Note particularly recurvatum deformity of PIP joint caused by increased stress on central slip of insertion of extensor tendon on base of middle phalanx due to proximal retraction of lateral bands.

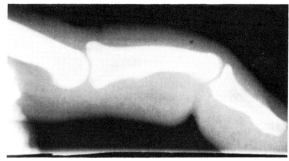

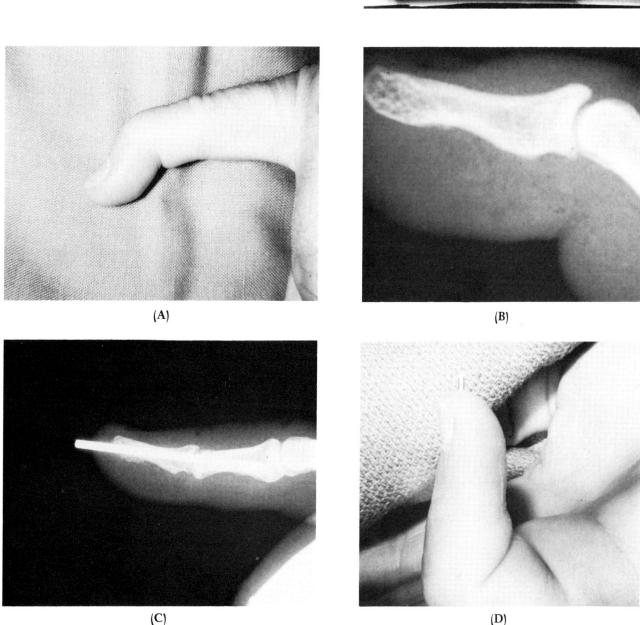

(A)

(B)

(C)

(D)

Figure 8-41 **(A)** Drop finger due to avulsion of extensor tendon insertion. **(B)** Lateral radiograph. **(C)** Lateral view after longitudinal Kirschner wire immobilization of DIP joint. **(D)** Lateral photograph shows nearly complete range of PIP flexion permitted during this type of immobilization of DIP joint. Extension (not shown) is normal.

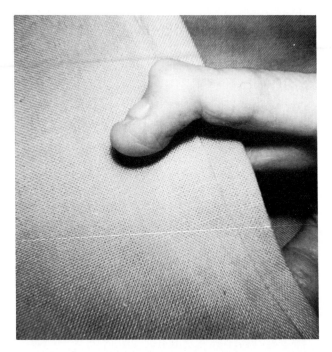

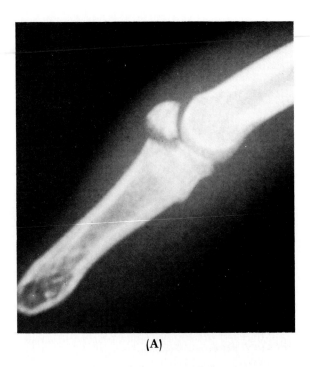

(A)

Figure 8-42   Drop finger due to erosion of extensor tendon by a giant cell tumor of tendon sheath.

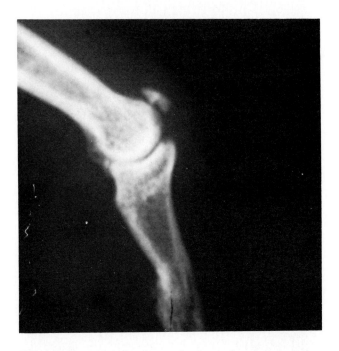

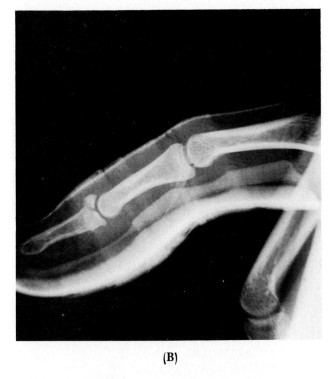

(B)

Figure 8-43   Lateral radiograph shows fracture avulsion of the extensor insertion.

Figure 8-44   **(A)** Dorsal articular fracture of distal phalanx slightly displaced causing a dropped DIP joint. **(B)** Conservative splint immobilization after closed reduction shows acceptable position at fracture site.

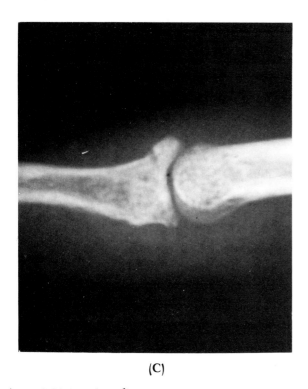

(C)

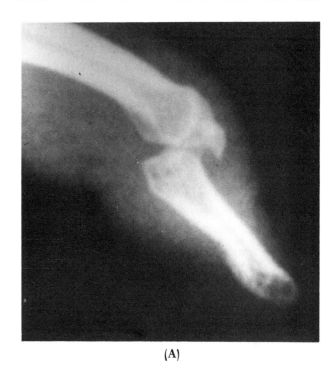

(A)

Figure 8-44 *(continued)*
(C) Lateral view 5 weeks after commencing splint im-
mobilization shows complete extension of DIP joint.
Flexion of 25° was obtained.

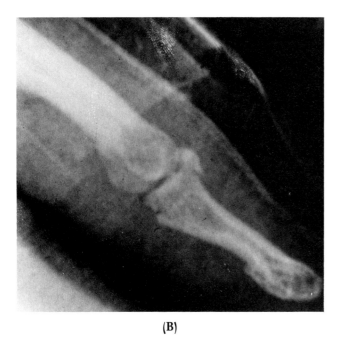

(B)

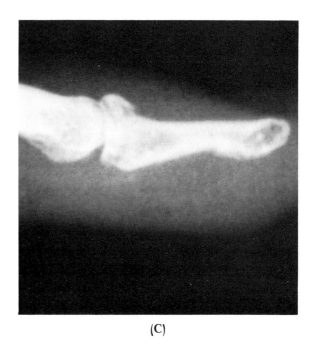

(C)

Figure 8-45   **(A)** Lateral view of fracture dislocation of DIP joint with resultant drop finger. **(B)** Acceptable position attained after closed manipulation and maintained by conservative splint immobilization. **(C)** Lateral view
6 weeks after injury shows complete extension with good union at fracture site. Flexion of 45° (not shown)
resulted.

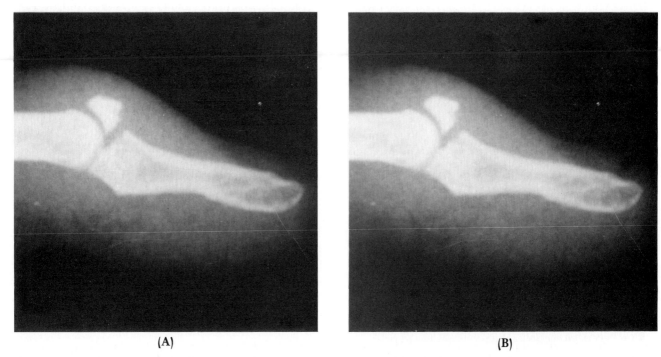

(A)   (B)

Figure 8-46 **(A)** Large articular fracture avulsion of the extensor tendon which was treated by conservative splint immobilization. **(B)** The third serial lateral radiograph 24 days after treatment commenced, revealed palmar subluxation of the DIP joint necessitating open reduction and internal fixation. The two previous radiographs at 7 and 17 days of splint immobilization showed normal anatomy of the DIP joint. This case emphasizes the importance in conservative treatment of this fracture or any articular fracture that periodic radiographs should be made to diagnosis possible subsequent loss of fracture reduction and/or joint subluxation for appropriate open reduction and fixation.

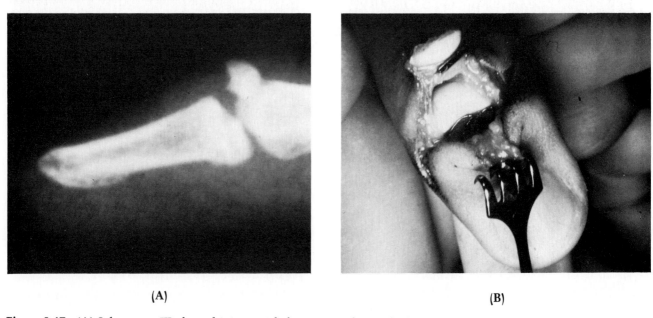

(A)   (B)

Figure 8-47 **(A)** Salter type III physeal injury with fracture avulsion of a large dorsal articular fragment from base of distal phalanx. Displacement results from proximal retraction of extensor insertion. **(B)** At surgery, avulsed fragment is seen superior to condyles of middle phalanx.

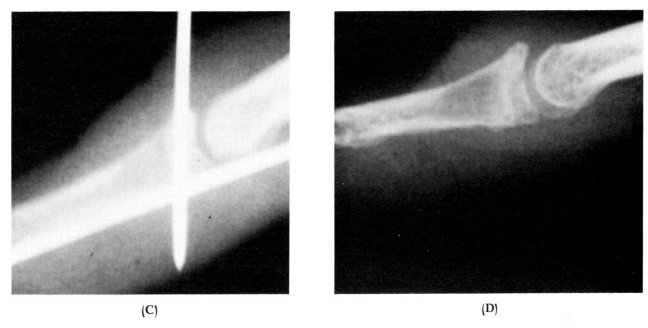

(C)   **(D)**

Figure 8-47 *(continued)*
(C) Lateral radiograph 3 weeks postoperative shows maintenance of position of open reduction by a single oblique Kirschner wire and temporary longitudinal fixation of DIP joint in extension by a similar wire. **(D)** Lateral radiograph 5 weeks after injury shows good contour of distal phalangeal articular surface and normal DIP joint cartilage space.

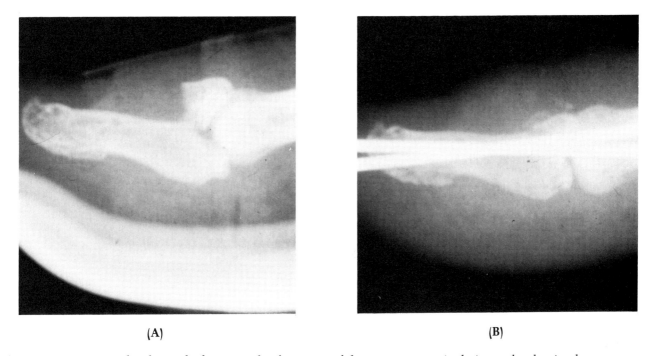

(A)   **(B)**

Figure 8-48 **(A)** Lateral radiograph shows result of unsuccessful attempt at manipulation and reduction by external immobilization of a large dorsal articular segment avulsed from distal phalanx with DIP joint palmar subluxation. **(B)** Lateral radiograph after open reduction and longitudinal Kirschner wire immobilization of fragment combined with temporary immobilization of DIP joint in extension.

(continued)

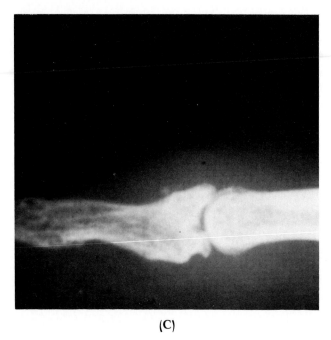

(C)

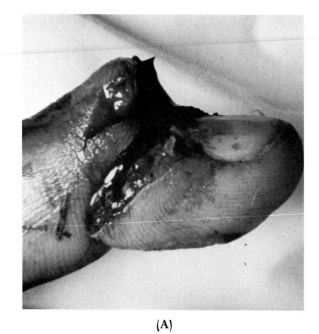

(A)

Figure 8-48 *(continued)*
(C) Lateral view after removal of Kirschner wires shows maintenance of complete extension of DIP joint with minimal damage to articular surface of distal phalangeal base. Flexion was 60°.

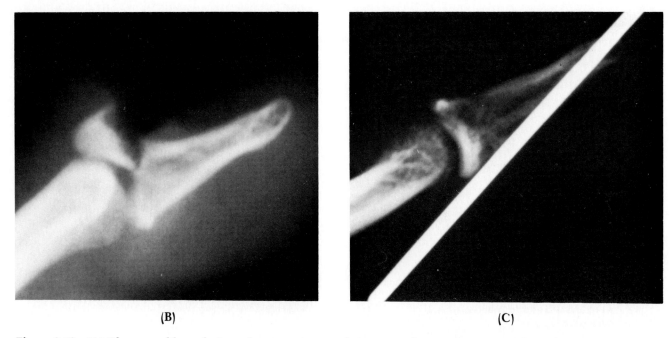

(B)   **(C)**

Figure 8-49 **(A)** Close-up of lateral view of severe open crush injury with near amputation through DIP joint level of ring finger in 14-year-old female. **(B)** Lateral radiograph shows palmar subluxation of distal phalanx and large avulsed articular segment of over 50% of articular surface of distal phalanx base. **(C)** After meticulous wound toilet, reduction of distal phalanx and large fracture fragment was accomplished by temporary fixation with a single Kirschner wire.

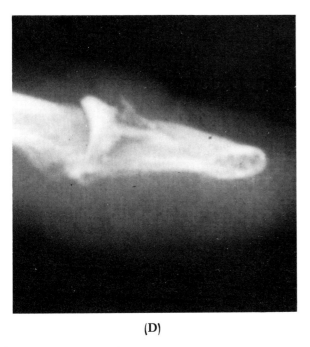

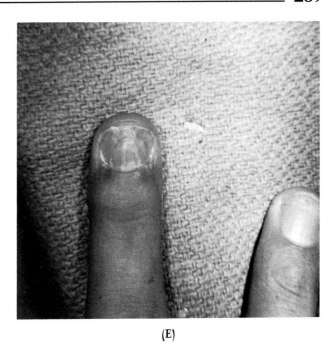

(D)   (E)

Figure 8-49 *(continued)*
(D) Lateral view 3 months after initial injury shows complete extension at DIP joint. Flexion was approximately 15° to 20°. **(E)** Dorsal view shows acceptable contour and cosmesis of nail plate. Regrowth of such a cosmetically acceptable nail seemed unlikely considering severe damage to germinal epithelium of nail plate.

In general, conservative management of all types of this injury yields similar or better results than surgical intervention (Figures 8-44A–C). The best prognosis is for the small chip avulsion fracture (No. 3 above) (Figure 8-43). Treatment for this lesion is immobilization of the DIP joint in extension for four weeks, either by external splint or by longitudinal Kirschner wire fixation across the DIP joint. A good functional recovery is expected in the vast majority of cases. One notable exception is the situation of a large displaced unstable or irreducible articular fracture fragment (No. 4 above), particularly with palmar subluxation of the distal phalanx at the DIP joint (No. 5 above). Proper treatment in this instance is open reduction and internal fixation of that large fracture fragment (Figures 8-47A–D, 8-48A–C, 8-49A–E, 8-50, 8-51A–C) if acceptable closed reduction cannot be accomplished and maintained by splint immobilization (Figures 8-44A–C, 8-45A–C, 8-52A).

Conservative palmar splint immobilization should incorporate both the PIP joint in 15° to 20° flexion and the DIP joint at neutral or in no more than 5° to 10° hyperextension, depending on the laxity of that joint. A convenient form of immobilization is the commercially available gutter type padded

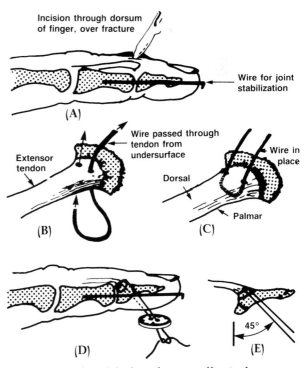

Figure 8-50 The Blalock technique effectively anatomically reduces and firmly fixes the majority of tendon or ligament fracture avulsions.

Figure 8-51 (A) Unsuccessful attempt at open reduction and internal fixation of a large articular fracture avulsion of the extensor insertion. A threaded Kirschner wire was used for longitudinal fixation which is definitely contraindicated. (B) The result after reduction and fixation by the Blalock technique. (C) Joint reduction was maintained and approximately 50% of DIP joint motion was restored.

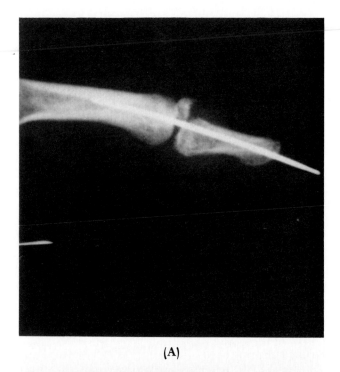

(A)

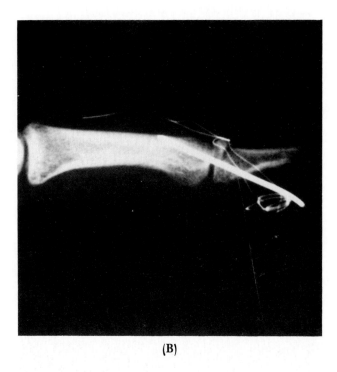

(B)

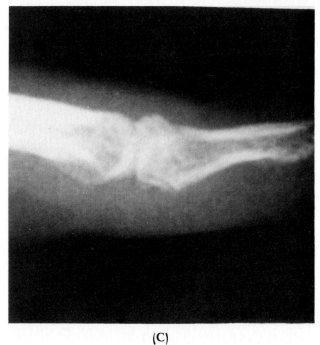

(C)

aluminum splint. *However, any metallic side attachments fabricated to hold the splint in position should be removed* (Figure 8-52). The splint should be maintained in position by tape only since the side attachments are extremely difficult to position and often cause discomfort and even skin damage. Tape should cover all skin to avoid points of window

edema either distally or between strips of tape (Figure 8-53); thin padding may protect the dorsal skin, if necessary. The patient must be carefully instructed to keep the immobilized digit absolutely dry at all times to avoid maceration and, possibly, secondary infection (Figures 8-54, 8-55). Unless the patient is most reliable, the physician should be responsible for

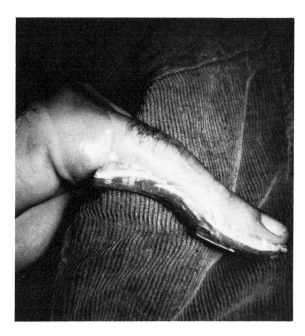

Figure 8-52 Method of immobilization for drop finger incorporating DIP and PIP joints for first 10 to 12 days. DIP joint shown in complete extension or slight recurvatum and PIP joint in slight (10° to 20°) flexion. Cellophane tape was used in this illustration for clarity, but in practice adhesive or paper tape is used on all skin surfaces to prevent "window edema."

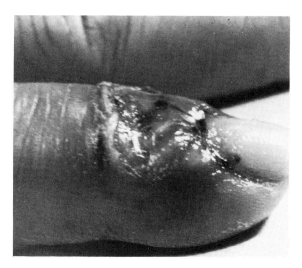

Figure 8-54 Severe maceration dorsal to DIP joint secondary to pressure from improper immobilization, compounded by maceration from wetness.

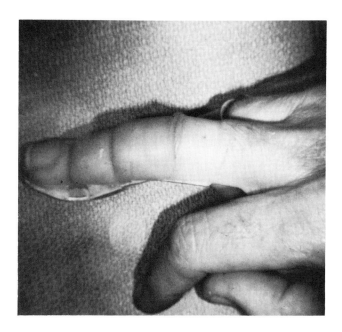

Figure 8-53 Improper application of splint immobilization shows window edema between the two strips of tape and edema of the distal phalanx.

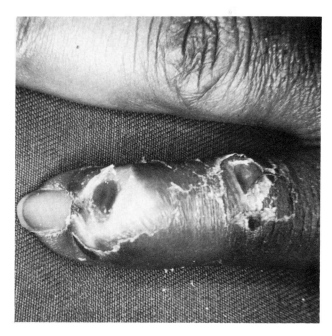

Figure 8-55 Excoriations dorsal to both PIP and DIP joints because of pressure from improper immobilization, compounded by maceration from wetness.

changing the splint at seven- to ten-day intervals to insure proper immobilization and to afford an attempt at hygiene. Comparable immobilization is effected by circular plaster cast, but this method is more difficult to apply and maintain.

A minimum of eight to ten weeks immobilization should be provided for tendon avulsions or lacerations. The PIP joint should remain immobilized for two weeks (Figure 8-52), except for the elderly patient in whom PIP joint immobilization should be discontinued at the end of 10 to 12 days; for the remainder of immobilization the DIP joint only should be kept in constant minimal hyperextension. The small padded splint used to immobilize the DIP joint may be attached palmarly or dorsally, as preferred by the patient. Immobilization for fractures should be maintained for approximately four weeks.

For tendon avulsion injuries in particular, the patient may be given an alternative of having conservative immobilization as described above or of having a longitudinal Kirschner wire drilled across the DIP joint for internal fixation (Figures 8-41A–D). With the latter method the patient is able to wash his hands at any time. A small aluminum splint across the DIP joint, however, should be maintained for external protection. The Kirschner wire should be allowed to protrude from the skin about 2 to 3 mm since this causes

fewer problems than a subcutaneous position. Complete mobility of the PIP joint is maintained with no loss of position of the reduced and percutaneously immobilized drop finger. If good personal hygiene is not possible, infection is a distinct possibility with this technique and may progress to osteomyelitis of the distal phalanx and septic arthritis of the DIP joint (Figures 8-56A,B). Approximately one in ten patients chooses the Kirschner wire method of immobilization. In the skeletally immature patient external immobilization is preferred to avoid possible damage to the physis of the distal phalanx.[3]

Treatment of the drop finger in the older child and adolescent results in a normal finger in over 90% of cases. However, in adults, particularly the elderly patient, the results are much less favorable, particularly when caused by tendon avulsion. The patient should be told that there is a 70% chance of a satisfactory result after either conservative splint immobilization or Kirschner wire fixation, defined as any result from complete active extension to loss of 15° to 20° active extension with some loss of complete DIP joint flexion.

Treatment of the drop finger caused by laceration of the extensor tendon insertion may be treated by appropriate tenorrhaphy if enough tendon material remains distally (Figure 8-57), supplemented by splint

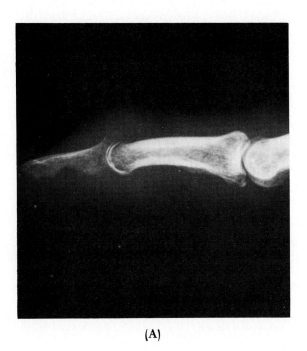

(A)

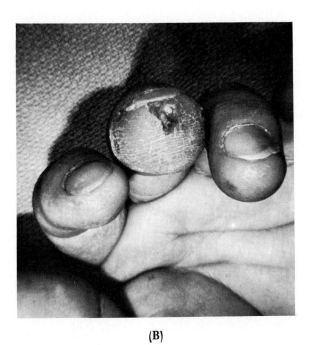

(B)

Figure 8-56 **(A)** Osteomyelitis of distal phalanx and distal end of middle phalanx, with pyarthrosis of DIP joint due to infection of pin tract of Kirschner wire used for temporary immobilization of drop finger. **(B)** Marked edema of the pulp and drainage of exudate from pin tract hole.

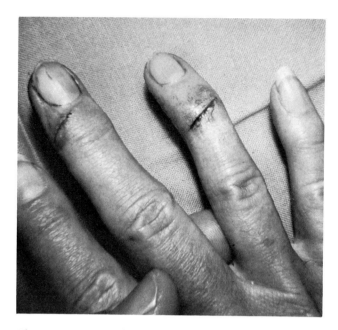

Figure 8-57 Dorsal laceration over DIP joint of ring finger with resultant drop finger from complete severance of extensor tendon.

or Kirschner wire immobilization, or it may be treated conservatively, as in the tendon avulsion treatment described above.

With a large displaced articular fracture fragment which is unstable or irreducible, particularly with palmar joint subluxation (refer to Figures 11-31A–C in Chapter 11, Physeal Injuries), open anatomic reduction and Kirschner or pull out wire fixation is indicated. However, one attempt at closed manipulation and reduction with splint immobilization should be performed prior to surgery (Figures 8-44A–C, 8-45A–C). A true lateral periodic radiograph at seven to 10 day intervals is necessary to reveal subsequent joint subluxation (Figure 8-46).

Anatomic reduction, maintained by Kirschner or pullout wire fixation of the reduced fragment, is the goal if surgery is performed (Figures 8-47–8-51).

The Blalock technique of temporary Kirschner wire fixation of a ligament or tendon fracture avulsion is particularly applicable in this case. This technique effectively anatomically reduces the fragment and securely fixes it by a pull-out wire which is removed five to six weeks postoperatively (Figures 8-50, 8-51). Temporary longitudinal Kirschner wire fixation across the DIP joint is a good adjunct to provide additional security during healing if the wire can be placed without distraction of fixation at the fracture site.

A severe open injury with almost complete amputation necessitates meticulous wound toilet before treatment of the fracture. Any method to maintain reduction without additional insult to vascularity may be employed (Figures 8-49A–D).

Drop IP Joint of the Thumb

Drop finger of the thumb IP joint is not encountered frequently (Figure 8-58). This may occur by the same mechanism of injury as the drop finger of other digits and is caused by tendon avulsion or laceration of the extensor insertion and fracture avulsions of the extensor insertion. Treatment is identical to that described above.

Subacute Drop Finger

Treatment of the subacute drop finger, defined as an injury first seen between two and ten weeks after trauma, is generally similar to treatment of the acute injury but one may elect to perform a secondary tenorraphy for a complete extensor laceration (Figure 8-59A–D).

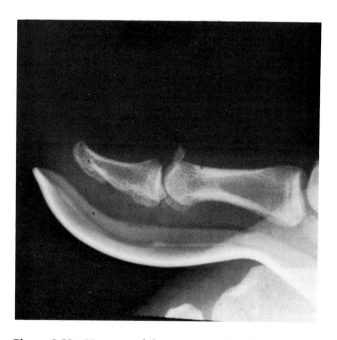

Figure 8-58 Unsuccessful attempt at closed manipulation, reduction, and splint immobilization of fracture avulsion of extensor pollicis longus from thumb distal phalanx. Open reinsertion of articular fragment with internal fixation was carried out. Complete extension of thumb IP joint resulted with flexion to 40°.

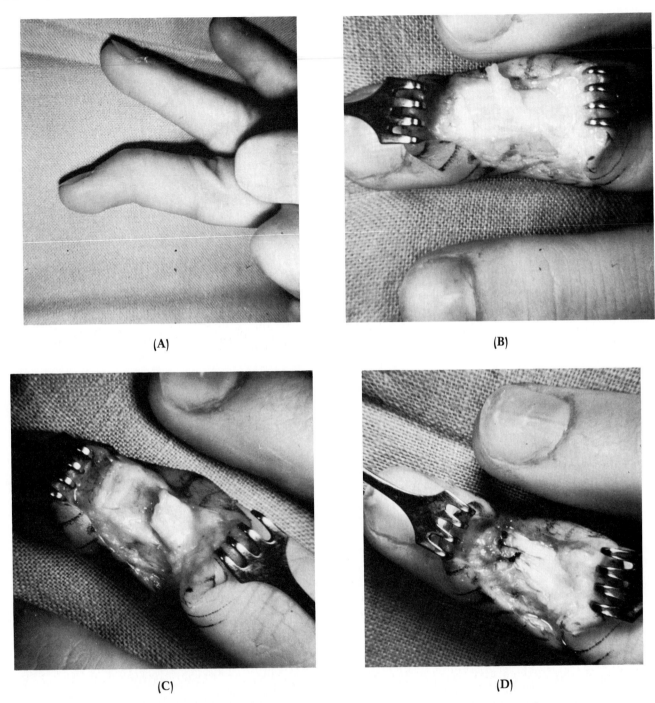

(A)

(B)

(C)

(D)

Figure 8-59 **(A)** Drop finger due to complete laceration of extensor insertion 4 weeks previously. **(B)** At surgery, clean laceration with tendon is visible adjacent to retractor with scar proximal to it. **(C)** After debridement of scar. **(D)** After extensor tenorrhaphy and temporary internal longitudinal fixation of PIP joint.

Figure 8-60 (A) Old fracture avulsion of extensor insertion incurred 6 months before. Note rounded edges of avulsed fracture fragment. (B) Lateral radiograph after excision of small articular fragment and reinsertion of extensor tendon into base of distal phalanx with pullout wire on pulp. Temporary longitudinal Kirschner wire fixation of DIP joint in complete extension for 7 weeks. (C) Lateral view following removal of pullout wire and longitudinal Kirschner wire fixation 7 weeks after surgery. Complete extension was maintained with flexion of 35°.

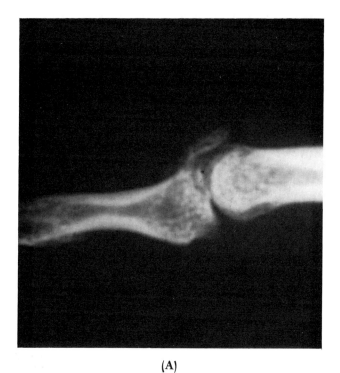

(A)

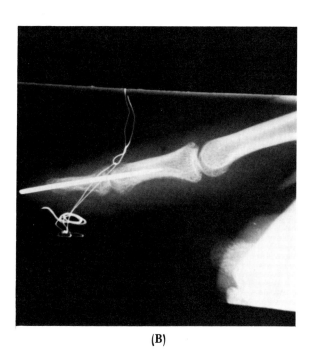

(B)

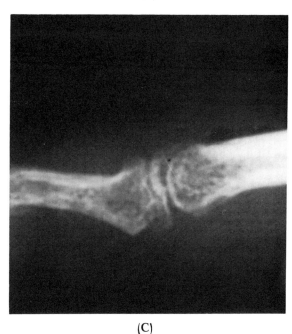

(C)

Chronic Drop Finger

The patient with a chronic drop finger is seen at approximately six to nine months after injury. Conservative treatment usually improves the condition only slightly (Figures 8-60A–C). Tendon reconstruction can be carried out by utilizing a portion of one lateral band reflected proximally to distally to bridge the extensor across the DIP joint.[4]

The chronic drop finger caused by a large displaced articular fracture may be treated by open reduction and internal fixation if there are only minimal degenerative arthritic changes. If post-traumatic degenerative arthritic changes are found, DIP fusion is indicated if symptoms warrant.

Reconstruction of old drop fingers is rarely indicated, unless arthrodesis of the DIP joint is performed to provide painless stability.

"Pseudomallet" Injuries

Various situations mimic drop finger at the DIP joint. Fracture of the distal phalanx through the junction of the base or proximal metaphysis and the diaphysis or shaft often results in palmar angulation of the shaft distal to the fracture (Figures 8-35A,B, 8-36A). The majority of these injuries are open and resemble a drop finger. Treatment includes proper wound toilet followed by reduction and longitudinal Kirschner wire fixation if the fracture is unstable. In the skeletally immature patient traumatic separation through the distal phalangeal physis, also usually open, mimics this situation in the adult (refer to Figures 11-6, 11-28A–C, 11-29A,B, 11-30A–D in Chapter 11, Physeal Injuries).

A condylar fracture of the middle phalanx or a transverse fracture at the junction of the shaft with the distal metaphysis may also resemble a drop finger. If necessary, appropriate surgery should be performed.

General References

Green DP, Rowland SA: Fractures and dislocations in the hand, in Rockwood CA Jr, Green DP (eds): *Fractures in Adults,* ed 2. Philadelphia, J.B. Lippincott Co., 1984, vol 1, pp 313–409.

O'Brien ET: Fractures of the metacarpals and phalanges, in Green DP (ed): *Operative Hand Surgery.* New York, Churchill Livingstone, 1982, vol 1, pp 583–635.

O'Brien ET: Fractures of the hand and wrist region, in Rockwood CA Jr, Wilkins KE, King RE (eds): *Fractures in Children,* ed 2. Philadelphia, J.B. Lippincott Co., 1984, vol 3, pp 229–272.

Sandzén SC Jr: Complex injuries of the wrist and hand, in Meyers MH (ed): *The Multiply Injured Patient with Complex Fractures.* Philadelphia, Lea & Febiger, 1984, pp 365–400.

References

1. Sandzén SC Jr: Treating acute fingertip injuries. *Am Fam Physician* 1972;5:68–79.
2. Sandzén SC Jr, Oakey RS: Crushing injury of the fingertip. *Hand* 1972;4:253–256.
3. Sandzén SC Jr: Management of the acute fingertip injury in the child. *Hand* 1974;6:190–197.
4. Snow JW: Surgical repair of mallet finger. *Plast Reconstr Surg* 1968;41:89–90.

Injuries to Digital Soft Tissue Structures

General Considerations

The severity of injury determines the degree of anatomic disruption of periarticular stabilizing ligamentous and capsular structures and the resultant severity of articular disruption.

Hyperextension injuries cause variable trauma to the palmar plate and lateral collateral and accessory collateral ligaments. The amount of dorsal angulation or recurvatum deformity is determined by the severity of injury and resultant extent of capsular and ligamentous trauma.

Dorsal joint subluxations and dislocations are the most severe manifestations of hyperextension injuries. A partial dislocation or subluxation is a joint injury in which the contiguous articular surfaces still retain some contact and some portion of the articulation persists. A complete dislocation is the result of a more severe injury and indicates severe disruption of the joint with complete displacement and loss of contact between the contiguous articular surfaces.

Dislocation of the metacarpophalangeal (MP), proximal interphalangeal (PIP), and distal interphalangeal (DIP) joints may be dorsal, lateral (radial or ulnar), or, infrequently, palmar. This classification indicates the position of the distal bone in reference to the proximal bone at the disrupted joint.

Palmar dislocation is infrequent due to the very secure fixation of the palmar plate and collateral ligament system, particularly the accessory collateral ligaments which resist the dislocating forces (see Chapter 1, Anatomy, section on Digital Joints, Similarities of Ligamentous Support and Figure 1-7). The dorsal aspect of the joint is much more vulnerable to disruption since only the capsule and the extensor apparatus resist dislocation.

Lateral dislocation or complete ligament avulsion which involves either collateral ligament of the thumb MP joint, the radial collateral ligament of the index finger MP joint, the radial collateral ligament of the index finger PIP joint, or the radial or ulnar collateral ligament of the little finger PIP joint is a serious injury and surgical repair is strongly recommended. Conservative management may be attempted for all other MP and PIP joint collateral ligament avulsions.

The most common dislocation involves the thumb MP joint (discussed in Chapter 6, The Thumb).

Next in frequency is dislocation of the PIP joints of the index, little, long, and ring fingers.

Fracture dislocations of all digits except the thumb most commonly involve the PIP joints which usually sublux or dislocate dorsally. Avulsion and displaced articular fracture of the thumb MP joint ulnar collateral ligament insertion, the most common collateral ligament injuries (discussed under Gamekeeper's Thumb—see Figures 6-10A–D), and fracture dislocation of the palmar beak of the thumb metacarpal base (discussed under Bennett's Fractures—see Figures 6-32A–C) are included in Chapter 6, The Thumb.

Acute ligamentous injuries are those diagnosed within two to two and one-half weeks from the time of injury. Subacute ligamentous injuries include those found between two and one-half to four or five weeks after injury. Chronic ligamentous injuries are those discovered four to six weeks after injury or later.

Radiographic documentation should be made prior to reduction of a dislocation to determine whether a concomitant fracture is present. The exception to this rule is immediate reduction of a dislocation or fracture dislocation to relieve severe vascular impairment of the digit distal to the injury in an attempt to restore circulation as soon as possible.

Open dislocation or fracture dislocation usually occurs at the PIP joint and may produce severe ischemic changes distal to the injury if caused by severe torsional force, with subsequent vascular avulsion, thrombosis, or a combination of both.

Meticulous wound toilet is mandatory prior to the reduction of an open dislocation or fracture dislocation. If immediate reduction was performed to relieve extreme vascular compromise, the joint should be redislocated and meticulously cleansed, irrigated, and debrided prior to its definitive reduction and wound closure.

Traumatic physeal separation often occurs in the skeletally immature individual rather than dislocation or ligamentous injury (see Chapter 12, Skeletal Remodeling, Figures 12-5A–E, Chapter 6, The Thumb, Figures 6-26A–D, and Chapter 11, Physeal Injuries).

Primary surgical reconstruction of either a tendon avulsion or fracture avulsion is strongly recommended in the following areas: flexor digitorum profundus and flexor pollicis longus, fracture avulsion of the central slip of insertion of the extensor tendon; and in certain cases, fracture avulsion of the extensor insertion from the base of the distal phalanx (discussed elsewhere in this chapter).

Capsular, Ligamentous, and Tendon Injuries of the Digits

Ligamentous injuries include attenuation or rupture of specific or multiple ligaments or ligamentous structures and may occur at any joint or joints of the wrist and digits. Also included are specific injuries to tendons, including avulsion or fracture avulsion of tendon insertions (flexor digitorum profundus) and boutonniere and swan neck deformities. (Ligamentous injuries to the thumb carpometacarpal, MP, and IP joints are discussed in Chapter 6, The Thumb; dislocations and fracture dislocations of the wrist are discussed in Chapter 4, Wrist Injuries.)

Metacarpophalangeal Joint

Acute rupture of an MP joint collateral ligament is possible at any location. Discussion of Gamekeeper's thumb (rupture of the ulnar collateral ligament of the thumb MP joint), the most common collateral ligament injury, and rupture of the radial collateral ligament of that joint are discussed in Chapter 6, The Thumb. The radial aspect of the index MP joint is the most susceptible of all the remaining digits because of its marginal position. The next most common injury is to the ulnar collateral ligament of the little finger MP joint.

The mechanism of injury is a severe direct lateral (radial or ulnar) blow to the proximal phalanx. If acute rupture of the radial collateral ligament of the index finger MP joint is suspected by specific tenderness on the radial joint line, swelling, and ecchymosis, it is most important to test the joint's stability. The radial stress test usually carried out under appropriate anesthesia will determine whether partial or complete ligament tear has occurred. Minor angulation amounting to no more than 10° to 15° abnormal laxity as compared to the normal contralateral index MP joint is acceptable for three to four weeks of conservative immobilization. If complete rupture is diagnosed by marked ulnar deviation on the stress test performed with the MP joint in maximum flexion, surgical repair is recommended as the most reliable treatment to provide the best ultimate stability.

If chronic instability of the index MP joint persists due to complete radial collateral ligament rupture, or if marked attenuation persists, symptomatic degenerative arthritic changes accompanied by secondary intrinsic atrophy (first dorsal interosseous) result (Figures 9-1A–D). Ulnar subluxation of the ex-

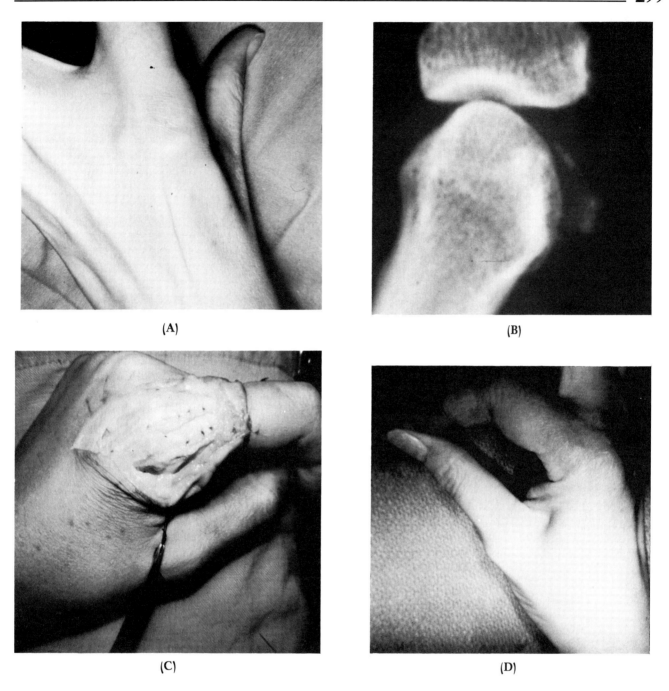

(A)

(B)

(C)

(D)

Figure 9-1 (A) Dorsal view of radial aspect of index finger MP joint. Patient had chronic instability of index finger due to avulsion of radial collateral ligament 12 years before. Note ulnar subluxation of extensor tendons of index finger (extensor indicis proprius and extensor digitorum communis) and atrophic skin over the dorso-radial aspect of MP joint, with marked intrinsic (first dorsal interosseous) muscle atrophy. (B) PA radiograph shows calcification in area of avulsion of proximal attachment of lateral collateral ligament at radial aspect of index finger MP joint. (C) Photograph after surgical reconstruction of the radial collateral ligament using available tissues and radial realignment of extensor tendons. (D) Photograph 1½ years after ligament reconstruction shows stable, painless thumb-index pinch and good muscle tone of first dorsal interosseous and adductor pollicis muscles. Chronic instability and pain caused disuse atrophy of muscles prior to the reconstructive procedures.

tensor digitorum communis and extensor indicis proprius tendons may be involved in the initial injury or may be a secondary manifestation of the ligamentous instability (Figure 9-1A).

Secondary reconstruction is not as predictable and is achieved by using either locally available tissue (Figure 9-1C) or a free tendon graft of the palmaris longus or other suitable tendon, threading the graft through drill holes in the distal metacarpal and base of the proximal phalanx to provide the necessary stability. If the extensor tendons are ulnarly subluxed, realignment should be effected simultaneously. After a stable asymptomatic thumb-index pinch is restored, increased use will produce hypertrophy of the atrophic first dorsal interosseous and adductor pollicis muscles (Figure 9-1D).

Acute rupture of the extensor aponeurosis and rupture or severe attenuation of a sagittal band (usually on the radial aspect of an MP joint) can occur either from a direct blow, which avulses the extensor tendon from that aponeurosis and the sagittal band, or by direct open trauma to that area. It usually involves the long or ring finger (Figure 9-2).

Physical examination discloses swelling and discrete tenderness at the site of the tear on one side of the MP joint (usually the radial aspect) and abnormal subluxation of the extensor tendon upon lateral pressure on that tendon away from that tear toward the opposite, normal side of the MP joint.

The most predictable result follows surgical repair for the closed injury but conservative immobilization for four weeks with the MP joint flexed 20° to 30° may achieve satisfactory healing. Occasionally symptoms of pain and tenderness are elicited in the area of rupture, and chronic extensor tendon subluxation persists, following conservative immobilization and secondary repair of this defect is indicated (Figure 9-2). Immobilization for four weeks postoperatively is the same as in the treatment of the acute injury.

In the open injury, primary fascial and tendon repair is advised in the clean wound; delayed primary repair is recommended should contamination be present.

Traumatic extensor tendon subluxation is rarely found in more than one MP joint area. When present it should be regarded either as a congenital laxity or as absence of the saggital band (usually radial) plus absence or attenuation of the extensor insertion at the base of the proximal phalanx or capsule of the MP joint (Figures 9-3A–C). If the chronic subluxation becomes symptomatic resulting in chronic recurrent subluxation of the extensor tendon or tendons associated with MP joint synovitis, reconstruction is indicated (Figures 9-3B,C). Plication of the radial sagittal bands in a "pants-over-vest" fashion without attachment of the extensor tendon to the proximal phalanx provides stability of the realigned extensor tendons in most cases (Figure 9-3C).

Ulnar nerve palsy or damage to ulnar nerve motor branches causes chronic stretching or attenuation of the MP joint palmar plate commonly in the little finger and to a lesser extent in the ring finger due to the loss of intrinsic muscle power to flex these joints (Figures 9-4A,B). In combined median and ulnar palsy all intrinsic muscles, including the first and second lumbrical and the thenar and hypothenar muscles, are paralyzed, and hyperextension deformity of all MP joints occurs following chronic stretching of the palmar plate (Figure 9-5B).

Numerous operative procedures have been advocated to restore flexion at the MP joint or a tenodesis effect to prevent hyperextension. The most effective active tendon transfer in ulnar palsy to correct recurvatum of the little finger MP joint is transfer of the extensor indicis proprius, routed from the dorsum of the hand (Figures 9-4C,D) on the radial aspect of the little finger, through the interossei and through the lumbrical canal, to be inserted into the periosteum, flexor sheath, or bone of the little finger proximal phalanx (Figures 9-4E–G). If recurvatum of the ring finger MP joint is severe enough, this tendon transfer may be split longitudinally with a similar routing and insertion into the ring finger proximal phalanx.

In combined low median and ulnar palsy many different procedures have been recommended — including use of the flexor digitorum superficialis of the long and ring fingers, each split longitudinally to be used for two contiguous digits, a wrist flexor, wrist extensor, or the brachio-radialis (all except the superficialis tendons prolonged by free tendon grafts) — in an attempt to supply active tendon transfers for MP joint flexion. The transfer to the index finger should be routed on the ulnar aspect of the MP joint rather than through the lumbrical canal (long through little fingers) to prevent radial divergence of that digit.

A tenodesis effect to correct MP recurvatum deformities may be performed using a tendon graft or fascia anchored to the metacarpal or flexor sheath proximally and to the proximal phalanx or flexor sheath distally. Advancement of the palmar plate of the MP joint (Zancolli procedure) is a good alternative but only if the procedure is precisely executed (Figures 9-5A–D). For best results with the Zancolli procedure the upper extremity should be diffusely weak since

Figure 9-2 (**A**) Traumatic avulsion of radial sagittal band from extensor tendon of long finger at MP joint area due to direct forceful, blunt trauma. (**B**) Surgical exposure shows acute traumatic avulsion of the radial sagittal band at the MP joint level of the long finger with ulnar subluxation of the extensor tendon. (**C**) Repair of the tear and realignment of the extensor tendon with four weeks post-operative immobilization holding the MP joint flexed 20°–25° restored tendon alignment and normal function.

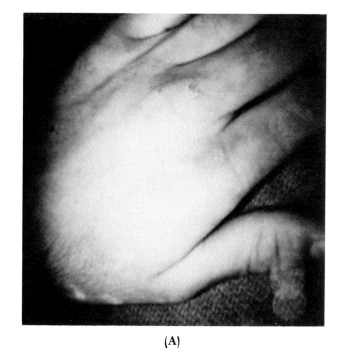

(A)

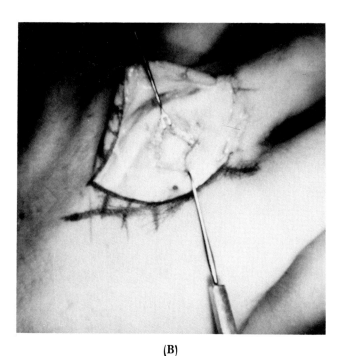

(B)

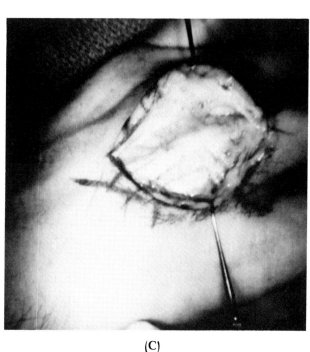

(C)

Figure 9-3 **(A)** Forced active MP flexion shows ulnar deviation of extensors of index, long, ring, and little fingers with the most severe deformities involving long and ring fingers. Patient noted increasing pain and swelling of long finger MP joint with subluxation of all extensors ulnarly over a period of 2 to 3 years. **(B)** Exposure at surgery shows ulnar deviation of long and ring finger extensors with MP flexion and synovitis of MP joints. Lesion found at surgery was chronic laxity of sagittal bands on radial aspects of MP joints. Attenuation or avulsion of extensor insertions or congenital absence of insertions from MP joint capsules or bases of proximal phalanges probably existed concurrently, but these areas were not explored. **(C)** Photograph after plication of radial sagittal bands to realign all extensor tendons at MP joints of index through little finger. No attempt was made to reconstruct extensor insertions, and no arthrotomies were performed. Normal painless motion resulted.

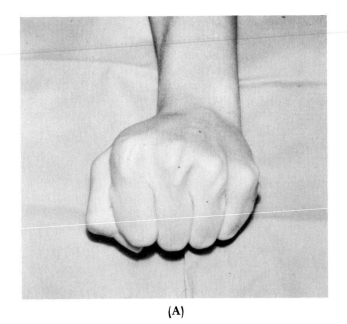

(A)

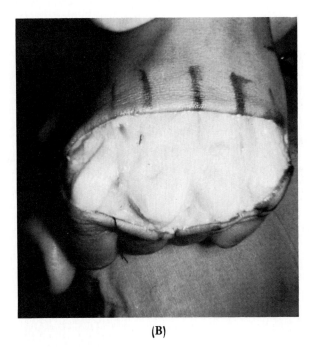

(B)

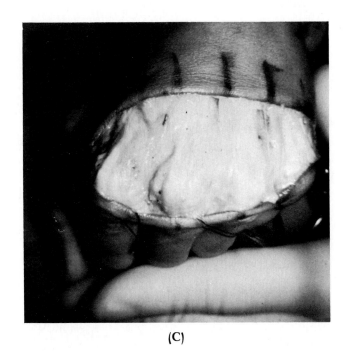

(C)

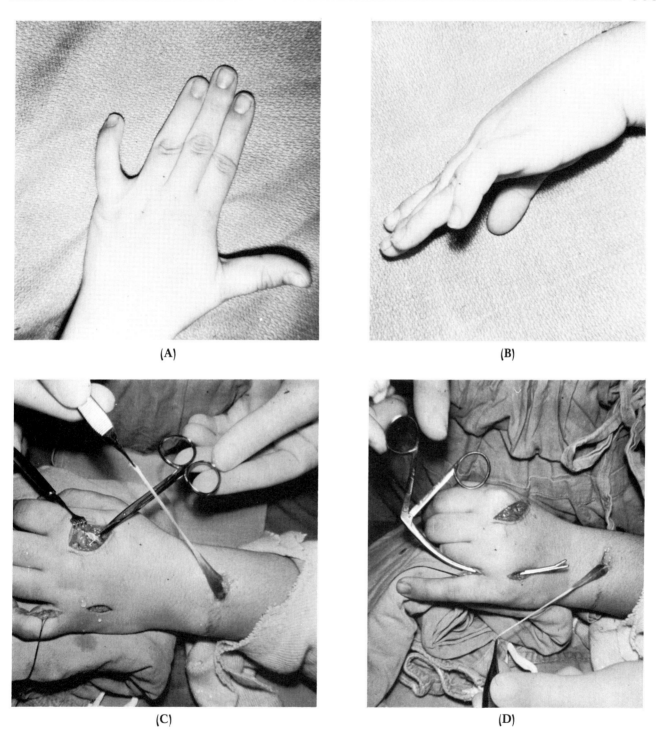

Figure 9-4 **(A)** Abduction of little finger proximal phalanx due to discrete penetrating injury which resulted in palsy of third palmar interosseous and fourth lumbrical muscles. **(B)** Another view, accentuating the recurvatum of MP joint and flexion of PIP joint due to discrete lesion of specific ulnar nerve motor branches. **(C)** Photograph at surgery illustrates indicis proprius tendon obtained for active tendon transfer. **(D)** Transfer of indicis proprius tendon rerouted through dorsal aspect of ring-little finger interosseous musculature, fourth lumbrical canal, and into flexor sheath at radial aspect of proximal phalanx of little finger.

(continued)

Figure 9-4 *(continued)*
(E) Dorsal view shows complete extension and adduction of little finger 10 weeks postoperatively. **(F)** Ulnar view also shows complete extension. **(G)** Complete flexion resulted. MP joint recurvatum, PIP joint flexion, and little finger abduction were all corrected by tendon transfer.

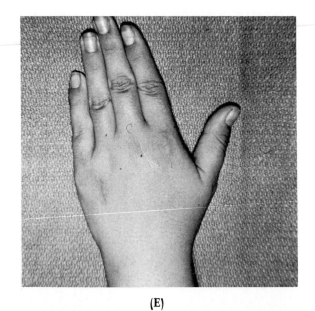

(E)

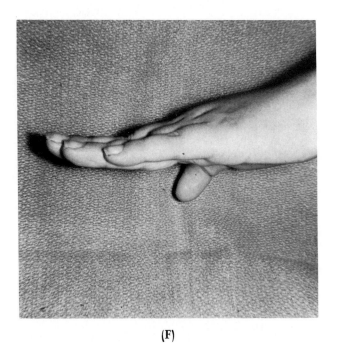

(F)

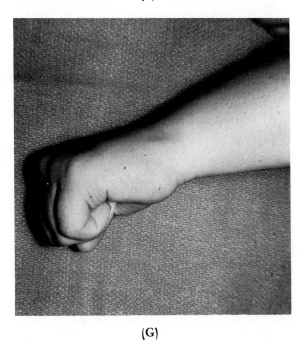

(G)

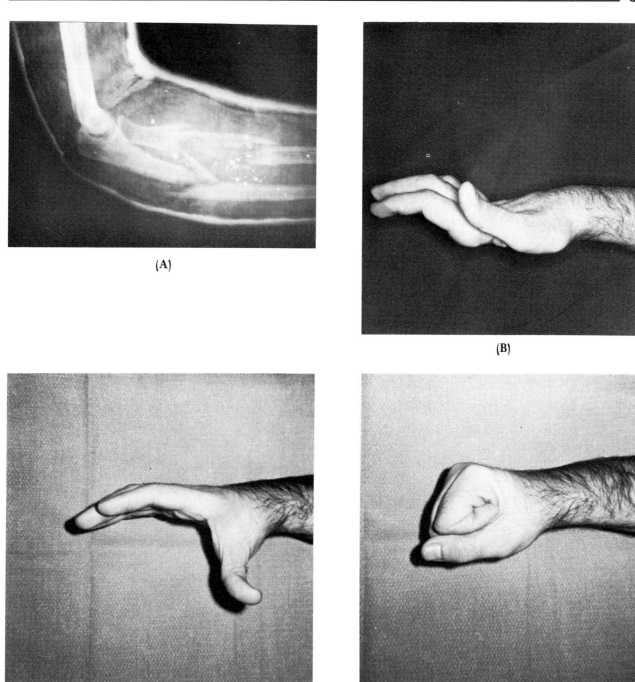

(A)

(B)

(C)

(D)

Figure 9-5 (A) Lateral radiograph of extremely comminuted open fractures of radius and ulna, sustained in high-velocity gunshot injury, after initial cleansing, irrigation, debridement, delayed primary closure, and long arm cast immobilization. (B) Lateral photograph. Diffuse upper extremity weakness persisted due to mixed, high partial nerve palsies involving ulnar, median, and radial nerves. Note extensive recurvatum deformity of all MP joints, inability to extend wrist, and inability to extend digital PIP joints. (C) Transfer of brachioradialis into extensor carpi radialis brevis performed to restore wrist extension. Photograph taken 5 years after subsequent Zancolli procedures (MP joint palmar plate advancements) of index through little fingers. Normal longitudinal arch of hand was restored, and good digital extension and wide thumb abduction resulted. (D) Good digital flexion and grasp of moderate power was restored.

normal digital extensors may gradually attenuate the palmar plate advancement and cause recurrence of the deformities. In Figures 9-5A–D the Zancolli procedure was used for this reason and because of lack of appropriate musculature for active transfers.

Proximal Interphalangeal Joint

Acute avulsion of a PIP joint collateral ligament is diagnosed by point tenderness and ecchymosis over the joint line or at the proximal or distal attachment of that ligament. To determine if complete or incomplete ligament rupture has occurred, stress examination of the ligament should be conducted under appropriate anesthesia (Figure 9-6A). A PA radiograph may disclose a fracture avulsed from the base of the middle phalanx, indicating collateral ligament fracture avulsion from its distal attachment (Figure 9-6B).

The radial collateral ligament of the index finger PIP joint is most frequently injured; next most frequently injured is either the radial or the ulnar collateral ligament of the little finger PIP joint. It is advisable to repair the completely avulsed ligament or fracture avulsion of the PIP joint collateral ligament in these marginal digits to guarantee the best possible stability. Complete tear of a PIP joint collateral ligament in other digits, except the thumb, and partial tear of any PIP joint collateral ligament are generally treated by conservative immobilization for three and one-half to four weeks with the PIP joint in 10° to 15° flexion. Complete laceration of any collateral ligament should be repaired primarily if possible (Figures 9-7A–C) and, if necessary, as a delayed primary procedure, particularly in the less protected index and little fingers.

Distal Interphalangeal Joint

Avulsion of the extensor insertion from the dorsal aspect of the distal phalanx base may manifest itself in various ways: avulsion of the tendon insertion alone, a small "flake" fracture avulsion of the tendon insertion, or a large articular fracture avulsion with or without DIP joint subluxation. Differentiation of these entities necessitates a thorough physical examination and radiographic evaluation for proper treatment of the cause of the "drop finger" (see Chapter 8, section Drop Finger).

Avulsion of the flexor digitorum profundus insertion from the palmar aspect of the distal phalanx is relatively common and should be easily diagnosed by the patient's inability to actively flex the DIP joint

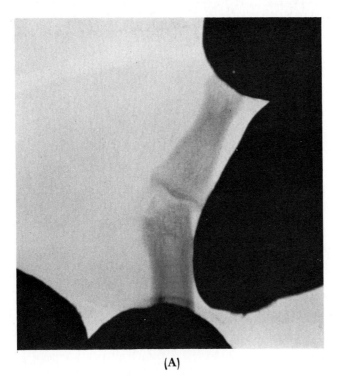

(A)

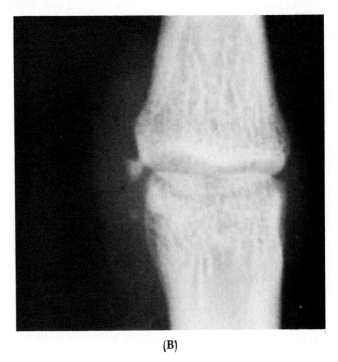

(B)

Figure 9-6 (A) PA view on stressed deviation of PIP joint under anesthesia demonstrates complete disruption of collateral ligament. (B) Close-up shows fracture avulsion of lateral collateral ligament from proximal phalanx.

Figure 9-7 (**A**) Saw injury to radial aspect of index finger with jagged dorsal skin flap laceration. (**B**) Complete laceration of index finger PIP joint radial collateral ligament. Primary surgical reconstruction of collateral ligament resulted in good joint stability but some limitation of PIP joint flexion. (**C**) PA radiograph shows soft tissue injury on radial aspect of index finger PIP joint with fracture avulsion of radial collateral ligament from base of middle phalanx.

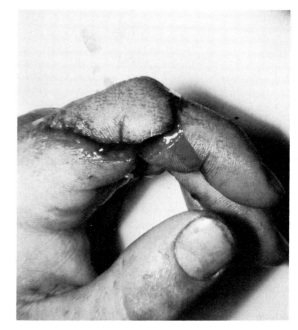

(A)

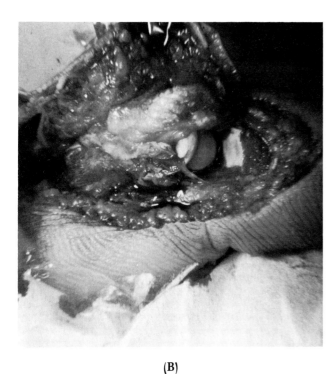

(B)

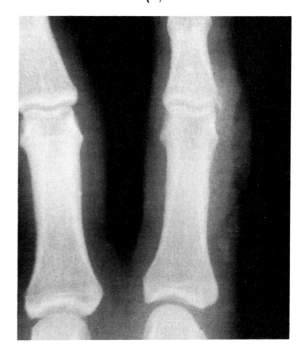

(C)

and by the unnatural extensor attitude of that joint at rest (Figure 9-8A). The ring finger is involved more often than any other digit because independent digital extension of that digit is the most restricted of all. A common history is entanglement of the ring finger in an opposing player's football jersey, associated with powerful DIP flexion and sudden violent, opposed hyperextension stress on that joint.

Three types of profundus avulsion are recognized[1]: Type I—tendon avulsion with proximal retraction into the palm; Type II—tendon avulsion remaining within the digital sheath, retracting only to the level of the PIP joint; and Type III—fracture avulsion. One should not be misled by the presence of an anterior interosseous nerve syndrome in which active index finger DIP joint and/or thumb IP joint flexion are absent or minimal. Electrodiagnostic evaluation should clinch that diagnosis.

Radiographs will accurately diagnose a fracture avulsion to differentiate it from a pure tendon avulsion.

Type I lesion must be reinserted within seven to 10 days of injury to prevent avascular necrosis of the tendon end. To prevent refractory flexion contracture of either PIP or DIP joint, tendon advancement and reinsertion of an avulsed flexor digitorum profundus of the ring and little fingers in a Type II lesion should be within two or three weeks from injury (Figure 9-8B) and for the index and long fingers, the flexor pollicis longus of the thumb, and for all Type III lesions within three to four weeks.

For displaced fracture avulsion (Type III lesion), particularly with concurrent joint subluxation, anatomic replacement of the fracture and fixation by Kirschner wires or the Blalock technique is recommended (Figure 9-9, and refer to Figure 16-20).

The earlier surgical reinsertion is carried out, the easier it is technically and the less probability there is of creating a flexion contracture.

If at surgical exploration the involved digit remains too flexed at the PIP and DIP joints after attempted reinsertion of the profundus tendon, tenodesis of the DIP joint with excision of the profundus tendon in the palm is the best treatment to avoid a persistent digital flexion contracture involving both joints.

In the majority of instances the profundus tendon is avulsed from the base of the distal phalanx; occasionally a segment of bone is simultaneously avulsed (Figures 9-9A,B, 9-10, 9-11). In addition to the patient's inability to actively flex the DIP joint, the lateral radiograph shows this avulsed bony fragment at any level in the digital sheath, depending upon the amount of proximal retraction of the profundus tendon. The avulsed fragment of bone may be a very small "flake" or a very large articular segment of the

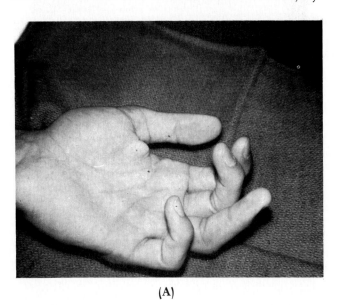

(A)

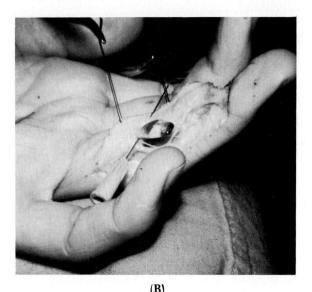

(B)

Figure 9-8 **(A)** Configuration of digits at rest shows abnormal extension of ring finger DIP joint, indicating loss of profundus action. Patient, a 17-year-old male, sustained this injury when his finger became tangled in a football jersey. **(B)** Exposure at surgery shows complete avulsion of flexor digitorum profundus tendon from distal phalanx insertion. Treatment consisted of profundus advancement with reinsertion into distal phalanx base by means of pullout wire. Light activity was commenced 7 to 10 days after surgery; pullout wire was removed 5 weeks after surgery.

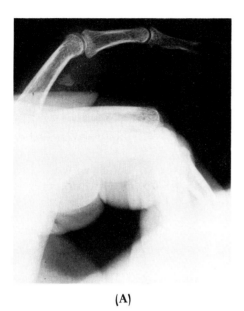

(A)

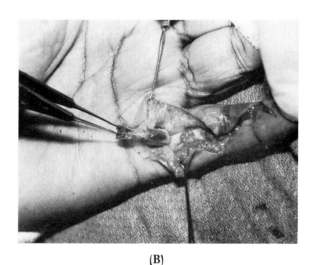

(B)

Figure 9-9 (A) Lateral radiograph shows a moderate-sized irregular bony fragment on palmar aspect of proximal phalanx in area of superficialis decussation, representing extraarticular fracture avulsion of profundus insertion caught at level of superficialis decussation, thus preventing profundus tendon from retracting proximally into the palm, a Type III lesion. Note irregular defect on palmar aspect of distal phalangeal base from which extra-articular fragment avulsed. (See Chapter 1 for description of profundus tendon insertion. (B) Exposure of little finger flexor area through palmar zigzag (Bruner) incision. Avulsed extraarticular bone fragment held in forceps and can be either anatomically reduced into defect on distal phalangeal base and firmly fixed or excised prior to reinsertion of tendon in this area. *(Illustrations 9-9A,B courtesy of J.B. Webber, M.D.)*

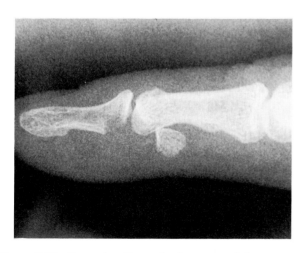

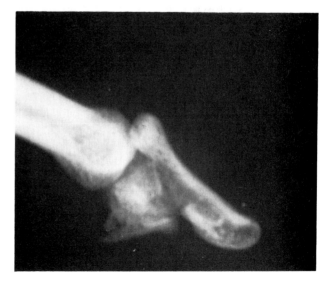

Figure 9-10 Lateral radiograph shows much larger segment of bone, avulsed from palmar aspect of distal phalangeal base which is proximally retracted by attached profundus tendon. Due to size of fragment and binding down of fragment in flexor sheath, proximal retraction is minimal. *(Illustration courtesy of S. Gunther, M.D.)*

Figure 9-11 Lateral view illustrates dorsal articular fracture dislocation of the distal phalanx. A very large articular fracture fragment is displaced and rotated from a corresponding defect on palmar proximal aspect of distal phalanx. Dorsal subluxation is due to gross instability owing to loss of large palmar fragment from distal phalangeal articular surface.

distal phalangeal articular surface. Usually the bony fragment is retained within the flexor sheath and is caught at the decussation of the superficialis tendon (Figure 9-9A), but occasionally it may be retracted proximally into the palm. Open reduction and internal fixation of the large avulsed articular fracture fragment (with the attached profundus tendon) is recommended as soon as possible, particularly if DIP joint subluxation is present. In unstable dorsal articular fracture subluxation or dislocation of the DIP joint (Figure 9-11), open anatomic reduction and internal fixation are usually necessary to restore the articular surface. If a stable reinsertion has been established, light range of motion exercises can be commenced in a responsible patient approximately seven days after surgery, as soon as generalized tissue edema and pain from both the injury and surgery have subsided. Excellent results of profundus tendon reinsertion are achieved with a 3–0 or 4–0 monofilament stainless steel pullout wire placed through the distal phalanx obliquely and fastened on a button dorsal to the nail plate; or with anatomic reduction and fixation of the avulsed large fracture fragment (Figures

9-10, 9-11) by a similar pullout wire technique (the Blalock technique may be especially useful—refer to Chapter 8, section on Drop Finger) (refer to Figure 16-20); or by Kirschner wire fixation. The small flake fracture avulsion is trimmed from the tendon and the tendon is then reinserted as noted (Figures 9-9A,B). Excellent but not normal powerful digital flexion across both DIP and PIP joints can be expected with nearly normal ranges of joint motion.

Occasionally profundus avulsion or fracture avulsion occurs simultaneously with a displaced articular fracture (Figure 9-12) necessitating anatomic reduction and fixation of both.

Fracture avulsion of the flexor pollicis longus tendon is an uncommon lesion and treatment is similar (Figure 9-13).

If both the palmar plate and flexor digitorum profundus insertion have been completely lacerated or avulsed, primary or delayed primary repair of both structures is recommended. Usually DIP joint range of motion is limited because of the severity of injury and extent of surgery necessary.

Gross instability of the DIP joint other than drop finger, collateral ligament or palmar plate and/or profundus tendon avulsion rarely occurs in a closed

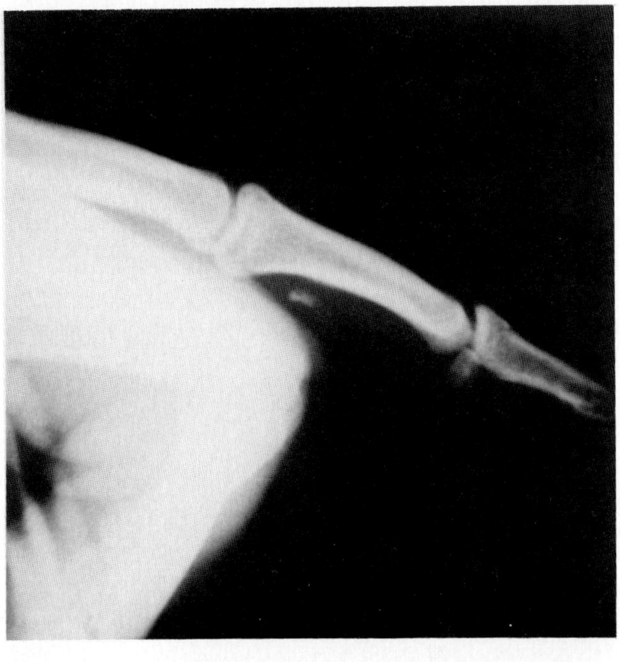

Figure 9-12 Combination of fracture avulsion of the profundus insertion and articular fracture of the base of the distal phalanx with dorsal DIP joint subluxation. Despite anatomic reduction of the DIP joint, the articular fracture, and profundus avulsion, limited DIP joint motion is expected. At worst, however, a stable asymptomatic tenodesis effect of the DIP joint is preferable to arthrodesis.

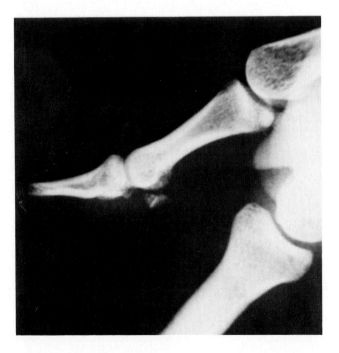

Figure 9-13 Fracture/avulsion of the flexor pollicis longus insertion is not a common injury and is treated similarly to profundus fracture avulsion by anatomic reduction and fixation of the fracture.

injury. Marked distraction of the DIP joint with an increased cartilage space indicates severe soft tissue trauma, probably including avulsion of both collateral ligaments and the palmar plate. Soft tissue interposition may persist. Conservative treatment is recommended for such a situation in the DIP joint unless soft tissue interposition is diagnosed. For the best functional result in this case, surgical exposure and release of the entrapped soft tissue, usually the palmar plate, is indicated (refer to Figures 9-62A–C and 9-63A,B). If chronic pain or instability of the DIP joint persists after conservative immobilization for three to four weeks, tenodesis or arthrodesis should be considered.

Boutonniere Deformity

Boutonniere deformity may occur either by acute laceration of the central slip of the extensor tendon insertion (which terminates on the dorsal aspect of the middle phalanx base) or, more commonly, by

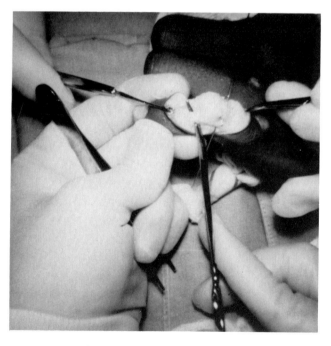

Figure 9-14 Photograph at surgery demonstrates mechanics of severe chronic boutonnierre deformity. Hemostat is beneath one lateral band, which is palmarly subluxed; central slip is proximally retracted; and material over PIP joint is a combination of cicatrix and thickened capsule. As seen here, it is impossible to extend PIP joint because central slip of extensor is ineffective and palmar displacement of lateral bands causes increased flexion.

blunt trauma avulsing that insertion. The central slip retracts proximally, and the adjacent lateral band on each side separates and eventually migrates palmarly. The lateral bands normally situated dorsal to the extensor-flexor axis of the PIP joint migrate palmar to that axis in the chronic lesion (Figure 9-14). Therefore any active attempt to extend the PIP joint proximally retracts the central slip further and progressively subluxes the lateral bands palmarly. The result is increase in the PIP joint flexion by the subluxed lateral bands, which also hyperextend the DIP joint due to increased tension on their insertions at the distal phalanx. Initial treatment of this injury must be aggressive, regardless of the etiology, to prevent the sequelae of PIP joint flexion contracture and DIP joint hyperextension contracture. The main disability of a chronic severe boutonniere deformity is fixed DIP joint hyperextension and inability to actively flex that joint.

The closed injury should be treated by splint immobilization with the PIP joint in complete extension for a minimum of five but preferably six weeks. The DIP joint is immobilized in extension at night but during waking hours active extension and flexion is encouraged to promote proximal and distal gliding of the lateral bands. If flexion contracture of the PIP joint is present, this must be passively relieved by stretching exercises prior to immobilization in order to relocate the lateral bands from their palmarly subluxed position to their normal anatomic position dorsal to the joint's flexion-extension axis. Only after the lateral bands are anatomically relocated and the PIP joint completely extended can the conservative immobilization be effective.

Acute laceration of the central slip should be surgically repaired (Figures 9-15A–E). Actually, more important than the initial surgery is the postoperative immobilization, which is identical to the conservative treatment previously described unless one or both of the lateral bands has also been lacerated which would necessitate DIP joint immobilization in extension also. Often temporary oblique Kirschner wire fixation of the PIP joint in extension is helpful postoperatively to protect healing and to prevent inadvertent flexion of that joint (Figure 9-15C).

Delayed primary reconstruction of a boutonniere deformity should provide results equally as good as primary repair. Delayed primary repair is recommended in any injury in which possible contamination is suspected. Secondary reconstruction of the boutonniere deformity provides the best results if normal anatomy can be restored by reinsertion or repair

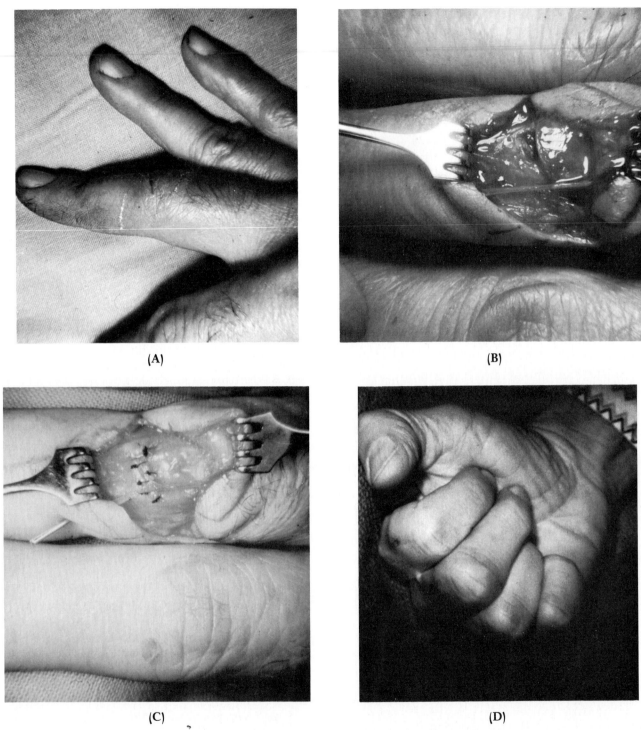

(A)

(B)

(C)

(D)

Figure 9-15 **(A)** Small transverse laceration just distal to PIP joint with resultant mild boutonniere deformity, including PIP flexion and DIP joint extension. **(B)** Exploration of wound by enlargement of laceration laterally and medially discloses discrete transverse laceration of central slip of insertion. It is interesting that this small discrepancy in the extensor slip of insertion caused a mild boutonniere deformity. **(C)** Primary repair of central slip laceration by interrupted 5–0 plain nylon sutures. **(D)** Excellent but not normal flexion of digit is seen 6 months after injury and repair.

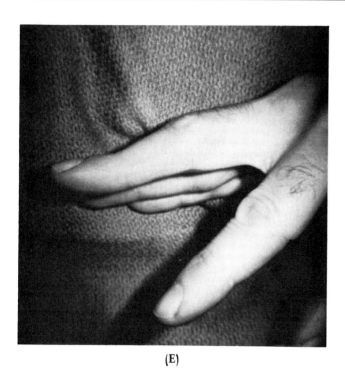

(E)

Figure 9-15 *(continued)*
(E) Slight flexion deformity of PIP joint persists.

of the central slip and by repositioning of the lateral bands to their proper position dorsal to the flexion-extension axis of the PIP joint. As noted, repair will not be successful unless complete passive PIP joint extension has been achieved prior to or at the time of reconstructive surgery. Surgical release of the PIP joint flexion contracture to replace the lateral bands is less satisfactory.

More complex procedures may utilize one lateral band transferred to substitute for an absent central slip to provide PIP joint extension.

Occasionally an open severe crushing avulsion injury destroys the majority of the central slip mass and results in a severe boutonniere deformity (Figures 9-16A–D). After appropriate wound toilet conservative immobilization may provide a satisfactory result in a cooperative patient. However, if infection occurs, resulting in a painful PIP joint with limited motion, arthrodesis is the best solution.

The worst functional impairment of the untreated boutonniere deformity is fixed hyperextension of the DIP joint, with very limited or absent DIP flexion handicapping digital dexterity. If active DIP joint flexion is present in a mild chronic boutonniere deformity, there is little reason to attempt reconstruction surgically (Figures 9-17A,B). In the more severe boutonniere deformity, reconstruction is warranted.

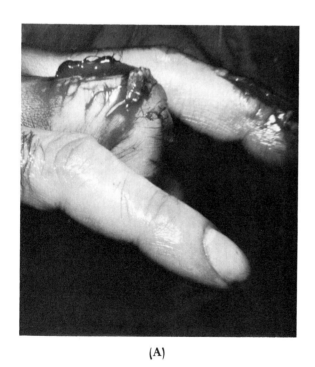

(A)

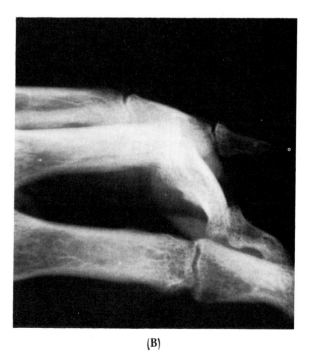

(B)

Figure 9-16 **(A)** Severe, acute boutonniere deformity with almost complete fragmentation and avulsion of central slip and injury of both lateral bands dorsal to ring finger PIP joint. **(B)** Radiograph shows marked flexion of ring finger PIP joint.

(continued)

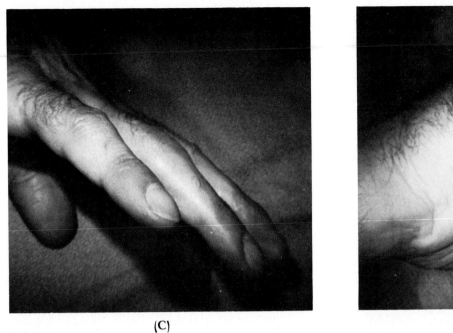

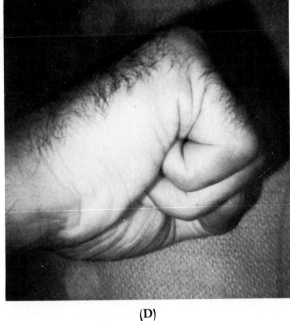

(C)   (D)

Figure 9-16 *(continued)*
(C) Initial meticulous wound toilet and loose skin closure were followed by conservative treatment of 8 weeks of external immobilization of PIP joint in extension. Excellent extension resulted. No tendon repair was possible initially due to severity of damage. Photograph taken 8 months postinjury. **(D)** Excellent flexion.

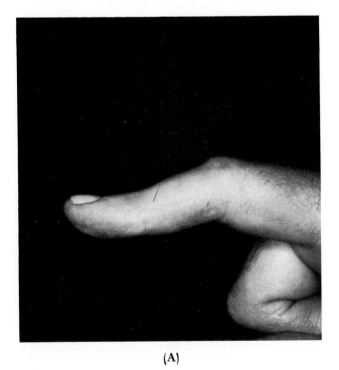

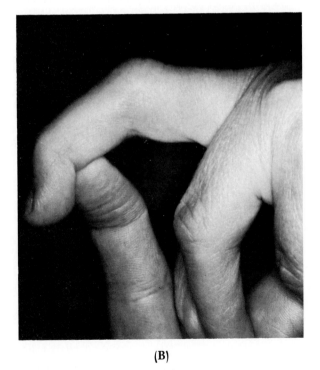

(A)   (B)

Figure 9-17 **(A)** Mild boutonniere deformity with incomplete PIP extension and mild DIP hyperextension. **(B)** Strong active DIP flexion. Reconstruction was not necessary in this case.

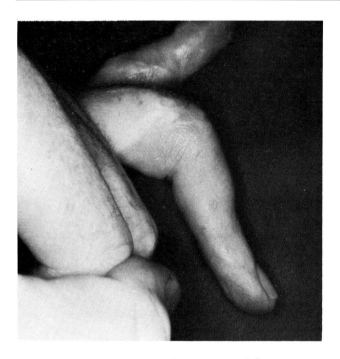

Figure 9-18 Severe chronic boutonniere deformity following multiple attempts at surgical repair. Recommended treatment is transverse sectioning of oblique fibers of lateral bands distal to PIP joint to allow active DIP joint flexion (Fowler procedure). PIP joint fusion might also be necessary.

Occasionally in a digit with severe boutonniere deformity with palmar subluxation of the middle phalanx and previously unsuccessful surgical repair, PIP joint arthroplasty incorporating a silastic implant with simultaneous extensor reconstruction may provide better function.

In a digit which has had multiple unsuccessful operations and which has severe chronic boutonniere deformity (Figure 9-18), transverse sectioning of the oblique fibers of the lateral bands distal to the PIP joint (Fowler procedure) permits active DIP joint flexion. If necessary, PIP joint fusion may be carried out.

Improper immobilization of an acute boutonniere deformity by temporary Kirschner wire fixation or aluminum splint immobilization of the PIP joint in flexion is an erroneous procedure and definitely contraindicated (Figures 9-19A,B).

Pseudoboutonniere deformities may result from numerous situations. A PIP joint dislocation erroneously treated by immobilization of that joint in excessive flexion for three to four weeks will result in a flexion contracture of that joint's palmar plate resembling a boutonniere deformity (Figure 9-20). Active and passive aggressive physical therapy sometimes corrects this problem.

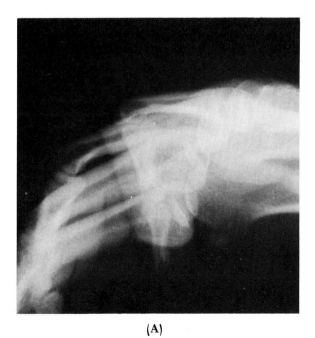

(A)

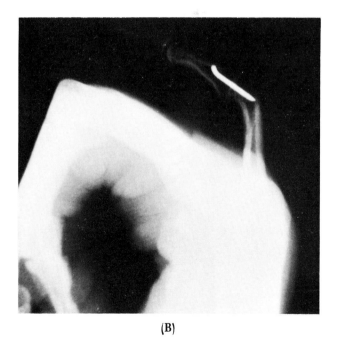

(B)

Figure 9-19 (A) Oblique radiograph of acute boutonniere deformity of little finger due to saw injury shows 90° flexion of PIP joint. (B) Improper temporary Kirschner wire immobilization of boutonniere deformity in 50° flexion. Result was an irreversible PIP joint flexion contracture of 45°.

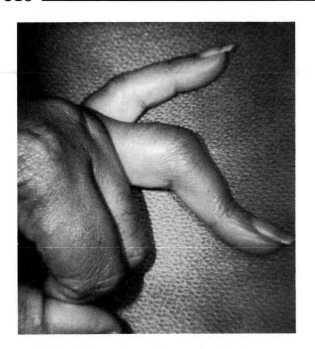

Figure 9-20 Flexion deformity from binding down of palmar plate due to improper immobilization of PIP joint in 35° flexion for 4 weeks following dorsal dislocation.

Articular displaced fracture of the insertion of the central slip on the dorsal aspect of the middle phalanx base with palmar PIP joint subluxation also mimics true boutonniere deformity (Figures 9-21A,B). Anatomic reconstruction, initially, of the articular surface is recommended.

Dorsal fracture subluxation of the PIP joint (Figure 9-22) also may mimic the boutonniere deformity and is treated as described elsewhere in the section on PIP joint dislocations.

Occasionally a marked flexion deformity of the PIP joint may be mistaken for a boutonniere deformity. However, in the former instance active strong DIP flexion is possible, whereas in a boutonniere deformity of this severity, hyperextension of the DIP joint is noted with inability to actively flex the DIP joint.

Severe degenerative joint disease occasionally results in prominence of the proximal phalangeal condyles and palmar subluxation of the middle phalanx base, also resembling a boutonniere deformity (Figure 9-23).

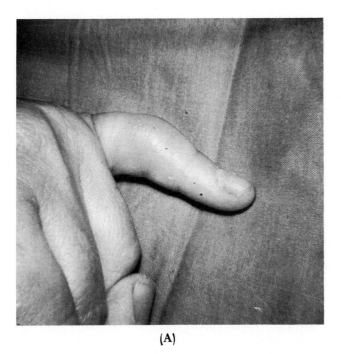

(A)

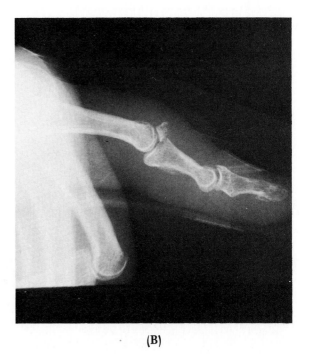

(B)

Figure 9-21 **(A)** Mild boutonniere deformity with swelling localized at PIP joint area 2½ weeks posttrauma. **(B)** Lateral radiograph shows a displaced dorsal fracture of base of middle phalanx, resulting in proximal retraction of central slip, palmar fracture subluxation of PIP joint, and boutonniere type deformity.

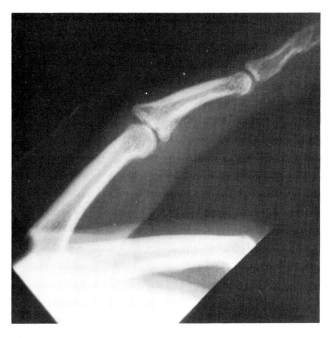

Figure 9-22 Lateral radiograph of comminuted dorsal fracture subluxation of PIP joint 4 weeks posttrauma with no treatment, resulting in PIP joint flexion and DIP joint extension.

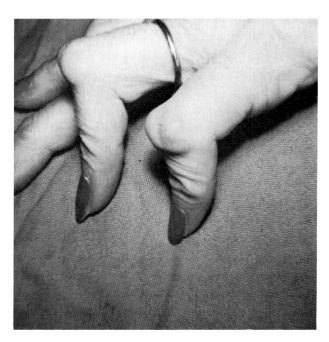

Figure 9-23 Prominent proximal phalangeal condyles with PIP joint flexion contractures and DIP joint hyperextensions of ring and little fingers resulting from severe degenerative joint changes.

Swan Neck Deformity

The swan neck deformity is the exact opposite configuration of the boutonniere deformity but usually does not result from an acute open injury (Figures 9-24A–F). It is usually the result of either avulsion or chronic laxity of the PIP joint's palmar plate, caused by an acute hyperextension injury, or from chronic attenuation. In the latter instance the palmar plate attenuation is usually secondary to loss of superficialis function. Therefore it is important, if the superficialis tendon is either excised from the digit or utilized as a tendon transfer, to tenodese the PIP joint in roughly 15° to 20° flexion, using the radial slip of the superficialis insertion tacked across the joint into the flexor sheath of the proximal phalanx.

The typical swan neck deformity includes hyperextension or recurvatum deformity of the PIP joint and flexion of the DIP joint (Figures 9-24A,B). The lateral bands in this instance are dorsal to the axis of extension-flexion of the PIP joint and together with the central slip cause hyperextension of that joint. The DIP flexion is caused primarily because of unphysiologic passive tension placed on the flexor digitorum profundus insertion by the PIP joint hyperextension. On the other hand, recurvatum of the PIP joint often occurs secondary to a drop DIP joint (mallet finger). The proximal retraction of the avulsed extensor insertion upsets the balance of the extensor mechanism, and hyperextension of the PIP joint occurs. Proximal retraction of the extensor insertion from the distal phalanx puts additional tension on the central slip of the extensor insertion on the middle phalanx, causing hyperextension of the PIP joint.

Reconstruction can be accomplished either by reinsertion of the palmar plate, tenodesis of the PIP joint in slight flexion using one slip of the superficialis insertion, or a retinacular ligament reconstruction (Figures 9-24C,D,E). The retinacular ligament reconstruction is performed by dividing the ulnar lateral band proximally in the web area (Figure 9-24C), dissecting that lateral band distally past the DIP joint level (Figure 9-24D), and rerouting it through Cleland's ligament to the flexor sheath or through a transverse hole in bone in the area of the proximal phalanx (Figure 9-24E). In this position it provides a tenodesis action of flexion for the PIP joint and extension of the DIP joint (method of Littler)[2] (Figure 9-24F).

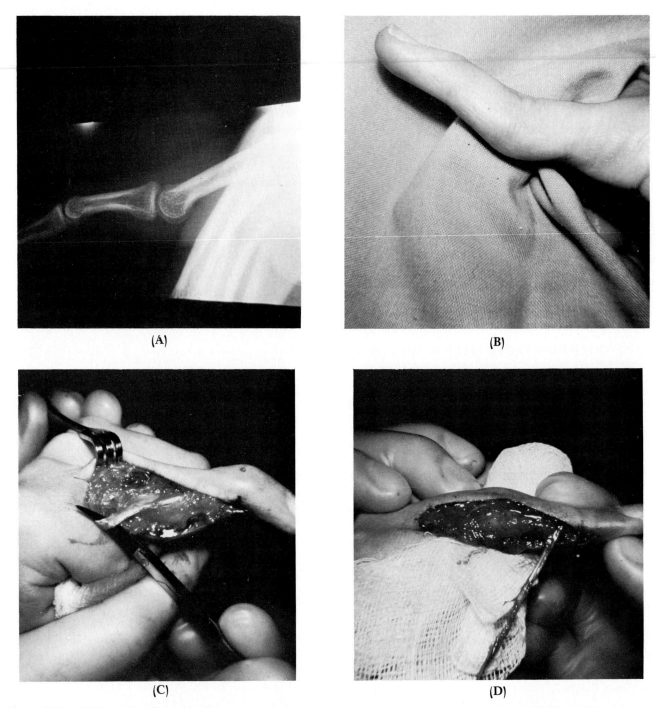

(A)

(B)

(C)

(D)

Figure 9-24 **(A)** Lateral radiograph shows swan neck deformity of PIP joint hyperextension and DIP joint flexion. **(B)** Clinical manifestation of swan neck deformity. Surgical reconstruction is indicated if PIP joint locks in hyperextension and prevents physiologic flexion. **(C)** Surgical exposure of similar case illustrates Littler procedure for retinacular ligament reconstruction of swan neck deformity. Photograph illustrates dissection of ulnar lateral band to a point just distal to DIP joint. **(D)** Proximal excision of lateral band and extension of DIP joint upon traction of this tendon is noted.

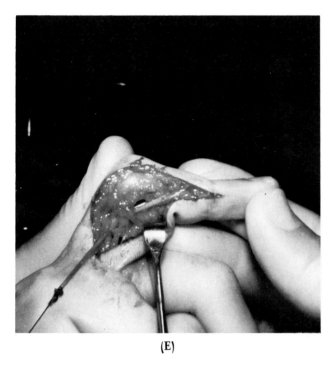

(E)

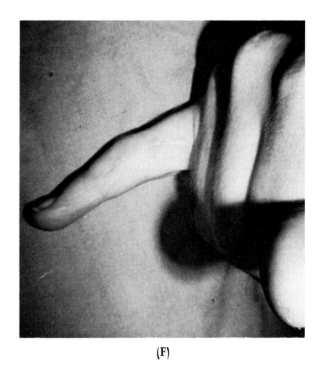

(F)

Figure 9-24 *(continued)*
(E) Rerouting of lateral band tendon transfer through Cleland's ligament to palmar aspect of proximal phalanx and through tunnel in flexor sheath (or through a tunnel in the proximal phalanx). **(F)** Postoperative extension 3 months after surgery is seen in case illustrated in Figures 9-24A,B. Radial view shows healed incision. PIP flexion of 90° and DIP flexion of 45° noted but not shown.

An injury which mimics the swan neck deformity is fracture avulsion of the PIP joint's distal palmar plate insertion with simultaneous dorsal subluxation of the middle phalanx base (Figure 9-25). This situation may be seen in the acute injury of acute dorsal fracture subluxation of the PIP joint or, chronically, as a result of improper initial treatment.

Both a dorsally angulated malunited fracture of the middle phalanx (Figure 9-26) and severe degenerative joint disease with chronic laxity of the palmar plate and recurvatum of the PIP joint (Figures 9-27A,B) may also mimic a swan neck deformity.

Voluntary dorsal subluxation of lateral bands, a normal congenital variant (Figure 9-28), must be differentiated from the pathologic swan neck deformity which it closely mimics.

Occasionally multiple swan neck or boutonniere deformities or combinations result posttraumatically from the same injury (Figure 9-29), and commonly occur in rheumatoid arthritis.

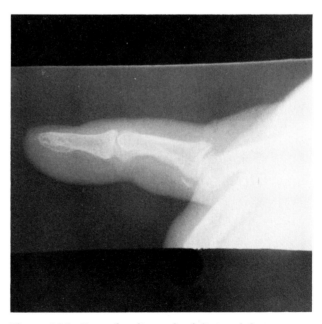

Figure 9-25 Lateral radiograph of digit exhibiting swan neck deformity shows dorsal subluxation of PIP joint with small fracture avulsion of palmar plate distal attachment.

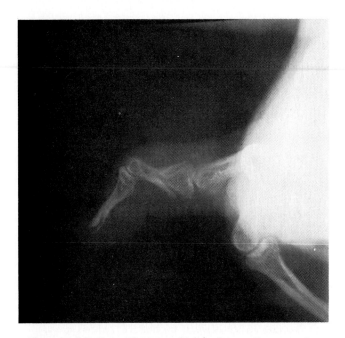

Figure 9-26 Lateral view of little finger shows malunion of middle phalanx with dorsal angulation and shortening, upsetting the delicate flexor-extensor mechanism of that digit and causing swan neck type deformity.

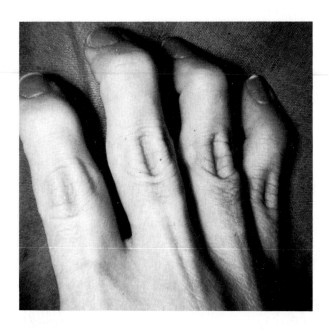

Figure 9-28 Prominent lateral bands dorsally are responsible for voluntary PIP joint hyperextension and DIP joint flexion in a normal variance of dorsally hypermobile lateral bands.

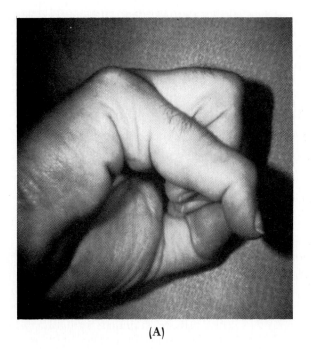

(A)

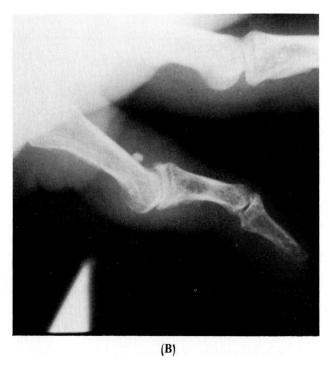

(B)

Figure 9-27 **(A)** No active or passive flexion of PIP joint and minimal active flexion in DIP joint found on examination. **(B)** Lateral view shows marked degenerative and posttraumatic changes in PIP joint with dorsal subluxation, which accounts for severe swan neck deformity.

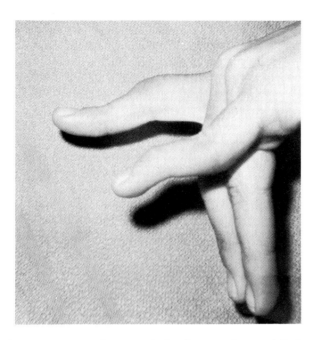

Figure 9-29 Simultaneous index boutonniere and little finger swan neck deformities due to trauma.

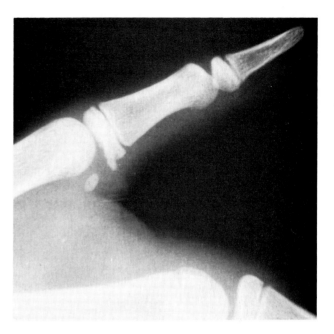

Figure 9-30 Lateral view of thumb in skeletally immature individual shows fracture avulsion from palmar aspect of proximal phalangeal epiphysis, indicating trauma to distal palmar plate attachment of thumb MP joint in hyperextension type injury. Conservative immobilization for 3 to 3½ weeks was recommended. Traumatic separation through physeal plate of proximal phalanx usually occurs rather than a ligamentous injury.

Hyperextension Injuries, Subluxations, Dislocations, and Fracture Dislocations

Metacarpophalangeal Joint (Refer to Figure 9-37)

Hyperextension injuries commonly occur to MP joints (Figure 9-30). The extent of ligamentous and capsular damage depends directly on the severity of injury which, however, is not severe enough to cause joint subluxation or dislocation. The history may reveal a diagnosis of subluxation or dislocation and radiography may be helpful, but physical examination is the most important factor. After examining active ranges of motion, passive ranges of motion and ligamentous and capsular stability are evaluated prior to anesthesia. Tenderness is centered on the palmar aspect of the joint, and abnormal hyperextension can usually be produced. Pain and tenderness may be found laterally and medially depending upon the amount of injury to the accessory collateral ligaments. Examination under anesthesia permits more accurate evaluation of ligamentous and capsular stability.

Treatment should include splint immobilization of the MP joint for about seven to ten days or until acute symptoms subside (usually no longer than two to three weeks). Some pain and limitation of motion will remain for many weeks after the injury, but proper initial treatment will decrease the severity of prolonged morbidity which often results from inadequate treatment of this relatively innocuous injury. Some chronic persistence of joint swelling may follow a severe hyperextension injury.

Dislocations of the MP joint other than the thumb are uncommon and involve most frequently the marginal rays—the index and little fingers. Isolated dislocation of the long or ring finger MP joint is uncommon due to the additional inherent support of the deep transverse intermetacarpal ligament attached firmly on each side of the respective joint to the palmar plate and to the accessory collateral ligament; also, these two digits (long and ring fingers) are obviously in a more protected position than the marginal rays.

Dislocation of the MP joint may occur dorsally (Figures 9-31A–E, 9-32A–E, 9-34A–C), laterally, and, rarely, palmarly (Figures 9-33A,B, 9-35A,B).

Index finger MP joint dislocation is by far the most frequent (Figures 9-31A–E) (excluding the thumb) and is caused by a severe hyperextension injury which avulses the tenuous proximal attachment of the palmar plate from the metacarpal. Eaton[3] states that actually the metacarpal head rather than the proximal phalanx is out of position. The metacarpal head ruptures through the radial aspect of the palmar plate, and the neck becomes constricted in a "purse string" fashion by the palmar plate distally and dorsally, the first lumbrical muscle radially, the flexor tendons ulnarly, and the palmar fascia and superficial transverse metacarpal ligament (natatory ligament) proximally. Closed manipulation is usually unsuccessful because any attempt at manipulation tightens the flexor tendon and lumbrical constriction about the metacarpal neck, wedging the disrupted palmar plate (which has remained attached to the proximal phalanx after its proximal avulsion from the metacarpal) more securely in its interposition between the metacarpal head and base of the proximal phalanx. Usually the radial collateral ligament is avulsed (due to the direction of force of trauma), and because of the more secure fixation of the ulnar collateral ligament (particularly its accessory collateral ligament portion firmly bound to the deep transverse intermetacarpal ligament), the ulnar aspect of the MP joint remains intact, acting like a hinge.

Physical examination (Figures 9-31A,B,D, 9-32B) discloses a shortened index finger with slight hyperextension and usually ulnar deviation of the digit due to the radial collateral ligament's avulsion. The dorsal displacement is not usually striking. Palmarly, the palmarly displaced metacarpal head is prominent, and puckering of the skin is usually evident (Figure 9-31D).

Radiographic evaluation discloses an abnormal incongruous joint articulation at the MP joint and a bayonet type deformity with the proximal phalanx dorsally displaced on the metacarpal head (Figures 9-31C, 9-32C). (Actually the proximal phalanx is more normally anatomically situated and the metacarpal head is inferiorly dislocated in relation to the proximal phalanx base.)

Ulnar deviation is usually seen subsequent to avulsion of the radial collateral ligament.

Gentle manipulation to attempt a closed reduction may be effected, although it is unsuccessful in the vast majority of instances. Open reduction is accomplished generally through an oblique palmar approach parallel to the distal palmar flexion crease. Great care must be taken to avoid damage to the very vulnerable palmar proper digital neurovascular structures to the radial aspect of the index finger which lie superficial to the first lumbrical muscle and are tented palmarly by the palmarly displaced index metacarpal head. The palmar fascia should be lysed proximally sufficiently to allow adequate surgical exposure. Findings to expect at surgery have been noted previously and include a protruding index metacarpal head (Figure 9-31E) caught between the first lumbrical on its radial aspect and the flexor tendons on the ulnar aspect. The partial rupture of the flexor sheath should be surgically extended to allow sufficient laxity of those flexor tendons to permit extraction of the interposed palmar plate and reduction of the metacarpal head onto the proximal phalangeal base. The anatomically replaced palmar plate may be reattached proximally by a single suture and the radial collateral ligament either reinserted or repaired anatomically. The findings illustrated in Figure 9-32E differ somewhat from the usual findings.

Kirschner wire temporary fixation to maintain reduction is not usually necessary in the acute injury, but it was used for three weeks in Figure 9-32E to provide stability. Immobilization of the MP joint in 35°

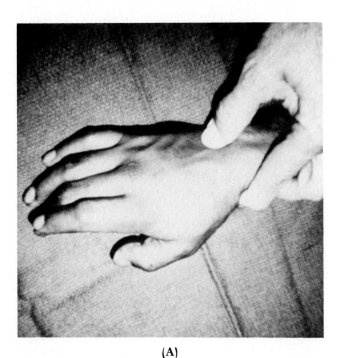

(A)

Figure 9-31 (A) Dorsal view of index MP joint dorsal dislocation: proximal phalangeal hyperextension, ulnar deviation of the digit and soft tissue depression proximal to the proximal phalangeal base are noted.

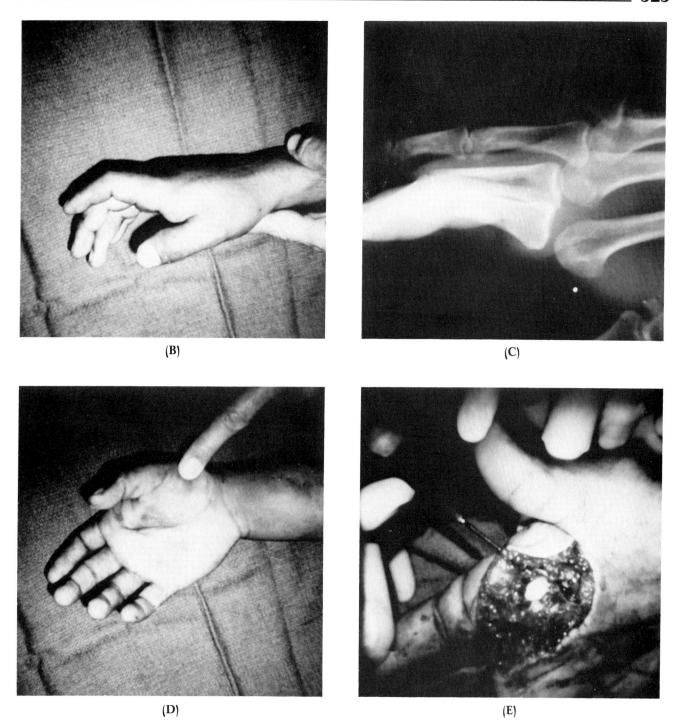

(B)

(C)

(D)

(E)

Figure 9-31 *(continued)*
(B) Lateral view demonstrates MP joint hyperextension, flexion of the PIP joint and prominence of the palmarly displaced index metacarpal head. **(C)** Corresponding radiograph illustrates dorsal dislocation. **(D)** Palmar view shows "puckering" of the skin at the dislocation site. **(E)** Operative exposure reveals the palmar protrusion of the metacarpal head in its dislocated position.

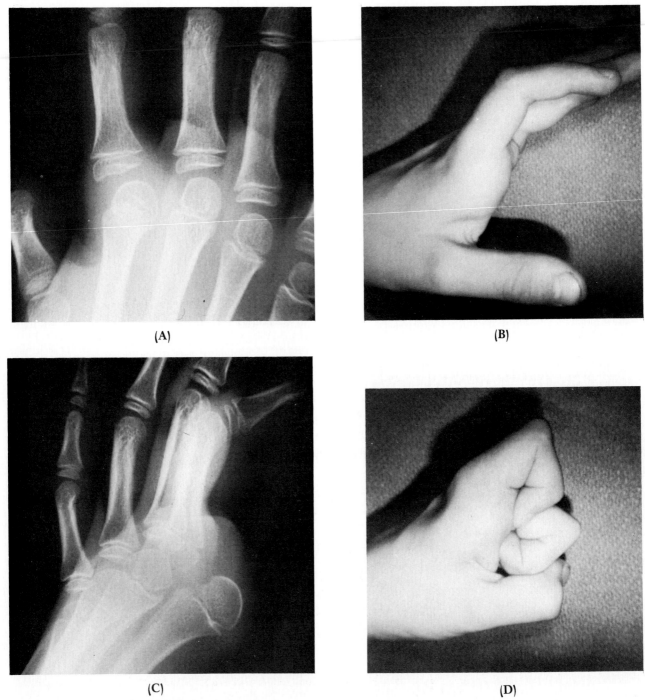

(A)

(B)

(C)

(D)

Figure 9-32 **(A)** PA view illustrates some malalignment of index finger proximal phalanx with metacarpal at MP joint in a 12-year-old boy who had sustained injury 10 weeks previously. **(B)** Hand in digital extension. Index MP joint is hyperextended 45° associated with PIP and DIP joint flexion. Note palmar protrusion of index metacarpal head. **(C)** Lateral view illustrates complete dorsal dislocation of index finger MP joint with marked palmar protrusion of index metacarpal head. Note that anatomic position of index finger proximal phalanx is essentially normal but that metacarpal is actually malpositioned. **(D)** Attempted active flexion of index finger MP joint attains only neutral position. Bayonet configuration of dorsal MP joint dislocation of index finger is particularly apparent here.

Figure 9-32 *(continued)*
(E) Surgical approach from oblique palmar incision parallel to distal palmar flexion crease reveals a rather tenuous first lumbrical muscle directly over the center of the metacarpal head, which protrudes palmarly. Palmar proper digital nerve to ulnar aspect of index finger is seen at ulnar aspect of metacarpal head.

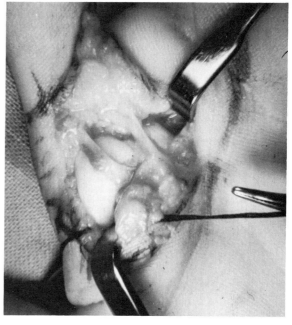

(E)

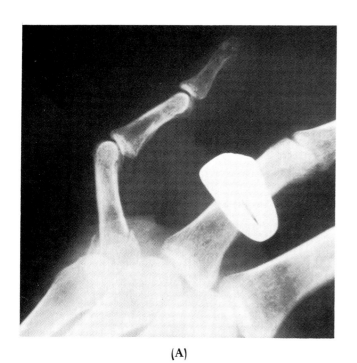

(A)

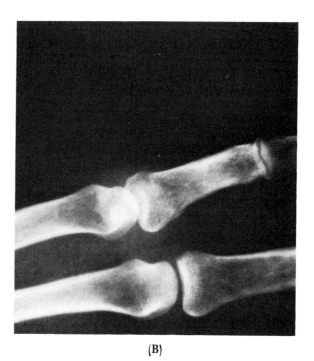

(B)

Figure 9-33 **(A)** Oblique view of palmar dislocation of little finger MP joint associated with dorsally angulated fracture of proximal phalanx. **(B)** Satisfactory reduction of both fracture and dislocation achieved by closed manipulation. Immobilization was continued for 3 weeks, followed by light activity. *(Illustrations 9-33A,B courtesy of D.C. Brown, M.D.)*

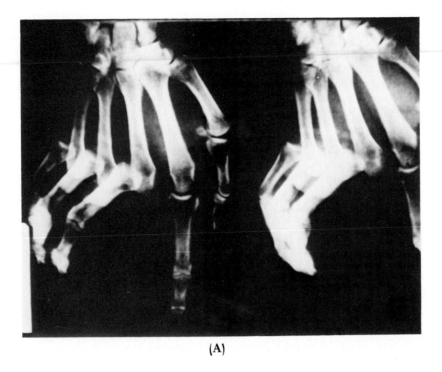

(A)

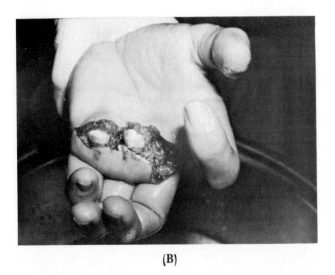

(B)

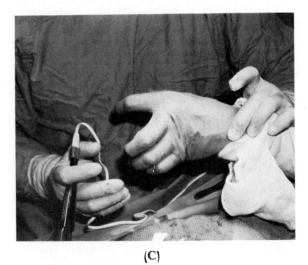

(C)

Figure 9-34 **(A)** Patient sustained open severe hyperextension injury of long, ring, and little finger MP joints in diving accident when he hit the bottom of the pool violently in a deep dive. Radiograph shows dorsal displacement of proximal phalangeal bases and recurvatum deformity of MP joints of those digits, characteristic of the dislocations. **(B)** Palmar view of injury illustrates jagged, open transverse laceration across palmar area of long, ring, and little finger MP joints, with protrusion of ring and little finger metacarpal heads from open wound and hyperextension of proximal phalanges of those three digits. **(C)** Dorsal view clearly shows proximal phalangeal hyperextension and ulnar deviation, together with PIP and DIP joint flexion of long, ring, and little fingers. Treatment included meticulous wound toilet, open reduction of the three dislocations, and repair of the palmar plates. Excellent strong, though incomplete, digital flexion and nearly complete digital extension of the involved fingers resulted 3 months after injury. *(Illustrations 9-34A–C courtesy of J.B. Webber, M.D.)*

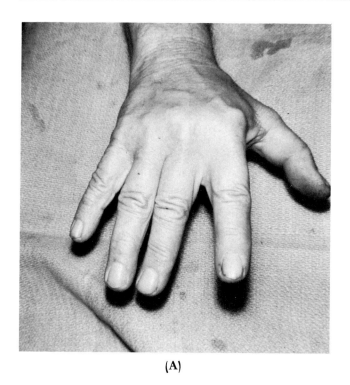

(A)

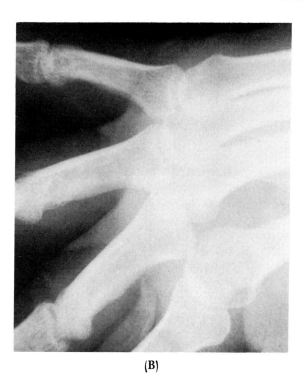

(B)

Figure 9-35 (A) Ulnar deviation, palmar subluxation, and flexion of long finger proximal phalanx at MP joint. This is an unusual manifestation of a traumatic palmar subluxation of the long finger MP joint. (B) Oblique radiograph shows palmar subluxation of long finger proximal phalanx base at MP joint. Gentle closed manipulation of MP flexion with palmar pressure and radial deviation on proximal phalanx base easily reduced the subluxation. Immobilization 2½ weeks posttrauma.

to 45° flexion should be maintained for three weeks postoperatively with no attempt at extension or ulnar deviation during the first week of light active and passive ranges of motion.

Chronic M-P joint dislocation is rarely seen and the longer the time interval of dislocation, the poorer the prognosis for acceptable motion after reduction (Figure 9-32 and refer to Figure 6-6 in Chapter 6, The Thumb).

The ultimate active motion achieved in the case illustrated in Figures 9-32A–E was 45° flexion in the physiologic range of motion.

Next in frequency of MP dislocations is dorsal dislocation of the little finger. This injury is usually a mirror image of the index MP joint dislocation anatomically. The little finger metacarpal head protrudes through the ulnar portion of the proximally avulsed palmar plate, and its metacarpal neck becomes constricted between the abductor digiti minimi ulnarly, the flexor tendons radially, the palmar plate dorsally and distally, and the palmar fascia and superficial transverse metacarpal (natatory) ligament proximally. A similar palmar surgical ex-

posure with similar precautions for reduction is likewise necessary in the majority of instances. Multiple MP joint dislocations, particularly in an open wound, indicate severe trauma to soft tissue as well as to the joints. Meticulous wound toilet is mandatory prior to reductions (Figures 9-34A–C).

Subluxation of an MP joint must be differentiated from true dislocation prior to any attempt at manipulation (Figures 9-35A,B). Subluxation indicates partial contact of the contiguous articular surfaces at the injured joint. Similar findings are noted at physical examination, but the radiographic evaluation discloses less deformity of the joint with hyperextension rather than true dislocation, less incongruity of the cartilage space, and usually no ulnar deviation, which indicates an intact radial collateral ligament. The bayonet type deformity of dorsal displacement of the proximal phalanx (actually palmar displacement of the metacarpal head) is not seen.

This important differentiation prevents conversion of a reducible subluxation into an irreducible complete dislocation. Gentle manipulation to flex the proximal phalanx on the metacarpal head will reduce the subluxation, but hyperextension and traction may terminate in a complete, irreducible dislocation. In a subluxation at least a portion of the radial collateral ligament remains intact, and by maintaining its connection to the palmar plate, prevents complete joint distraction and the drawing of the palmar plate into the joint with consequent impingement. If during aggressive manipulation of the subluxation the radial collateral ligament is completely avulsed and the palmar plate is drawn completely into the joint, then closed reduction of this impinged structure usually will be impossible and open reduction necessary.

Lateral MP joint dislocation, other than the thumb, occurs most commonly to the index finger and is caused by avulsion of the radial collateral ligament by a strong ulnar deviating force on the proximal phalanx. Physical examination after spontaneous or manipulative reduction is not as clear-cut and discloses tenderness, ecchymosis, and swelling on the radial aspect of the MP joint. Stress, with the MP joint in maximal flexion and the patient under appropriate anesthesia, shows marked laxity at the radial aspect of the joint when compared to the contralateral normal index MP joint.

Tear of one collateral ligament in lateral dislocation of an MP joint often avulses the sagittal fibers of the extensor hood at the MP joint level on the same side of the joint. This results in subluxation of the extensor tendons away from the site of ligamentous and sagittal band avulsion. Therefore, deviation toward the intact side of the joint is aggravated, and relocation of the subluxed extensors is important during either conservative immobilization or surgical reconstruction.

Definite diagnosis of complete avulsion of the index finger MP joint radial collateral ligament is best treated by surgical exploration and anatomic repair or reinsertion of that completely avulsed ligament. Chronic laxity of the radial aspect of the index finger MP joint predisposes that joint to degenerative arthritic changes, chronic pain, and relative disuse of the digit (Figures 9-1A–D).

Complete rupture of the little finger MP joint radial collateral ligament or ulnar collateral ligament may be treated conservatively by four weeks immobilization of the MP joint in 45° flexion, but the best and most consistent results will follow surgical exploration and ligamentous repair carried out initially.

Palmar dislocation of the proximal phalanx is rare (Figures 9-33A,B) and is usually encountered in a severe open injury, following infection (Figures 9-36A,B), or as a consequence of rheumatoid arthritis due to chronic ligamentous and capsular attenuation. Ulnar deviation is an important disabling component of this chronic entity and is due to a great many fac-

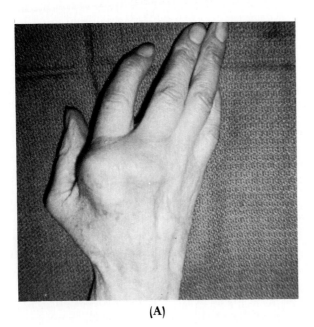
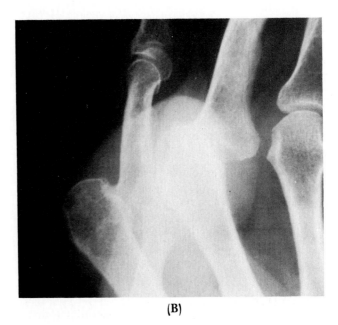

(A)   (B)

Figure 9-36 **(A)** Dorsal view of hand of woman who previously suffered infection of both index and long finger MP joints after steroid injections into those joints. Note prominence of both index and long finger metacarpal heads. **(B)** Radiograph illustrates palmar dislocation and ulnar deviation of index finger MP joint and subluxation and ulnar deviation of long finger MP joint.

tors but primarily to the natural ulnar deviating force exerted by the long flexors and extensors. Surgical reconstruction of the MP joint or joints often incorporating silastic implant arthroplasty and release or transfer of ulnar lateral bands is necessary to anatomically replace the proximal phalanx and to restore function as well as possible in the chronic situation.

A long-standing (greater than three weeks) MP joint dislocation usually means an unfavorable prognosis with limitation of joint motion (Figures 9-32A,E). In addition to the palmar approach, a dorsal approach is often necessary to release exuberant cicatrix and to release the ulnar collateral ligament which is contracted due to prolonged extension or hyperextension of the index finger MP joint. After reduction of the dislocation, reconstruction of the palmar plate should be attempted, if possible. In this instance, temporary Kirschner wire fixation of the MP joint in 45° flexion is indicated for two to three weeks postoperatively to prevent redislocation. Only 30° to 45° of active MP motion is anticipated following reduction of a long-standing dislocation. It is important, therefore, to immobilize the involved MP joint in 45° flexion to be sure the expected 30° to 45° of anticipated active motion will be within the physiologic range for maximal use of that joint.

(Ligamentous instability of the MP joint is discussed in that section of this chapter.)

Proximal Interphalangeal Joint

General Discussion. The diagnosis of "strain" or "sprain" of the proximal interphalangeal joint, or "jammed finger," should not be made unless diagnoses of PIP joint hyperextension injury, subluxation, dislocation, fracture dislocation, or ligamentous avulsion can be definitely excluded. Inadequate treatment of a seemingly innocent PIP joint injury which is actually an undiagnosed or misdiagnosed more severe injury results in prolonged morbidity and often permanent partial disability, with consequences of limited joint motion, pain, and degenerative and posttraumatic arthritic changes.

Hyperextension or recurvatum injury to the PIP joint (Figure 9-37A) results from either acute avulsion or chronic attenuation of the palmar plate. The severity of dorsal angulation (recurvatum) is determined by the degree of injury to the capsular and ligamentous structures, including the palmar plate, and the lateral collateral and accessory collateral ligaments. Most frequently the palmar plate is avulsed from its distal (middle phalangeal) attach-

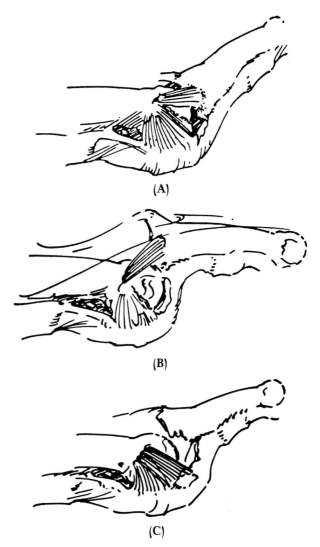

Figure 9-37 Pathology of dorsal PIP joint hyperextension injury and dislocations. **(A)** Hyperextension lesion: palmar plate is avulsed, incomplete longitudinal split occurs in the collateral ligaments and the articular surfaces remain in contact. **(B)** Dorsal dislocation: complete palmar plate avulsion with complete split in the collateral ligaments occurs with the base of the middle phalanx dislocated dorsal to the head of the proximal phalanx. **(C)** Fracture/dislocation (refer to Figure 9-41C and text). *(Courtesy of Richard Eaton, M.D.[3])*

ment in the hyperextension injury or in dorsal dislocation (Figures 9-37, 9-38).[3]

Reattachment of the avulsed palmar plate in the open injury is effected primarily if the wound is clean or, if contamination is suspected, as a delayed primary procedure. Delayed primary or secondary reconstruction of the palmar plate distal attachment may be effected utilizing local tissue (Figures 9-39A–C). However, stabilization of the joint may be

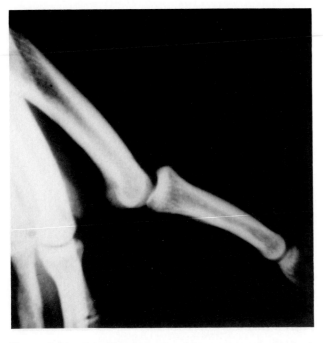

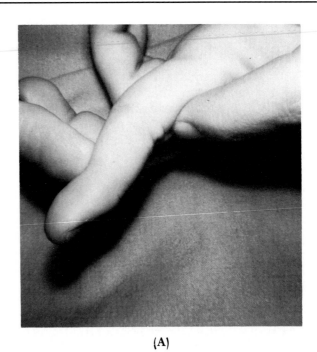

(A)

Figure 9-38 Dorsal PIP joint subluxation with the findings noted in Figure 9-37A. The articular surfaces remain in contact.

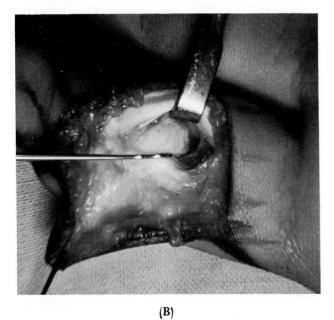

(B)

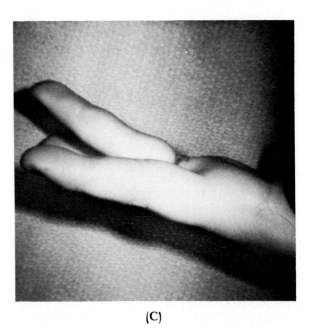

(C)

Figure 9-39 (A) Recurvatum deformity of PIP joint sustained in hyperextension injury demonstrated by palmar pressure on middle phalanx and dorsal pressure on proximal phalanx. DIP flexion due to tenodesis effect on profundus tendon owing to PIP joint hyperextension. (B) Surgical exposure made through palmar incision with flap based on dominant ulnar aspect of little finger and retraction of superficialis and profundus tendons after excision of portion of flexor sheath over PIP joint area. Rent in palmar plate can be seen held by hook retractor. Surgical repair of defect was easily accomplished. (C) Minimal hyperextension of PIP joint upon maximum active motion was noted 4 months after surgical reconstruction of palmar plate. Normal flexion of the digit at all joints resulted.

necessary by using one slip of the superficialis insertion tethered across the joint or a retinacular ligament reconstruction (Figures 9-24A–F; see also Swan Neck Deformity in this chapter).

A lateral radiograph showing a small fracture on the palmar aspect of the middle phalangeal base (Figure 9-40), which may be either undisplaced or displaced to any degree, indicates damage to the insertion of that palmar plate. Very often a history of recurvatum injury, subluxation, or dislocation is discovered upon closer questioning of the patient who originally was thought to have a "jammed finger" (Figures 9-41B,C).[4,5] Three weeks of immobilization of the PIP joint in nearly complete extension (10° to 25° flexion) is advised to guarantee the best stability, particularly if it is suspected that dislocation occurred at the time of original injury. Displaced or undisplaced fracture avulsions on the dorsal aspect of the PIP joint indicate a probable avulsion of the central slip of the extensor insertion from the base of the middle phalanx, particularly if the PIP joint cannot be completely extended actively. This injury must be treated as an acute boutonniere deformity (Figures 9-21A,B; see also section Boutonniere Deformity in this chapter). If this injury is associated with a fracture on the palmar aspect of the middle phalanx base,

it becomes obvious that a severe injury to that joint has occurred (Figure 9-42).

In the skeletally immature individual a similar finding of a displaced or undisplaced fracture avulsion of the palmar aspect of the epiphysis also indicates damage to the palmar plate insertion (Figure 9-30). The palmar plate inserts distally into the palmar aspect of the epiphysis of the middle phalanx, and a similar anatomic arrangement exists for all digital joints. This insertion is therefore proximal to the physis. Usually traumatic physeal separation occurs (see also Chapter 11, Physeal Injuries) rather than ligament or palmar plate avulsion or fracture avulsion in the child and adolescent.

The primary physician often can deduce by history alone that PIP joint subluxation or dislocation, which has undergone spontaneous reduction, was the actual injury. The patient may state "the joint was out of place and popped back by itself" or "the trainer pulled the joint back into position." Often the patient knows precisely that there was marked deformity and angulation at the site of joint injury even though at the time of examination in the emergency room both radiographic and physical findings disclose equivocal evidence of dislocation. Sometimes, particularly on a lateral radiograph, a small fracture can be noted. If the fracture is dorsal to the joint, it indicates fracture avulsion of the insertion of the central slip of the extensor tendon; if it is palmar, it indicates avulsion of the palmar plate insertion. PA radiographs occasionally show a fracture avulsion of a collateral ligament insertion.

Physical examination usually discloses a diffusely swollen PIP joint with generalized tenderness as well as specific tenderness at the area of soft tissue avulsion. If some hours or days have elapsed since the injury, rather marked generalized edema of this digit is seen centralized about effusion and ecchymosis of the PIP joint (Figure 9-43A). A dorsal dislocation of the PIP joint is most frequently seen (Figure 9-43B). The palmar plate usually ruptures from its attachment on the base of the middle phalanx and is associated with partial rupture of at least one collateral ligament (Figure 9-41B) or fracture of the middle phalangeal base (which includes the insertion of the palmar plate and the lateral collateral ligaments) (Figure 9-41C). The accessory collateral ligaments remain in normal position attached to the palmar plate which, in turn, retains its normal position in relation to the proximal phalanx by the strong proximal attachments of its two check ligaments. A tear in the collateral ligament occurs parallel to the fibers in the area of the indefinite boundary between the lateral

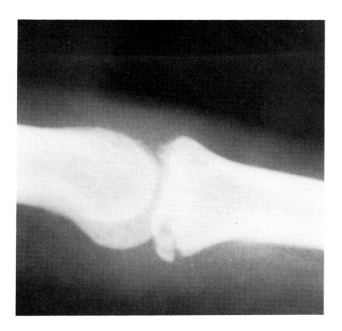

Figure 9-40 Lateral view shows minimally displaced palmar fracture of middle phalanx base, indicating hyperextension injury fracture avulsion of palmar plate distal attachment.

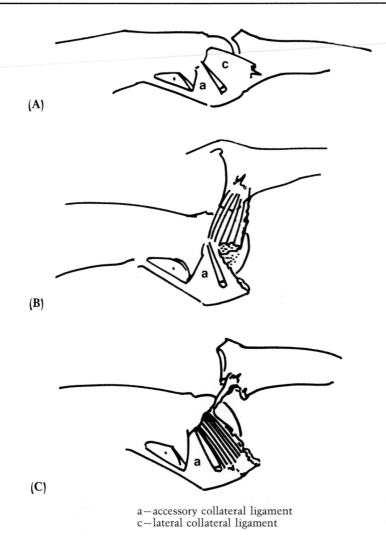

(A)

(B)

(C)

a—accessory collateral ligament
c—lateral collateral ligament

Figure 9-41 A,B,C Diagrammatic representation of the anatomy of proximal interphalangeal (PIP) joint dorsal dislocation and fracture dislocation:
(A) Normal anatomy of ligaments surrounding the PIP joint (see Figure 1-7 in Chapter 1, Anatomy).
(B) Dorsal dislocation of the PIP joint. The palmar plate is avulsed from the base of the middle phalanx, and the tear in the collateral ligaments occurs parallel with fibers in the area of the indefinite boundary between the lateral collateral ligament and the accessory collateral ligament. The palmar plate retains its normal anatomic relationship to the head of the proximal phalanx, secured by its strong proximal attachments, the two check ligaments, and the accessory collateral ligaments. Joint should be stable after reduction because of the normal buttress of the articular surface of the base of the middle phalanx.
(C) An unstable dorsal fracture dislocation of the proximal phalanx at the PIP joint. Reduction is unstable because the palmar portion of the middle phalangeal articular surface is avulsed and no longer can serve as a buttress to prevent redislocation. The major portion of the lateral collateral ligament remains attached to this avulsed articular fragment and the palmar plate. If a few fibers of the lateral collateral ligament retain their attachments to the base of the middle phalanx, reduction usually can be accomplished easily, and occasionally stability may be achieved. In the vast majority of instances, whether a few fibers of the lateral collateral ligament remain attached to the base of the middle phalanx or whether they are completely avulsed from the middle phalanx, reduction is unstable. Surgical intervention usually is advised to restore skeletal stability to the palmar aspect of the middle phalangeal base, necessary to act as a buttress to prevent redislocation. *(Reprinted, by permission, from Richard G. Eaton, M.D. and J. William Littler, M.D., Joint Injuries of the Hand, Fig. 6, 1971, Springfield, Ill., Charles C Thomas, Publisher.)*

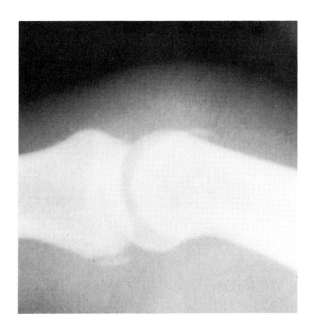

Figure 9-42 Small fracture avulsion dorsal to proximal phalangeal condyles, indicating avulsion of central slip of insertion from dorsal aspect of middle phalanx base, and minimally displaced avulsion fracture of palmar aspect of middle phalangeal base indicate severe soft tissue trauma. Complete immobilization of PIP joint in extension for a minimum of 4 weeks to prevent boutonniere deformity.

collateral and accessory collateral ligaments, thus permitting separation of these ligaments and the dorsal dislocation (Figure 9-41B).

Treatment. A hyperextension injury with good joint contact of the contiguous surfaces of the distal end of the proximal phalanx and base of the middle phalanx is indicative of a rupture of the palmar plate and partial rupture of one or both of the proper collateral ligaments. Reduction is effected by gentle flexion, followed by three and one-half weeks of external immobilization with the PIP joint flexed approximately 15°. Dorsal subluxation indicates a more severe hyperextension injury even though there is still some contact between the contiguous articular surfaces. Ligamentous rupture is more severe, but incomplete rupture of a proper collateral ligament or ligaments permits easy reduction and external immobilization for four weeks, as above.

Complete dorsal dislocation with a bayonet type deformity on physical examination and on lateral radiograph, with dorsal displacement of the middle phalanx base on the distal end of the proximal phalanx (Figure 9-43B), indicates severe injury to both proper collateral ligaments. Reduction, however, should be easily effected by gentle traction, pressure

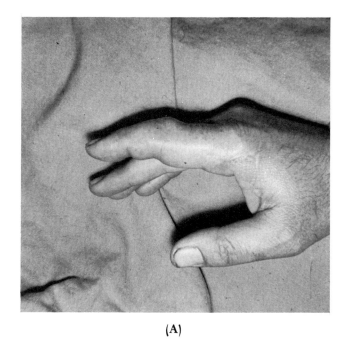

(A)

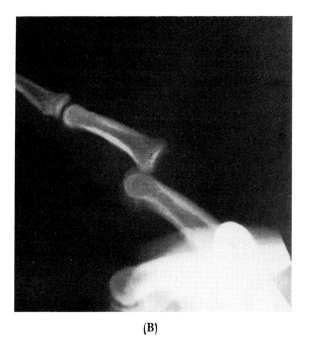

(B)

Figure 9-43 (A) PIP joint dorsal dislocation 4 days after injury. Moderately severe uniform swelling of index finger and dorsal prominence of middle phalanx base are evident. (B) Lateral radiograph shows a complete dorsal dislocation of index finger PIP joint. Excellent extension, lacking only 10° to 15°, and active flexion to 80°, was obtained 3 months after reduction.

distally and palmarly on the dorsal aspect of the displaced middle phalanx base, and pressure on the palmar aspect of the distal end of the proximal phalanx.

Radiographs should always be taken prior to treatment to determine whether a fracture is associated with the dislocation. Before attempted reduction of any dislocation, adequate anesthesia usually should be provided by blocking the appropriate proper and common digital nerves in the palm, combined with infiltrative anesthesia on the dorsal aspect of the hand. Peripheral nerve block anesthesia of the ulnar nerve at the elbow or wrist, or median and radial nerves at the wrist, or by injection of a few cc of 1% plain local anesthetic agent directly into the dislocated joint under aseptic technique may be preferred. Axillary block anesthesia or general anesthesia is rarely necessary unless multiple injuries have been sustained.

Reduction will be stable only if a portion of the proper collateral ligament has remained attached to the palmar plate. These intact fibers of the proper collateral ligament serve to guide the base of the middle phalanx around the proximal phalangeal articular surface back into its proper position, very similar to the lowering action of a knight's visor or the closing of an automobile convertible top. The reduction is unstable, however, if the complete proper collateral ligament attachments are avulsed from their insertions on the base of the middle phalanx, or because of a fracture, together with their attached insertions displaced from the base of the middle phalanx. In this case there is no stabilizing element, either ligamentous or osseous, to maintain the base of the middle phalanx in the reduced position. Unstable fracture dislocation of the PIP joint will be discussed later.

The unstable dorsal dislocation may be treated by percutaneous Kirschner wire fixation of the PIP joint in 15° flexion after reduction or, preferably, by palmar exploration of the joint, repair of the proper collateral ligament avulsions, and reattachment of the palmar plate to the middle phalanx.

After closed reduction it is important to examine PIP joint stability both by the patient's active flexion and extension and by stress testing the collateral ligaments. If recurrent subluxation or dislocation occurs, or if marked lateral instability is demonstrated, particularly on the radial aspect of the index finger or radial or ulnar aspect of the little finger, operative intervention as noted above is recommended.

In the adult the range of motion following treatment of joint dislocation will not be normal, par-

ticularly if reduction was delayed some time after trauma. After immobilization for two and one-half to three weeks in approximately 15° flexion, physical therapy is commenced with emphasis on active flexion and extension at hourly intervals during waking hours. The involved digit may be strapped to an adjacent digit (buddy technique) to aid in regaining motion and to protect the digit. The patient should be advised that he must involve himself energetically in physical therapy for many weeks in order to regain as much active motion as possible and warned that some chronic swelling of the joint will be permanent.

Lateral dislocation of the PIP joint naturally involves complete avulsion of the proper collateral ligament and the palmar plate insertion on the involved side of the joint (Figures 9-44A,B). The gross deformity prior to reduction is pathognomonic in the complete avulsion. Following reduction, either spontaneous or manipulated if necessary, stress of the damaged collateral ligament under appropriate anesthesia determines whether the ligament was completely ruptured or only partially avulsed. Complete collateral ligament avulsion from the radial aspect of the index finger or the radial or ulnar aspect of the little finger PIP joint should be treated primarily by surgical repair for the best ultimate functional stability. Immobilization, whether or not surgery has been carried out, should continue for three and one-half to four weeks with the PIP joint in about 10° to 15° flexion. An avulsion fracture associated with the disruption noted on a PA radiograph is occasionally helpful in the diagnosis (Figure 9-6B).

Palmar subluxation or dislocation is the least common of PIP joint dislocations[6] (Figure 9-45). Spinner[7] believes the mechanism of injury involves two separate actions: first, the initial force ruptures one collateral ligament and the palmar plate by a lateral force similar to the injury sustained in a lateral PIP joint dislocation; second, dorsal force ruptures the insertion of the central slip of the extensor tendon and dislocates the middle phalanx palmarly. For this reason a boutonniere deformity invariably ensues (Figure 9-46). Immobilization after reduction must be continued for a minimum of five to six weeks with the PIP joint in extension to allow proper healing of the central slip and lateral bands and thus prevent a chronic boutonniere deformity (Figure 9-46).

Occasionally an irreducible PIP joint palmar dislocation occurs because of impingement of the proximal phalangeal head between one lateral band and the central slip of the extensor. These tendons act as a "purse string" around the proximal phalangeal neck which is dorsal to the base of the middle phalanx

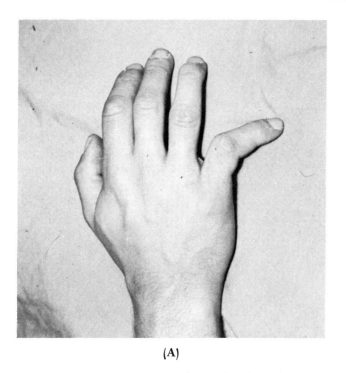

(A)

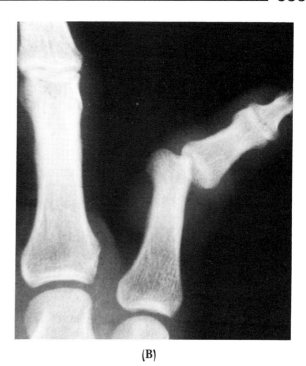

(B)

Figure 9-44 **(A)** Dorsal view of complete lateral dislocation of right little finger PIP joint sustained in a football injury. For this injury to occur there must be complete avulsion of the radial collateral ligament of the PIP joint and at least partial avulsion of the palmar plate. **(B)** Complete lateral dislocation of little finger PIP joint.

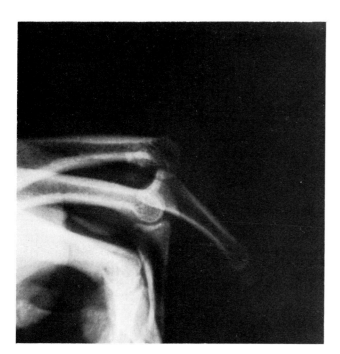

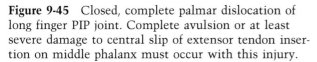

Figure 9-45 Closed, complete palmar dislocation of long finger PIP joint. Complete avulsion or at least severe damage to central slip of extensor tendon insertion on middle phalanx must occur with this injury.

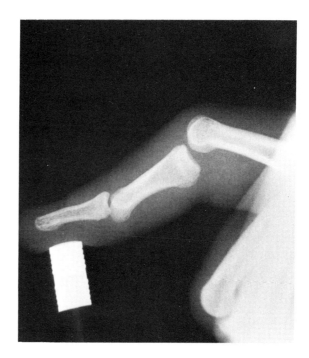

Figure 9-46 PIP joint palmar subluxation with flexion contracture and boutonniere deformity following 3½ weeks of improper immobilization of PIP joint in 60° flexion after reduction of palmar dislocation.

and often prevent closed reduction. Surgical exploration and open reduction are necessary for an irreducible PIP joint dislocation due to soft tissue interposition.

Dorsal fracture subluxation or fracture dislocation of the PIP joint is not uncommon[4,5] (Figures 9-47, 9-48, 9-49). It is usually caused by a direct blow on the tip of the involved digit which is flexed at the PIP joint. The fracture involves the palmar aspect of the middle phalangeal base. If the fracture is small, a portion of the lateral collateral ligaments usually remains attached to the middle phalanx and provides stability after reduction. However, if a large articular segment of the palmar lip of the middle phalanx base is displaced, then nearly the entire insertions of the lateral collateral ligaments are detached from the middle phalanx and the fracture dislocation becomes unstable because the palmar buttress is lost (Figure 9-41C).

Stable closed reduction may be treated by splint immobilization in PIP joint extension or 15° to 20° flexion for three to four weeks (Figure 9-47).

If closed reduction achieves normal PIP joint anatomy, but reduction is unstable, temporary percutaneous Kirschner wire fixation in extension may or may not be successful (Figure 9-48).

If the PIP joint redislocates in complete or nearly complete extension, but is stable otherwise, dynamic splint immobilization which blocks extension in the unstable ranges may be applicable.[8] If the joint must be maintained in marked flexion for stability (Figure 9-49A), whether or not a temporary Kirschner wire is utilized across that joint (Figure 9-50), it is preferable to perform open reduction and reconstruction. Maintenance of the PIP joint in marked (70° or more) flexion for a prolonged time (longer than two and one-half to three weeks) will create a severe flexion contracture, quite refractory to rehabilitation (Figures 9-49A, 9-50). Figure 9-50 is a good example of this.

Surgical exposure for the unstable dorsal fracture dislocation utilizes a palmar flap type incision, with the flap based on the dominant aspect of the digit, carefully executed to avoid damage to proper neurovascular structures. A segment of the flexor sheath overlying the PIP joint is excised to allow retraction of both the profundus and superficialis tendons in order to expose the palmar plate. The palmar plate is elevated sufficiently to expose the palmar

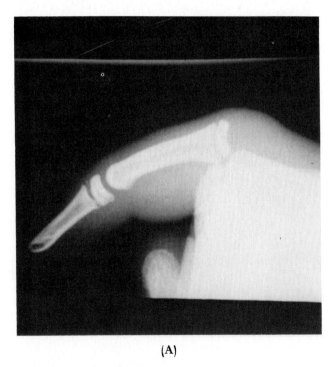

(A)

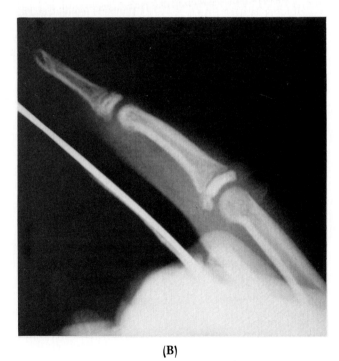

(B)

Figure 9-47 **(A)** Dorsal fracture dislocation of the PIP joint in a skeletally immature patient. **(B)** Stable reduction illustrates the fracture, a Salter III physeal injury; treated for three weeks by splint immobilization with the PIP joint flexed to 10°.

Figure 9-48 (**A**) Dorsal fracture subluxation of the PIP joint. (**B**) Closed reduction and percutaneous oblique Kirschner wire fixation of the PIP in 10° flexion. (**C**) 4½ weeks later malunion is associated with hyperextension and dorsal subluxation of the PIP joint.

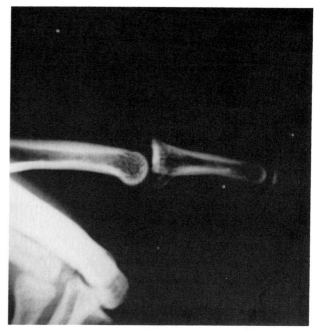

(A)

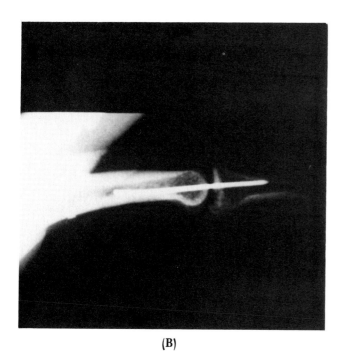

(B)

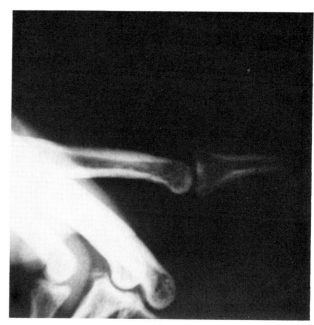

(C)

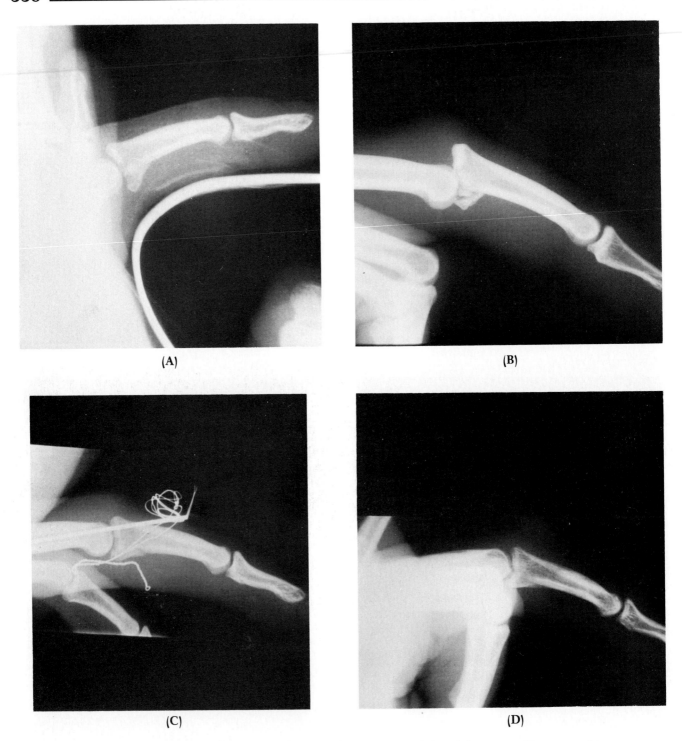

(A)

(B)

(C)

(D)

Figure 9-49   **(A)** Lateral radiograph illustrates reduction of a comminuted dorsal fracture subluxation of ring finger PIP joint with immobilization on an aluminum splint in 70° to 80° flexion. **(B)** After removal of splint a comminuted palmar articular fracture of middle phalangeal base, associated with dorsal subluxation of ring finger PIP joint, is seen. **(C)** Following open reduction and internal fixation of comminuted fracture, palmar plate advancement, reduction of PIP joint dorsal subluxation, and temporary oblique Kirschner wire fixation of joint in 5° to 10° flexion. **(D)** Six weeks after surgery. The temporary Kirschner wire fixation and pullout wire have been removed, and the joint is in anatomic position.

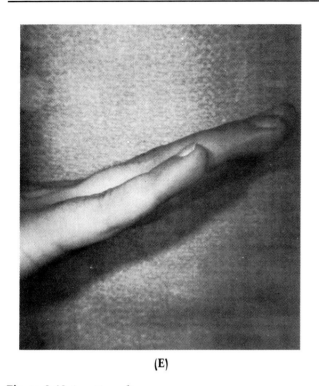

(E)

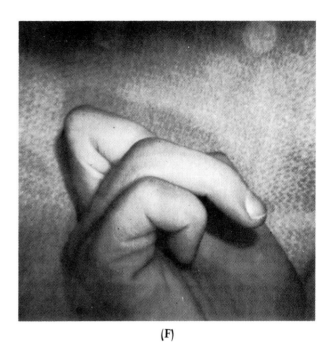

(F)

Figure 9-49 *(continued)*
(E) Complete extension of PIP joint noted 5 months after surgery. **(F)** PIP joint flexion of 75° noted. With aggressive self therapy of active PIP joint flexion, better motion can be expected in the cooperative patient.

Figure 9-50 Comminuted articular displaced fracture of palmar 50% of middle phalangeal base with dorsal PIP joint subluxation from crushing injury. Good reduction of both PIP joint subluxation and articular fracture with incorrect percutaneous Kirschner wire temporary immobilization of PIP joint in 85° flexion; marked flexion contracture owing to continued immobilization of PIP joint in marked flexion for 2½ weeks. However, if stable reduction of PIP joint subluxation and the articular fracture can be achieved with PIP joint in nearly complete extension by temporary Kirschner wire fixation or external splint immobilization, either of these methods is acceptable.

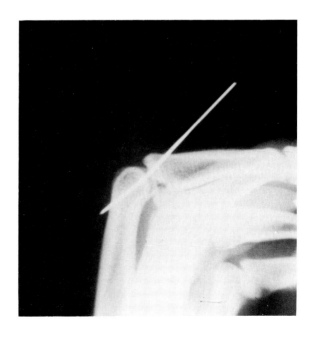

aspect of the PIP joint by parallel longitudinal incisions, usually connected distally by a transverse incision, thus forming a trap door of the palmar plate based proximally. If a large articular fracture fragment is responsible for the unstable dorsal fracture dislocation, it should be anatomically replaced to provide a normal articular surface of the middle phalangeal base and should be maintained in reduction by a stainless steel monofilament pullout wire routed through the palmar plate insertion, through drill holes placed in the fracture fragment, and obliquely through the middle phalanx, avoiding damage to the extensor ten-

don, to be tied over a padded button on the dorsal aspect of the middle phalanx. The pullout wire is routed laterally through the skin for later retrieval (Figures 9-49A–F).

If the fracture fragment is small or if there is gross comminution with instability (Figure 9-51A), the fracture fragments should be removed and the palmar plate advanced into the defect on the palmar aspect of the middle phalanx base to provide stability for the joint and to prevent recurrent dorsal dislocation. A similar pullout wire is used to attach the palmar plate to the defect thus created (Figure

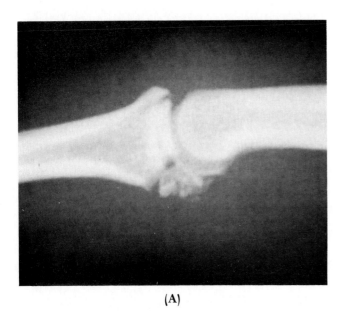

(A)

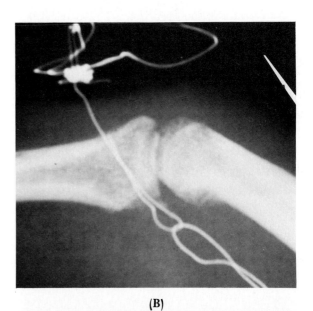

(B)

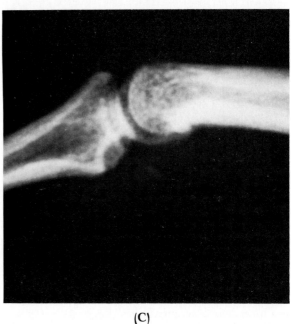

(C)

Figure 9-51 (A) Extremely comminuted fracture of palmar aspect of little finger middle phalangeal base, associated with undisplaced dorsal fracture of base and marked instability. (B) Close-up lateral radiograph following removal of bony fragments and palmar plate advancement into raw defect created on palmar aspect of middle phalangeal base. Note pullout wire utilized to hold palmar plate advancement temporarily in position. (C) Nearly complete extension of little finger PIP joint and 90° flexion resulted 4 months after surgery.

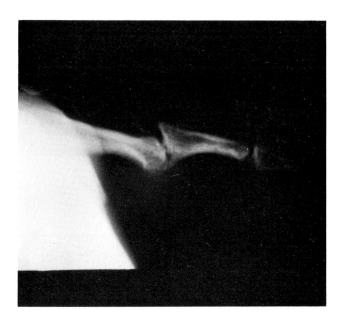

Figure 9-52 Lateral radiograph illustrates severe post-traumatic changes due to chronic dorsal subluxation of PIP joint resulting from inadequate treatment of comminuted unstable fracture of palmar aspect of middle phalangeal base, with dorsal PIP joint subluxation.

9-51B). In both the case of reduction of a large articular fracture fragment or palmar plate advancement, temporary oblique or longitudinal Kirschner wire fixation across the PIP joint in extension or 10° flexion is recommended for a period of three and one-half weeks. At the end of this time the temporary Kirschner wire fixation is removed and active flexion and extension of the joint is commenced. Seven to ten days later the pullout wire is removed (Figures 9-51A–C).

If chronic subluxation of the PIP joint remains following an untreated or inadequately treated dorsal fracture subluxation, posttraumatic arthritic changes invariably develop with marked loss of PIP joint function (Figures 9-22, 9-52). The only recourse then is PIP joint reconstruction incorporating silastic implant arthroplasty or arthrodesis.

Palmar subluxation or dislocation of the PIP joint is much less common (Figures 9-53A, 9-54, 9-55A). This injury is a mirror image of the dorsal fracture subluxation and is caused by a proximally directed blow on the dorsal aspect of the middle phalanx with the PIP joint extended or slightly flexed. The flexor digitorum superficialis tendon causes

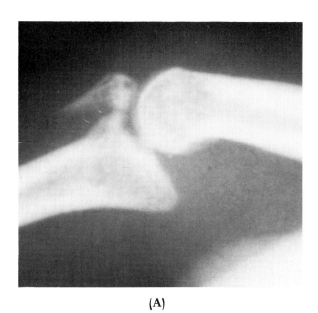

(A)

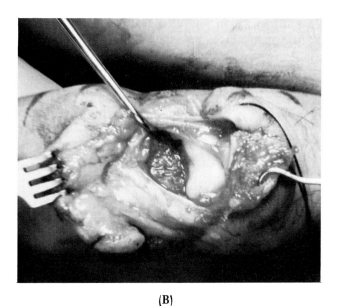

(B)

Figure 9-53 **(A)** Close-up lateral radiograph illustrates palmar subluxation of PIP joint due to unstable displaced fracture of dorsal aspect of base of middle phalanx. **(B)** Exposure of PIP joint made through dorsal incision between central slip of extensor insertion and ulnar lateral band, displaced inferiorly in operative field. Retraction of completely avulsed fracture fragment is proximal (to the right); raw bone of middle phalangeal base is just distal (to the left) to area from which displaced dorsal articular fragment was avulsed; articular cartilage of proximal phalangeal condyles is seen just proximally (to the right). *(continued)*

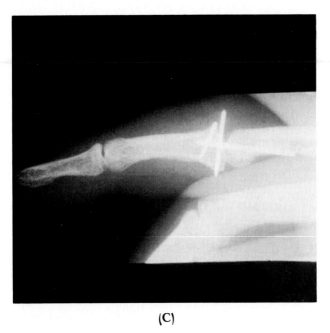

(C)

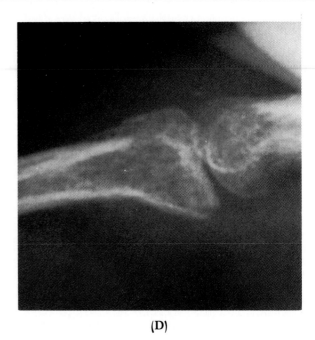

(D)

Figure 9-53 *(continued)*
(C) Lateral radiograph after open reduction and internal fixation of displaced articular fracture fragment and temporary oblique Kirschner wire fixation of PIP joint in extension shows reduction of both PIP joint subluxation and of dorsal articular fracture fragment with PIP joint in extension. **(D)** Close-up lateral view 9 weeks after injury shows maintenance of PIP joint reduction and good healing of large dorsal fracture fragment in an acceptable position.

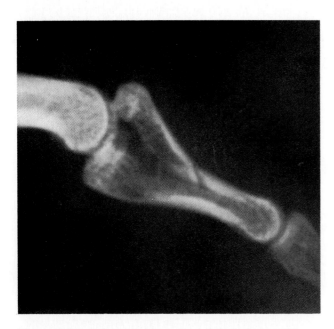

Figure 9-54 Palmar subluxation of little finger PIP joint with large dorsally displaced articular fracture fragment and comminution of middle phalangeal proximal metaphysis. Regardless of treatment, this joint will be limited in active and passive ranges of motion, and posttraumatic arthritic changes are inevitable.

palmar subluxation of the PIP joint because it is unopposed both by loss of the insertion of the central slip of the extensor tendon and by loss of the dorsal lip of the middle phalanx base which normally provides skeletal architectural stability as a buttress to the dorsal aspect of the middle phalanx base.

Treatment consists of dorsal exposure of the joint to anatomically reposition the displaced articular fracture fragment and to reinsert the fracture avulsion of the central slip of the extensor tendon insertion (Figure 9-53B). The skin incision may be oblique, transverse, or flap type, with the flap based on the dominant aspect of the digit. Sharp longitudinal incision through the extensor mechanism between the central slip and the lateral band on one side permits exposure of the fracture fragment and the joint for irrigation and anatomic fracture reduction. The postoperative treatment is identical to that described under dorsal fracture subluxation. By anatomically reestablishing the dorsal lip of the middle phalanx base, the reduced palmar PIP joint subluxation should be permanently corrected (Figures 9-53A–D). Chronic untreated or inadequately treated palmar fracture subluxation results in marked disability and arthritic changes (Figures 9-21A,B,

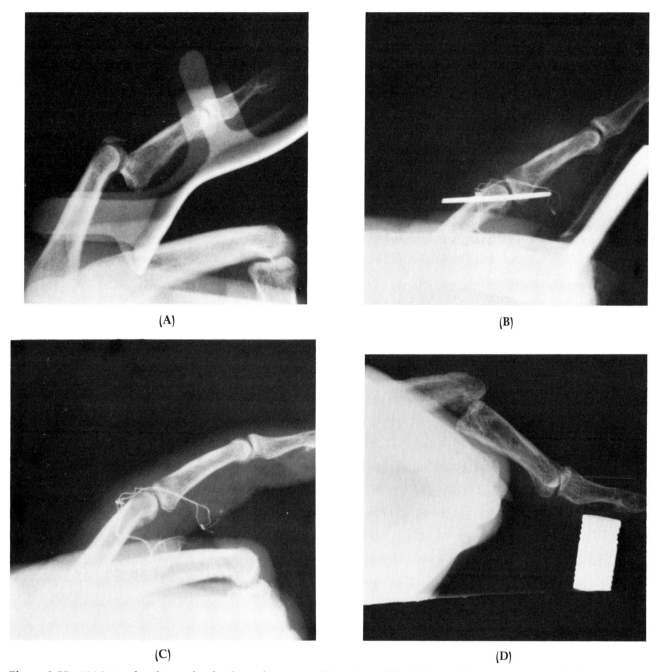

(A)

(B)

(C)

(D)

Figure 9-55 (A) Lateral radiograph of palmar fracture subluxation of little finger PIP joint. Fracture fragment which has been avulsed from dorsal aspect of middle phalangeal base can be seen, indicating complete loss of central slip of insertion from that area. Inadequate temporary aluminum splint immobilization is noted. (B) Lateral radiograph after open reduction of fracture subluxation and temporary oblique Kirschner wire fixation of joint, with pullout wire fixation of fracture fragment. (C) Lateral view 3 weeks postoperatively at which time oblique Kirschner wire across PIP joint was removed. There is some question as to whether fracture fragment of dorsal aspect of middle phalangeal base remains reduced. (D) Lateral radiograph 4 months later (pullout wire removed 3½ weeks postoperatively). Palmar subluxation of PIP joint has recurred and is chronic. Internal fixation was discontinued too early, allowing resubluxation of PIP joint.

9-55A–D). The case in Figures 9-55A–D illustrates this point well. Internal fixation was discontinued too early, allowing resubluxation of the PIP joint. The capsular structures and insertion of the central slip of the extensor tendon had not healed sufficiently after three and one-half weeks to prevent recurrence of the deformity. The dorsal fracture fragment and insertion of the central slip of the extensor tendon perhaps were not anatomically reduced at the time of surgery, which would contribute to the later loss of position.

Occasionally a comminuted "Y" or "T" type fracture of the middle phalanx base involves fractures of both the dorsal and palmar portions of the articular surface, resulting in gross deformity or instability of the PIP joint. In such cases the most unstable segment should be operatively fixed to the shaft of the middle phalanx to provide the necessary stability to maintain reduction (Figure 9-56). If the fracture is extremely comminuted with no single segment large enough for accurate reduction and fixation, then balanced skeletal traction by transverse Kirschner wire fixation through the middle phalangeal shaft should be considered (Figure 9-56).

The primary objective in the treatment of an open dislocation or fracture dislocation is meticulous wound toilet. If joint reduction has been accomplished previously to prevent irreversible ischemic changes distal to the dislocation, the joint must be redislocated prior to the definitive reduction to allow adequate exposure for meticulous cleansing, irrigation, and debridement.

Often when the patient is first seen the joint has already been reduced (Figures 9-57A–I). The force necessary to literally tear or burst the palmar or lateral skin should make one highly suspicious that open joint dislocation was present initially (Figure 9-57A). Often this suspicion can be verified by radiographs which on the lateral view may show a small fracture avulsion on the palmar aspect of the PIP joint accompanied by recurvatum deformity of that joint, indicating acute avulsion of the palmar plate insertion (Figure 9-57B). On the PA view fracture avulsions laterally indicate avulsion of one or both lateral collateral ligament insertions (Figure 9-57C). Occasionally a complete dorsal dislocation can be documented on a lateral radiograph prior to spontaneous reduction in the interval between radiographic evaluation and

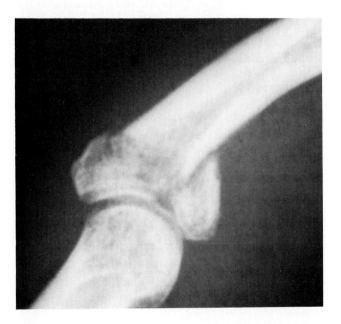

Figure 9-56 Comminuted "T" or "Y" fracture of middle phalangeal base with large dorsal fragment and large palmar fragment. Displacement of palmar fragment is accompanied by flexion deformity (palmar angulation) of middle phalangeal shaft 45° to 50°. Treatment is very difficult; early operative intervention should attempt to align shaft of middle phalanx with dorsal fracture fragment and then to reduce the palmar fragment.

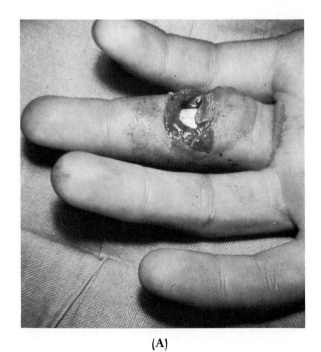

(A)

Figure 9-57 (A) Bursting transverse wound on palmar aspect of long finger PIP joint with exposure of flexor tendons. Photograph taken after spontaneous reduction of an open dislocation and before meticulous wound toilet.

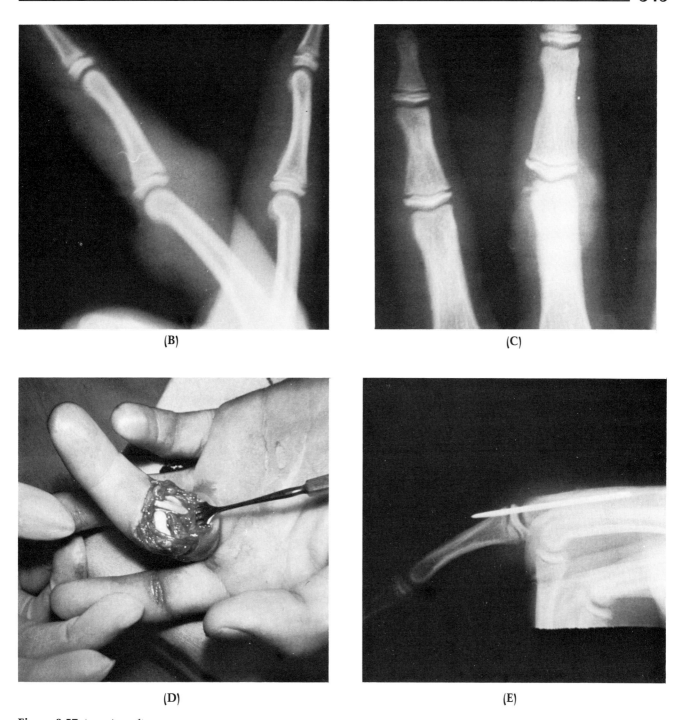

(B)

(C)

(D)

(E)

Figure 9-57 *(continued)*
(B) Lateral view shows hyperextension at PIP joint, soft tissue injury on palmar aspect of joint, marked swelling on dorsum of joint, and, possibly, a few flecks of bone on palmar aspect. Findings indicate severe trauma to joint and adjacent soft tissues, with complete avulsion of palmar plate. **(C)** PA view illustrates fracture avulsion of radial collateral ligament at PIP joint. **(D)** Proximal retraction of skin shows clearly radial condyle of proximal phalanx and palmar proper digital nerve to radial aspect of long finger. At time of wound toilet PIP joint was redislocated to permit proper cleansing prior to definitive palmar plate reduction, reattachment, and loose skin closure. **(E)** Postoperative lateral radiograph shows temporary oblique Kirschner wire fixation of PIP joint in 10° to 15° flexion. At surgery, approximation of completely avulsed distal attachment of palmar plate was achieved after joint reduction and temporary Kirschner wire immobilization.

(continued)

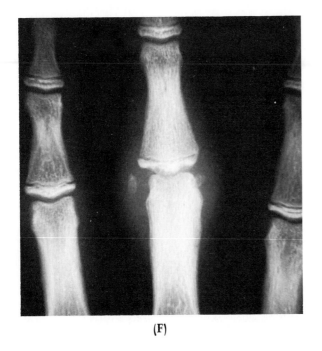

(F)

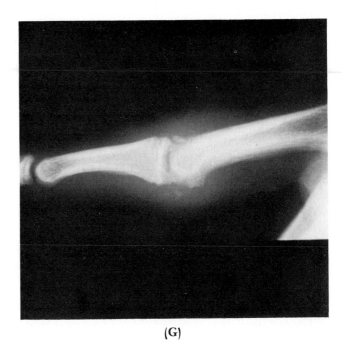

(G)

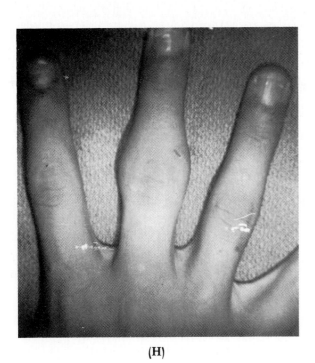

(H)

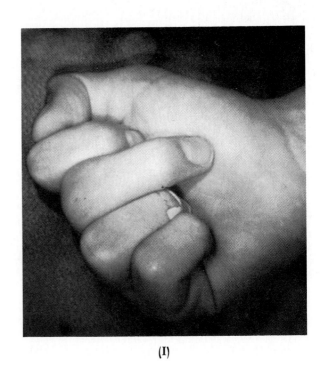

(I)

Figure 9-57 *(continued)*
(F) PA radiograph 8 months after original injury illustrates good PIP joint cartilage space and calcification in origins of both collateral ligaments of PIP joint. **(G)** Lateral radiograph shows similar findings, with calcification also noted on dorsal and palmar aspects of joint. **(H)** Eight months after injury there is persistent swelling of PIP joint. **(I)** Palmar view shows excellent PIP flexion but somewhat restricted DIP flexion due to adhesions. Extension of both joints (not shown) was normal.

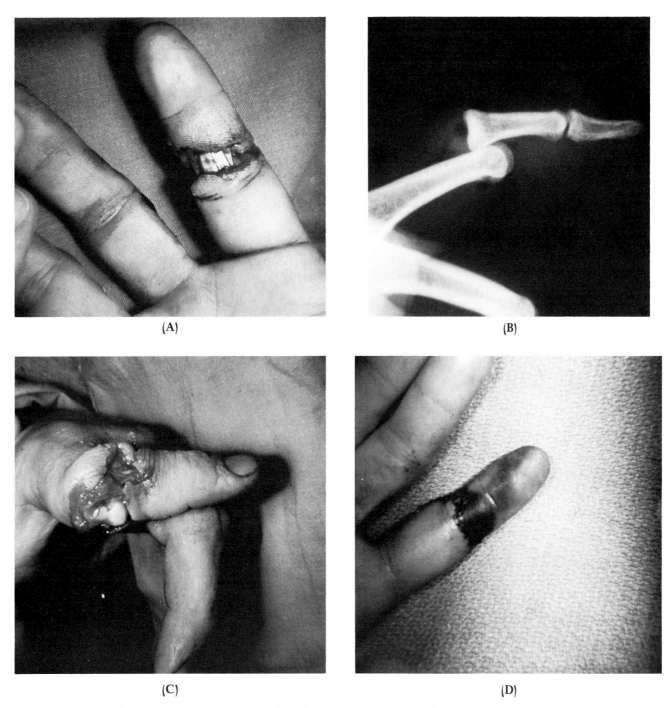

(A)   (B)

(C)   (D)

Figure 9-58 (A) Palmar view of severe torsional avulsion injury with ragged transverse laceration at PIP joint level and exposure of flexor tendons. No dislocation was seen at this time. (B) Lateral radiograph taken before primary wound care shows complete dorsal dislocaton of PIP joint with overriding of base of middle phalanx dorsal to condyles of proximal phalanx. Dislocation had been reduced some time between radiographic evaluation and initial care. (C) Redislocation of little finger PIP joint was necessary to allow meticulous wound toilet. Note poor circulation distal to PIP joint open dislocation. Complete avulsion of proper neurovascular supply to ulnar aspect of little finger and marked contusion to radial proper vascular supply were found at exploration. (D) Gangrenous changes resulted from diffuse thrombosis of vascular supply to radial aspect of digit.

the physician's initial care of the wound (Figure 9-58B).

Open dislocation of the PIP joint is a serious injury and requires:

1. Meticulous wound toilet (often the flexor tendons are exposed and protrude into the open wound)
2. Reduction of the dislocation
3. Evaluation of the vascular status distal to the injury
4. Loose closure or delayed primary closure of the wound
5. Constant immobilization and evaluation of the extremity postoperatively (Figures 9-57A–I, 9-58A–D)

Approximation of the avulsed palmar plate and/or collateral ligament repair may be performed if additional exposure is not necessary and if the vascularity of the digit distal to the dislocation is acceptable following reduction. Prolonged surgery involving multiple soft tissue reconstructions or additional surgical exposure is contraindicated if any vascular impairment is noted. Temporary oblique Kirschner wire fixation of the reduced PIP joint may often be useful to maintain reduction and help prevent additional vascular impairment in a very unstable situation (Figure 9-57E).

Occasionally, because of severe torsional injury sustained by the proper neurovascular bundles, consequent arterial and venous thrombosis results in irreversible vascular changes and tissue death (gangrene) (Figures 9-58A–D).

If initial reconstruction is contraindicated and ligamentous instability persists, collateral ligament reconstruction may be performed at a later date if joint instability produces symptoms or impairs functional use of the digit.

Distal Interphalangeal Joint

Acute palmar plate avulsion of the DIP joint sustained in a hyperextension injury usually involves the proximal attachment. Diagnosis may be difficult and is based on physical findings of tenderness, primarily on the palmar aspect of the joint, and abnormal hyperextension of the DIP joint on stress testing under appropriate anesthesia as compared to the normal contralateral digit. If the profundus tendon insertion is intact and active DIP joint flexion can be demonstrated, the palmar plate avulsion should be treated by complete immobilization of the DIP joint in 10° to 15° flexion for three and one-half to four weeks.

Occasionally rupture or laceration of the profundus insertion may accompany a similar injury to the palmar plate. Treatment should include advancement of the profundus insertion into the base of the distal phalanx and repair of the palmar plate. Naturally there will be abundant scar formation during healing of such a serious injury, and DIP joint ranges of motion will be diminished, although stability should be acceptable.

Chronic DIP joint hyperextension instability is best treated by repair with local palmar plate tissue if possible, or by using a portion of the profundus insertion. This segment of profundus is left attached distally at its normal insertion and fixed proximally to the sheath or periosteum or into the bone of the middle phalanx (Figures 9-59A,B).

Chronic hyperextension instability due to old profundus laceration or avulsion with DIP joint palmar plate attenuation is best treated by tenodesis rather than DIP joint fusion. With the former, resiliency of the DIP joint is retained upon strong pinch of that digit, giving better proprioception, and with full digital flexion the patient can passively flex the involved DIP joint with the adjacent digit or digits, "getting it out of the way." Fusion of the DIP joint is an excellent procedure but eliminates the dexterity of passive DIP joint flexion. Resection of the profundus tendon in the palm should accompany either DIP tenodesis or arthrodesis, since the mass of that proximally retracted, often curled-up tendon is often the patient's main concern.

The most stable tenodesis is provided by a segment of the profundus insertion placed into a prepared cavity in the middle phalanx and retained there by a pullout wire for four to five weeks with the DIP joint flexed 25° to 30°. If no profundus tendon is available, a free tendon graft may also be inserted into bone, both at the base of the distal phalanx and at the distal end of the middle phalanx, and retained by pullout wires. A more complicated dynamic tenodesis procedure can be used if preferred.

If active DIP flexion is desired and profundus advancement is not possible, the only alternative is a free tendon graft. *It is of utmost importance that an intact superficialis tendon never be sacrificed.* Also, the extremely important PIP joint motion should not be endangered and possibly impaired in an attempt to regain active DIP joint flexion. Therefore great discretion must be used to select the proper patient for this meticulous procedure. The

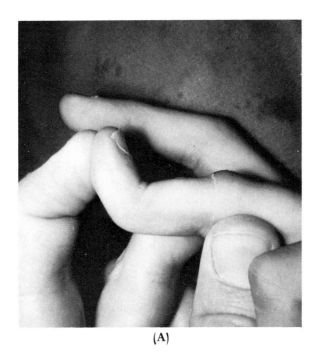

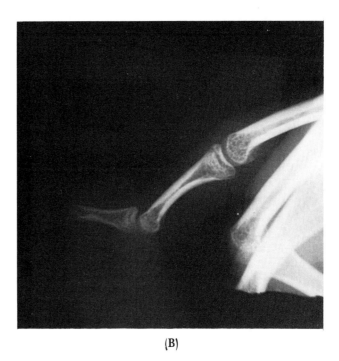

(A)

(B)

Figure 9-59 (A) Marked hyperextension of ring finger DIP joint secondary to flexor digitorum profundus attenuation subsequent to DIP joint palmar plate avulsion in severe hyperextension injury. (B) Radiograph shows DIP joint hyperextension. Treatment consisted of use of segment of flexor digitorum profundus tendon to tenodese DIP joint. Nine months after surgery and reconstruction of palmar plate, DIP joint could be actively flexed 30° and extended to neutral.

only candidate for a free tendon graft with an intact functioning superficialis tendon and good DIP joint motion is someone who absolutely requires independent DIP joint active flexion. A free tendon graft to restore profundus action may be routed anatomically through the normal decussation of the intact superficialis, or the tendon graft may be routed around the superficialis tendon in the distal palm.

Subluxation, dislocation, and fracture dislocation of the distal interphalangeal joint are relatively infrequent because of the strong, short collateral ligaments, the strong palmar plate, and the added security of the extensor and the flexor digitorum profundus tendon insertions. The lever arm of the distal phalanx at the DIP joint is so short and security of ligamentous attachments at the DIP joint so secure, that fracture dislocation or fracture subluxation or dislocation of the PIP joint is far more likely to occur.

Palmar fracture subluxation is most commonly associated with avulsion fracture of a large dorsal articular fragment, including the extensor tendon insertion (discussed in section Drop Finger in Chapter 8). Occasionally pure palmar dislocation occurs, invariably avulsing or attenuating the extensor insertion from the base of the distal phalanx (Figure 9-60).

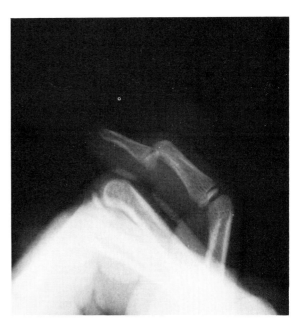

Figure 9-60 Complete palmar dislocation of DIP joint includes avulsion of extensor insertion from base of that distal phalanx. After reduction, immobilization should be continued for a minimum of 8 weeks, maintaining DIP joint in complete extension for treatment of tendon avulsion (drop finger).

Dorsal dislocation occurs by avulsion or partial avulsion of the palmar plate from its attachment to either the middle or distal phalanx (Figures 9-61A,B). Dorsal dislocation of the phalanx can also occur after a large displaced articular fracture avulsion (including the profundus insertion) has occurred (refer to Figure 9-11). If palmar plate rupture occurs at its distal attachment, the accessory collateral ligaments retain their connection to the palmar plate. Both the extensor and flexor insertions usually remain intact.

Physical examination is often not remarkable (Figure 9-61A), but dorsal displacement of the distal phalanx and transverse skin dimpling may be noted with inability to flex the DIP joint. Relocation is accomplished simply by dorsal pressure on the distal phalanx and palmar pressure on the middle phalanx, with slight distraction at the joint by traction. External splint immobilization should be continued for about three weeks to insure adequate healing. A large displaced articular fracture from the palmar aspect of the distal phalanx associated with profundus tendon insertion (refer to Figure 9-11) should be anatomically replaced at surgery. A large displaced articular fracture of the dorsal aspect of the distal phalanx base is discussed in section on Drop Finger in Chapter 8; see also Figures 8-47–8-51.

Subluxation may be persistent because of an avulsed deep segment of the palmar plate attachment to the distal phalanx (Figures 9-62A–C) and/or a small displaced fracture fragment (Figures 9-63A,B) which becomes impinged within the joint, very similar to a medial meniscus tear (bucket handle tear) which becomes locked in the knee joint. Surgical exploration, extraction of the soft tissue and/or the fracture fragments, and reconstruction of the palmar plate is indicated in such cases. In Figures 9-63A,B, exploration through a palmar approach disclosed avulsion of the palmar plate from its distal attachment, associated with a small fracture avulsion. A deep layer of the palmar plate interposed between the base of the distal phalanx and the condyles of the middle phalanx prevented closed reduction. After removal of the deep segment of the palmar plate from the joint and its reattachment to the distal phalanx, splint immobilization was maintained for three weeks.

Unstable dorsal fracture subluxation of the DIP joint should be treated similarly to the same injury of the PIP joint of index through little fingers and of the IP joint of the thumb or severe arthritic changes and minimal motion will result (Figure 9-64).

Lateral dislocation occurs secondary to lateral force on the distal phalanx, avulsing the collateral ligament complex (proper and accessory collateral

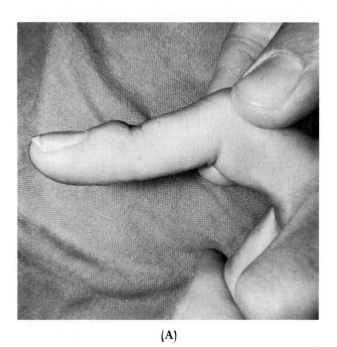

(A)

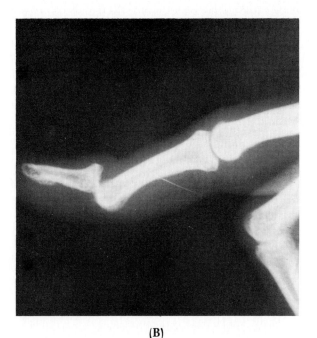

(B)

Figure 9-61 (A) Dorsal dislocation of DIP joint of ring finger. Note dorsal protuberance of distal phalangeal base and indentation of dorsal skin. (B) Lateral radiograph illustrates complete dorsal dislocation of DIP joint. Following closed reduction complete extension and 55° active flexion were obtained 8 weeks after injury.

Figure 9-62 (A) Lateral view of distal end of middle phalanx of 8-year-old girl shows dorsal fracture subluxation of DIP joint which proved to be irreducible by closed manipulation. (B) Lateral view after open reduction from palmar approach and temporary longitudinal Kirschner wire fixation of DIP joint in extension. A deep layer of palmar plate interposed within DIP joint prevented closed reduction. Injury is rare since physeal separation is the usual occurrence in this age group. (C) Lateral radiograph 4 weeks after surgery shows good cartilage space of DIP joint and maintenance of reduction. Essentially normal DIP joint motion was achieved.

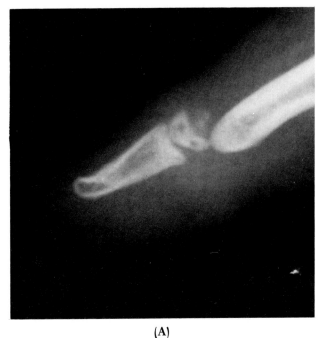

(A)

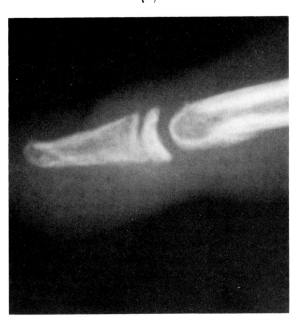

(B)   (C)

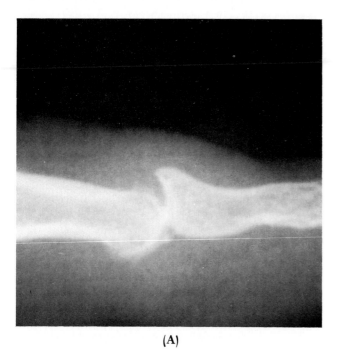

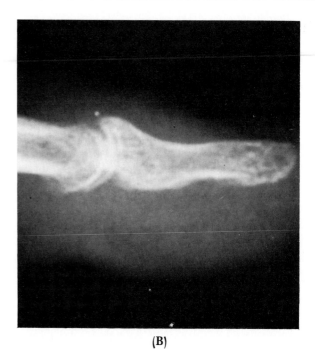

(A)   (B)

Figure 9-63 **(A)** Dorsal subluxation of little finger DIP joint seen approximately 2 weeks after the original injury. Note small avulsion fracture just inferior to distal phalangeal base. **(B)** Lateral radiograph 2 months after surgery shows narrowed cartilage space of DIP joint but maintenance of reduction. Though extension was complete, only 35° active and passive flexion resulted.

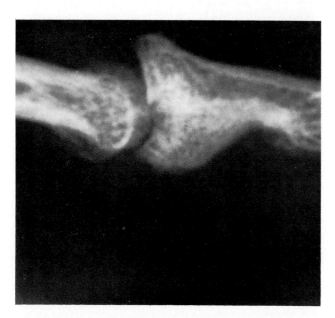

Figure 9-64 Lateral radiograph illustrates untreated DIP joint injury with chronic dorsal fracture subluxation 4 weeks postrauma. Note dorsal subluxation, incongruity of distal phalangeal articular surface, and early changes of degenerative arthritis.

ligaments) and the palmar plate attachment either to the middle phalanx or to the distal phalanx. This type of injury is almost always open because of the limited pliability of the skin in this area due to the vertical septal fibers, extending from the periosteum of the distal phalanx to the dermis of the skin, which allow little mobility.

Treatment is similar to that for any open fracture dislocation and includes meticulous wound toilet followed by repair of the avulsed collateral ligament and palmar plate as indicated.

Occasionally pain and/or instability of the DIP joint persists and may be best relieved by either tenodesis or arthrodesis of the DIP joint.

Multiple dislocations in different digits may occur at times. Each dislocation should be evaluated individually and treated accordingly, as in Figures 9-65A–C, which illustrate a simultaneous lateral subluxation of the long finger PIP joint and dorsal dislocation of the ring finger PIP joint. Both injuries were treated successfully by closed reduction and immobilization of the involved PIP joints in extension for three weeks. Rarely, multiple dislocations occur in the same digit (Figure 9-66).

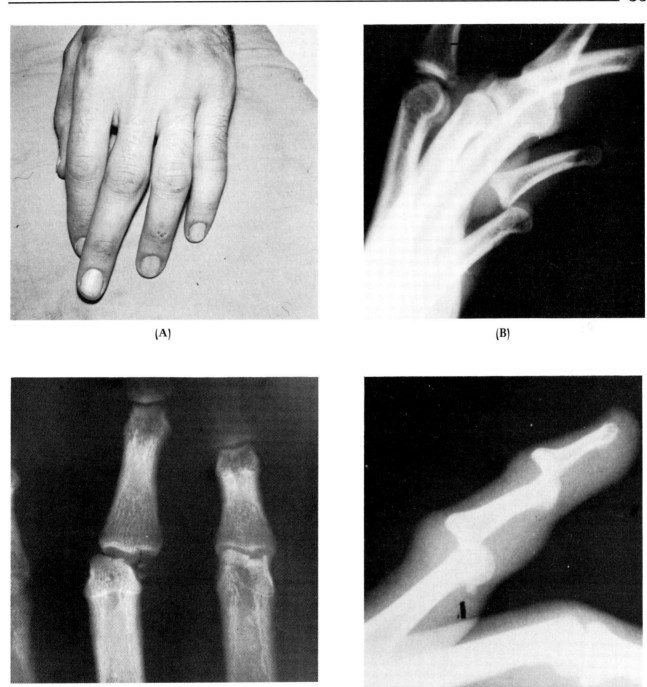

(A)

(B)

(C)

Figure 9-65 (A) Photograph illustrates obvious deformity of long finger PIP joint with radial deviation. Some fullness of ring finger PIP joint is noted, but no evident deformity can be seen on this dorsal view. (B) Radiograph shows an obvious complete dorsal dislocation of ring finger PIP joint. (C) Close-up of PA view shows lateral subluxation (radial) of long finger PIP joint.

Figure 9-66 Simultaneous complete dorsal dislocation of both PIP and DIP joints of same digit. This rare injury was treated by closed manipulation, reduction, and immobilization for 3 weeks in extension, with acceptable, but not normal, digital flexion resulting. *(Illustration courtesy of S. Leiner, M.D.)*

References

1. Leddy JP: Flexor tendons—acute injuries, in Green DP (ed): *Operative Hand Surgery*. New York, Churchill Livingstone, 1982, vol 2, pp 1347–1373.
2. Littler JW: The finger extensor mechanism. *Surg Clin North Am* 1967;47:415–432.
3. Eaton RG, Littler JW: Joint injuries and their sequelae. *Clin Plast Surg* 1976;3:85.
4. Eaton RG: *Joint Injuries of the Hand*. Springfield, Ill, Charles C Thomas, 1971.
5. Eaton RG, Malerich MM: Volar plate arthroplasty of the proximal interphalangeal joint: A review of ten years' experience. *J Hand Surg* 1980;5(3):260–268.
6. Peimer CA, Sullivan DJ, Wild DR: Palmar dislocation of the proximal interphalangeal joint. *J Hand Surg* 1984;9A:39–48.
7. Spinner M, Choi BY: Anterior dislocation of the proximal interphalangeal joint. *J Bone Joint Surg (Am)* 1970;52-A:1329–1336.
8. McElfresh EC, Dobyns JH, O'Brien ET: Management of fracture-dislocation of the proximal interphalangeal joints by extension-block splinting. *J Bone Joint Surg (Am)* 1972; 54-A:1705–1711.

General References

Eaton RG, Dray GJ: Dislocations and ligament injuries in the digits, in Green DP (ed): *Operative Hand Surgery*. New York, Churchill Livingstone, 1982, vol 1, pp 637–668.

CHAPTER 10

Articular Fractures

For proper evaluation of articular fractures, multiple good quality radiographs centered precisely at the fracture site are often necessary. Trauma to an articular surface, particularly if a displaced fracture is involved, will predispose that surface to posttraumatic arthritic changes and will accelerate degenerative joint changes during aging.

Articular fractures must be differentiated from periarticular fractures for successful treatment (Figures 10-1A–D, 10-2A,B). Displaced articular fractures often require surgery (Figures 10-1A–D), whereas displaced periarticular fractures may be treated conservatively by closed manipulation with adequate reduction (Figures 10-2A,B) (refer to Figures 6-20, 6-30–6-41 in the section Articular Fractures in Chapter 6, The Thumb).

Essentially normal ranges of motion can be expected in children and young adults after proper treatment of articular fractures if anatomic reduction is achieved and maintained, but in the older age groups some limitation of motion is to be expected. The adult patient should be warned that with any articular fracture, particularly if it is displaced and reduced, whether conservatively or operatively, normal ranges of motion may not be achieved, and that the joint will probably remain somewhat swollen and chronically bulbous.

An undisplaced articular fracture is treated conservatively by appropriate cast or splint immobilization for two and one-half to three weeks. Radiographic reevaluation is made at seven- to ten-day intervals. This is followed by progressive light activity for 10 to 14 days and then full activity (Figures 10-3A,B).

If an articular surface has suffered a markedly comminuted fracture, such as from a severe crush injury, surgery is usually contraindicated (Figure 10-4; also refer to Figure 13-10 in Chapter 13, Crush Injuries). The position of function is maintained by accurate immobilization to adjacent digits to prevent rotation and angulation deformities for approximately ten days. Light motion is then stressed in an attempt to remold the comminuted joint articular surface for ultimate maximal possible motion. Occasionally dynamic skeletal traction may be used to maintain anatomic configuration as well as possible after reduction.

Displaced articular fractures, regardless of whatever joint involved, should be anatomically reduced, unless the fragment involved is merely a

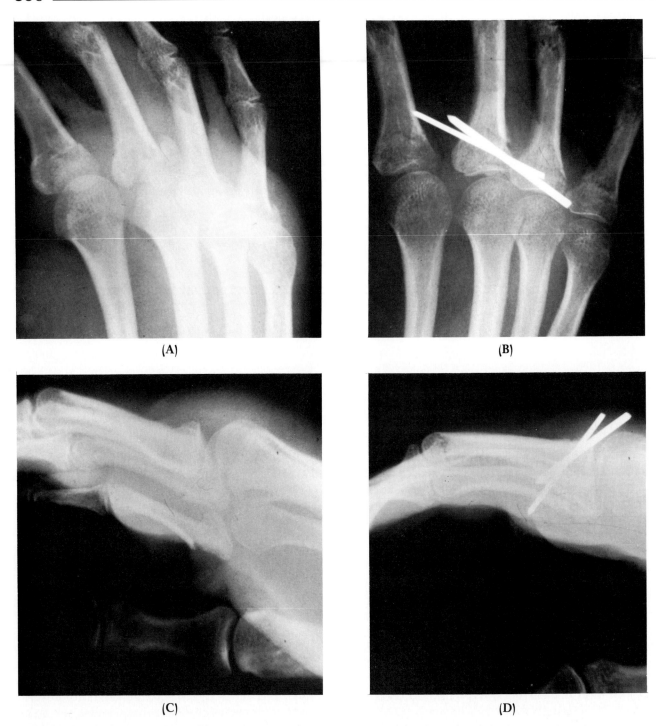

(A)

(B)

(C)

(D)

Figure 10-1 (A) Oblique radiograph shows crush fractures of index, long, ring, and little finger proximal phalanges. Index proximal phalangeal fracture is undisplaced, but ring and little finger fractures are angulated, and fracture of long finger proximal phalanx is articular and displaced. (B) Oblique radiograph after closed manipulation and reduction of ring and little finger fractures and open reduction and internal fixation of displaced condylar fracture of long finger. (C) Lateral radiograph prior to manipulation and closed and open reductions. (D) Lateral view shows restored anatomy after both closed and open reductions with internal fixation as described. Complete extension and flexion of all MP joints resulted.

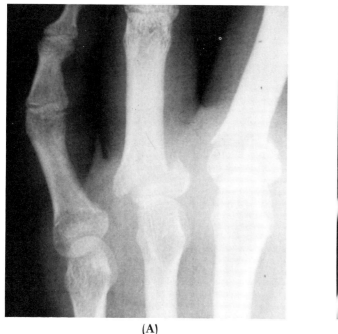
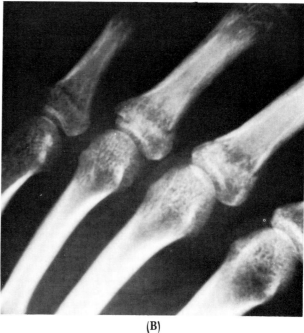

(A) (B)

Figure 10-2 (A) Oblique view shows proximal phalangeal fractures of long, ring, and little fingers with palmar radial angulation at long finger fracture site and ulnar displacement at ring finger fracture site. Fractures are all extraarticular. **(B)** Oblique view 5 weeks after closed manipulation and reduction of fractures. Normal flexion and extension resulted. Figures 10-1A–D and 10-2A,B illustrate the importance of differentiating between displaced extraarticular and displaced articular fractures to determine proper management.

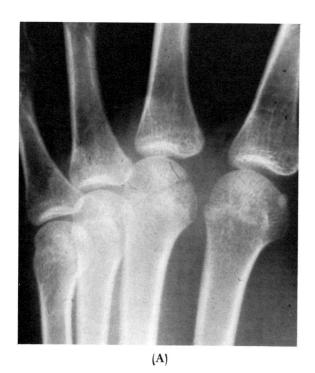
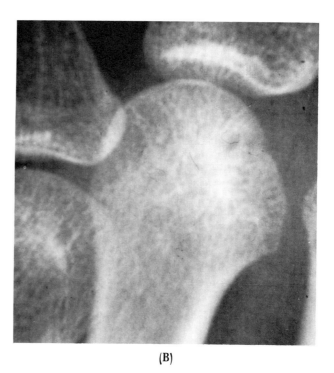

(A) (B)

Figure 10-3 **(A)** Oblique view shows undisplaced oblique fracture of long finger metacarpal head. **(B)** Close-up, same view, 6 months later shows healed fracture with good contour of metacarpal head, with no evidence of avascular necrosis, and essentially normal cartilage space of joint.

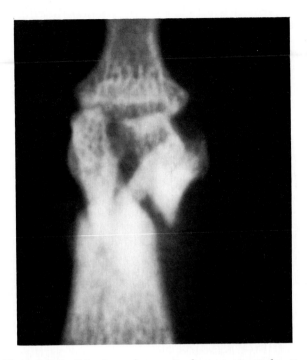

Figure 10-4 PA view of extensively comminuted articular crush fracture of DIP joint. Treatment consists of either conservative splint immobilization or, possibly, dynamic skeletal traction, depending on surgeon's preference and severity of vascular impairment distal to site of injury. Early motion should be encouraged with either treatment.

small chip avulsion such as that resulting from a palmar plate avulsion or avulsion of a profundus insertion. (In the latter instance immediate reinsertion of the flexor digitorum profundus tendon into the base of the distal phalanx is recommended.)

If an articular fracture is undisplaced or if closed manipulation has achieved satisfactory reduction, radiographic follow-up evaluations at seven- to ten-day intervals for three weeks are extremely important to note whether the fracture displaces. Such fractures are often inherently unstable, and anatomic reduction may be lost easily. If an articular fracture is unstable, either closed reduction and percutaneous fixation, if possible, or open reduction and internal fixation is strongly recommended. One should strive for normal anatomic restoration of the joint surface to guarantee the best functional result. Obviously it is far easier to correct surgically the acute articular injury initially than to reconstruct a malunion by osteotomy.

Small avulsions of articular surfaces, if intraarticularly displaced, should be surgically removed to prevent joint damage, particularly if the fragment is unattached to soft tissue. If the small fragment is contiguous to the ligamentous structure, the ligament

insertion, or origin, should be reconstructed (or reinserted) to provide adequate joint stability after excision of the fragment.

An important part of treatment during open reduction and internal fixation of an articular fracture is meticulous irrigation and debridement of the joint. Any small loose fragments of bone and articular cartilage must be removed to decrease the possibility of posttraumatic arthritis.

The importance of proper care (either conservative or surgical) for articular fractures cannot be overemphasized. Normal anatomic configuration of a joint surface guarantees the best prognosis for an ultimately functional result, including maximal ranges of motion and decreased propensity for posttraumatic and degenerative arthritic changes in future years.

Metacarpophalangeal Joint

Fractures of the metacarpal head are usually sustained by closed blunt trauma with the fist clenched, as might occur during an altercation. If the wound is open, it must be considered to be grossly contaminated.

If the extensor tendon has been lacerated and particularly if a joint has been violated (usually MP or PIP joint) this is a true surgical emergency mandating hospitalization, radical surgical debridement with open wound treatment, intravenous antibiotics, appropriate tetanus prophylaxis, immobilization and elevation.

Significant functional impairment usually results if treatment is delayed more than eight hours after this type of wound (refer to Figure 2-26 in Chapter 2).

If a fracture is undisplaced, healing may be expected to proceed with no difficulty (Figures 10-3A,B), but there is always the possibility of avascular necrosis due to a compromised vascular supply.

Occasionally a large single segment of metacarpal articular surface becomes displaced; it is almost always irreducible by closed methods. Open reduction and internal fixation are mandatory for optimal care (Figures 10-5A–D).

A significantly proximally displaced distal metaphysis of a metacarpal resulting from an oblique unstable fracture should be anatomically reduced, surgically if necessary, and fixed by Kirschner wires to preserve joint function (Figures 10-6A,B).

Comminuted undisplaced fractures of the proximal phalanx base are treated conservatively with

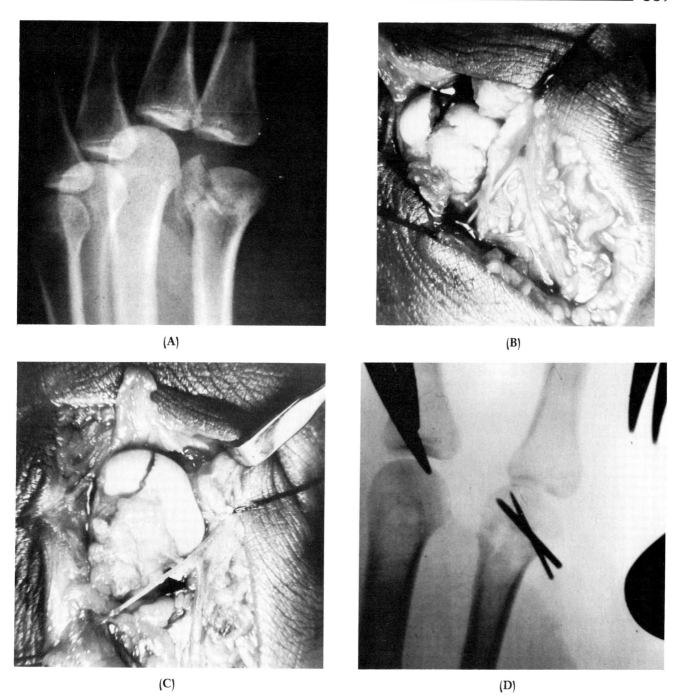

(A)

(B)

(C)

(D)

Figure 10-5 (A) Oblique view shows displaced articular fracture of index metacarpal head. (B) Close-up of operative exposure through curvilinear incision transversely across dorsum of index MP joint shows displaced articular fragment on left and most of metacarpal head on right. (C) Anatomic restoration of displaced articular fragment. (D) Radiograph following open reduction of displaced articular fragment shows its fixation to metacarpal head by two Kirschner wires. Complete MP joint extension and nearly normal flexion resulted 4 months after injury and surgery.

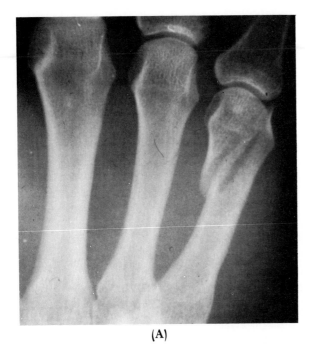
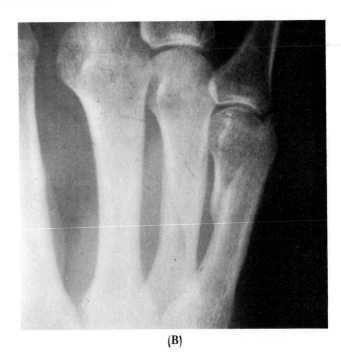

(A)   (B)

Figure 10-6 **(A)** Oblique fracture of little finger distal metacarpal shaft and metaphysis with proximal displacement of metacarpal head. **(B)** Malunion noted 4 months later with impingement of spicule at end of proximal fragment into MP joint resulting in decreased motion. Although this fracture is not articular, it manifests a distinct effect on the adjacent articulation. Proper initial treatment should consist of anatomic reduction, and fixation.

early range of motion after approximately ten days of immobilization (Figure 10-7). A single undisplaced (Figure 10-8) or relatively undisplaced (Figure 10-9) fracture of a condyle of the proximal phalanx base should be treated by immobilization in the functional position with the MP joint flexed for two and one-half weeks to insure maintenance of a satisfactory position. If the fragment is relatively undisplaced (Figure 10-9), surgery is not indicated. However, with more significant displacement or angulation of the fragment, open reduction and internal fixation by the appropriate method is advised to insure the best possible phalangeal articular surface (Figures 10-10A,B, 10-11A,B). The condylar fragment may be exposed and fixed to the proximal phalanx or vice versa. Often a condylar fragment is found to be palmar as well as lateral, making operative exposure difficult. If a displaced or rotated fragment is small, it may be surgically excised with reconstruction of the ligament insertion, particularly if this injury occurs at the radial aspect of the index finger MP joint. Malunion of a moderately displaced condylar rracture of the proximal phalanx base results in a deformed articular surface, which is certainly more prone to develop posttraumatic and degenerative arthritic changes with age (Figures 10-10A,B, 10-11A,B).

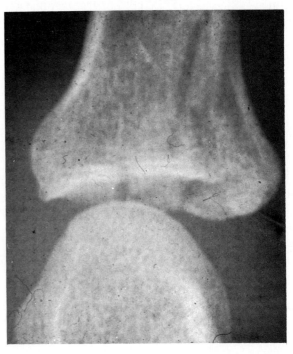

Figure 10-7 Comminuted articular undisplaced fracture of proximal phalanx base. Treatment consisted of conservative immobilization for 12 days, after which light activity was permitted.

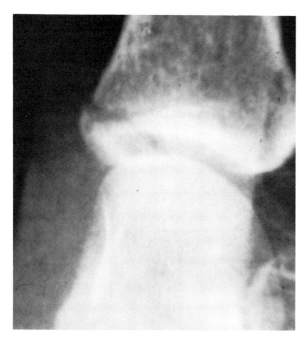

Figure 10-8 Essentially undisplaced fracture of condyle of proximal phalanx base. Treatment consisted of immobilization for 3 weeks before light activity was allowed.

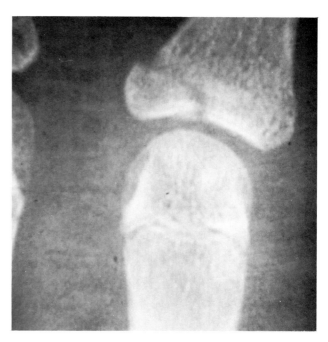

Figure 10-9 Minimally displaced condyle of proximal phalanx with slight angulation representing approximately 40% of articular surface. Treatment was conservative immobilization for 2½ weeks.

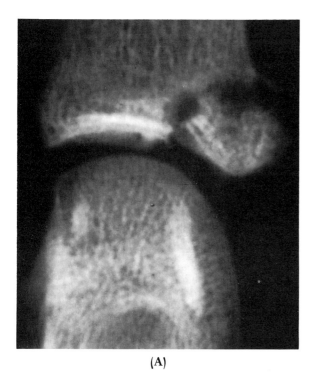

(A)

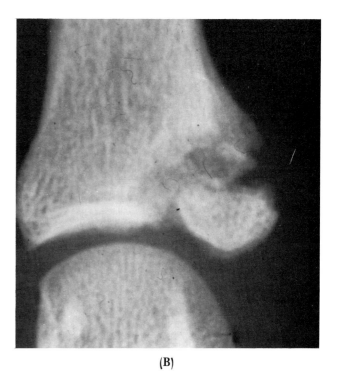

(B)

Figure 10-10 (A) Displaced rotated condyle of proximal phalanx involving approximately one-third of articular surface. As injury was 3 weeks old, it was treated conservatively rather than surgically. (B) Same lesion 8 months later shows irregular articular surface and malunion with approximately 90° rotational deformity of fragment, in addition to cystic changes of metaphysis adjacent to area of healing. This type of displaced articular fracture should be treated by open reduction and internal fixation as soon as possible after injury.

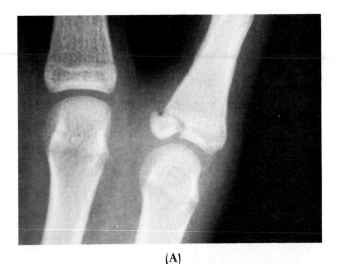

(A)

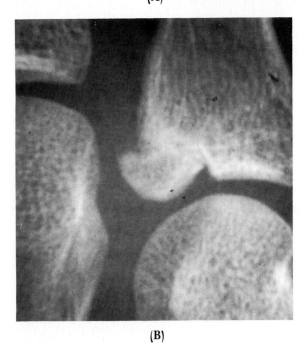

(B)

Figure 10-11 **(A)** Moderately displaced condylar fracture of proximal phalanx base with rotation of approximately 25° to 30° and some displacement. **(B)** Conservative treatment resulted in nearly normal flexion and extension, despite malunion, 10 weeks after injury, as seen on follow-up radiograph. The probability of posttraumatic and degenerative arthritic changes, however, makes debatable the question of conservative treatment versus initial open reduction and internal fixation. In an injury with this amount of displacement and rotation, the patient should be allowed to choose between alternatives.

Proximal Interphalangeal Joint

(For fracture dislocations of the PIP joint, refer to Chapter 9, Injuries to Digital Soft Tissue Structures section on hyperextension injuries, subluxations, and dislocations of the PIP joint.)

Trauma may cause a rather insignificant undisplaced crushing of the dorsal area of the middle phalangeal base. This is treated by aluminum splint immobilization until the signs of acute injury have subsided (Figure 10-12). Immobilization is continued for seven to ten days to allow edema and ecchymosis to subside prior to commencing light activity. If this dorsal segment is displaced, the insertion of the central slip probably has been avulsed; without proper treatment of PIP joint extension for three to four weeks, incomplete extension of the PIP joint with resultant boutonniere deformity is to be anticipated (refer to Boutonniere Deformity in section Capsular, Ligamentous, and Tendon Injuries of the Finger, Chapter 9).

Undisplaced or minimally displaced fractures of the palmar base of the middle phalanx (Figure 10-13) should be splinted for approximately two and one-half weeks before the patient begins light activity, since the insertion of the PIP joint palmar plate

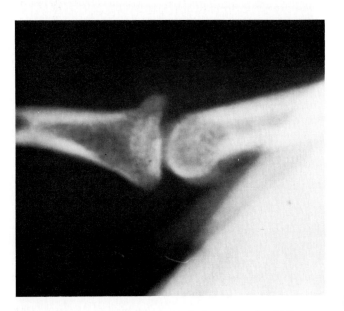

Figure 10-12 Undisplaced crush fracture of middle phalangeal dorsal lip of base. Treatment was conservative immobilization for 10 days, followed by light activity.

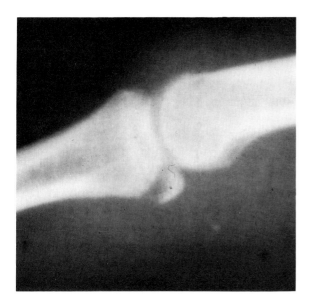

Figure 10-13 Relatively undisplaced avulsion fracture of palmar aspect of middle phalanx base. Treatment consisted of immobilization for 2½ weeks before light activity was begun, since palmar plate attaches in this area and displacement could lead to PIP joint instability.

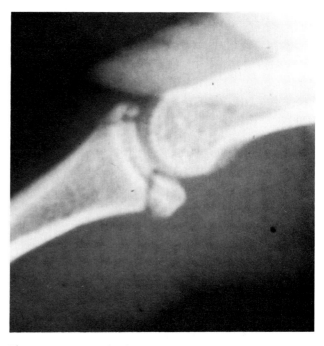

Figure 10-14 Undisplaced large segmental fractures of dorsal and palmar articular surface of middle phalanx base treated by conservative immobilization for 2½ weeks to prevent displacement of the fragments.

also has been avulsed with the fragment. Immobilization practically guarantees proper healing of this important structure.

If both dorsal and palmar lips of the middle phalangeal base have been injured, gentle ranges of motion should be commenced after about ten days to remold the articular surface, particularly if the fracture resulted from a crushing injury. If the fragments are minimally displaced, immobilization should be continued for approximately two and one-half to three weeks to insure early healing of the insertion of the central slip dorsally and of the palmar plate palmarly. If the fractures involve a fair percentage of the articular surface of the middle phalanx base (Figure 10-14), immobilization also should be continued for two and one-half to three weeks before light activity is allowed to prevent displacement of these fragments.

Open reduction and internal fixation are indicated if the fracture fragment involves 25% to 30% of the articular surface and is displaced (Figures 10-15A–F), or if both condyles are displaced (a bicondylar fracture). If it is impossible to restore anatomically a small articular fragment, the fragment should be excised; a ligamentous or tendinous structure can then be reattached into its proper insertion. If malunion of such a fragment occurs, the range of joint

motion is impaired, which often necessitates later excision of the malunited fragment (Figures 10-16A–C). Attempted reduction and internal fixation of a large articular fragment occasionally may be effected up to three or three and one-half weeks posttrauma (Figures 10-17A–E). If reduction is achieved, a far better functional result is attained than with a malunion (Figures 10-17A–E, 10-18A,B).

Distal Interphalangeal Joint

Undisplaced fractures of the condyles of the middle phalanx or base of the distal phalanx are treated as noted in the introductory general discussion (see also Figure 10-19).

Displaced condylar fractures of the middle phalanx should be surgically explored for anatomical reduction and internal fixation if closed reduction is impossible (Figures 10-20A–C).

An oblique condylar fracture regardless of the joint involved is essentially unstable and is prone to displace proximally (Figures 10-17A–E to 10-19). With

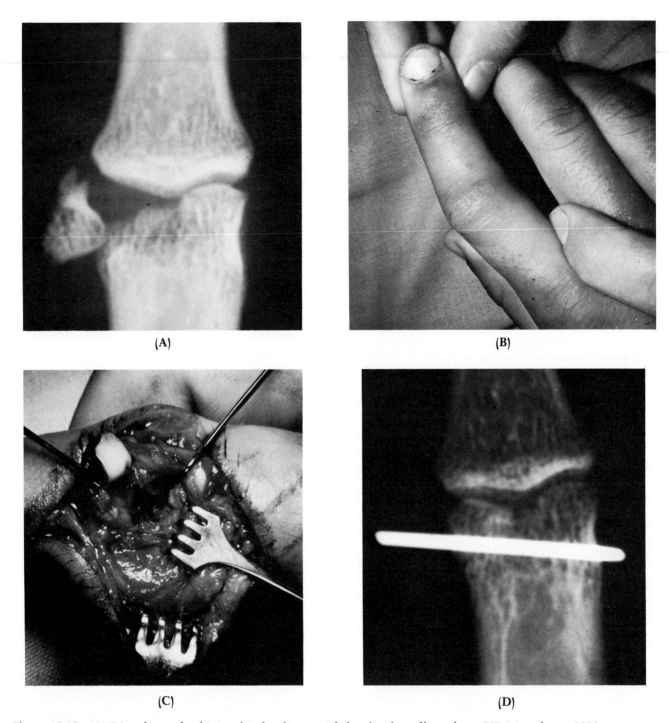

(A)

(B)

(C)

(D)

Figure 10-15 **(A)** PA radiograph of injured index finger with localized swelling about PIP joint shows 180° rotation of displaced radial condyle of proximal phalanx. **(B)** Stress placed on radial aspect of index finger PIP joint shows instability. **(C)** Lateral photograph of open reduction (and internal fixation) shows displaced radial condyle and bed from which it was avulsed. **(D)** PA radiograph after open reduction and internal Kirschner wire fixation.

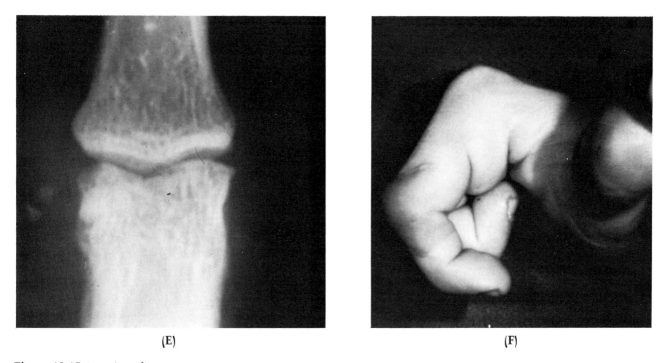

(E) (F)

Figure 10-15 *(continued)*
(E) PA radiograph 4 months after initial surgery. Note acceptable articular surfaces of both proximal phalangeal condyles and base of middle phalanx, with a good cartilage space intervening. **(F)** Nearly complete PIP joint extension (not shown) and flexion of 75° resulted. Open reduction and internal fixation proved far superior to conservative treatment or excision of the fragment, which undoubtedly would have necessitated arthroplasty or arthrodesis.

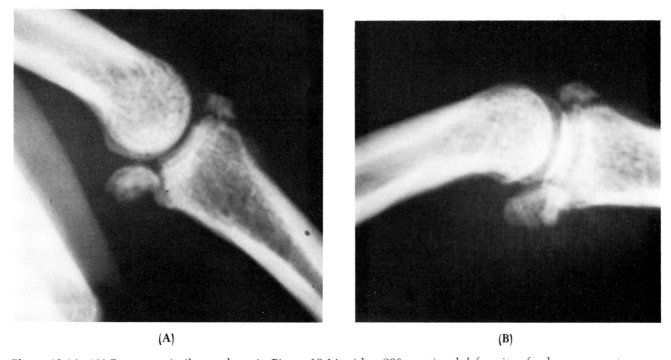

(A) (B)

Figure 10-16 **(A)** Fractures similar to those in Figure 10-14 with a 90° rotational deformity of palmar segment were initially untreated. **(B)** Same case 3 months after injury shows malunion of displaced palmar fragment which impinged on inferior aspect of proximal phalangeal head to prevent full flexion. *(continued)*

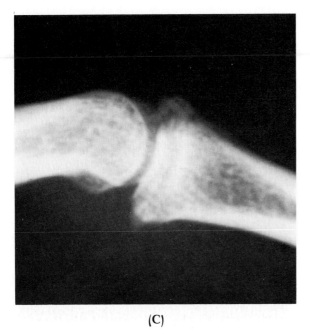

(C)

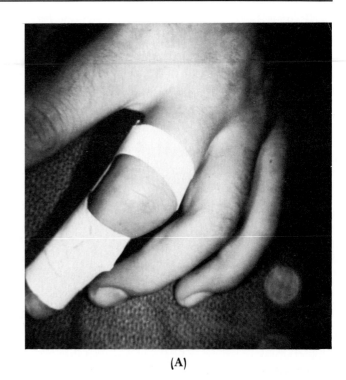

(A)

Figure 10-16 *(continued)*
(C) Lateral radiograph after surgical excision of malunited palmar articular segment, which allowed increased flexion.

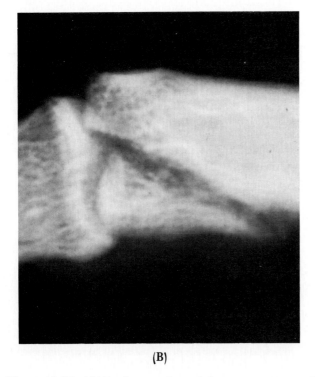

(B)

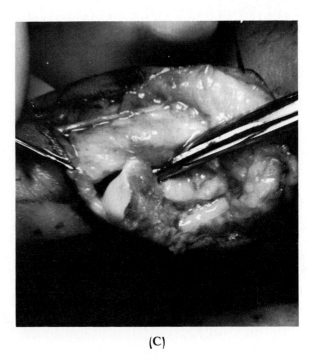

(C)

Figure 10-17 **(A)** Inadequate immobilization at 3½ weeks posttrauma for displaced ulnar condyle of long finger proximal phalanx. **(B)** PA radiograph prior to surgery demonstrates displaced ulnar condyle. **(C)** Close-up of surgical exploration shows completely displaced ulnar condyle of long finger proximal phalanx. Surprisingly, minimal union was found at site of displaced fracture despite interval of 3½ weeks.

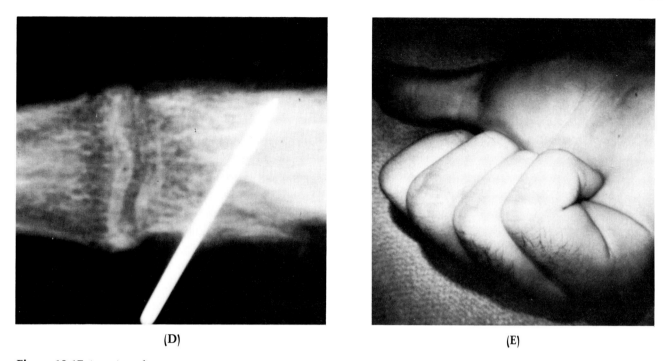

(D) (E)

Figure 10-17 *(continued)*
(D) PA radiograph after anatomic reduction of ulnar condyle. **(E)** Virtually normal flexion of long finger PIP joint and nearly complete extension (not shown) resulted 10 weeks after injury.

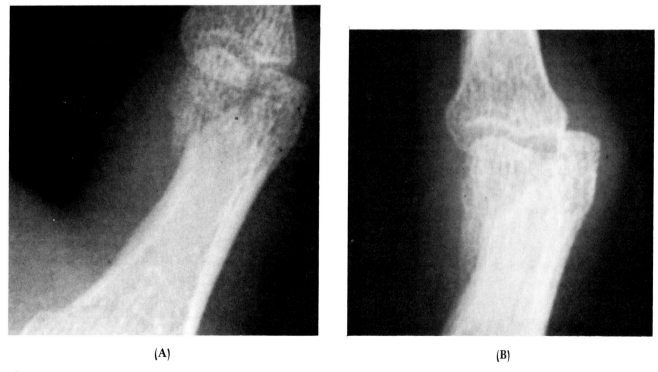

(A) (B)

Figure 10-18 **(A)** Oblique radiograph of minimally displaced condylar fracture of proximal phalanx. **(B)** Same patient 10 weeks later shows malunion at fracture site with proximal displacement of condyle and gross incongruity of articular surface. Case demonstrates importance of adequate immobilization and radiographic follow-up examinations of such a potentially unstable fracture at 7- to 10-day intervals to detect and correct any displacement should it occur.

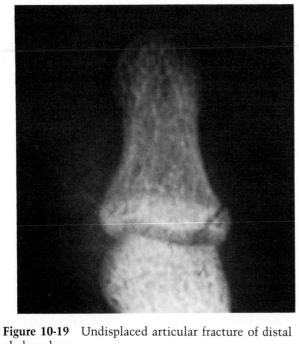

Figure 10-19 Undisplaced articular fracture of distal phalanx base.

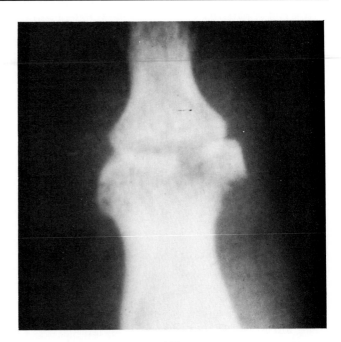

(A)

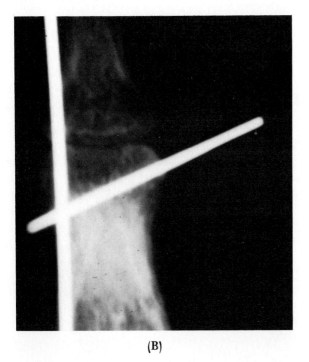

(B)

(C)

Figure 10-20 **(A)** PA view of displaced condylar fracture of middle phalanx. At surgery, completely displaced condyle was found to be firmly attached to its corresponding lateral collateral ligament of DIP joint. **(B)** PA radiograph after open reduction and internal fixation with temporary longitudinal Kirschner wire fixation across DIP joint to maintain extension and allow proper healing of extensor tendon. **(C)** PA view 12 weeks after surgery shows essentially normal DIP joint articular contour, except for small defect at site of union.

proximal displacement a distinct "step off" of the articular surface results, with malalignment and malrotation responsible for subsequent limitation and abnormal ranges of joint motion. An incongruous articulation certainly will be more prone to posttraumatic and degenerative arthritic changes (Figures 10-18A,B). (Refer to Chapter 11, Physeal Injuries and section Drop Finger in Chapter 8 for additional information and examples of displaced articular fractures of the distal phalanx causing drop finger or "mallet finger.")

Extremely comminuted articular fractures are treated as noted above (Figure 10-4), but occasionally open reduction and internal fixation will provide a more satisfactory articulation, as in the case of a comminuted bicondylar fracture. The time and effort involved to obtain a satisfactory reduction and to provide stable fixation are rewarded by better physiologic joint motion.

Open reduction and internal fixation of a displaced unstable or irreducible articular fracture may be best undertaken after initial edema and ecchymosis have subsided some seven to ten days posttrauma. Occasionally a lesion of this type is encountered two and one-half to three and one-half weeks after injury. At this time, even if early union has commenced, open reduction and fixation are recommended (Figures 10-17A–E). The only alternative is later osteotomy, which will not refashion the incongruous articular surface but will merely correct malrotation and malalignment. The only alternative then is arthroplasty or arthrodesis of the joint if chronic joint changes produce severe enough symptoms (Figure 10-21).

Most important is the restoration of normal anatomy to a joint's articular surface to provide the best physiologic function. If a displaced articular fragment is irreducible or unstable, open reduction and internal fixation are strongly recommended within seven to ten days after trauma, before shortening of an attached ligament or contraction of other soft tissue (e.g., capsule, tendon insertion and so forth) develops and makes reduction more difficult. If a fragment is small and impinges on joint surfaces, ligament or tendon reconstruction is advised after excision of the fragment.

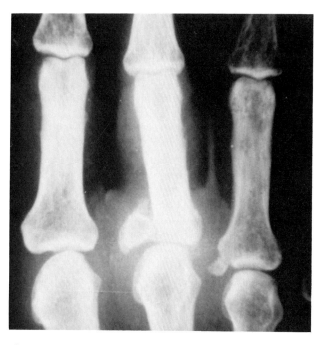

Figure 10-21 Old ununited radial condylar fracture of long finger proximal phalanx base with posttraumatic arthritic changes of MP joint. MP joint arthroplasty is indicated if symptoms and limited motion warrant.

General References

Beasley RW: *Hand Injuries.* Philadelphia, W.B. Saunders, 1981.

Flatt AE: *The Care of Minor Hand Injuries,* ed 4. St. Louis, C.V. Mosby Co., 1979.

Gelberman RH, Menon J: The vascularity of the scaphoid bone. *J Hand Surg* 1980;5(5):508–513.

Green DP: *Operative Hand Surgery.* New York, Churchill Livingstone, 1982, vol 1.

Hollinshead WH: *Anatomy for Surgeons: Volume 3 The Back and Limbs,* ed 3. New York, Harper Medical, 1982.

Littler JW: The hand and upper extremity, vol 6, in Converse JM (ed): *Reconstructive Plastic Surgery,* ed 2. Philadelphia, W.B. Saunders, 1977.

Milford L: The hand, ed 2, in: *Campbell's Operative Orthopaedics*, ed 6. St. Louis, C.V. Mosby Co., 1982.

Moore DC: *Regional Block*, ed 4. Springfield, Ill, Charles C Thomas, 1965.

Rockwood CA Jr, Green DP: *Fractures in Adults*. Philadelphia, J.B. Lippincott Co., 1984, vol 1.

Sandzén SC Jr: *Current Management of Complications in Orthopedics: The Hand and Wrist.* Baltimore, Williams and Wilkins, 1985.

Spinner M: *Kaplan's Functional and Surgical Anatomy of the Hand*, ed 3. Philadelphia, J.B. Lippincott Co., 1984.

Weeks PM, Wray RC: *Management of Acute Hand Injuries: A Biological Approach*, ed 2. St. Louis, C.V. Mosby Co., 1978.

CHAPTER
11

Physeal (Epiphyseal Growth Plate) Injuries

Significant injuries to the distal forearm and hand which may cause fracture of the long bone diaphyses (shafts) and/or metaphyses in children or adolescents may instead cause physeal (epiphyseal growth plate) injuries.

Anatomy and Pathology

The radius and ulna each have two physes, one located proximally and the other distally. The distal physis contributes approximately 60% to 70% of the longitudinal growth of these bones. All metacarpal physes are based distally with the exception of the thumb metacarpal and all phalangeal physes are located proximally (Figure 11-1).

Histologically, a physis is composed of four contiguous integrated zones or layers (Figure 11-2): 1) The zone resting cartilage; 2) zone of proliferating cartilage; 3) zone of hypertrophy or vacuolization, and 4) zone of calcification.

Longitudinal growth of all long bones is centered in the physes and at skeletal maturity — approximately age 14 in males and 16 in females — this growth ceases and the physes become ossified.

Various diseases, commonly endocrine abnormalities can accelerate or decelerate physeal growth, hasten or retard skeletal maturity or cause an irregular growth pattern.

Accelerated physeal growth may occur with an excess of androgens or estrogens, and with infection or trauma (e.g., fracture) near to but not involving the physis. Conversely, decreased physeal growth results from a deficiency of androgens or estrogens, and infection or trauma, causing damage to the zones of resting or proliferating cartilage of the physis.

Premature physeal ossification results from excess androgens or estrogens, Cushing's disease and prolonged administration of corticosteroids (for example, in treatment of juvenile rheumatoid arthritis). Skeletal maturity is retarded and the physeal plate persists abnormally long in hypopituitarism, Turner's syndrome (Figure 11-3), hypothyroidism and deficiency of androgens or estrogens.

Irregular growth may occur from metabolic diseases (scurvy and rickets), trauma to all or a portion of a physis, tumor (for example, osteochondroma involving the distal ulna causing growth aberration of the distal radius — see Figure 11-35) and unknown etiologies (for example, Madelung's deformity — Figure 11-4).

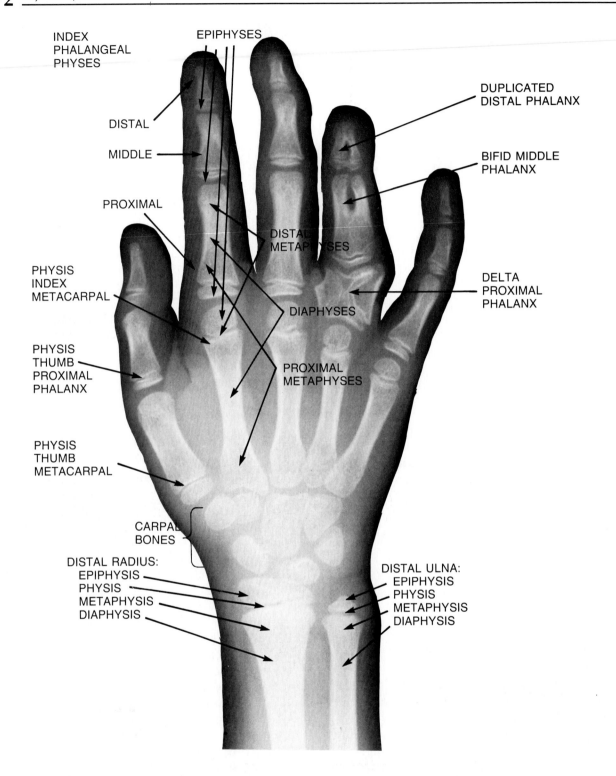

Figure 11-1 PA radiograph illustrates physes of the distal radius and ulna, metacarpals, and phalanges. All metacarpal physes are distal except for the thumb and all phalangeal physes are proximal. Note the congenital abnormalities of the delta proximal phalanx and bifid middle and distal phalanges of the ring finger.

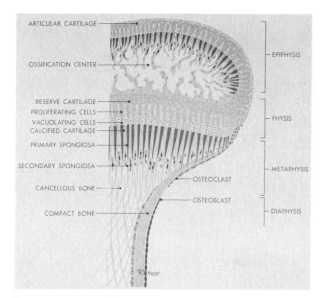

Figure 11-2 Histologic anatomy of the physis with its relationship to epiphysis and metaphysis. *(Reprinted, by permission, from Philip Rubin, M.D., Dynamic Classification of Bone Dysplasias. YearBook Medical Publishers, Chicago, Ill., 1964, p4.)*

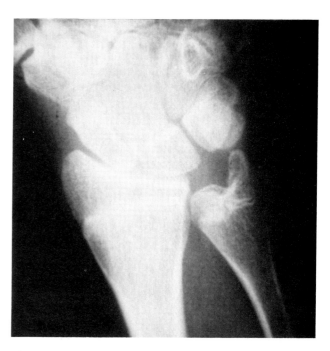

Figure 11-3 Turner's syndrome. The area of physeal line of the distal radius still remains visible in this 27-year-old woman.

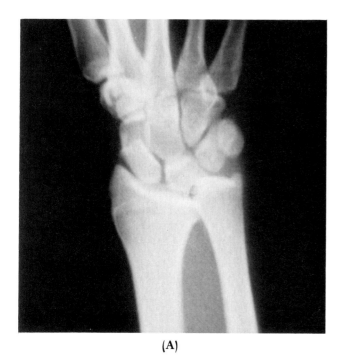

(A)

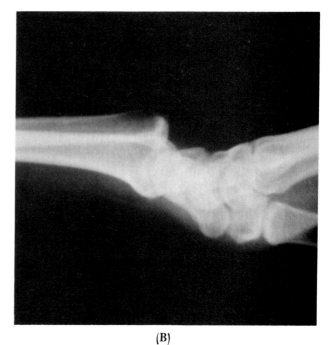

(B)

Figure 11-4 **(A)** AP view of Madelung's deformity with exaggerated ulnar angulation of the distal radius responsible for relative ulnar lengthening. **(B)** Lateral view demonstrates palmar angulation of the distal radius and dorsal protrusion of the relatively long distal ulna.

Classification of Physeal Injuries

Though "epiphyseal slip" is a common term for physeal injuries, physeal separation or epiphyseal growth plate injury and/or separation is more correct. Structurally the weakest zones of the normal functioning physis are those of hypertrophic cartilage cells and of calcification because of the relatively sparse intercellular protecting framework. Physeal injury occurs through these two areas but fracture of a contiguous segment of metaphysis and/or epiphysis may be associated.

The Salter-Harris classification of physeal injuries (Figure 11-5) is the most useful, although other authors have provided more complicated categorizations with numerous sub-classifications.

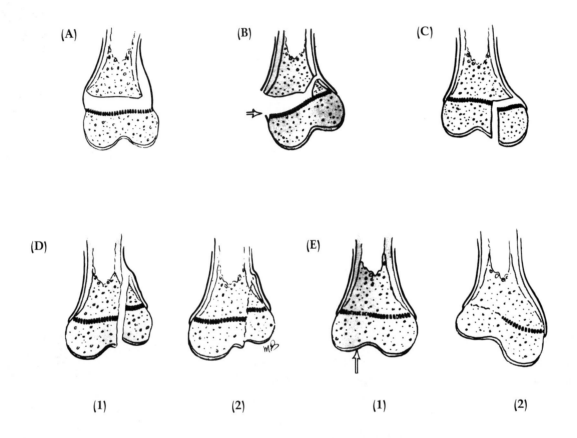

Figure 11-5 (A–E) Salter-Harris classification of types of physeal separation injuries:
(A) Type I physeal injury is complete separation through the physeal plate, usually occurring through the zone of hypertrophic cartilage cells.
(B) Type II injury is a fracture separation through the physeal plate, with a variable amount of metaphyseal bone remaining attached to the physis.
(C) Type III injury is partial separation through the physeal plate combined with a longitudinal fracture through the bone of the epiphysis.
(D) Type IV injury is a longitudinal fracture which extends through a portion of the metaphysis, the physeal plate, and the epiphysis.
(E) Type V injury is a severe crushing injury either to a portion of or to the entire physeal plate.
    Anatomic reduction should be strived for in all physeal injuries but is mandatory in types III and IV. Anatomic reduction is necessary to restore the normal configuration of the articular surface in both injuries. Inability to restore normal anatomy results in malunion, incongruous articular surfaces (D-2), and often premature cessation of growth plate activity in the area of injury.
    Type V physeal trauma is the most severe because of diffuse crushing damage to physeal cells with resultant abnormal and/or premature cessation of growth of a portion of or the entire physeal plate (E-2).
(Reprinted, by permission, from Robert B. Salter, M.D., Injuries involving the epiphyseal plate, American Academy of Orthopaedic Surgeons Instructional Course Lecture, JBJS, 45A, #3, Figures 13, 19, 22, 25, 28, 1963.)

Type I physeal separation is a clear cut separation transversely through the zone of hypertrophic cartilage cells and/or the zone of calcification (Figure 11-6).

Type II physeal separation combines a transverse separation through the physis with a fracture of the metaphysis which remains attached to the epiphysis (the Thurston-Holland sign on radiograph—Figure 11-7).

Type III physeal separation combines a longitudinal fracture through the epiphysis with a partial transverse separation through the physeal plate (Figure 11-8).

Type IV physeal separation is a longitudinal fracture including a segment of metaphysis, physis and epiphysis, all attached as one free segment (Figure 11-9).

Type V Physeal injury is a longitudinal compressive injury (e.g., crush injury) partially or completely involving the physis (Figures 11-10, 11-11).

Injury to the growth area of the physis and severity of the resulting pathology depend upon five factors:

1. The type of physeal injury
2. The severity of the injury
3. The extent of interruption of blood supply to the physeal plate

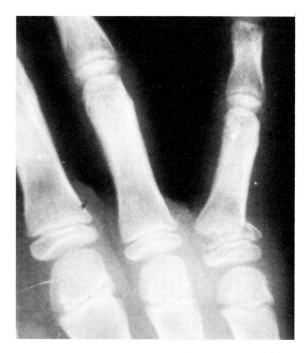

Figure 11-7 Salter type II physeal separation with metaphyseal fragment retained with physis.

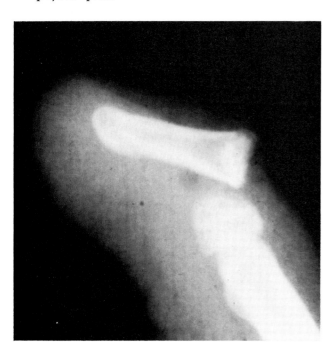

Figure 11-6 Salter type I physeal separation (lateral radiograph of distal phalangeal physeal separation with no metaphyseal component).

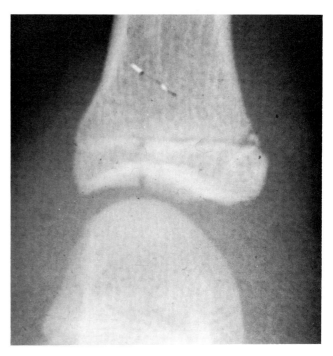

Figure 11-8 Salter type III physeal injury with no displacement.

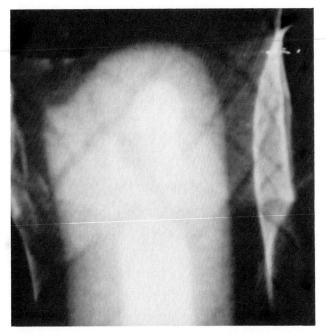

Figure 11-9 Salter IV displaced physeal injury of the distal phalanx.

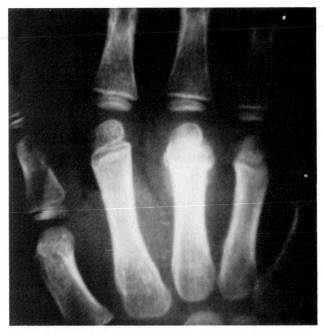

Figure 11-11 Salter V injury to the long finger metacarpal physis with retarded growth.

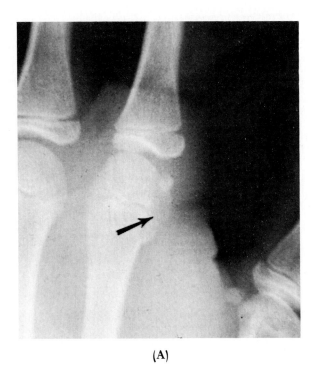

(A)

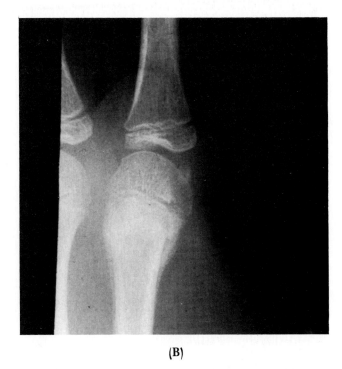

(B)

Figure 11-10 **(A)** Salter type V physeal injury, generalized crush injury to entire physeal plate of index metacarpal. **(B)** Same case, 3½ weeks after injury, showing progressive healing with obliteration of physeal plate.

4. The quality of reduction of physeal separation (inadequate, improper or none)
5. Infection

Type V physeal injury has the worst prognosis since the growth of a portion of or the complete physis will either cease or be aberrant (Figures 11-10, 11-11).

Unreduced Types III and IV physeal injuries cause later joint problems (e.g., posttraumatic and degenerative arthritis) because of persisting joint surface incongruity. However, the innocuous appearing reduced Types I and II injuries may be deceiving and result in abnormalities.

Obviously the more severe the injury and the greater the interruption of blood supply to the physeal plate, the greater the potential for aberrant or halted physeal growth.

Although all physeal separations should be reduced anatomically, it is the most important in Types III and IV injuries since an articular surface is involved.

Whereas infection in the diaphysis or metaphysis adjacent to a physis may accelerate growth, involvement of the physis itself can be disastrous.

The most common physeal injuries are Types I and II involving the distal phalanges (often open wounds) proximal phalanges (predominantly the little finger), the thumb metacarpal base and the distal radius.

Clinical Findings and Treatment

Anatomically the insertion of each long extensor tendon is on the dorsum of an epiphysis, and the long flexors insert on the palmar metaphysis or diaphysis. Therefore, extensors and flexors insert on opposite sides of the physis. This fact is very important in understanding the mechanism of injury and the characteristic deformities of physeal separations since these muscle-tendon units act antagonistically on the site of injury, causing predictable pathologic skeletal configurations.

However, physeal injuries should be suspected with joint effusion and tenderness but no skeletal deformity. A "chip fracture" is usually an incorrect radiographic diagnosis (Figure 11-12)!

Types I and II physeal separations generally are easily reduced under adequate anesthesia. Displaced

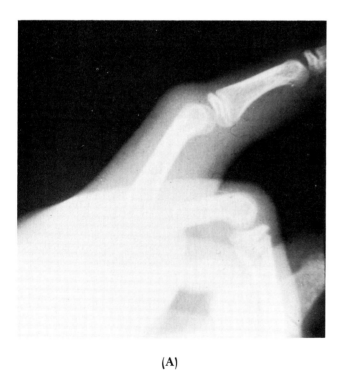 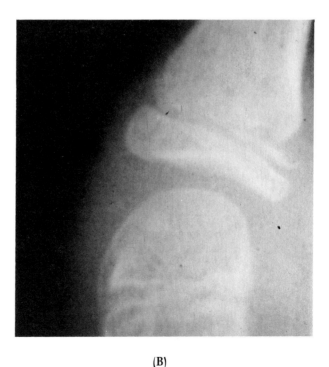

(A)   (B)

Figure 11-12 (A) Lateral radiograph of PIP joint showing soft tissue swelling in that area. (B) Close-up PA view of similar injury shows physeal damage to proximal phalanx and indicates Salter type II physeal separation. An erroneous diagnosis of "chip fracture" would lead to improper treatment of this injury.

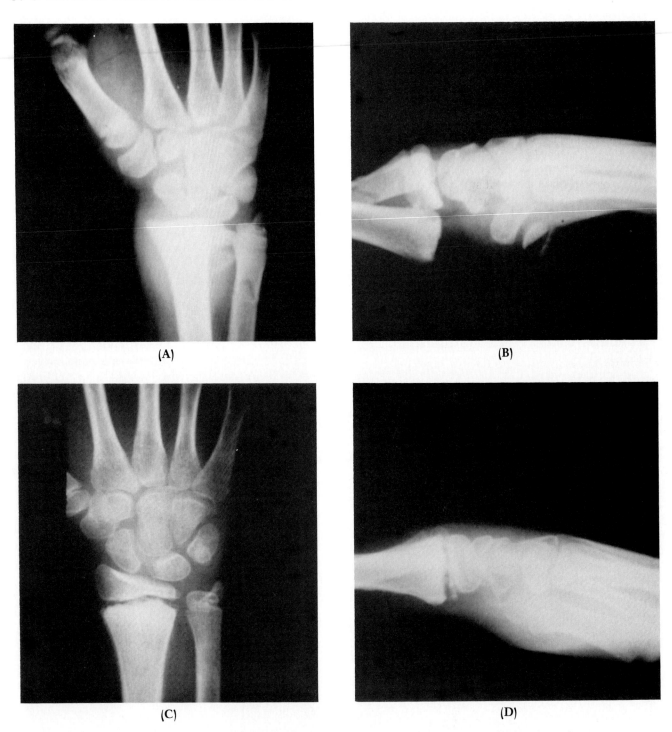

(A)   (B)

(C)   (D)

Figure 11-13 **(A)** Severe injury to the wrist area in a 13-year-old boy with complete Salter II physeal separation of the distal radius and diastasis of the distal radioulnar joint. **(B)** Lateral view demonstrates the complete dorsal and proximal displacement at the radial physis and dorsal dislocation of the distal ulna. **(C)** Closed manipulation and reduction restored satisfactory anatomy on this PA view. **(D)** Lateral view shows acceptable anatomy restored.

Types III and IV physeal injuries, however, and irreducible and unstable Types I and II lesions often require open reduction and either internal or percutaneous Kirschner wire fixation. Smooth Kirschner wires are used as few as possible and technically should be placed centrally through the physis since peripheral fixation of a physis may cause aberrant growth or cessation of growth in that area.

Discussion of physeal injuries will be in anatomic sequence beginning with the distal radius and ulna and ending with the phalanges. Emphasis is placed on the most common lesions encountered in each particular anatomic area.

Distal Radius

Physeal separation of the distal radius is comparable to a dorsal distal metaphyseal fracture of the radius (Colles' fracture) in the adult (Figure 11-13). Dorsal angulation and/or displacement of the distal radial epiphysis at the physeal injury produces a characteristic "silver fork" deformity, usually accompanied by either fracture of the ulnar styloid process or, in severe injuries, damage to the distal radial ulnar joint.

Treatment is identical to that for a dorsal distal metaphyseal fracture of the distal radius (refer to Chapter 3, Injuries to the Distal Radius and Ulna).

Immobilization, however, is usually not necessary for longer than four weeks, at which time the patient is asymptomatic and there is radiographic evidence of sufficient healing. Despite the ease of anatomic reduction and rapid healing, the parents must be advised that aberrant growth, though rare, may be a later complication (Figures 11-14, 11-15).

Distal Ulna

Physeal separation of the distal ulna is rare and usually results from massive open trauma and requires meticulous wound toilet prior to reduction and im-

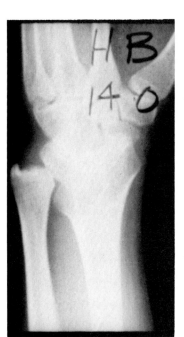
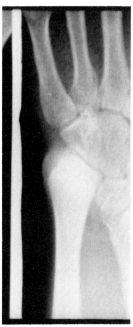

Figure 11-14 This oblique and PA radiograph of the wrist area was made 14 years after an uncomplicated Salter I physeal separation of the distal radius. Marked distortion of the distal radius occurred because of partial cessation of physeal growth on the ulnar aspect. *(Courtesy of William Rhangos, M.D.)*

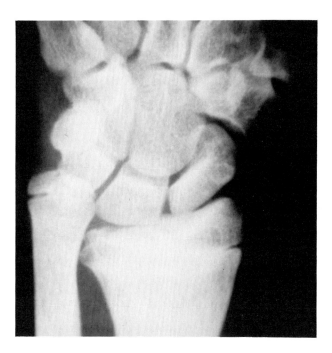

Figure 11-15 PA radiograph 8 years after a Salter I physeal injury of the distal radius shows marked shortening of the entire radius due to complete cessation of physeal growth.

Figures 11-14 and 11-15 demonstrate the importance of informing parents that aberrant growth or actual cessation of physeal growth may occur with any physeal injury regardless of the initial innocuous-appearing lesion. In both these cases most likely there was a crushing component causing altered and terminated physeal growth, respectively.

mobilization. Since injury to the distal radial physis is usually associated, reductions of both injuries are carried out simultaneously by the same technique.

Metacarpals

Physeal separation of the index through little finger metacarpals is uncommon and is caused by rather severe direct trauma. Ulnar and either palmar or dorsal displacement usually occur and Types I, II and V lesions are the most common (refer to Figure 12-5 in Chapter 12, Posttraumatic Skeletal Remodeling).

Anesthesia is best achieved with hematoma injection with or without peripheral nerve block anesthesia of the radial, median and/or ulnar nerves at the wrist or proper and common digital nerves in the distal palm supplemented with dorsal infiltrative anesthesia.

Thumb metacarpal physeal injury is more common and if displaced produces the characteristic deformity of metacarpal shaft adduction and/or flexion (Figure 11-16 and refer to Figure 6-26 in Chapter 6, The Thumb: Dislocations, Ligamentous Injuries and Fractures), mimicking the configuration of a displaced transverse fracture of the proximal metacarpal metaphysis in an adult. The adduction is caused by the adductor pollicis and the deep head of the flexor pollicis brevis and flexion by the combined pull of the thenar muscles plus the flexor pollicis longus.

Closed reductions, although usually easy, may be impossible because of soft tissue impingement in which case open reduction and often Kirschner wire internal fixation are necessary.

Immobilization of injuries to index through little finger metacarpal physes is by a palmar splint extending from the tip of the involved digit and the adjacent digit or digits on either side which should extend to the proximal forearm and maintain a position of wrist extension, metacarpophalangeal joint flexion and proximal and distal interphalangeal joint extension (Figure 11-17). For the thumb, immobilization is from the tip to the proximal forearm maintaining physiologic thumb metacarpal abduction and opposition. After subsidence of edema and congestion five to seven days after treatment, a snug, well-fitting short arm cast or long arm cast in a young child provides better security for an additional two weeks. For the thumb, however, immobilization is one week in a splint and then in a thumb spica cast for an additional three or four weeks to prevent recurrence of the deformity.

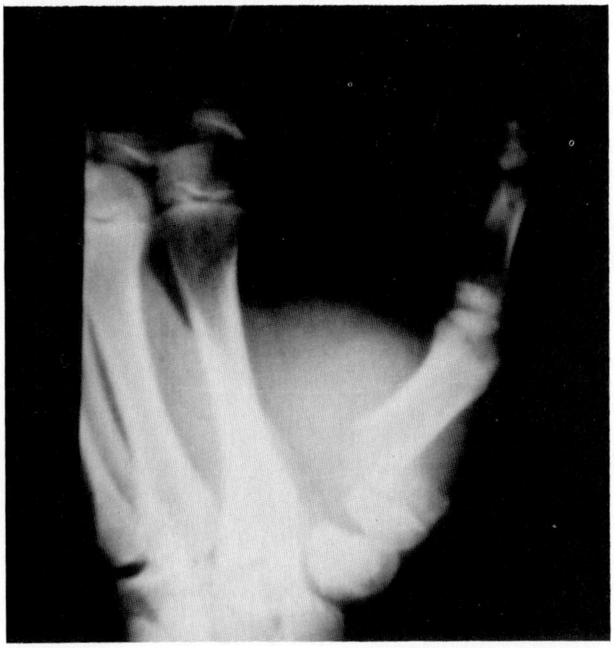

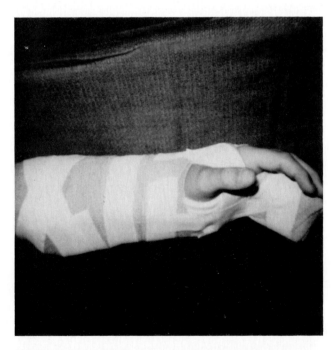

Figure 11-16 Characteristic adduction deformity of the thumb metacarpal following Salter II physeal separation.

Figure 11-17 Initial recommended immobilization includes the injured digit and normal digits on either side from the fingertips to the proximal forearm. In the infant and young child the splint should extend to the axilla and should be incorporated into a soft velpeau dressing.

Phalanges

Although a single attempt to mani͟r͟ ͟͟.c and reduce
a displaced phalangeal physeal injury with no anesthesia may be preferred by some physicians "to
reduce a slip," this technique is condemned. If the initial attempt is unsuccessful, the treating physician
is placed in the embarrassing position of reattempt-
ing reduction on a screaming apprehensive child in
pain or resorting to some type of anesthesia.

Instead, anesthesia should be provided before
any attempt to manipulate and reduce a displaced
phalangeal physeal injury. A simple method is to
anesthetize the palmar digital nerves with a few
milliliters of 1.5% lidocaine at the bifurcation of the
common into the two proper digital nerves in the
distal palm. The least painful approach is by skin
penetration dorsally in the web area supplemented
by dorsal subcutaneous infiltrative anesthesia. A
direct palmar approach to the digital nerves is preferred by some, but this is more painful.

For a closed proximal phalangeal physeal separation a few milliliters of lidocaine can be injected
directly into the fracture hematoma. This converts
a closed wound into an open wound but has not been
a problem.

Fracture hematoma anesthesia alone is insufficient, however, for the technique of manipulation
and reduction described here and must be augmented
by peripheral nerve blocks or by subcutaneous infiltrative anesthesia of the contiguous aspects of the
injured digit and adjacent normal digit including the
intervening web space.

Occasionally an ulnar nerve block either at the
wrist or the elbow may be preferred for reduction of
a proximal phalangeal physeal injury to the little
finger. Medial and radial nerve blocks may be instituted at the wrist for other digits (combined with
ulnar nerve block for the ring finger).

Proximal Phalanx

The most common physeal injuries of the proximal
phalanx are Types I and II. Type III injuries may involve the thumb (Figure 11-18) and index proximal
phalanges, most commonly the bony insertion of the
appropriate metacarpophalangeal joint collateral ligament, and Type V injuries are always a possibility in
crushing trauma.

The characteristic configuration both on
physical examination and radiographs is either radial

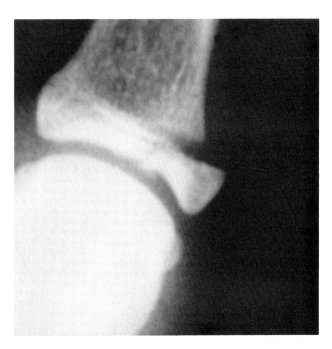

Figure 11-18 Salter III physeal injury of the ulnar
aspect of the thumb proximal phalanx with minimal
displacement. This is a "gamekeeper's injury" in a
skeletally immature patient since the MP joint ulnar
collateral ligament attaches to this segment of the
epiphysis. Stress testing, therefore, is contraindicated
since the articular fragment could be displaced.

or ulnar angulation with dorsal angulation of the
diaphysis on the epiphysis (Figure 11-19).

Reduction of the proximal phalanx is achieved
by repositioning the displaced angulated and often
rotated diaphysis onto the epiphysis which remains
in its normal anatomic position. The epiphysis must
be stabilized by flexion of the metacarpophalangeal
joint which tightens the lateral collateral ligaments
and/or by wedging a well-padded, firm, thin object
(pen or pencil) into the web space between the injured
digit and the adjacent normal digit (Figure 11-19C).
This padded, firm object serves as a fulcrum to lever
the diaphysis onto the stabilized epiphysis.

Minimal persistent ulnar angulation (e.g., 10°
to 15° may be accepted in a little finger (Figure 11-20)
but any significant angulation in any digit (Figure
11-21) and any malrotation (Figure 11-22) must be corrected. Reduction is particularly important in the
proximal phalanges of other digits. Even a minor, persistent lateral angulation of the proximal phalanx of
the index, long and ring finger (Figure 11-23) will
cause either a rather significant divergence or cross
over of the injured digit on adjacent digits when
synergistic digital flexion is attempted.

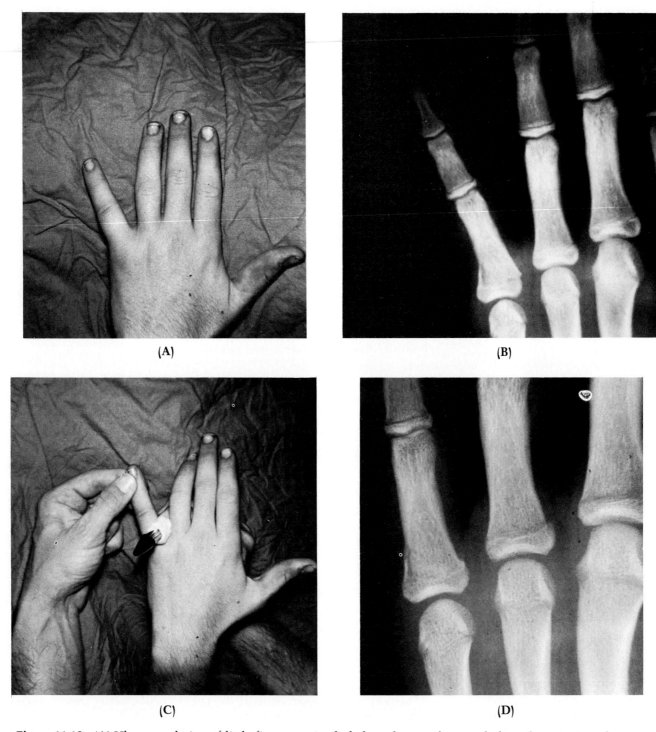

(A)

(B)

(C)

(D)

Figure 11-19 **(A)** Ulnar angulation of little finger proximal phalanx due to edema and physeal separation of proximal phalanx. **(B)** PA view shows Salter type II physeal separation of little finger proximal phalanx. **(C)** Padded, firm implement (pencil) wedged securely into ring-little finger web space provides fulcrum for stability of small proximal epiphysis segment at reduction of diaphysis and metaphysis to this segment. **(D)** PA view after anatomic reduction.

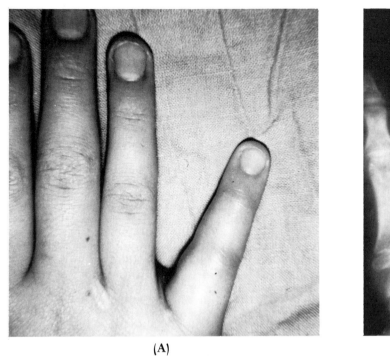
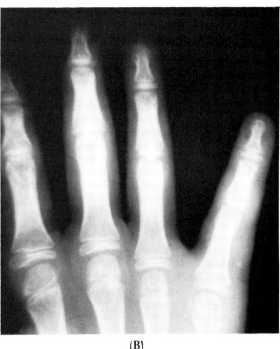

(A)   (B)

Figure 11-20 **(A)** Close-up dorsal view shows marked angulation of little finger proximal phalanx. **(B)** Minimal angulation of physeal separation of little finger proximal phalanx. Appearance of rather marked angulation of little finger proximal phalanx is primarily due to edema and congestion of soft tissue and not to actual skeletal angulation. No reduction was necessary.

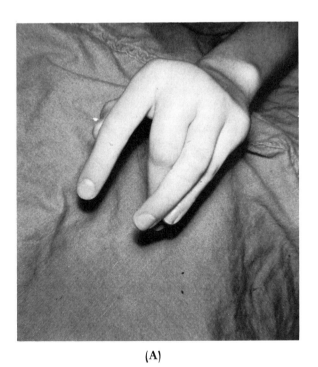
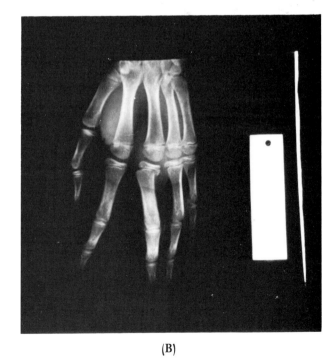

(A)   (B)

Figure 11-21 **(A)** Ulnar angulation of long finger proximal phalanx, dorsal view. **(B)** Radiograph shows physeal separation of long finger proximal phalanx with ulnar deviation at site of separation.

Figure 11-22 (A) Malrotation of long finger upon attempted full flexion 16 days after injury. (B) Radiographs show a Salter type II injury of long finger proximal phalanx physis with malrotation. (C) Physiologic anatomic flexion after open reduction with no internal fixation 2½ weeks after original trauma. No postreduction radiograph is shown since there is no apparent discrepancy from Figure 11-22B.

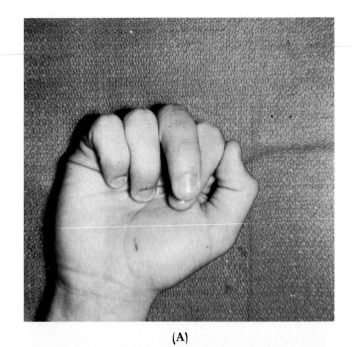

(A)

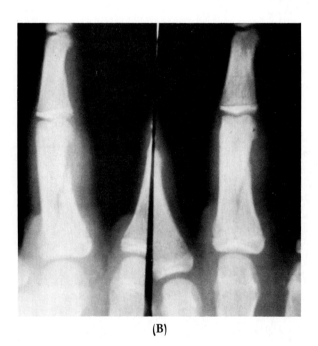

(B)

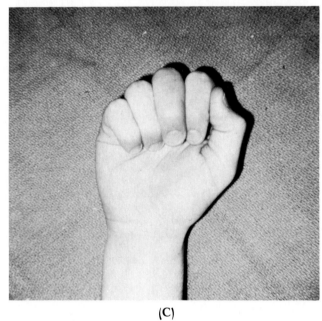

(C)

Radiographic evaluation may not be helpful in disclosing a persistent minor angulation or malrotation (Figures 11-22, 11-23). This type of injury can be detected only by careful clinical assessment using the following methods: 1) Comparison of the anatomic configuration of the injured digit to the adjacent normal digits and 2) comparison of the relationship of the injured digit and the adjacent normal digits (Figure 11-22A) to the comparable digits of the contralateral normal hand. To assure satisfactory reductions, the comparisons must be carried out in maximal flexion and extension and by comparison of the planes of the nail plates.

The injured digit and adjacent digit should be immobilized for two and a half to three weeks initially in a palmar plaster splint as noted above (refer

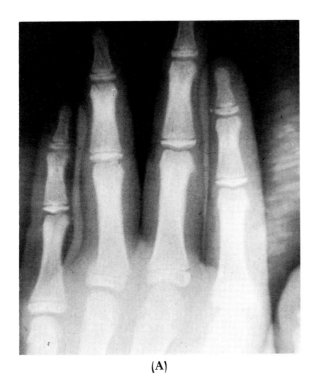
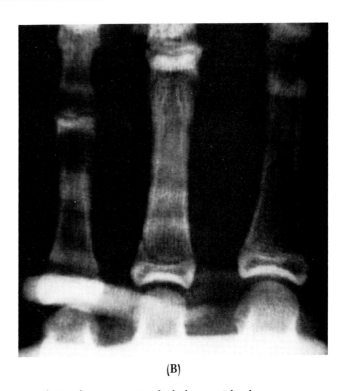

(A)   (B)

Figure 11-23 **(A)** Radiograph shows minimal physeal separation of ring finger proximal phalanx with ulnar deviation. Note divergence of tips of ring and long fingers, necessitating anatomic reduction. **(B)** PA radiograph after reduction shows anatomic alignment of ring finger to long and little finger proximal phalanges.

to Figure 11-17) (for the first week) and for the remainder of immobilization a palmar splint may be applied to the injured digit alone extending from the fingertip to the proximal palm.

If gamekeeper's injury (avulsion or fracture/avulsion of the ulnar collateral ligament insertion of the thumb MP joint) or reverse gamekeeper's injury (mirror image of the former involving the radial collateral ligament) is suspected (refer to Figure 11-18), stress test of the collateral ligament is contraindicated prior to radiographic evaluation. If a Type III physeal injury of the proximal phalangeal base attached to either the ulnar or radial collateral ligament insertion is not recognized prior to stress testing, that stress may displace the bone fragment and necessitate open reduction and internal fixation.

Middle Phalanx

Middle phalangeal physeal injuries (Figure 11-24) are extremely uncommon because of the unique anatomic stability of the collateral ligaments and periosteum and also the broad wide stable configuration of the phalanx.[1] The mechanism of injury is

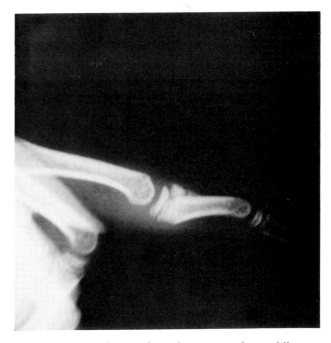

Figure 11-24 Salter II physeal injury to the middle phalanx which is an extremely rare lesion. *(Courtesy of Jack Tupper, M.D.)*

usually a severe crush. Instead, trauma usually involves other injuries of the digit (distal phalanx, the distal interphalangeal joint, the proximal phalanx, the proximal interphalangeal joint or the metacarpal).

Distal Phalanx

Distal phalangeal physeal separation is very common in all digits. Though all types of injury may occur, the most common are open Types I and II injuries. Since the articular surface is involved in Types III and IV injuries, any such displaced unstable or irreducible fracture must be reduced anatomically to prevent aberrant or partial cessation of physeal growth (Figures 11-25, 11-26, and refer to Figure 11-9).

In a closed injury, displacement or angulation of the metaphysis on the epiphysis produces a deformity equivalent to a drop, mallet or baseball injury in the adult (Figure 11-27A). A secondary hyperextension (recurvatum) of the PIP joint often occurs (Figure 11-27B). However, this very often is an open wound with palmar angulation of the diaphysis and avulsion of the nail plate from its cul de sac which is dorsally displaced with the proximal metaphysis (Figures 11-28, 11-29).

The single most important aspect in treating this injury is to provide meticulous wound toilet of the open wound: debriding any devitalized tissue and foreign matter, gentle mechanical cleansing to avoid damage to the germinal epithelium, and irrigating copiously with sterile normal saline solution. Any avulsed segment or the complete avulsed nail plate should be removed, but if the nail plate remains firmly attached to the nail bed and the proximal metaphysis, it should be retained.

Reduction of a Type I or II injury is achieved by immobilization of the epiphysis and reduction of the metaphysis by pressure on the dorsum. Reduction may be difficult or even impossible without surgical incisions proximally to provide appropriate skin laxity. The germinal epithelium must be protected and anatomic reduction achieved to prevent aberrant nail plate regrowth and persistent palmar angulation of the diaphysis (Figure 11-30).

Inattention to meticulous wound cleansing may result in infection, often with subsequent partial or complete cessation of physeal growth (refer to Figures 2-25A–E in Chapter 2, General Principles of Management).

A Salter Type III physeal injury may occur in the older child and adolescent at the distal inter-

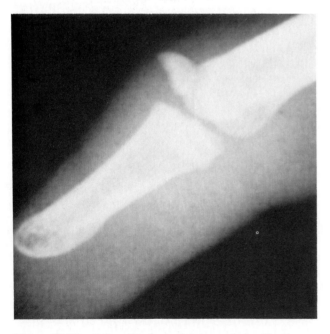

Figure 11-25 Salter III physeal injury of the distal phalanx demonstrating the displaced articular fragment which must be anatomically reduced.

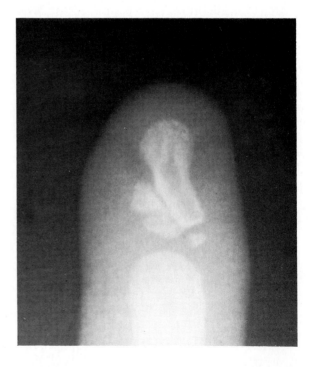

Figure 11-26 Salter type IV physeal injury, displaced.

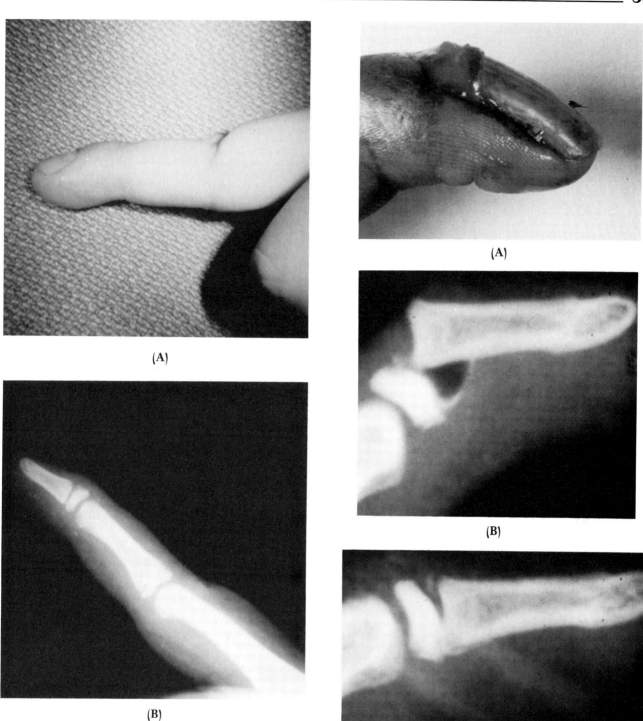

(A)

(B)

(A)

(B)

(C)

Figure 11-27 **(A)** Hyperextension of the PIP joint and what appears to be a mallet finger of the DIP joint. **(B)** Corresponding radiograph shows a Salter I physeal injury of the distal phalanx with palmar angulation, which is responsible for the secondary PIP joint hyperextension.

Figure 11-28 **(A)** Palmar angulation of distal phalanx with protrusion of base of distal phalangeal metaphysis and nail plate avulsed from cul-de-sac. **(B)** Radiograph shows Salter type I open physeal separation of distal phalanx. **(C)** Lateral radiograph after open reduction following meticulous cleansing, debridement, and irrigation of wound.

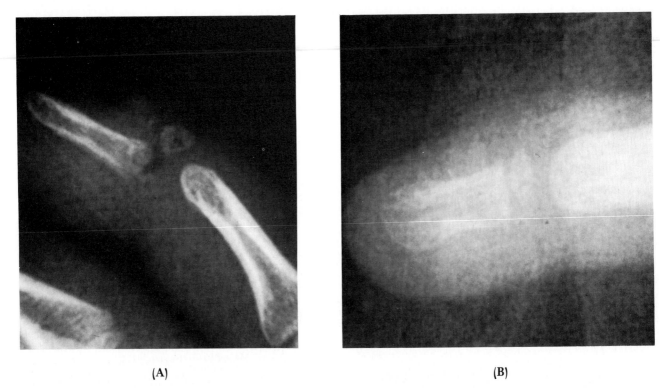

(A)   (B)

Figure 11-29 **(A)** Lateral radiograph shows complete physeal separation of distal phalanx. Injury is in person younger than patient shown in Figure 11-28A–C **(B)** Lateral view after meticulous wound toilet and anatomic reduction.

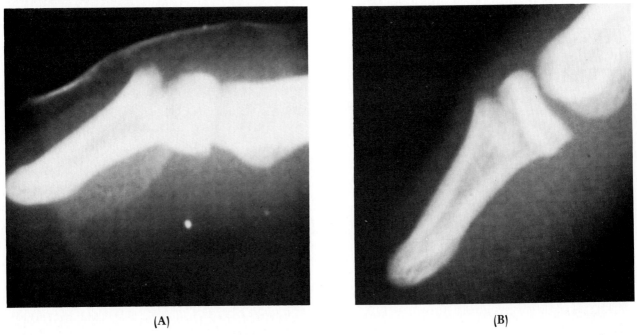

(A)   (B)

Figure 11-30 **(A)** Lateral radiograph shows complete physeal separation of distal phalanx with palmar angulation. **(B)** Lateral view shows continued palmar angulation of distal phalanx at physeal plate area after attempted reduction.   *(continued)*

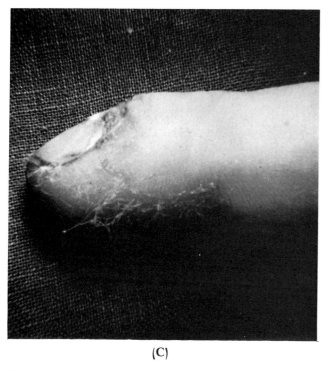

(C)

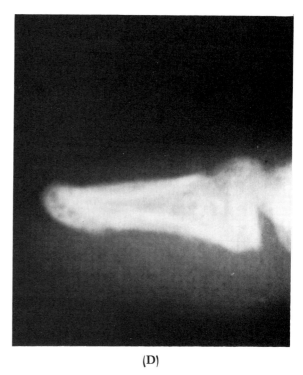

(D)

Figure 11-30 *(continued)*
(C) Lateral photograph shows persistence of slight palmar angulation (20° to 25°), indicating incomplete reduction of distal phalangeal physeal separation. **(D)** Lateral radiograph shows successful reduction after second manipulation of this distal phalangeal physeal separation.

phalangeal joint. A dorsal segment of the epiphysis in continuity with the extensor tendon insertion is fractured from the distal phalanx causing a true drop finger. If the fracture is associated with palmar subluxation of the joint, open reduction and fixation may be necessary to prevent post traumatic arthritic changes (Figure 11-31 and refer to Figure 11-25).

The Thumb

Physeal injuries of the thumb proximal and distal phalanges are treated similarly to those injuries in other digits (Figure 11-32).

Multiple Physeal Injuries

Multiple physeal trauma is relatively uncommon (Figure 11-33) and usually occurs in massive open injuries (Figure 11-34). If internal fixation is necessary (unstable closed reduction, open reduction and open wound, or for an irreducible fracture), smooth Kirschner wires are recommended—as few and as small a caliber as possible placed through the central area of the physis as noted above.

Later Treatment of Physeal Injuries

Effective anatomic reduction of Types I and II injuries usually is achieved easily within the first 24 to 36 hours after injury. However, after approximately five days it is often impossible to change the position due to rapid healing, particularly in the young child. Approximately one week after the injury, the position should be accepted except for any malrotation or pronounced lateral angulation. However, angulation deformities in the flexion/extension plane will usually remodel and spontaneously correct themselves (refer to Figures 12-2, 12-3, 12-4 in Chapter 12, Post-traumatic Skeletal Remodeling).

Figure 11-31 **(A)** Moderately displaced dorsal articular fracture of the base of the distal phalanx with minimal palmar DIP joint subluxation in a 14-year-old child—the equivalent injury of a Salter III physeal injury. Conservative splint immobilization was the treatment. **(B)** Three weeks after injury with no interval radiograph this lateral view shows palmar subluxation of the DIP joint and more displacement of the fracture fragment. **(C)** Six weeks after injury posttraumatic arthritic changes are evident, combined with complete palmar DIP joint subluxation. A prominent dorsal protuberance remains and there is minimal painful DIP joint motion. This case emphasizes the need to obtain serial radiographs at 7- to 10-day intervals to diagnose displacement of an articular fracture and possible subsequent joint subluxation.

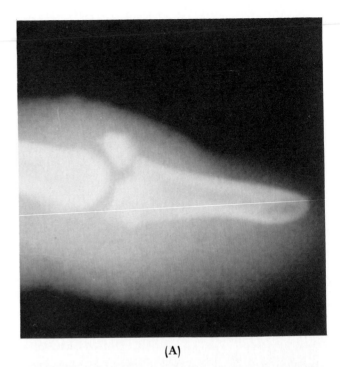

(A)

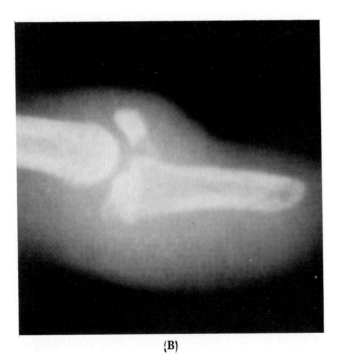

(B)

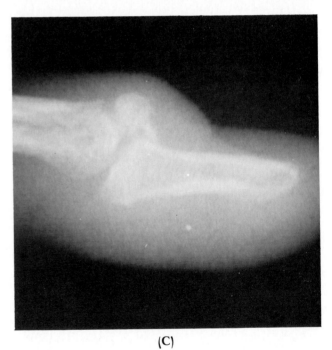

(C)

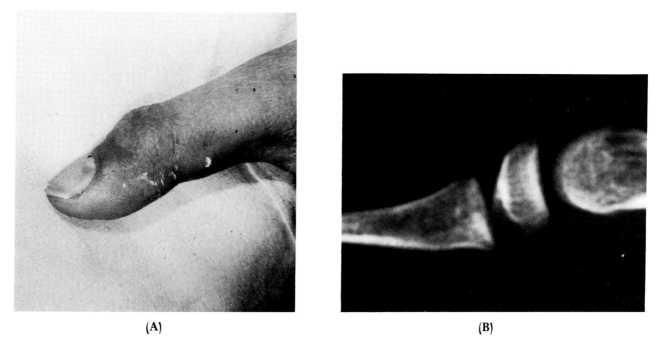

Figure 11-32 **(A)** Oblique view shows some loss of extension of thumb distal phalanx at IP joint, with swelling in that area. **(B)** Lateral view shows Salter type I complete physeal separation of thumb distal phalanx. No manipulation or reduction was necessary; immobilization continued for three weeks with DIP joint in extension.

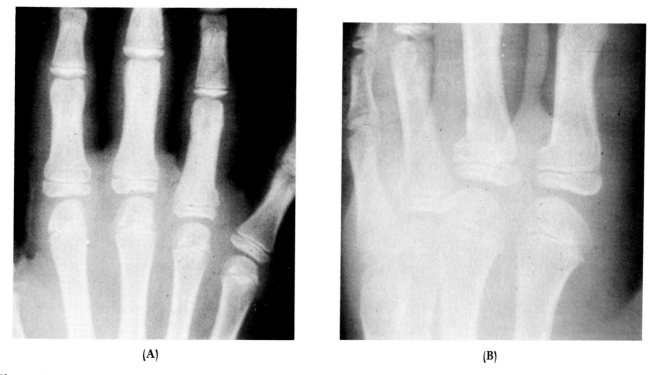

Figure 11-33 **(A)** PA radiograph shows minimal pathology involving the proximal phalanges. **(B)** Oblique view shows Salter type II physeal injuries to index, long, and ring finger proximal phalanges, indicating multiple physeal trauma. Treated conservatively with no manipulation.

Figure 11-34 (**A**) Almost complete amputation of thumb and index fingers with open Salter type II physeal separation of thumb metacarpal and proximal phalanx and Salter type I open complete separation of index finger proximal phalanx physis. Note protruding shaft of index finger proximal phalanx. (**B**) Corresponding radiograph. (**C**) Open reduction and Kirschner wire fixation of thumb metacarpal and proximal phalangeal fractures after meticulous wound toilet. No fixation of index proximal phalangeal physeal separation necessary since injury was stable after reduction. Emphasis must be placed on meticulous cleansing, irrigation, and debridement prior to any attempted reductions.

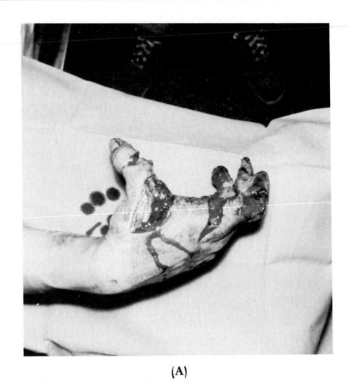

(A)

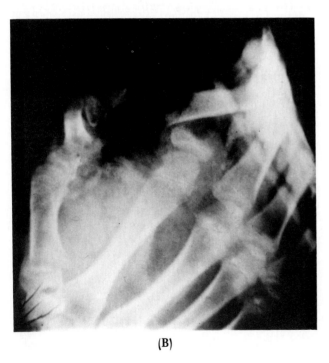

(B)

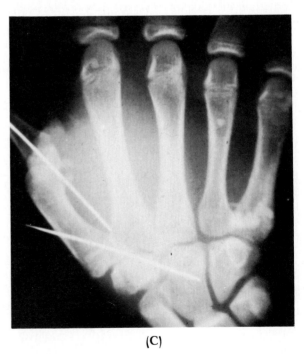

(C)

Reconstruction

Regardless of the type of physeal trauma, parents must be advised that there is the possibility of aberrant growth or complete growth cessation even in the innocuous appearing reduced Types I and II lesions (refer to Figures 11-14, 11-15).

Any persistent malrotation and any significant persistent lateral angulation after healing must be corrected by surgery if physiologic synergistic digital

Figure 11-35 (A) Osteochondroma of the distal ulna which has retarded growth of the distal ulnar physis causing traction on the wrist and marked ulnar deviation of the distal radial articular surface. Also evident is an osteochondroma of the distal radial diaphysis. (B) Decrease in ulnar angulation of the distal radius followed excision of the osteochondroma of the distal ulna and stapling of the radial aspect of the distal radial physis to retard growth. (C) Two years after surgery acceptable realignment of the distal radius and the wrist are noted.

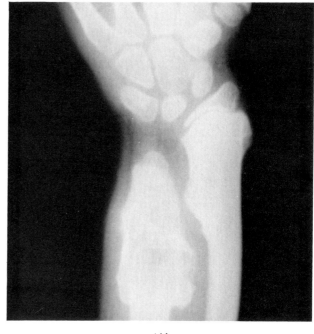

(A)

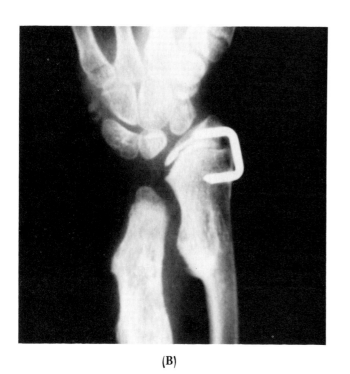

(B)

(C)

flexion and extension are impaired. At the time of osteotomy, great care should be taken to be as gentle as possible in the area of the physis to prevent inopportune early partial or complete physeal growth arrest (refer to Figures 11-22 and 12-3 in Chapter 12).

Rarely, physeal arrest or partial arrest by surgery may be indicated to either correct the existing injury or to prevent further deformity (Figure 11-35). Differential growth rate of a physis following crush trauma or other pathology (e.g., tumor) with delayed physeal growth or partial physeal growth arrest can be treated by surgical arrest of the remaining viable portion of the physis to prevent overgrowth and angulation (refer to Figures 11-14, 11-15).

Arthroplasty is sometimes indicated for marked irregularity of an articular surface causing painful post traumatic arthritic changes, deformity and persistent instability and arthrodesis may occasionally be necessary.

Therapy is usually not indicated or necessary in rehabilitation because of the age of these patients. The child and adolescent will progressively use the digit or extremity in direct relation to subsidence of pain and the desire for social interaction with his (her) peers.

References

1. Bogumill GP: A morphologic study of the relationship of collateral ligaments to growth plates in the digits. *J Hand Surg* 1983;8:74–79.

General References

Blount WP: *Fractures in Children*, ed 1. Baltimore, Williams and Wilkins, 1955.

Ogden JA: *Skeletal Injury in the Child*. Philadelphia, Lea & Febiger, 1982.

Rang M: *Children's Fractures*, ed 2. Philadelphia, J.B. Lippincott Co., 1983.

Rockwood CA Jr, Wilkins KE, King RE: *Fractures in Children*. Philadelphia, J.B. Lippincott Co., 1984, vol 3.

Sandzén SC Jr: Growth plate injuries of the wrist and hand. *Am Fam Physician* 1984;29(6): 153–168.

CHAPTER
12

Posttraumatic Skeletal Remodeling

Wolff's law best applies to posttraumatic skeletal remodeling. The principle of this law is that adaptive dynamic skeletal remodeling responds to functional stresses and demands placed on the involved area. Such stresses include muscle contractions across the involved area, normal architectural stress pattern in that area of bone, effectiveness of fracture immobilization, and longitudinal compression due to muscle exertion or weight bearing.

The changes brought about by adaptive remodeling of bone are particularly evident in fracture healing in the long bones of children. *Rotational deformities are permanent if untreated, and any malrotation should be corrected at the initial manipulation, if possible* (refer to Figure 11-22 in Chapter 11, Physeal Injuries).

At the site of an angulation deformity, remodeling causes accretion of bone on the concave side of the angulation due to stress of pressure and compaction as well as resorption on the convex side due to distraction stresses. Interestingly, the angulation at the malunion remains in situ and is actually incorporated into the remodeling process (Figure 12-1).

Angulation deformities will spontaneously correct themselves depending on the following factors:

1. The age of the child
2. If the angulation is in line with the motion of an adjacent hinge joint
3. If the angulation is toward the midshaft of the bone or if it is within or close to the metaphysis
4. The severity of the angulation

The younger the child, the more rapid and better the correction will be. If the angulation is not in the plane of motion of an adjacent hinge joint or a joint in which motion is primarily flexion and extension (e.g., elbow, wrist, MP and IP joints), some angulation is likely to persist. The closer the angulation is to the metaphysis adjacent to the hinge joint of the long bone, the better the correction will be. Naturally the less severe the angulation, the more correction will result (Figures 12-2A–F).

Therefore, in the older child with a severe angulation in the midshaft of a long bone which is not in the plane of flexion and extension of a nearby

Figure 12-1 (A) Lateral radiograph of a completely displaced Salter I fracture of the thumb metacarpal base with palmar angulation in an 8-year-old boy two-and-one-half weeks after injury. Osteotomy, realignment, and fixaton were not advised. (B) Six weeks later the lateral radiograph shows progressive healing with remodeling at the fracture site. (C) The same thumb metacarpal at age 20 shows excellent remodeling with normal thumb carpometacarpal joint function.

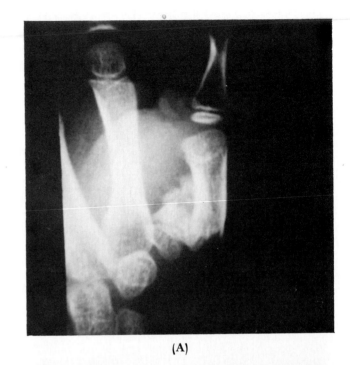

(A)

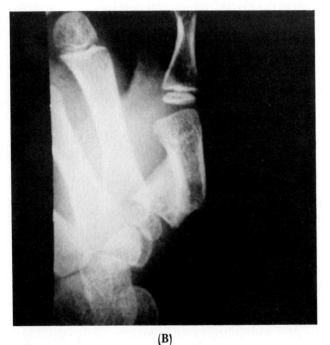

(B)

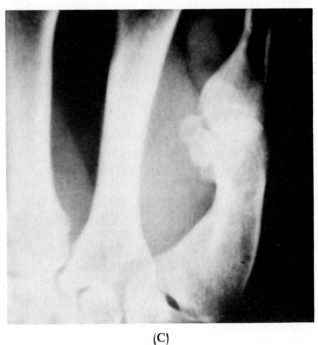

(C)

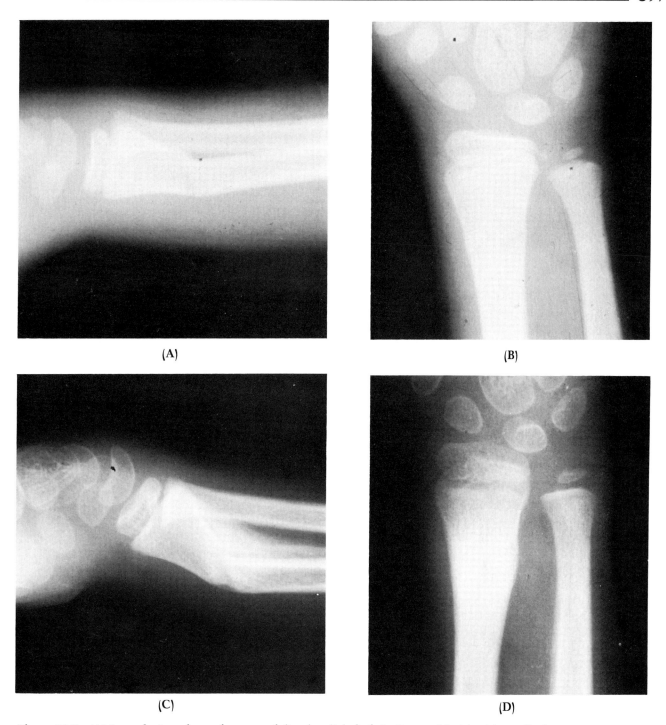

(A)

(B)

(C)

(D)

Figure 12-2 (A) Lateral view shows fracture of distal radial shaft in 8-year-old girl with no displacement seen and dorsal angulation of about 10° to 15°. (B) PA view. (C) Radiograph taken 3½ weeks after injury shows loss of position at fracture site, with dorsal angulation of 35° and an established stable malunion. (D) PA view shows good healing.

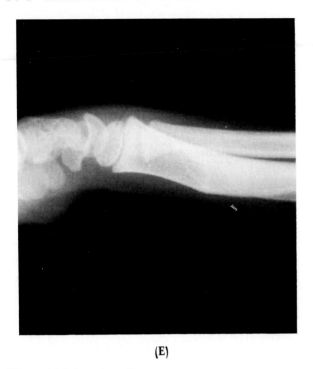

(E)

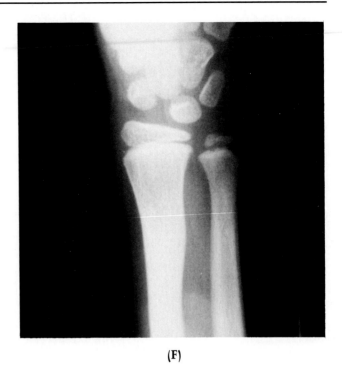

(F)

Figure 12-2 *(continued)*
(E) Lateral view 2 years after initial injury shows acceptable remodeling at site of previous dorsal angulation of radius. Persistent dorsal angulation is about 10° to 15°. **(F)** PA view shows excellent healing. Normal function resulted.

hinge joint, adaptive changes of growth and remodeling will not significantly alter the deformity. It is particularly important to achieve reduction of such a fracture initially to lessen the need for later correction by refracture or osteotomy (Figure 12-3).

A younger child sustaining a fracture in the proximal or distal shaft or metaphyseal areas of a long bone which is moderately angled in the line of flexion and extension of a nearby hinge joint has an excellent chance for adaptive remodeling if the fracture was not treated initially or if it was treated and angulation resulting in malunion recurred (Figures 12-4A–E). A traumatic physeal separation (Salter type I or II) should be reduced anatomically; but if circumstances prevent ideal treatment, the result may be satisfactory (Figures 12-5A–E).

End-to-end apposition of bones at the site of a long bone fracture should be achieved in the older adolescent and the adult. Though some shortening can be accepted, apposition of at least a portion of the opposing bone surfaces at the fracture site should be attempted.

In younger children bayonet apposition or parallel side-to-side apposition at the site of a long

bone fracture is acceptable in all locations, even the phalanges. Anatomic reduction should be strived for in fractures of the proximal and middle phalanges to prevent functional distortion of the intricate balance between the flexors and the extensor apparatus but in the younger child, adaptive remodeling may be surprisingly good (Figure 12-6). Side-to-side apposition is permissible in other areas since there will be accelerated growth in the fractured long bone. This sometimes also causes accelerated growth in the bone distal to it.

Inadequate immobilization of any fracture results in the formation of redundant callus which contains much cartilage (refer to Figure 2-16).

Infection may accelerate bone growth at the site of an open fracture or may arrest it, either partially or completely, if an epiphyseal growth plate is damaged severely enough to cause death of either a portion of or the complete germinal layer. Physeal arrest, partial arrest or growth retardation may be necessary with aberrant growth posttraumatically or subsequent to other pathology (e.g., tumor-osteochondroma, refer to Figure 11-35 in Chapter 11, Physeal Injuries) or juvenile rheumatoid arthritis.

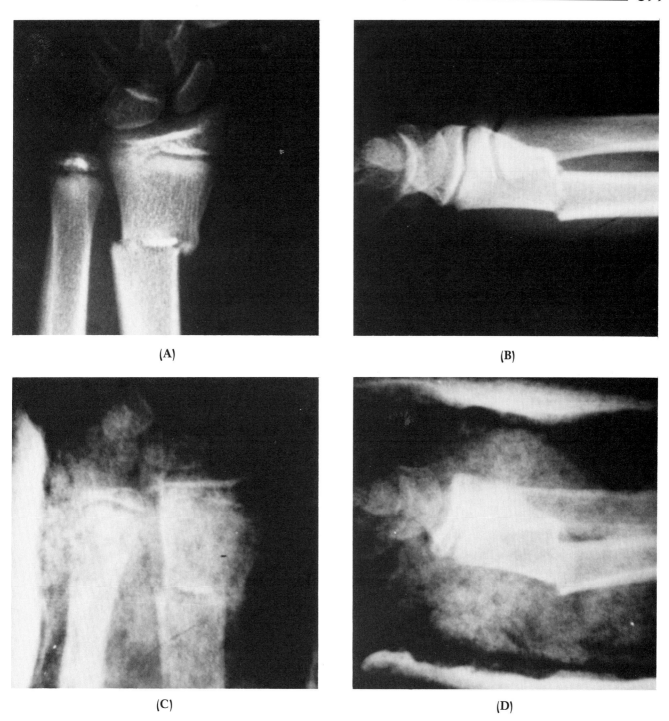

(A)

(B)

(C)

(D)

Figure 12-3 (**A**) Transverse fracture of the radius at the junction of the diaphysis with the distal metaphysis in a 10-year-old girl. (**B**) Lateral radiograph shows minimal dorsal angulation and dorsal displacement. (**C**) One week later the PA view in a long-arm plaster cast is unchanged. (**D**) The lateral view in plaster, however, shows progressive dorsal angulation which now is approximately 25° to 30°.

(continued)

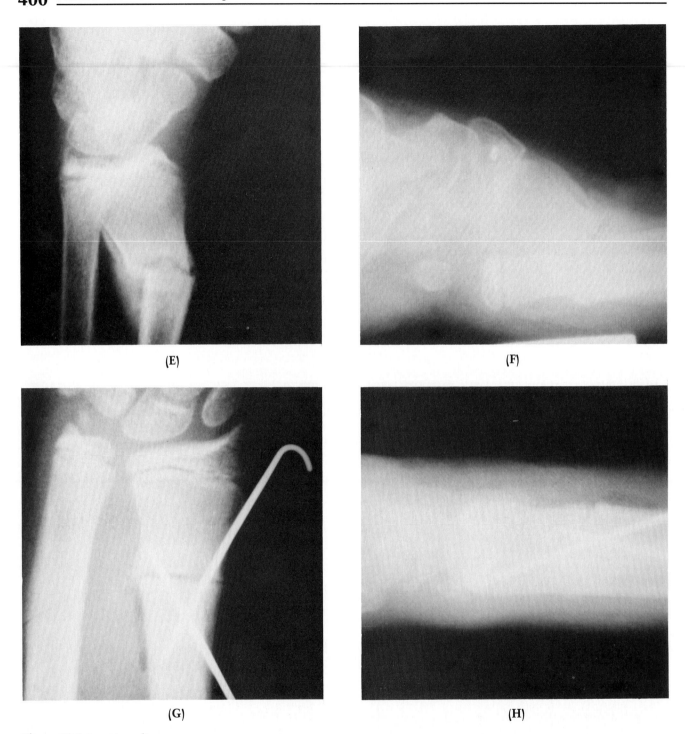

(E)

(F)

(G)

(H)

Figure 12-3 *(continued)*
(E) Four weeks after injury an oblique view shows ulnar angulation at the site of malunion. **(F)** The lateral view shows dorsal angulation of 50° and palmar dislocation of the ulnar head. **(G)** Osteotomy and realignment of the malunion of the radius was necessary because of the significant distal radioulnar joint pathology, including palmar dislocation of that ulnar head. Two Kirschner wires provided adequate skeletal fixation. **(H)** The lateral view shows anatomy of both the distal radius and the distal radioulnar joint restored.

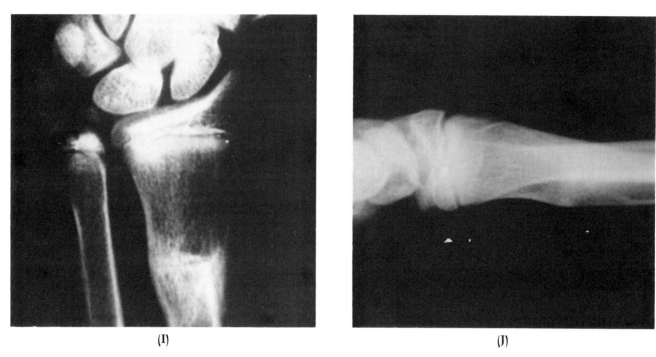

(I)   (J)

Figure 12-3 *(continued)*
(I) PA view four months after osteotomy shows an essentially normal radius but some diastasis of the distal radioulnar joint. **(J)** The lateral view shows good alignment of the distal radius and the ulna. *(Figures 12-3A–J courtesy of Marybeth Ezaki, M.D.)*

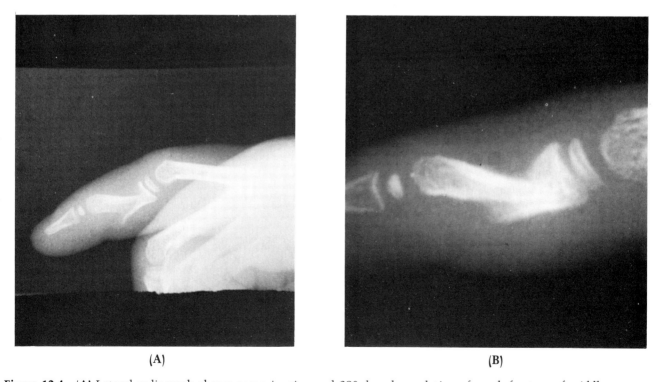

(A)   (B)

Figure 12-4 **(A)** Lateral radiograph shows comminution and 30° dorsal angulation of crush fracture of middle phalanx in a 6-year-old boy. **(B)** Lateral radiograph 5 weeks later shows persistence of dorsal angulation, and good healing occurring.

(continued)

Figure 12-4 *(continued)*
(C) Lateral radiograph 1½ years later shows excellent correction of dorsal angulation and remodeling of entire middle phalanx. Approximately 10° to 15° of dorsal angulation persists. **(D)** Complete extension of index finger shows some recurvatum in area of middle phalanx. **(E)** Complete normal flexion.

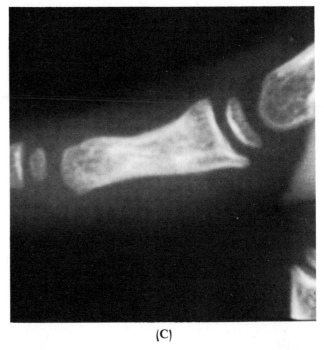

(C)

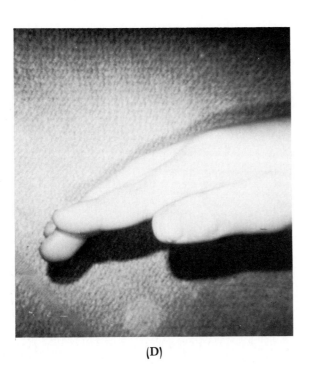

(D)

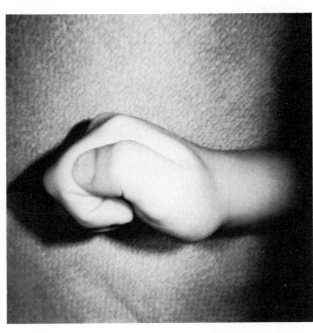

(E)

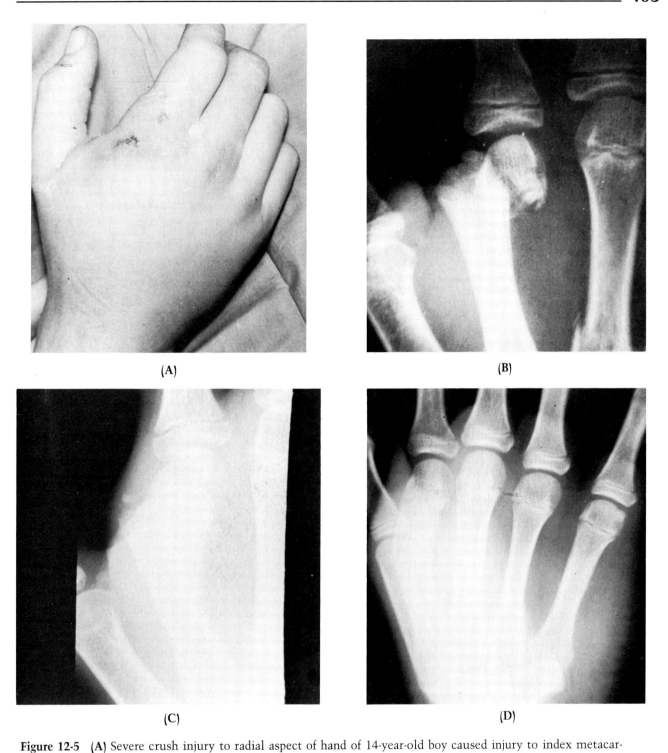

(A)

(B)

(C)

(D)

Figure 12-5 (A) Severe crush injury to radial aspect of hand of 14-year-old boy caused injury to index metacarpal and diffuse swelling of dorsum of hand and all digits. Seen here 6 days after injury. (B) Complete ulnar and palmar displacement of traumatic Salter type II physeal separation of index metacarpal. (C) Attempt at closed reduction 10 days after injury was unsuccessful. Open reduction was impossible because of patient's poor general condition. Oblique view 9 weeks after injury shows good healing of displaced malunion. (D) Oblique view 1½ years after injury shows excellent correction at site of malunion due to growth and corrective remodeling, with minimal persistent palmar angulation.

(continued)

Figure 12-5 *(continued)*
(E) Radial view shows 60° to 65° MP joint flexion of injured index finger on right compared to 80° flexion of normal contralateral joint. Extension was normal and patient had normal use of involved index finger.

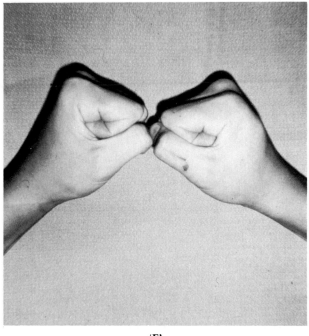

(E)

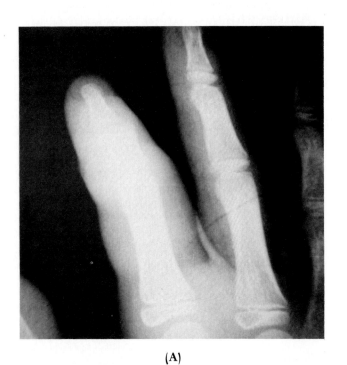

(A)

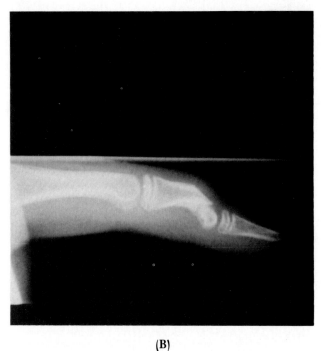

(B)

Figure 12-6 **(A)** Because of injury to the index finger this oblique radiograph was made and shows an undisplaced fracture of the index finger proximal phalanx. Not noted at that time was the displaced distal metaphyseal fracture of the middle phalanx of that digit. **(B)** Three-and-a-half weeks later this true lateral radiograph shows complete palmar displacement of the condyles of that index finger middle phalanx with malunion. At that time it was advised not to intervene surgically and to rely on skeletal remodeling for correction.

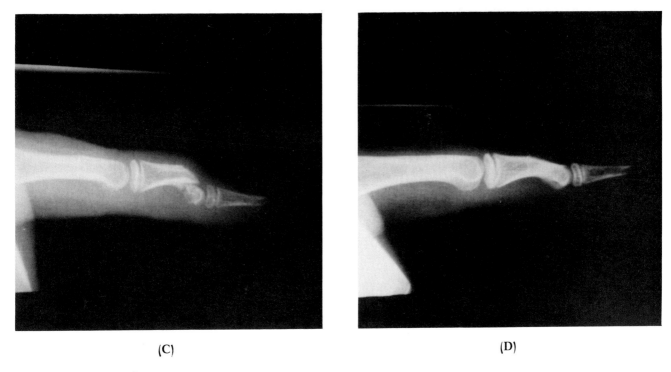

(C)   (D)

Figure 12-6 *(continued)*
(C) Three months after injury remodeling is progressing well and normal digital function was noted. **(D)** One-and-a-half years after injury excellent skeletal remodeling has produced a nearly normal middle phalanx.

General References

Blount WP: *Fractures in Children*, ed 1. Baltimore, Williams and Wilkins, 1955.

Ogden JA: *Skeletal Injury in the Child*. Philadelphia, Lea & Febiger, 1982.

Rang M: *Children's Fractures*, ed 2. Philadelphia, J.B. Lippincott Co., 1983.

Rockwood CA Jr, Wilkins KE, King RE: *Fractures in Children*. Philadelphia, J.B. Lippincott Co., 1984, vol 3.

Sandzén SC Jr: Growth plate injuries of the wrist and hand. *Am Fam Physician* 1984;29(6): 153–168.

CHAPTER
13

Crush Injuries

Crush injuries are included as a separate section both because of particular distinguishing characteristics inherent in the injury and specific important aspects of treatment which differ from that for other types of trauma. These injuries are much more damaging than pure lacerations causing more marginally viable soft tissue and abundant scar formation with decreased joint mobility (Figure 13-1 and refer to Figures 2-27A,B of Chapter 2, General Principles of Management).

In crush injuries often one can judge the massive trauma sustained by soft tissues by evaluating the history (e.g., hydraulic press, trash compactor) and radiographically reviewing the skeletal damage often including multiple fractures, dislocations and fracture dislocations (Figure 13-1). Precise radiographs are a prerequisite to accurately assess that skeletal damage and include minimally for the hand and wrist four views (PA, lateral and two obliques) of good technical quality centered directly on the pathology.

Most severe crush injuries are open wounds necessitating meticulous wound toilet. However, an extensive closed crushing injury must be closely observed to diagnose a progressive closed compartment or closed space compression syndrome for timely fascial lysis to prevent irreversible muscle and nerve ischemia.

The crush syndrome is the systemic and worst consequence of massive crush trauma of a single extremity or multiple extremities and must be properly diagnosed to prevent acute renal failure. This syndrome, however, would be rare following a severe crush injury to a single hand and wrist alone.

Crush Syndrome

The crush syndrome must be suspected if one extremity and certainly if multiple extremities have been subjected either to massive acute crushing trauma (e.g., pinned beneath a collapsing building or wall) or have sustained prolonged compression (e.g., prolonged immobility of an extremity pinned beneath the body of a comatose person)[1] (Figure 13-2).

Acute crush or chronic pressure applied directly to muscle mass, augmented by vascular com-

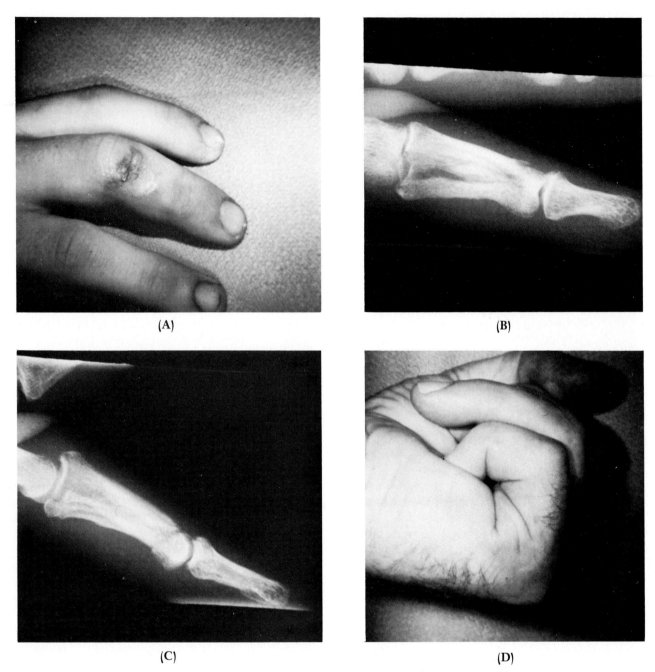

(A)

(B)

(C)

(D)

Figure 13-1 (**A**) Severe crush injury of ring finger middle phalanx. Note edema and ecchymosis of dorsoradial skin of middle phalanx base. (**B**) Oblique radiograph shows severely comminuted longitudinal fracture of ring finger middle phalanx with PIP joint articular involvement. (**C**) Lateral radiograph shows a spreading out of middle phalanx base due to effects of injury. (**D**) Flexion of PIP joint is 85°, but flexion of DIP joint is only 15°due to binding down of extensor apparatus in cicatrix at area of healed middle phalangeal crush fracture. Extensor tenolysis can improve digital flexion of DIP joint, but nature of articular PIP joint fracture points to poor prognosis for increase in function.

pression, causes muscle breakdown (rhabdomyolysis) with myoglobulinuria which may cause acute renal failure. Rhabdomyolysis may cause hyperkalemia, particularly with concurrent oliguria or anuria to cause sudden death.

Surprisingly, the quantity of myoglobin released from damaged muscle is not directly related to the probability of acute renal failure. The acute failure is most likely caused by a combination of pigmented casts obstructing renal tubules; obstruction of renal vasculature; the direct toxic effect of myoglobin; and other related systemic factors, including shock, hypothermia, fever, and acidosis.

Helpful diagnostic laboratory determinations center on urinalysis and serum analysis. Urinalysis shows myoglobulinuria with its distinctive characteristic brownish discoloration and pigmented urinary casts, and is orthotoluidine (Hematest) positive (dip stick test). Serum analysis shows marked elevation of CPK (serum creatine phosphokinase), LDH (lactic dehydrogenase), SGOT (serum glutamic oxaloacetic transaminase) and aldolase. These enzyme elevations are absent with hemoglobulinuria. In acute renal

failure with tissue necrosis, creatinine and BUN are also elevated.

Early treatment of any suspected case of "crush syndrome" mandates aggressive hydration and alkalinization of the urine to prevent acute renal failure monitored by accurate intake and output by indwelling catheter and repeated serum electrolyte determinations.

Open Crush Injuries

Most severe crush injuries are open. Typically the skin is burst apart and avulsed like the skin of a grape or tomato when squashed or after impacting against a hard surface. The extreme pressure causes extrusion of the underlying muscle and subcutaneous tissues through the avulsive laceration much like tooth paste squeezed from a ruptured tooth paste tube. The web spaces are particularly vulnerable especially the thumb-index web containing the muscle mass of the adductor pollicis, the first dorsal interosseous and the

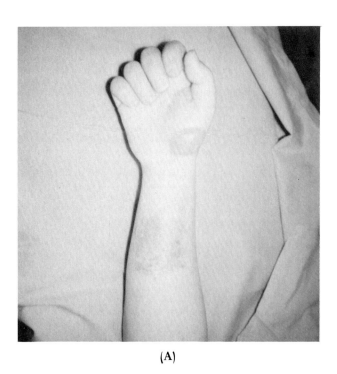 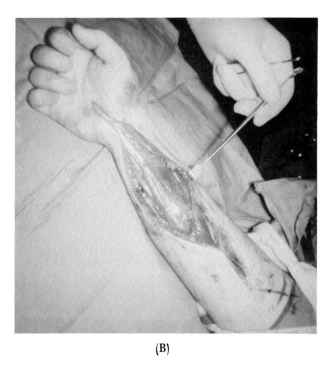

| (A) | (B) |

Figure 13-2 **(A)** Closed space compression injury of the forearm shown five days after injury. This 22-year-old male was in diabetic coma for several hours with his entire body weight impinging on his forearm. Tense non-pitting edema of the forearm and hand with blister formation ("kissing lesions") are noted with intrinsic minus position of the fingers. **(B)** Radical fascial lysis from the palm to the proximal forearm included sectioning of the transverse carpal ligament. *(continued)*

Figure 13-2 *(continued)*
(C) Five days after fascial lysis, partial necrosis of the forearm muscles is seen proximal to the musculotendinous junctions. **(D)** Approximately three weeks after initial fascial lysis and median neurolysis and secondary debridement of necrotic muscle, split thickness skin graft resurfacing was provided. **(E)** Status six months after initial treatment shows cavitation in the area of muscle loss at the time of partial split thickness skin graft excision.

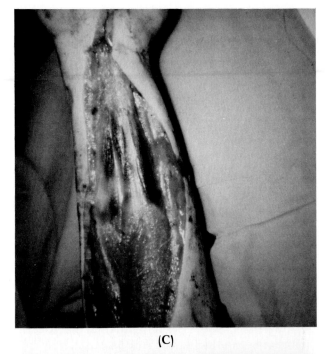

(C)

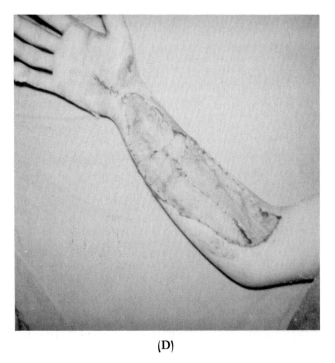

(D)

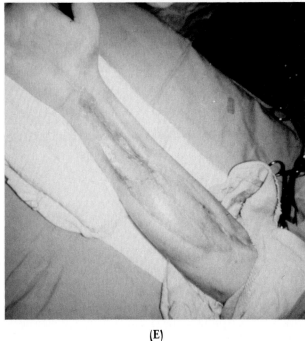

(E)

deep head of the flexor pollicis brevis muscles[2] (Figure 13-3).

Appropriate tetanus prophylaxis should be administered and, in severe wounds which may be contaminated or in which much marginally viable soft tissue remains, prophylactic antibiotics are recommended. (E.g., 1 gm IV of a cephalosporin in the emergency room, a second gram before elevation of the tourniquet in surgery and continued administration for 48 to 72 hours postoperatively.)

Localized digital injuries may be safely treated in an adequately equipped emergency suite, but any extensive wound and usually multiple digital injuries are best treated in the operating room. Safe, adequate anesthesia for wounds of any magnitude is an axillary block with appropriate supplemental peripheral nerve

Figure 13-3 (A) Severe crush injury causing nearly complete amputation at wrist, with dorsal protrusion of ulna and fracture of radius. Bursting type wound of thumb-index web space caused by severity of crush injury which literally burst skin and extruded soft tissue (first dorsal interosseous and adductor pollicis muscles) through rent in skin. (B) Marked edema of dorsum of hand and digits despite compressive dressing, constant elevation, and immobilization of extremity 10 days after injury. (C) Palmar view after reconstructive surgery involving deletion of completely functionless little finger. Patient showed strong grasp and release, fairly good thumb opposition, and strong pinch. Ring finger retained for strong functional grasp despite a 45° flexion contracture of MP joint.

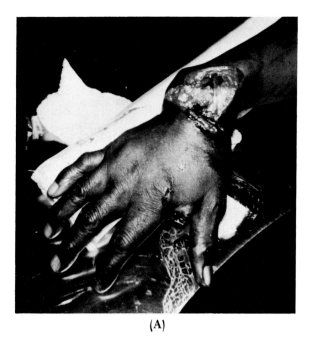

(A)

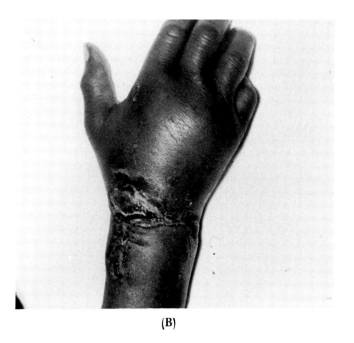

(B)

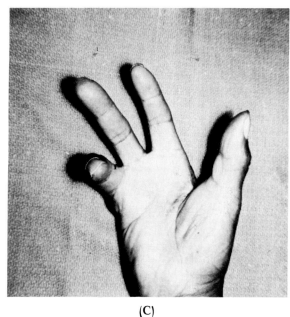

(C)

blocks. A tourniquet should always be placed on the upper arm after administration of the axillary block though inflation to 280 mm of pressure may be unnecessary.

Despite the profound ischemia and minimal remaining vascularity, conservative initial treatment often will provide a viable functioning digit (Figure 13-4).

In primary treatment of an open crush injury the most important aspect is meticulous wound toilet, performed twice if indicated, with sterile glove changes between, including copious irrigation with sterile physiologic solution down to and including the depth of the wound (Figure 13-5). Prior to wound toilet, however, cultures and tissue cell counts should be taken from appropriate areas including the deepest portion of the wound.

The wound must be debrided down to clean viable vascularized tissue (Figure 13-6). Because demarcation between viable and nonviable tissue may not be clearly evident at the time of initial treatment, debridement should be limited to only definitely non-

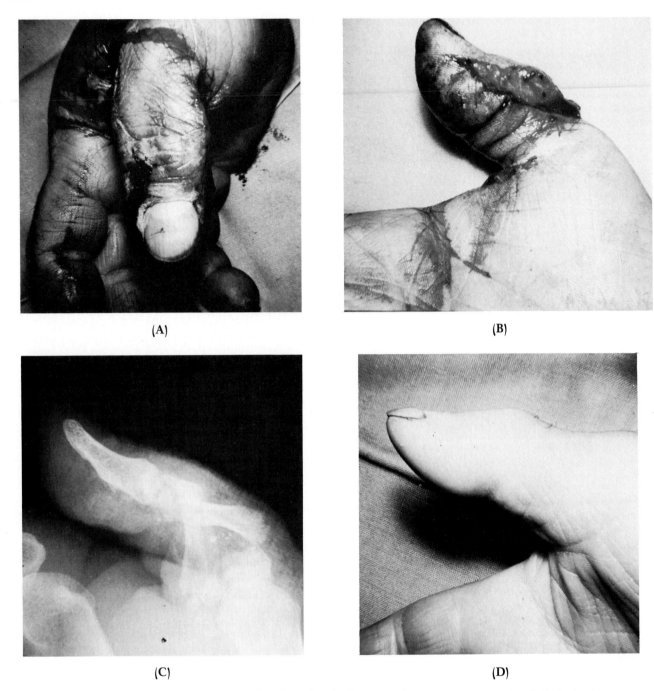

(A)

(B)

(C)

(D)

Figure 13-4 (A) Thumb caught between truck axle and jack shows crush injury to its proximal phalanx, with obvious flattening of digit. (B) Oblique palmar view shows bursting skin lesion resulting from excessive crushing pressure on soft tissues. Note minimal bleeding. (C) Lateral view shows extremely comminuted displaced proximal phalangeal fracture with complete destruction of thumb MP joint. Initial treatment was meticulous wound toilet followed by gross positioning of fracture fragments and open treatment of wound. Thumb viability was maintained. (D) Three months after injury shows complete wound healing and satisfactory position of thumb with some persistent recurvatum of proximal phalanx.

Figure 13-4 *(continued)*
(E) Radiograph shows malunion of proximal phalangeal fractures and complete destruction of MP joint. Patient declined reconstructive surgery since he achieved a stable, powerful thumb with sensibility.

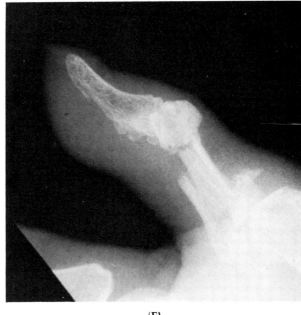

(E)

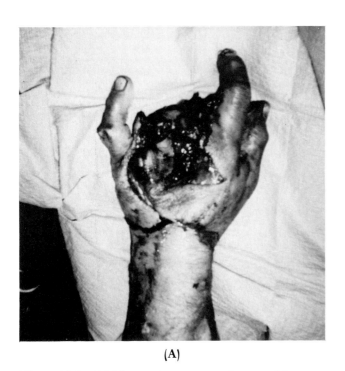

(A)

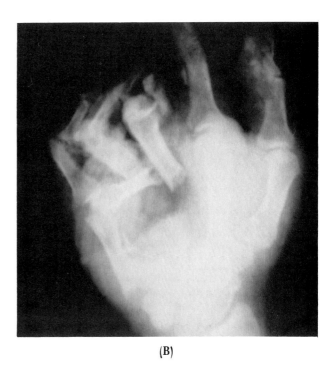

(B)

Figure 13-5 **(A)** This patient sustained severe blast injury to his left hand 72 hours prior and wound toilet including debridement of the now foul smelling necrotic central portion of the hand was erroneously not carried out until this time. **(B)** Simultaneous radiograph shows marked destruction of the central portion of the hand with displaced fractures of the index and little finger metacarpal bases. *(continued)*

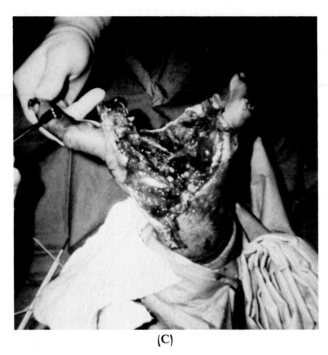

(C)

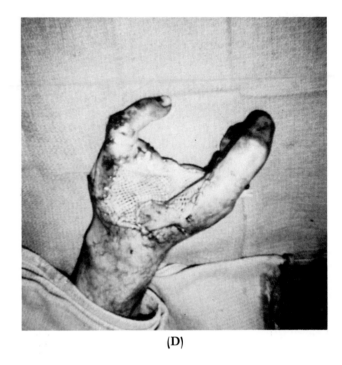

(D)

Figure 13-5 *(continued)*
(C) The remaining viable elements included skin tags, the little finger, the thumb, and an index ray of very precarious viability. **(D)** After four staged debridements, a meshed split thickness skin graft was applied to the clean wound approximately three weeks after injury. Despite the 72 hour delay of debridement which caused over two weeks additional morbidity, severe sepsis, particularly clostridial invasion, fortunately did not occur.

Figure 13-6 **(A)** Massive crush injury to the radial aspect of his hand sustained by a 64-year-old man in a press injury. Thumb was split open from distal metacarpal area to distal phalanx with loss of most of latter. Index and long fingers were virtually filleted from the metacarpus distally. Oblique view after meticulous wound cleansing and irrigation shows the situation prior to amputation of the index finger through the PIP joint area.

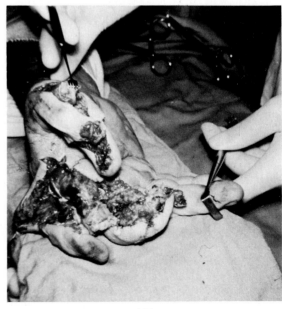

(A)

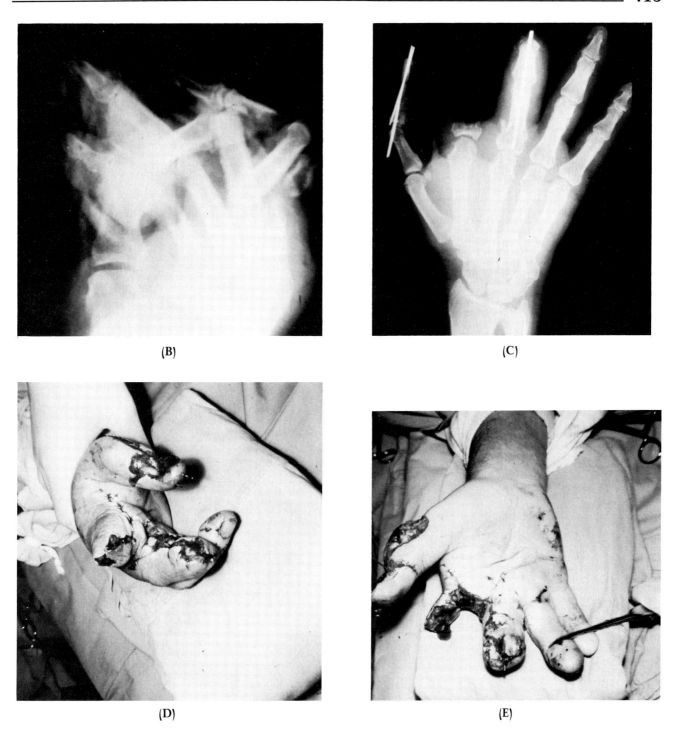

(B)

(C)

(D)

(E)

Figure 13-6 *(continued)*
(B) Oblique radiograph illustrates complete displacement of long finger middle phalangeal fracture and diffuse soft tissue and skeletal injuries. **(C)** PA radiograph after primary wound care shows longitudinal Kirschner wire fixation of thumb and long finger and point of amputation of index finger at base of proximal phalanx. **(D)** Four days after injury, at second debridement after initial surgical procedure, oblique view shows necrosis of distal skin at index amputation site. **(E)** Palmar view illustrates radial pedicle of skin maintained from index finger after debridement of gangrenous soft tissue distally. Pulp of distal phalanx and massively traumatized soft tissue of long finger are viable.

(continued)

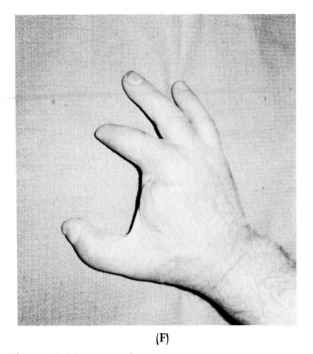

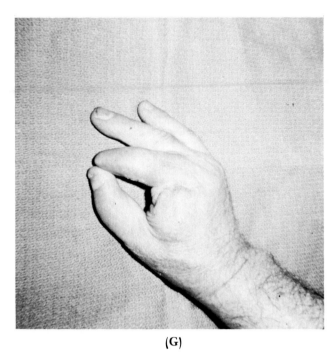

(F)

(G)

Figure 13-6 *(continued)*
(F) PA view 6 weeks after injury shows maintenance of viability of important pulp of thumb distal phalanx and also of severely crushed long finger out to its amputation at DIP joint. **(G)** Grasp is good, and there is strong, sensible thumb-to-finger pinch possible at this time.

viable tissue and foreign material. All marginally viable tissue must be handled delicately and preserved and protected for use either in primary, delayed primary or secondary reconstruction (Figures 13-6C–G).

Skeletal fragments attached to soft tissue and large segmental bone fragments whether attached to soft tissue or not should be retained. Bone fragments in exposed areas of an open fracture are debrided by rongeur down to clean, bleeding, normal appearing bone regardless of the skeletal defect created. In crush injuries to the distal phalanx there should be no attempt to remove any of the comminuted fragments of the tuft or distal metaphysis of the distal phalanx unless the fragments literally fall out during wound irrigation (refer to Figure 8-28, phalangeal fractures).

Primary excision of damaged germinal epithelium in severe crush or partial amputation of a distal phalanx is contraindicated. Excision of any viable segment of soft tissue including a portion of the nail bed and/or germinal epithelium may prevent primary or delayed primary closure under no tension because of insufficient tissue. Eradication of a ger-

minal epithelial remnant which causes symptomatic aberrant nail plate regrowth should be performed under magnification as a secondary reconstructive procedure.

Reestablishing skeletal stability to as near normal as possible is next in importance in primary or delayed primary treatment (Figure 13-7) and often includes internal or percutaneous fixation (Figures 13-8, 13-9). Fractures of one or both bones of the forearm, and distal radius are treated as recommended elsewhere (refer to Chapters 3, 16).

Anatomy of the radiocarpal joint (wrist joint) and carpus must be restored to as near normal as possible by reduction (usually open) and appropriate internal or percutaneous fixation. At the time of open reduction, ligamentous structures should be repaired if additional extensive surgical exposure is unnecessary (refer to Chapters 4, 16).

Fractures of the long bones of the hand (metacarpal, proximal, middle and distal phalanges) also are treated as recommended elsewhere (refer to Chapters 7, 8, 16). The most important consideration in fractures of these long bones is to prevent malrota-

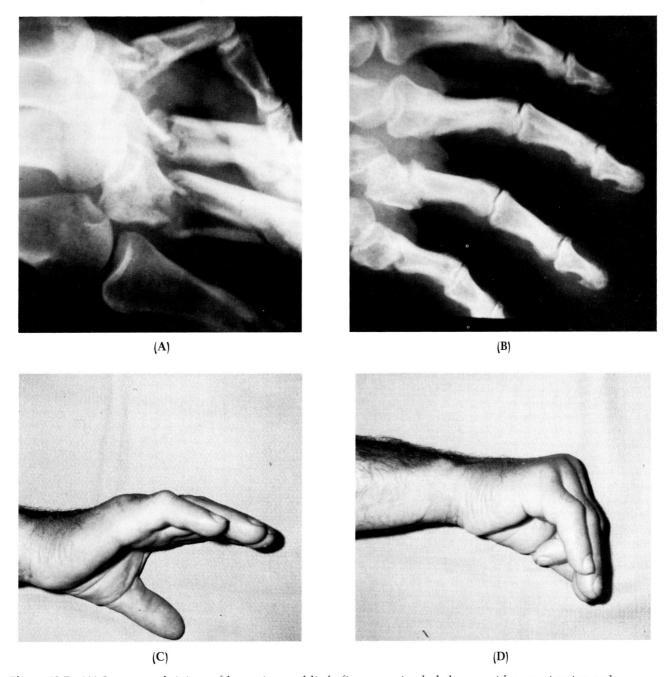

(A)

(B)

(C)

(D)

Figure 13-7 (A) Severe crush injury of long, ring, and little finger proximal phalanges with comminution and characteristic dorsal angulation at fracture sites. (B) Oblique view emphasizes persistent dorsal angulations 6 months after injury. (C) Ulnar view showing extent of digital extension. (D) Extent of flexion. Little finger in particular illustrates well recurvatum deformity of healed proximal phalangeal fracture, with extensive cicatrix of flexor and extensor tendons preventing adequate flexion. Reconstructive surgery may include lysis or excision of superficialis tendons and lysis of profundus and extensor tendons to regain some active digital flexion, as demonstrated in Figures 13-11A–E.

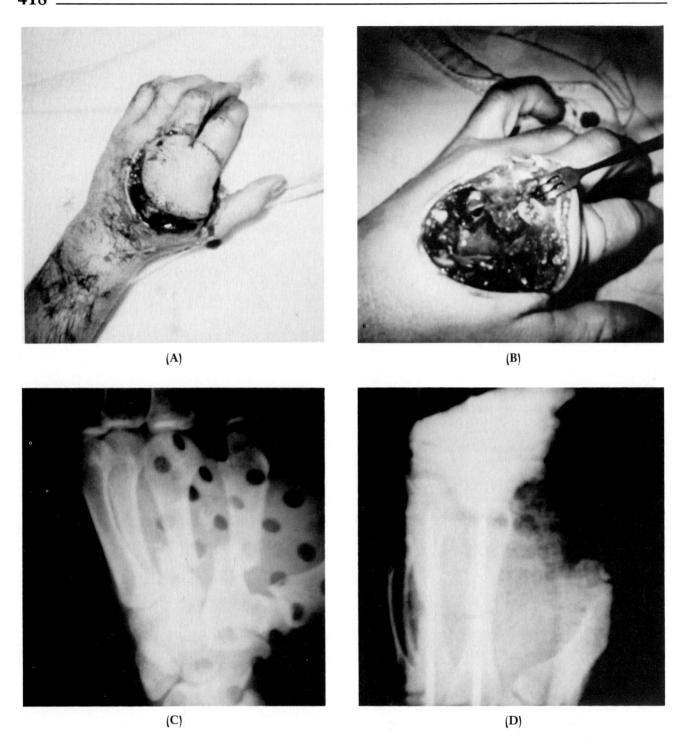

(A) (B)

(C) (D)

Figure 13-8 **(A)** Die press crush injury of the hand with circular outline noted on the index and long metacarpals proximally and proximal phalanges of those digits distally. The area contained within that circle was essentially undamaged. **(B)** Retraction shows complete transverse laceration of extensors to those digits and fracture of both metacarpals in the midshaft with laceration of all adjacent interossei. Additionally, extensor tendons were cut at the proximal phalangeal lacerations. **(C)** Corresponding radiographs of the metacarpal fractures. **(D)** The metacarpal diaphyseal fractures were treated by primary longitudinal intramedullary Kirschner wire fixation.

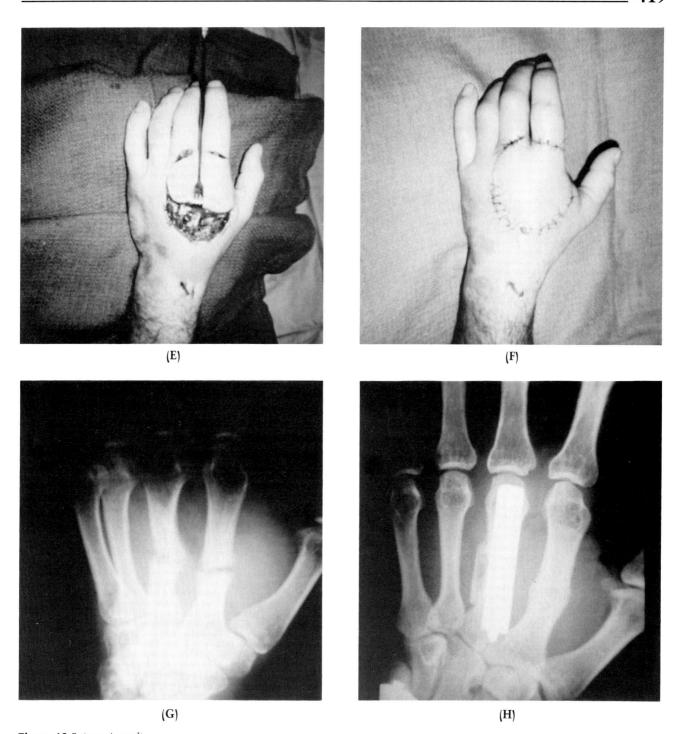

(E)

(F)

(G)

(H)

Figure 13-8 *(continued)*
(E) Two days later minimal redebridement was necessary and the distally based pedicle of skin and subcuta-neous tissue was entirely viable. Delayed primary tenorrhaphies of six lacerated tendons (common extensor to index and long fingers at two sites, and the proprius tendon of the index finger at two sites), with delayed primary wound closures were effected. **(F)** Twelve days after delayed primary reconstruction moderate edema of the hand, index and long fingers is seen but all soft tissues are viable. **(G)** Radiograph approximately four months after injury shows delayed healing at both fracture sites following Kirschner wire removals two months previously.**(H)** The index metacarpal healed satisfactorily but plate fixation and bone graft of the long finger metacarpal was necessary because of nonunion.

(continued)

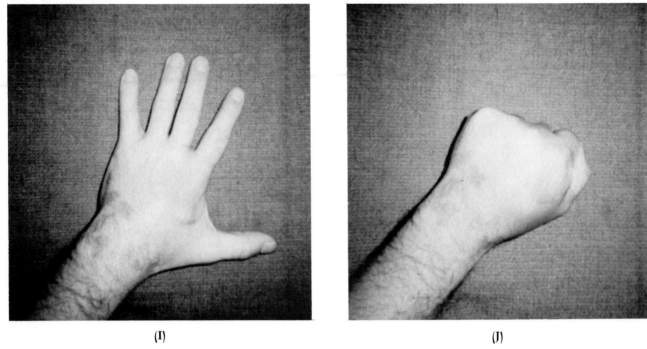

(I)   (J)

Figure 13-8 *(continued)*
(I) Essentially normal digital extension is seen approximately 8 months after injury. **(J)** Normal digital flexion.

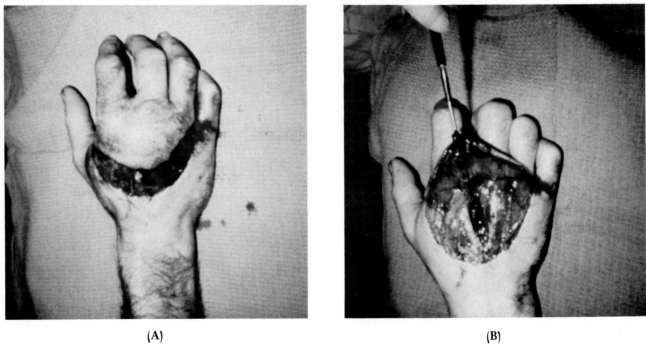

(A)   (B)

Figure 13-9 **(A)** Similar type injury with distally based pedicle but in this case all soft tissues involved were crushed in a press injury. **(B)** Examination of the wound shows damage to the extensors of index and long fingers and interossei avulsions as well as fracture of the long finger distal metaphysis.

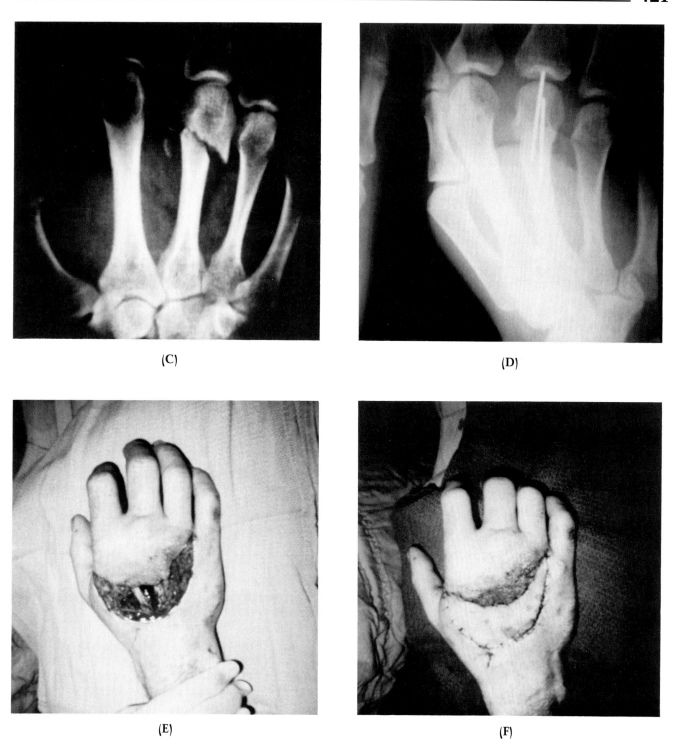

(C)

(D)

(E)

(F)

Figure 13-9 *(continued)*
(C) Corresponding radiograph shows the oblique fracture of the long finger distal metaphysis. **(D)** Initial treatment included meticulous wound toilet and internal Kirschner wire fixation of the long finger metacarpal fracture. **(E)** Four days later at redebridement the periphery of the distally based pedicle of skin and subcutaneous tissue is necrotic. Elevation of the distally based pedicle reveals the delayed primary repair of the extensor tendons. **(F)** Following debridement of the necrotic skin and subcutaneous tissue, split thickness skin graft augmentation closed the wound.

(continued)

Figure 13-9 *(continued)*

(G) Four months after injury complete digital extension is noted and (not shown) complete digital flexion.

These two cases demonstrate the importance of initial open wound treatment in massive crush injuries with re-debridement at two to three day intervals and appropriate skin closure or split thickness skin graft coverage. Initial skeletal fixation is followed by delayed primary soft tissue repairs.

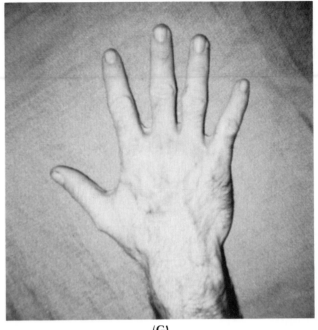

(G)

tion since malrotation of a single metacarpal or proximal phalanx can destroy the function of the entire hand.

Initial open treatment of a crush injury is strongly recommended particularly in the more severe wounds (Figures 13-6, 13-8, 13-9). It is much more acceptable to delay wound closure or coverage than to attempt primary closure which may result in further gangrenous changes from vascular compromise with prolonged morbidity deferring reconstructive procedures until healing is complete.

Any partial tissue avulsion, particularly distally pedicled, must be treated open because of precarious viability from marginal arterial supply and interruption of venous and lymphatic drainage.

Occasionally, a free split-thickness skin graft may be applied primarily. An excellent alternative either initially or delayed primarily is to use a meshed, split-thickness skin graft with a ratio of 1.5:1.0 (length/width) in the event of any persistent edema or hemorrhagic oozing, or to use a physiologic temporary resurfacing by a homograft (cadaver skin) or heterograft (porcine-xenograft).

Local and distant pedicles are rarely used in initial treatment unless an attached skin segment can be preserved after deletion of an irreparable digit (Figure 13-6). Bone from the deleted segment can be used to replace skeletal deficits in other areas.

If the tourniquet was inflated to control hemorrhage at the time of initial wound treatment it must be deflated prior to dressing and immobilization to assess vascularity and tissue viability.

Any procedure requiring additional surgical exposure, traction or repetitive attempts of fracture reduction generally is contraindicated because of additional insult to already severely traumatized tissue.

There is absolutely no indication to attempt primary tenorrhaphy or neurorrhaphy in a severe crush injury at the time of primary treatment. The necessary immobilization postoperatively binds down the repaired structure(s) in massive scar, preventing any perceptible functional return.

Physiologic immobilization includes a non-constrictive compressive dressing reinforced by palmar or dorsal plaster splint. A circumferential plaster cast is contraindicated to prevent the possibility of external compression triggering a progressive closed space or closed compartment syndrome. The physiologic position for immobilization includes wrist extension, MP joint flexion, PIP and DIP joint extension and physiologic thumb metacarpal abduction and opposition.

Constant vertical elevation of the hand and forearm decrease edema and hemorrhage (refer to Figure 13-3B) and gentle progressive mobilization of all joints is encouraged as soon as possible without endangering fracture or joint reduction. Comminuted articular fractures require early motion (utilizing dynamic skeletal traction occasionally) to remold the joint surfaces as congruously as possible for best ultimate function (Figure 13-10). All uninjured and minimally injured digits should be unrestricted by dressings and mobilized immediately.

Dressings should be changed and redebridements effected at two to three day intervals until all nonviable tissue has demarcated and has been debrided.

Delayed primary closure or resurfacing by split-thickness skin graft is ideally performed three days to one week post injury if the wound remains clean with no evidence of contamination, infection or further necrosis (Figures 13-8, 13-9).

Figure 13-6 is an excellent example emphasizing all aspects of treating a massive open crush injury of the hand. The basic concepts of meticulous wound toilet and salvage and protection of viable tissue are most important in these most severe injuries. In Figure 13-6A the wound has been me-

ticulously cleansed and irrigated prior to amputation of the index finger through the PIP joint area. The distal phalanx of the long finger has been comminuted and split longitudinally, and the skin irreparably crushed. This distal phalangeal bone was used to stabilize the pulp of the thumb distal phalanx in an attempt to provide enough stability to retain the precarious viability of the pulp tissue. Care was taken to position the injured parts in order to prevent additional vascular impairment by torsion or pressure on the minimal existing blood supply (Figures 13-6A, D,E). After meticulous debridement loose approximation of tissues was accomplished but there was no attempt at definitive closure. The skin of the index finger was fashioned into a tube to prevent infolding of the soft tissue at the time of dressing application. The bone graft to the thumb distal phalanx was fixed by a single longitudinal Kirschner wire and the completely displaced transverse fracture of the long finger middle phalanx was reduced and fixed by a single longitudinal wire.

Eight days after injury at the third and final

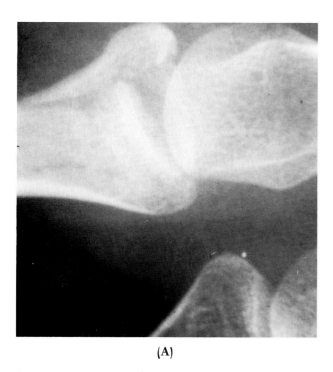

(A)

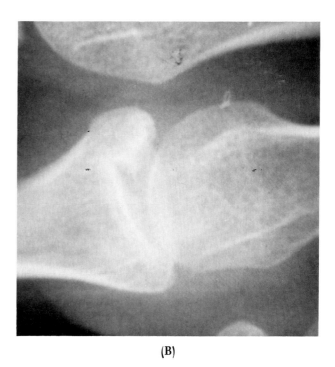

(B)

Figure 13-10 (A) Ring finger MP joint crush injury. Articular surface of base of proximal phalanx is incongruous, and a portion is depressed, or crushed, into metaphysis. Treatment is early (5 days postinjury) light range of motion to attempt to mold incongruous surface and achieve best functional result. (B) 10 weeks after injury MP joint range of motion was about 80% of normal. Posttraumatic arthritic changes should be expected and cannot be prevented.

redebridement wound closure was accomplished using the pedicled index skin remnant to resurface the thumb-long finger web space.

Eventually good grasp and strong pinch with nearly normal sensation resulted with complete thumb length and functional long finger length maintained at the DIP joint amputation.

A distant pedicle (e.g., supraclavicular, cross arm, abdominal, groin, and those derived from the hand and digits themselves—dorsal cross finger and palmar pedicles) occasionally may be indicated in the late primary treatment in a clean wound.

The general rule is to employ pedicled resurfacing only in a controlled situation in which infection and further tissue necrosis are not anticipated since either complication creates an extremely unpleasant situation.

Periodic radiographs at seven to 10 day intervals will diagnose any loss of fracture or joint reduction early enough for correction, particularly if skeletal fixation was not used initially.

Reconstructive procedures are carried out only after subsidence of edema and after joint ranges of motion have reached their maximum active and passive ranges. It is the responsibility of the physician to retain all viable tissue initially and to revise elements

of the hand reconstructively, according to the patients' desires and functional needs, in order to provide a functioning hand with the best possible sensation, stability, motor power and joint mobility.

Crushing injuries involving the proximal phalanges invariably bind down the flexor tendons in the scar (Figures 13-11A–E, 13-7A–D). The superficialis tendon is particularly vulnerable since it is deep to the profundus at this point and becomes intimately adherent to fracture callus and soft tissue cicatrix. Reconstructive tenolysis of the profundus tendon may be accomplished by either tenolysis or excision of the superficialis tendon to regain some increase in active flexion of the involved digit or digits (Figure 13-11D). In crushing injuries of the middle phalanx either or both the superficialis and deep flexor may be bound down by scar (Figures 13-1A–D).

In the reconstruction of a severely crushed digit or hand only the severely functionally impaired digit with ischemic changes, markedly limited motion, and decreased sensation should be sacrificed. Such a digit will impair the general function of all other digits. Reconstructive surgery should include deletion of obviously irreparable digits with use of portions to augment remaining functional digits (Figures 13-3A–C). Osteotomy to correct skeletal

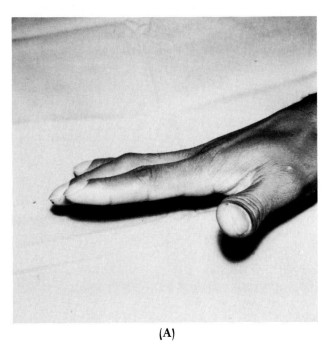

(A)

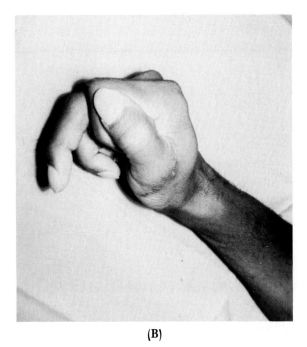

(B)

Figure 13-11 **(A)** Patient sustained oblique displaced crushing fracture of long finger proximal phalanx 10 months prior to photograph. PIP joint lacks 25° extension. **(B)** Flexion of PIP joint is approximately 60°, flexion of DIP joint is approximately 20°.

Figure 13-11 *(continued)*
(C) PA view of healed oblique crush fracture of long finger proximal phalanx 10 weeks after manipulation and reduction. (D) View at surgery shows excision of superficialis tendon of long finger and its extraction from wrist, combined with tenolysis of flexor digitorum profundus tendon, with care being taken to preserve flexor pulleys. In addition, extensor tenolysis was carried out through a separate dorsal incision. (E) Nine weeks after surgery, long finger digital flexion has improved, with 85° of PIP joint flexion and 45° of DIP joint flexion. PIP joint extension remains essentially unchanged.

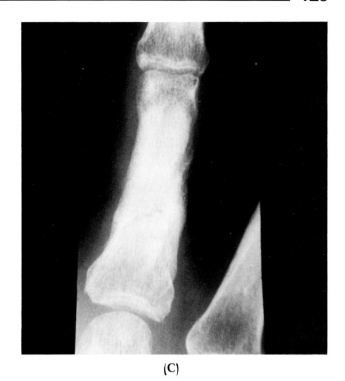

(C)

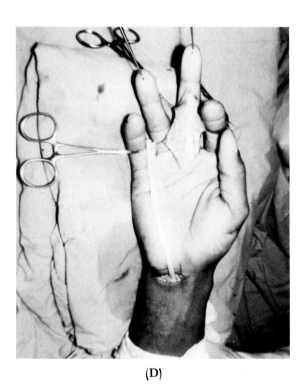

(D)

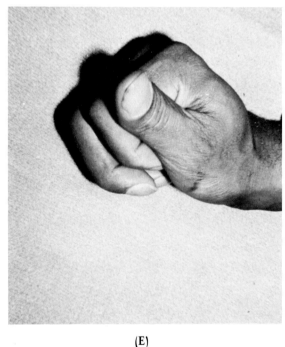

(E)

realignment or arthrodesis to provide stability may be combined with, or follow, resurfacing procedures. If reconstruction will be a prolonged affair and the functional result far from normal, the patient may prefer amputation of the severely injured digit.

Closed Crush Injuries

In the closed injury with stable fracture(s), compression dressing, immobilization, and elevation are followed by active and passive ranges of motion as soon as subsidence of edema permits (Figures 13-1A–D).

Early mobilization of a joint which has sustaiₙed a crush injury is essential to restore acceptable motion (Figure 13-10). As soon as the acute pain has somewhat subsided (plus or minus five days postinjury) the patient should be encouraged to actively and passively move the involved joint(s).

Closed crush injuries may, however, present an entirely different situation. The diagnosis of a progressive closed space or closed compartment compression syndrome depends upon intelligent correlation of history, physical examination and radiographs. Determinations of intracompartmental tissue pressure are also helpful.

The best clue to suspect this syndrome is the history either of significant acute crushing trauma (e.g., heavy industrial rollers, punch press) or chronic prolonged pressure on an extremity (e.g., an upper extremity trapped for an extended period of time beneath the body weight of a comatose person) (refer to Figures 13-2, 13-12A).

Radiographs of acute injury may reveal multiple skeletal pathology including fractures, dislocations and fracture dislocations often correlating with gross skeletal distortion (Figure 13-12C).

Physical examination discloses a uniformly swelled extremity with diffuse, tense, non-pitting edema and often decreased temperature from circulatory impairment. Pain is centered in the involved muscles not at the site of fracture(s) (Figure 13-12) if present and limits any attempt at active motion.

Initially, the hand assumes the "intrinsic plus" position of MP joint flexion, PIP and DIP joint extension and thumb adduction because of muscle irritability. However, with progressive denervation of the intrinsic muscles, the digits gradually assume the "intrinsic minus" position of MP joint extension or hyperextension, PIP and DIP joint flexion and flattening and adduction of the thumb with no power of opposition (Figure 13-12).

Progressive neurapraxia and vascular impairment identified by pain on attempted passive motion opposite to the normal action of the ischemic muscle or muscles, decreasing sensibility manifested first by paresthesia and then hypesthesia verify the diagnosis.

Pain on attempted passive digital extension indicates Volkmann's phenomenon in the palmar forearm musculature. Symptoms on passive wrist and digital flexion indicate dorsal forearm compartment syndrome. If passive abduction and adduction of the digits with MP joints extended and PIP joints flexed produces pain, interosseous compartment ischemia is suspect. Thenar compartment involvement results in pain on attempted passive extension, adduction and abduction of the thumb and for the hypothenar compartment on extension, adduction and abduction of the little finger.

"Kissing lesions" of blisters, bullae or actual tissue necrosis can be found in the chronic compression syndrome on the extremity and the areas of torso or head which have been in direct contact for a prolonged period of time (refer to Figure 13-2). Obviously absence of the radial and/or ulnar pulse forbodes a bad prognosis. However, the presence of either or both of these pulses does not exclude the development of any compartment syndrome of the forearm or hand.

Though evaluation of patency of the superficial palmar arch by the Doppler ultraflow technique may be very important to diagnose forearm compression syndrome, particularly Volkmann's, it is not helpful to diagnose intrinsic muscle ischemia of the hand (interosseous, thenar, hypothenar and central compartment syndromes). In the equivocal case serial intracompartmental pressures over 30 ml by either the Whitesides[3] method or the Wick catheter[4] help clarify the diagnosis and decision to explore.

However, progressive neurapraxia of increasing paresthesia and decreasing sensibility combined with increasing circulatory impairment noted on periodic examinations at 10 to 15 minute intervals mandates surgical intervention. *The necessity of appropriate fascial lyses cannot be overemphasized* and may be compared to the decision to perform a tracheostomy. If the treating physician thinks either procedure may be indicated then it should be performed (Figure 13-12)!

Fasciotomies must be extensive enough to completely relieve the constrained internal pressure and therefore must extend into normal tissues proximally.[5] If a burn has been sustained, escharotomy alone is usually insufficient and fasciotomy also must be performed. Physiologic skin incisions are performed with care to avoid damage to deeper structures (the ulnar nerve at the elbow and the median and ulnar nerves at the wrist) and to prevent unnecessary secondary scar contractures (Figure 13-13). Occasionally, compartmental fasciolysis must be supplemented by lysis of individual muscle fascial coverings (epimysium). Decompression of the interossei is by dorsal longitudinal incisions between each pair of metacarpals (Figure 13-12D). Decompression of the thenar, hypothenar and central compartments is by the standard incision used for carpal tunnel exploration which extends from the distal forearm

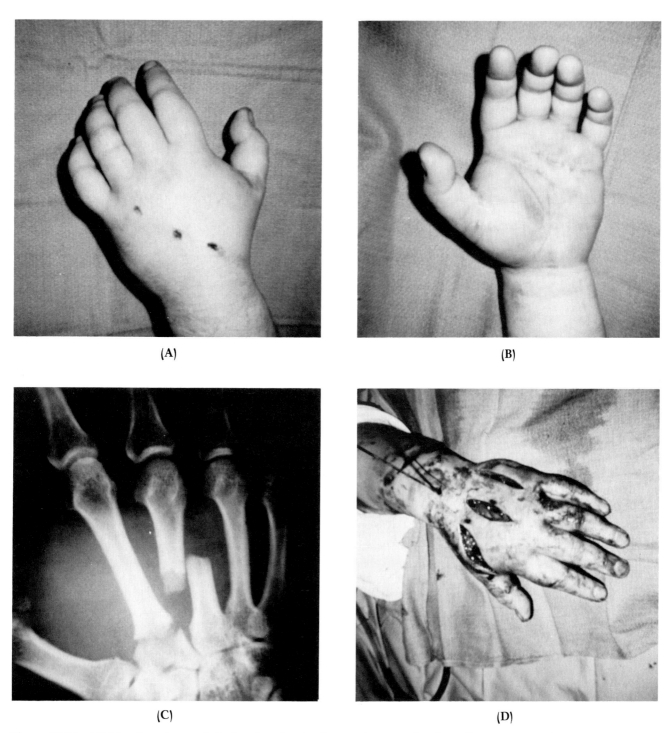

(A)

(B)

(C)

(D)

Figure 13-12 **(A)** Massive edema of the hand and wrist from a discreet closed crushing injury to the metacarpus in a press. All the signs and symptoms of a closed compartment syndrome dorsally involving the metacarpus (interossei) and palmarly (the thenar, hypothenar and central compartments) were present. Note the intrinsic minus position of the hand. **(B)** Palmar view. **(C)** Corresponding radiograph illustrates undisplaced transverse proximal metaphyseal fracture of the index metacarpal and displaced transverse diaphyseal fracture of the long finger metacarpal. **(D)** Dorsal incisions for evacuation of massive hematoma subcutaneously and intramuscularly of all dorsal interossei are noted. The extent of decompression can be appreciated by comparing this to Figure 13-12A.

(continued)

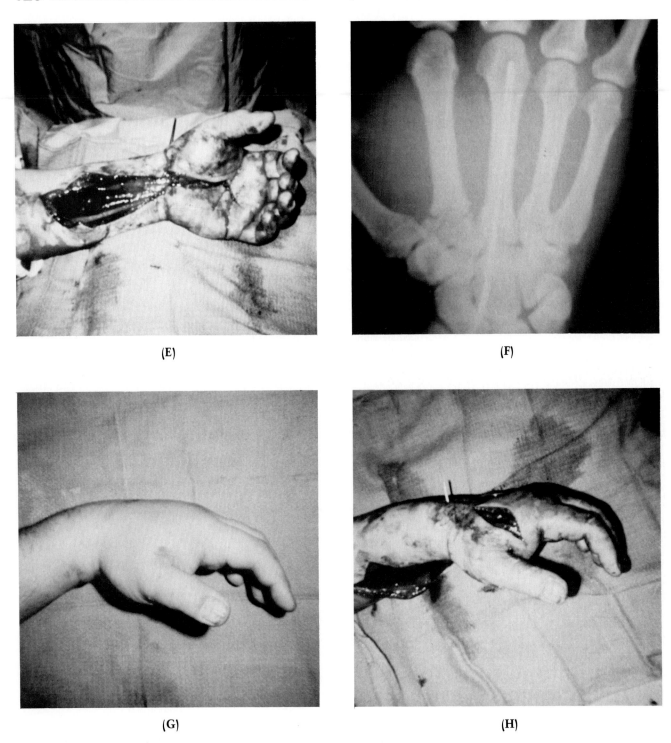

Figure 13-12 *(continued)*
(E) Release of thenar, hypothenar and central compartments and the palmar aspect of the distal forearm was by incision from the midforearm into the distal palm with sectioning of the transverse carpal ligament. **(F)** Anatomic reduction and stable longitudinal intramedullary Kirschner wire fixation of the long finger metacarpal diaphyseal fracture.
(G) Radial view of the hand prior to fascial lysis and decompression shows intrinsic minus position of the digits and the antalgic position of the wrist and hand. **(H)** After fascial lysis and decompression (compare to Figure 13-12G preoperatively).

Figure 13-12 *(continued)*
(I) Three months after injury and delayed primary closure of dorsal incisions seven days after fascial lysis—normal digital extension. **(J)** Three months after injury, palmar view after partial delayed primary closure seven days after injury and complete closure three days later. **(K)** Normal digital flexion.

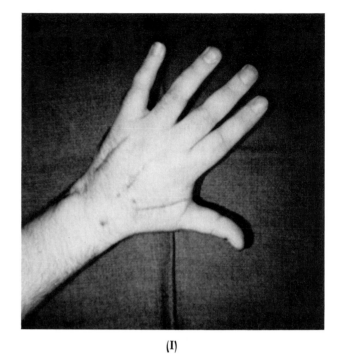

(I)

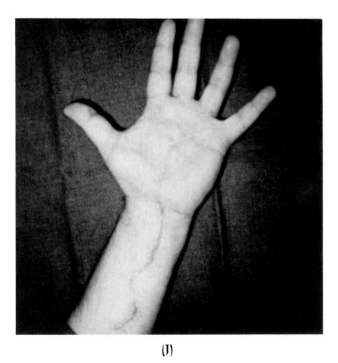

(J)

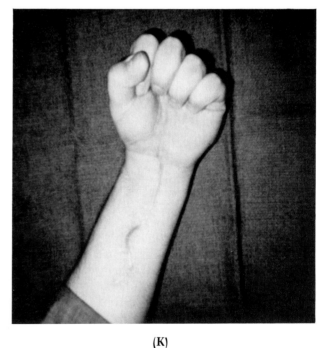

(K)

centered between the flexor carpi radialis and flexor carpi ulnaris tendons and connects to a curvilinear incision at the base of the thenar eminence by a small transverse incision at the wrist. Through this incision, decompression of all three compartments on the palmar aspect of the hand is easily accomplished combined with transection of the transverse carpal ligament (Figure 13-12E).

Release of a closed space compression syndrome of the distal phalangeal pulp is by an incision similar to that used to decompress and evacuate an extensive pulp space abscess (refer to Figures 8-38 and 8-39 in Chapter 8, Phalangeal Injuries). The incision extends from the distal end of the nail plate at the midline down to the distal phalanx extending as far proximally as necessary toward the midaxial line on

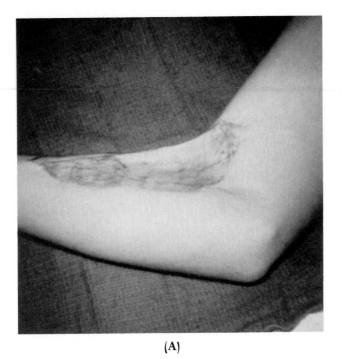

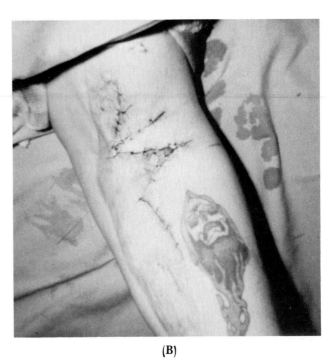

(A) (B)

Figure 13-13 **(A)** Hypertrophic longitudinal scar with flexion contracture following fascial lysis of closed compartment syndrome from both bone forearm fracture. Split thickness skin graft was applied 10 days after fascial lysis. **(B)** Status following modified Z-plasty release of flexion contracture and partial split thickness skin graft excision.

the non-dominant aspect of the digit.[6] In this manner all septal fibers can be lysed for decompression of the pulp. Decompression of an entire digit is by longitudinal midaxial incision on the non-dominant side of that digit.

One must remember, however, that a compartment syndrome can develop in an open wound if that skin laceration is insufficient to successfully decompress increasing edema and/or hemorrhage. This is particularly true if significant muscle injury has been sustained (e.g., stab wound of either the extensor or flexor muscle mass in the proximal forearm) and following vascular injury (e.g., complete or incomplete laceration of a significantly large artery or vein).

Postoperatively, the upper extremity is elevated vertically and immobilized by sterile compressive dressing and splint immobilization. All incisions remain open until they can be closed after subsidence of edema and congestion or are resurfaced by split thickness skin graft coverage. Active ROM (range of motion) exercises are commenced as soon as symp-

toms subside sufficiently (e.g., two to three days postsurgery) even with wounds remaining open.

Burn-Crush Injuries

Burn-crush injuries of any magnitude are disastrous (Figure 13-14). Initial debridement down to bleeding tissue is followed by redebridement at two to three day intervals until no further tissue necrosis is seen and then resurfacing, by split thickness skin grafts, is usually indicated. Pedicled resurfacing generally is reserved for reconstruction later after complete initial healing (Figure 13-14F).

Rarely, delayed primary resurfacing may incorporate a distant pedicle if the wound is clean with no evidence of contamination or marginally viable tissue. Certainly, an infected necrosing flap is an extremely unpleasant, sometimes dangerous situation.

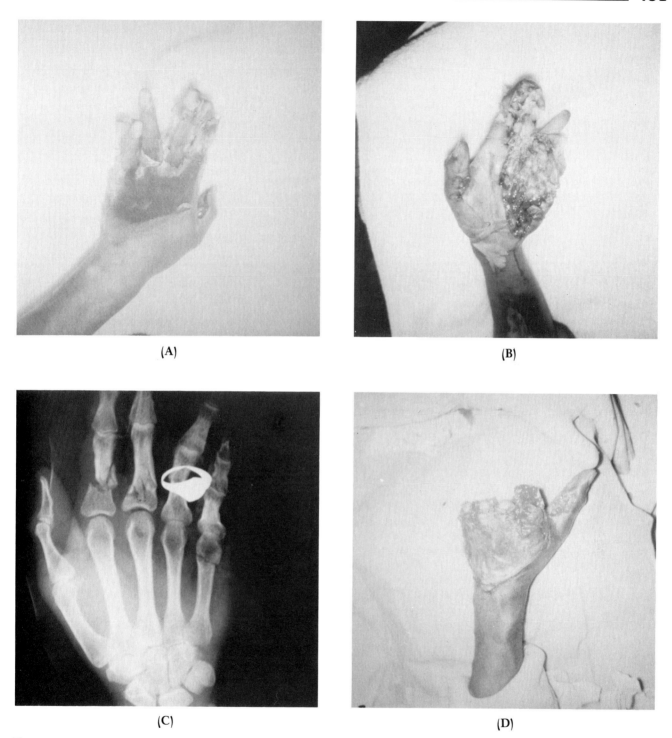

(A)

(B)

(C)

(D)

Figure 13-14 **(A)** Pressure crush burns of the hand sustained in an industrial laundry mangle. Lack of hemorrhage indicates the severe thermal coagulation of vessels. **(B)** Palmar view. **(C)** Corresponding radiographs show multiple fractures of proximal phalanges. **(D)** Viable tissue seen after debridement of completely ischemic burn tissue.

(continued)

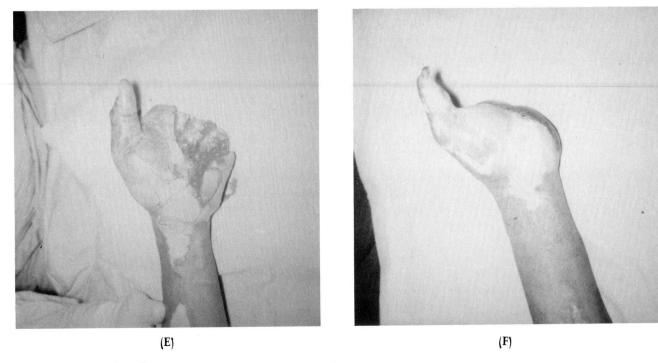

(E) (F)

Figure 13-14 *(continued)*
(E) Palmar view. **(F)** Four months later following secondary application of abdominal pedicle for metacarpal resurfacing.

References

1. Sandzén SC Jr: Surgery of the hand and upper extremity. *Shumpert Med Q* 1984;3:73–79.
2. Sandzén SC Jr, Britton JA: Crush injuries of the upper extremity. *Orthopaedic Audio-Synopsis Foundation*, tape no. 66A, 1984.
3. Whitesides TE, Haney TC, Morimoto K, et al: Tissue pressure measurements as a determinant for the need of fasciotomy. *Clin Orthop* 1975;113:43–51.
4. Mubarak SJ, Hargens AR: *Compartment Syndromes and Volkmann's Contracture.* Philadelphia, W.B. Saunders, 1981.
5. Rowland SA: Fasciotomy, in Green DP (ed): *Operative Hand Surgery.* New York, Churchill Livingstone, 1982, vol 1, pp 565–581.
6. Sandzén SC Jr: Closed space compression injury of the fingertip. *Bull Hosp Joint Dis* 1974;35:162–167.

CHAPTER 14

Retained Foreign Bodies and Through-and-Through Injuries

Retained metallic foreign bodies resulting from a low-velocity projectile injury or a blast injury may be difficult to localize without multiple radiographic views. With only one view, the metallic fragment may often appear to be embedded in bone when, in reality, it remains in soft tissue (Figures 14-1A,B). If the foreign body is easily accessible, it may be localized and removed with relatively little difficulty (Figures 14-1A,B). However, if the foreign body is deeply embedded in either soft tissue or bone but does not impinge upon or lie within a joint, it would be best left in situ (Figures 14-2A,B). After appropriate anesthesia the point of entrance should be well cleansed, and postoperative immobilization should be provided to permit soft tissue healing without difficulty. If infection does develop, a wide incision and drainage become mandatory, but this is usually not necessary. With low-velocity projectile injuries of small calibre (e.g., 22-calibre), foreign matter is rarely driven in with the projectile. If there is suspicion that either fragments of clothing or wadding from a shotgun shell have been driven into the wound, wide exploration and debridement are necessary and the wound should be packed open. If initial exploration was not necessary, mobility is stressed after signs of acute trauma have subsided and there is no evidence of infection. The foreign body is removed later only if it impinges upon neurovascular structures, tendons, or a joint. If the foreign body is intraarticularly located and was not removed at the time of initial treatment, joint motion should not be allowed before arthrotomy and removal of the fragment have been effected (Figure 14-3).

Unnecessary morbidity and occasional infection do result from prolonged exploration at the initial treatment for a small foreign body which would have caused no difficulty had it been left in situ.

A separate category is devoted to projectile through-and-through injuries because of:

1. The massive local destruction of skeleton and soft tissues produced by a low-velocity large-calibre projectile (e.g., 45-calibre bullet) or shotgun blast
2. The tremendous damage caused by a high-velocity missile (1,500 or 2,000 ft/sec or faster) to tissues both in the direct area of the bullet's passage and also circumferentially in soft tissue and skeleton along the course of the projectile

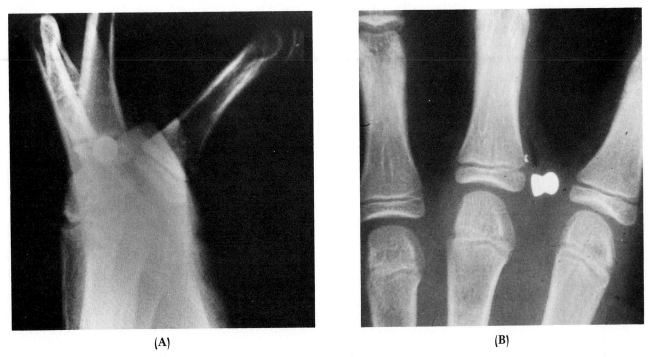

(A)   (B)

Figure 14-1 **(A)** Lateral view showing metallic foreign body apparently embedded in proximal third of index finger proximal phalanx. **(B)** PA view shows foreign body to be actually in web space between index and long finger proximal phalangeal bases.

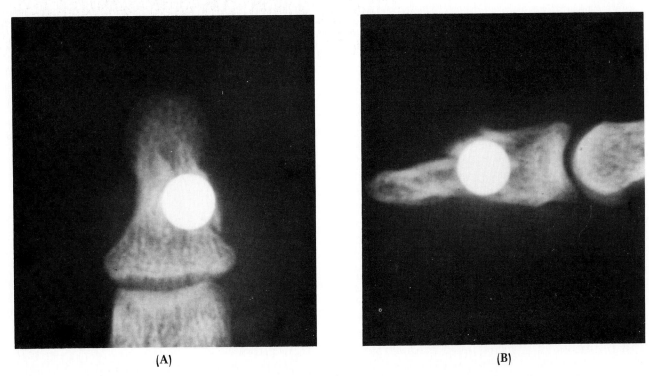

(A)   (B)

Figure 14-2 **(A)** PA radiograph of a BB pellet apparently retained in center of distal phalanx. **(B)** Lateral radiograph shows foreign body to be actually embedded in distal phalanx and illustrates also comminuted fracture. Removal of foreign body unnecessary.

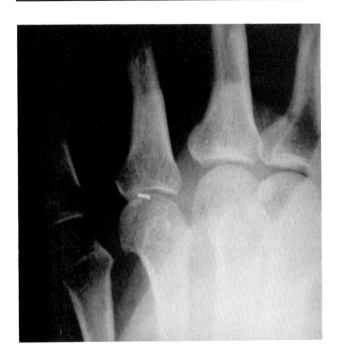

Figure 14-3 Metallic foreign body retained in ring finger MP joint. Surgical exploration and removal are mandatory.

Low-velocity missiles of small calibre, such as 22-calibre bullets, shrapnel, or other exploded material, usually cause damage only in the immediate area of the projectile's path. Meticulous wound toilet at the point of entrance and the point of exit should be followed by irrigation of the wound tract, if possible, using physiologic sterile saline (Figures 14-4A–C). It is best to defer deeper exploration of the injury unless it is suspected that foreign matter such as clothing might have been driven in with the projectile, not usually the case with small-calibre low-velocity projectiles. It is much safer to perform delayed primary or secondary repair of deep structures as indicated at that time of exploration. Primary closure of the skin either at the point of entry or exit is contraindicated (Figures 14-5A,B, 14-6A,B).

The amount of permanent functional impairment caused by a through-and-through low-velocity small-calibre projectile injury depends primarily on whether a joint has been violated and, if so, how much damage has been sustained by articular surfaces. Also involved in the prognosis is the amount of damage sustained by flexor and extensor tendons and neurosvascular structures.

Due to the comminution of a shaft fracture of a long bone in the hand (e.g., metacarpal or phalanx) (Figures 14-4A, 14-5C, 14-6C), conservative treatment

is usually indicated, which rarely may incorporate longitudinal dynamic skeletal traction.

Arthrotomy is indicated for joint damage, particularly if foreign bodies or bone fragments are retained intraarticularly (Figures 14-5A–F). Primary, delayed primary, or secondary surgery depends on the degree of wound contamination and is necessary to cleanse the joint of foreign particles as well as possible. In Figures 14-5A–F arthrotomy of the MP joint was performed through a palmar approach to irrigate and debride the joint completely of free metallic fragments and small free bone spicules.

Tenolysis may be necessary after healing has occurred to provide as much unrestricted tendon gliding as possible (Figures 14-6A–D). If bony spurs impinge upon a joint's range of motion, these should be removed simultaneously.

Low-velocity wounds caused by large-calibre projectiles and shotgun wounds cause much more localized trauma and increase the possibility of foreign bodies being driven in with the projectile, e.g., clothing or wadding from the shotgun shell.

Meticulous wound toilet and initial packing of the wound open is followed by delayed primary closure, split thickness skin graft resurfacing, or secondary closure.

High-velocity missile injuries are the most destructive type and cause great damage to the skeleton and soft tissue circumferentially around the projectile's passage (Figures 14-7A–C). Wide exposure of the path of the high-velocity missile is usually necessary to permit adequate debridement of nonviable soft tissue and bone and to decompress internal pressure. Lysis of all restricting structures, including fascia and skin, may be necessary to prevent ischemic changes due to vascular constriction in a closed compartment compression syndrome. The point of entrance is generally much smaller than the point of exit (Figures 14-7A,B), which is true also for large-calibre low-projectile missiles. Definitely contraindicated is a primary attempt to close the wound or to repair deeper structures initially. The primary treatment may include application of a split thickness skin graft to cover a large denuded area (Figure 14-7D).

If large bone fragments have been lost, skeletal length of a metacarpal, in particular, may be maintained either by dynamic skeletal traction (if vascularity is not impaired), transverse Kirschner wire fixation of the distal metacarpal shaft to the adjacent metacarpal or metacarpals, or by a metal spreader placed longitudinally in the area of bone loss exerting pressure on the proximal and distal metacarpal remnants.

Figure 14-4 (A) PA radiograph shows a comminuted, shortened fracture of index finger metacarpal shaft due to through-and-through 22-calibre projectile injury. MP joint does not appear to be violated. Note metallic fragments retained in soft tissue and bone. (B) PA radiograph 14 months after injury shows good healing of index metacarpal fracture with good alignment, some shortening, and retention of metallic fragments in soft tissue and skeleton. (C) Photograph shows excellent, although incomplete index MP flexion. Nearly complete extension (not shown).

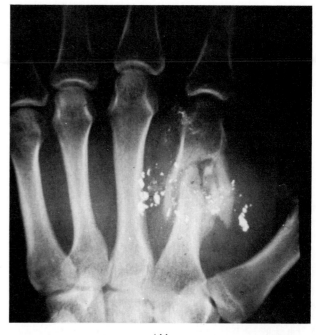

(A)

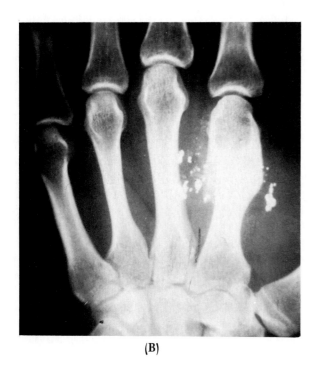

(B)

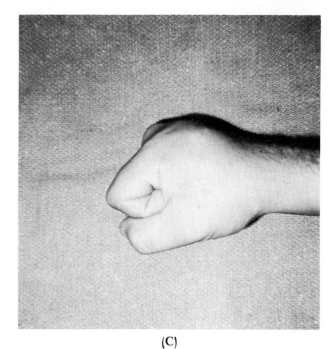

(C)

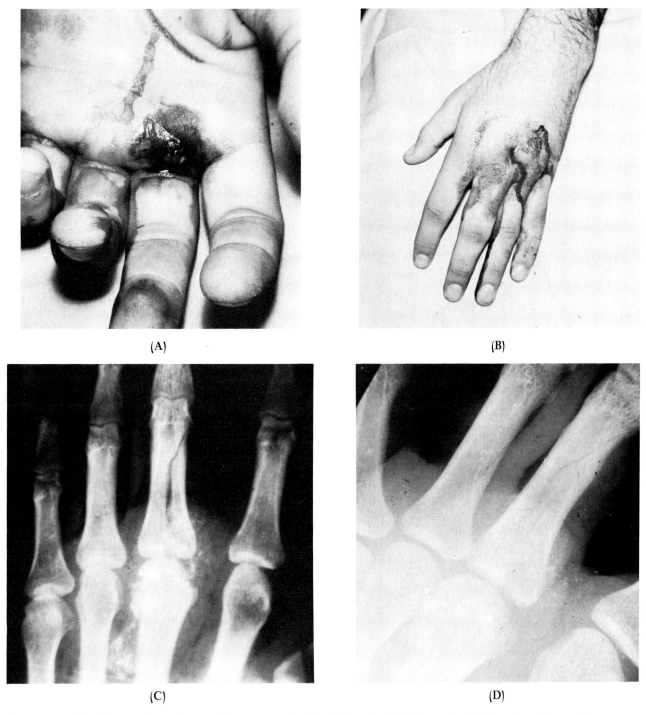

(A)

(B)

(C)

(D)

Figure 14-5 (A) Palmar view of point of entrance of a 38-calibre pistol bullet at level of proximal finger flexion crease of long finger. (B) Dorsal view showing point of exit at MP joint of long finger. Wound of exit is not larger than wound of entry, probably because of the close range, as indicated by powder burns on palmar view. (C) PA radiograph shows comminuted undisplaced fractures of long finger distal metacarpal and proximal phalanx, with long undisplaced articular oblique shaft fracture of proximal phalanx extending into MP joint. Multiple metallic foreign bodies are distributed through soft tissue and are retained in area of MP joint itself. (D) Oblique radiograph 2 weeks after surgery shows a diminished number of metallic fragments in soft tissue and none in MP joint. Healing of all fractures is progressing well, with no displacement.

(continued)

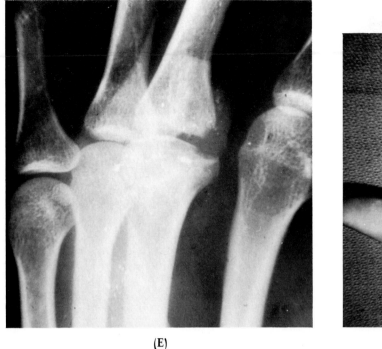

(E)

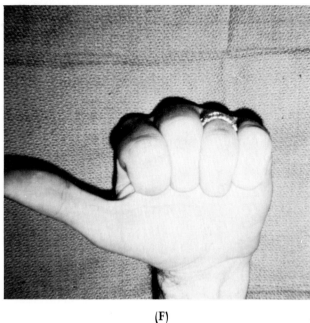

(F)

Figure 14-5 *(continued)*
(E) Oblique view one year later shows osteophyte protrusion on palmar radial aspect of long finger metacarpal metaphysis and a well-maintained cartilage space of MP joint. **(F)** Excellent flexion noted despite osteophyte visible in previous radiograph. Case illustrates importance of meticulous debridement of any joint involved in through-and-through projectile injury if foreign bodies and/or free bone fragments are retained intraarticularly. Initially no attempt was made to close either wound of entry or exit.

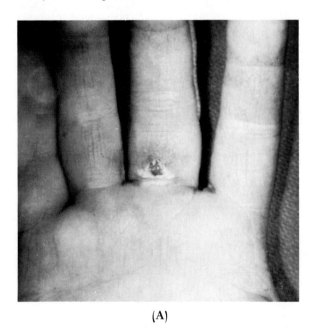

(A)

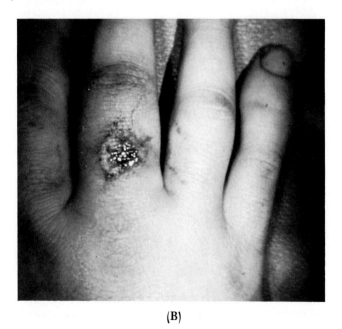

(B)

Figure 14-6 **(A)** Palmar view showing point of entrance of a 22-calibre pistol bullet at level of proximal finger flexion crease of long finger. **(B)** Characteristic larger point of exit on dorsal aspect of long finger proximal phalanx in midshaft.

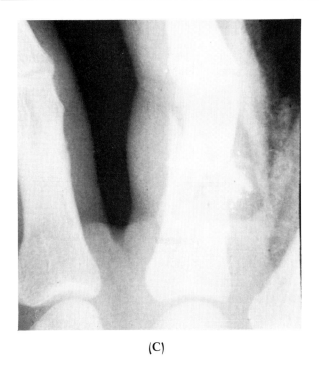

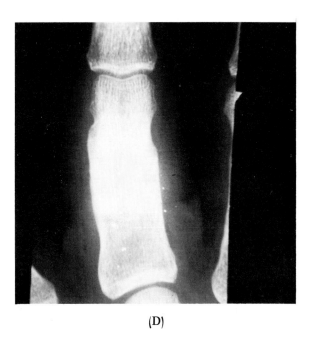

(C)   (D)

Figure 14-6 *(continued)*
(C) Radiograph shows comminuted, somewhat displaced fracture of long finger proximal phalanx with metallic fragments buried in bone and debris dorsal to shaft of phalanx. Initial treatment included cleansing, debridement, irrigation, and immobilization of long finger and index finger in functional position. **(D)** Reconstructive surgery 2½ months after injury included tenolysis of extensor, since incomplete extension and flexion resulted from binding down of this tendon in cicatrix, and debridement of bone spicules and metallic foreign bodies impinging on and binding extensor tendon. PA view shows solid healing of proximal phalangeal fractures.

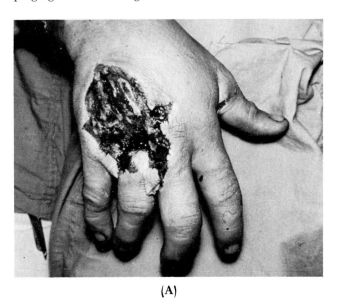

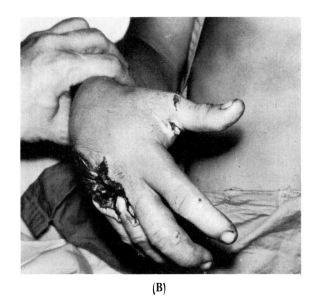

(A)   (B)

Figure 14-7 **(A)** Dorsal view of severe high-velocity through-and-through injury of hand. Small point of entrance noted on ulnar aspect of thumb in thumb-index web area. Large avulsive point of exit centered over ring finger metacarpal shaft area. Loss of extensor and flexor tendons and palmar proper digital nerve and vessels to ulnar aspect of ring finger; also large segmental bone loss of ring finger metacarpal. **(B)** Oblique view shows more clearly point of entrance in thumb-index web.

(continued)

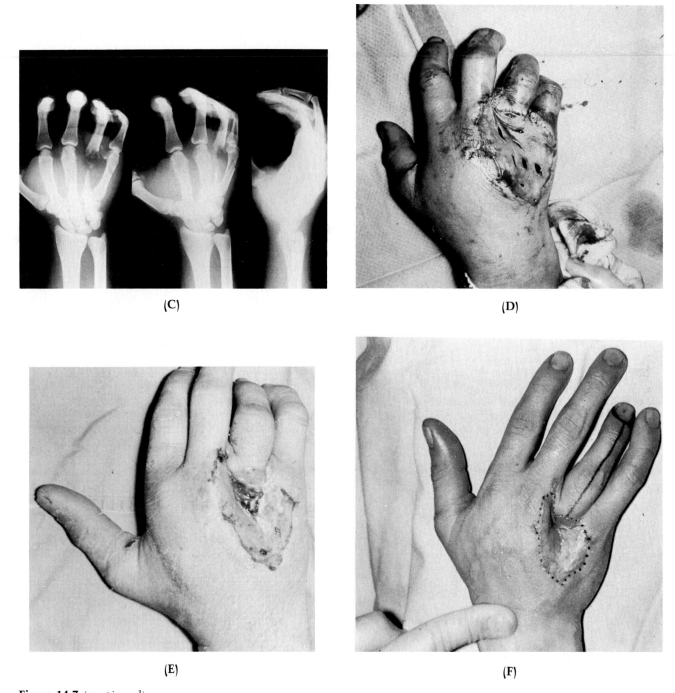

(C)

(D)

(E)

(F)

Figure 14-7 *(continued)*
(C) PA, oblique, and lateral radiographs illustrating absence of most of ring finger metacarpal and portion of base of proximal phalanx, and essentially undisplaced fractures of long and little finger metacarpals. **(D)** Initial treatment consisted of meticulous cleansing, debridement, and irrigation of wounds with application of a fenestrated split thickness skin graft as primary coverage. Note generalized edema of hand and digits. **(E)** Nearly complete wound healing 3 weeks after initial treatment. Generalized edema is still present but diminished. **(F)** Three months after initial injury this view shows complete subsidence of edema prior to reconstructive surgery. Note healed split thickness skin graft coverage, which has contracted about 40%, and marked shortening of ring finger.

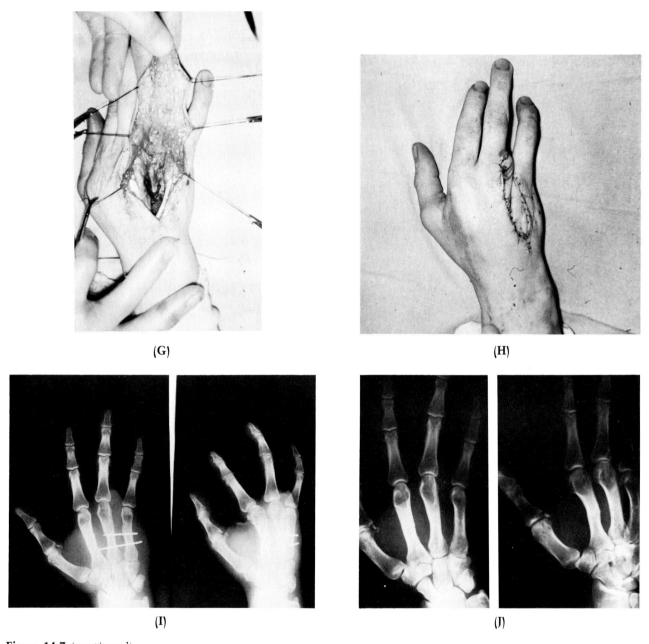

(G)

(H)

(I)

(J)

Figure 14-7 *(continued)*
(G) Filleted skin after deletion of entire ring finger ray (metacarpal, proximal, middle, and distal phalanges) and excision of split thickness skin graft. **(H)** Use of filleted skin to cover dorsal skin defect and transposition of entire little finger metacarpal into ring finger position with temporary internal transverse Kirschner wire fixation. No attempt was made to remove the "dog ear" at base of pedicle of filleted skin. **(I)** Transposed little finger metacarpal with transverse Kirschner wire temporary fixation. **(J)** Good alignment of all metacarpals after removal of temporary transverse Kirschner wire fixation 2½ months following deletion of ring ray.

(continued)

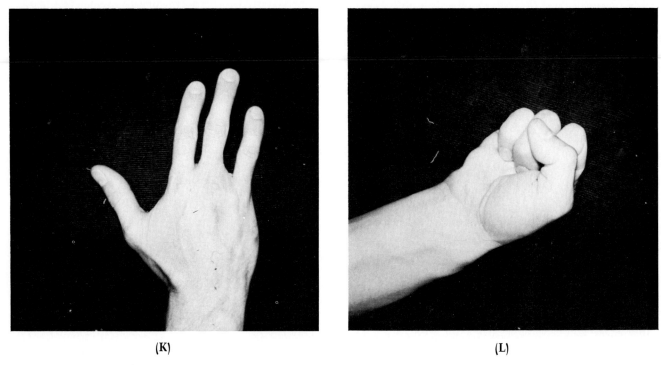

(K)　　　　　　　　　　　　　　　　　(L)

Figure 14-7 *(continued)*
(K) Dorsal view 10 months after reconstruction shows complete extension of all digits and good alignment of little finger with index and long fingers. **(L)** Palmar view illustrates essentially normal digital flexion.

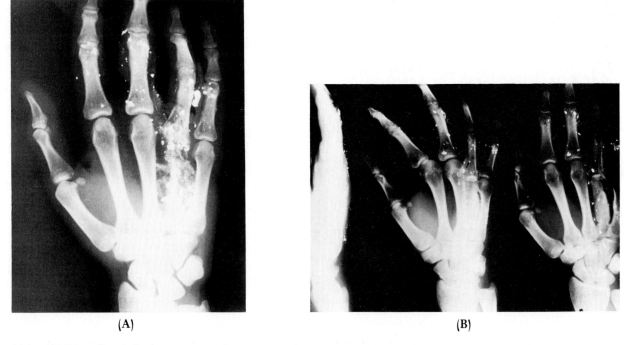

(A)　　　　　　　　　　　　　　　　　(B)

Figure 14-8 **(A)** PA radiograph shows severe destruction of ring finger with loss of much of its metacarpal, severe damage of MP joint, and fractures of proximal phalanx, with multiple retained metallic foreign bodies. Through-and-through injury was caused by a high-velocity projectile (AK 47 round). **(B)** Lateral, oblique, and PA radiographs of hand after reconstructive surgery show large iliac bone graft which was used to replace nearly absent ring finger metacarpal. There is shortening of ring finger and absence of MP joint.

Extensive bone and soft tissue reconstruction is deferred for secondary care until there has been satisfactory initial wound healing, subsidence of edema, and after maximum active and passive joint ranges of motion have been achieved (Figures 14-7E–L).

Some metacarpal shortening is acceptable (see Chapter 7, Metacarpal Fractures) but very large deficits must be treated by an autogenous bone graft as in Figures 14-8A,B, where an iliac bone graft replaced the ring finger metacarpal. Further reconstruction of this severely damaged digit would include arthroplasty and insertion of a silastic implant to fabricate a ring finger MP joint and extensor and flexor tendon grafts or tendon transfers to restore digital motion. Here reconstruction of the severely mutilated digit was chosen rather than deletion, with transfer of the little finger metacarpal into the ring finger position (Figures 14-7A–L). Many operative procedures are needed to restore a mutilated digit with gross lesions of multiple systems (skin, bone, tendon, and nerve) to even limited functional use.

If multiple systems have been irreparably damaged (flexor and extensor tendons, one or both neurovascular bundles, skeleton, and skin), deletion of the involved digit may be the best alternative. Deletion of either the long or ring finger ray is best managed by transposition of the adjacent marginal ray to correct the gap created (Figures 14-7A–L). If the little finger ray is deleted, it is most important to reinsert the hypothenar muscles onto the base of the ring finger proximal phalanx. If this muscle mass cannot work across a joint, the entire hypothenar muscle compartment will atrophy. The same is true for index ray deletion and transfer of the first dorsal interosseous insertion into the base of the long finger proximal phalanx.

General References

Burkhalter WE, Butler B, Metz W, et al: Experiences with delayed primary closure of war wounds of the hand in Vietnam. *J Bone Joint Surg* 1968;50-A:95.

DeMuth WE, Smith JM: High velocity bullet wounds of muscle and bone: The basis of rational early treatment. *J Trauma* 1966;6:744–755.

Jabaley ME, Peterson HD: Early treatment of war wounds of the hand and forearm in Vietnam. *Ann Surg* 1973;177:167–173.

Swan KG, Swan RC: *Gunshot Wounds Pathophysiology and Management.* Littleton, MA, PSG Publishing Company, Inc, 1980.

CHAPTER
15

Multiple Fractures

In the hand or digit which has sustained multiple injuries, each fracture, dislocation, or fracture dislocation must be treated appropriately as a separate entity (Figures 15-1A–D, 15-9C–G).

Mismanagement of multiple hand injuries results in prolonged morbidity, malunion, infection, and limited motion both of the injured digit(s) and adjacent normal digits. Reconstructive procedures are often necessary to restore function as well as possible (Figures 15-2A–H, 15-3A–F).

The responsibility for the ultimate functional result of a multiply injured digit, hand, extremity, or bilateral upper extremities often lies with the physician who treats the injury initially. This is particularly true with open injuries involving primary open reduction and internal fixation of fractures. The physician who provides initial definitive treatment is responsible for accurate diagnosis of the injury or injuries and the appropriate management (Figures 15-4A–C). The case illustrated in Figures 15-3A–F is an example of unnecessary surgery of a long finger metacarpal shaft fracture, complicated by improper external immobilization with all MP joints in exten-

sion. Results would have been much better with no medical care at all.

Multiple skeletal injuries must be suspected in a severely injured digit (Figures 15-5A,B, 15-8A–E, and Figure 8-11B in Chapter 8), a severely injured hand (Figures 15-3A–F, 15-4A–C, 15-7A,B, 15-9A–G, 15-11A–E), and elsewhere in the ipsilateral upper extremity (refer to Figures 2-28A–D in Chapter 2) and the contralateral (refer to Figures 5-5A–E in Chapter 5).

Multiple articular fractures are not common but the general rules of treatment apply. Undisplaced or relatively undisplaced articular fractures are treated conservatively (Figure 15-6); large displaced articular fractures (usually over 25% to 30% of the articular surface) should be anatomically reduced, usually by surgical exposure and internal fixation.

Before definitive treatment of multiple fractures in a severely injured hand, a waiting period of five to six days is often indicated to permit subsidence of edema and congestion (Figure 15-7A). Initially a large, bulky compressive dressing with appropriate plaster splint or cast immobilization and constant elevation achieves this result and allows later applica-

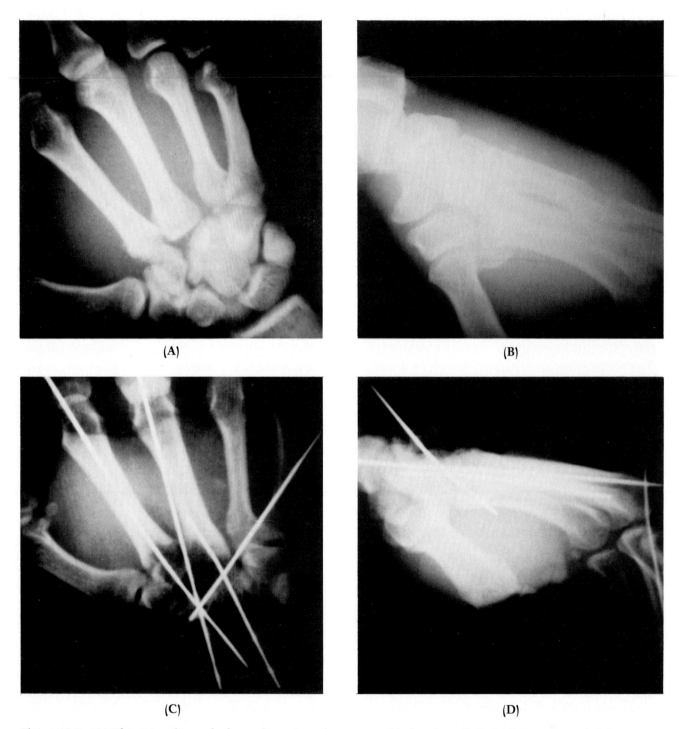

(A)

(B)

(C)

(D)

Figure 15-1 **(A)** This PA radiograph shows distortion of anatomy of index through little finger metacarpal bases with disorientation of trapezium and trapezoid as well as palmar subluxation of the long finger MP joint. **(B)** Corresponding lateral radiograph illustrates complete anterior fracture dislocation of index and long metacarpal bases with a segment of the trapezoid. **(C)** Anatomic relocation of the segmental fracture of the index metacarpal proximal metaphysis; the trapezium; the trapezoid; long, ring, and little finger metacarpal bases; and long finger MP joint, stabilized by multiple Kirschner wire fixations. **(D)** Corresponding lateral view shows same anatomic reductions with skeletal fixations. This case demonstrates the importance of accurate radiographs to properly diagnose multiple skeletal injuries for anatomic reductions and appropriate fixations.

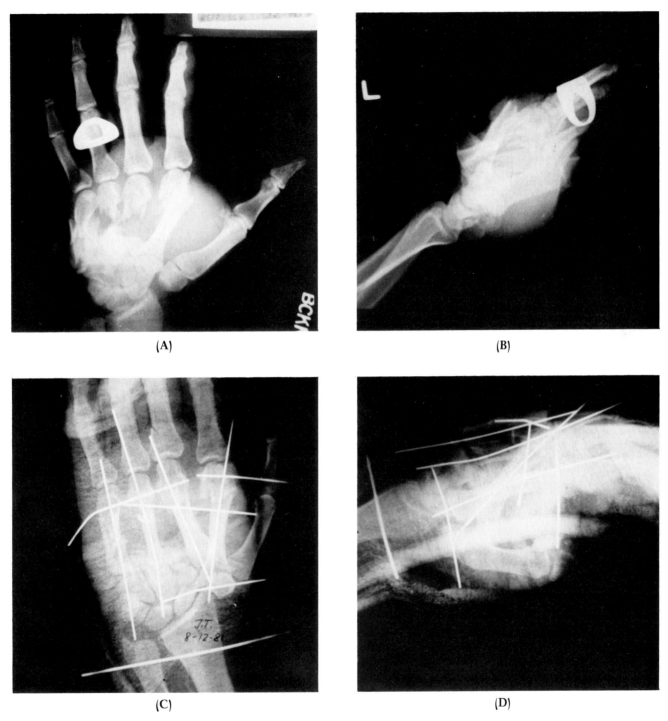

(A)

(B)

(C)

(D)

Figure 15-2 (A) Massive skeletal trauma to the metacarpus sustained in a motor vehicle accident including multiple metacarpal fractures and loss of segments of the long and ring finger metacarpals. (B) Corresponding lateral view. (C) Status after "reduction and fixation" of the multiple fractures. It should be noted that there is absolutely no change in the positions of the metacarpals when compared to Figure 15-2A. (D) Corresponding lateral view. This is an example of ill advised inadequate treatment of a severe injury in which fracture and joint reductions were never achieved and immobilization techniques not only were ineffective but technically ill-conceived and erroneous.

(continued)

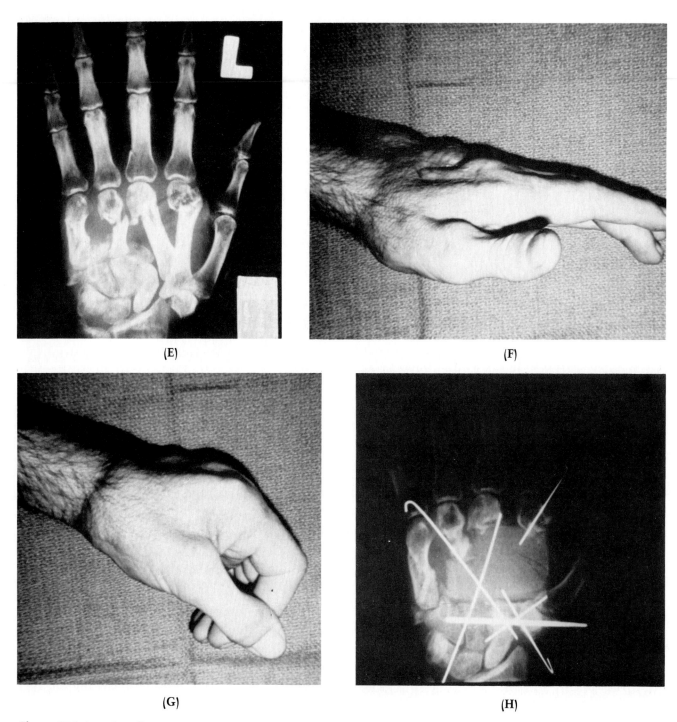

(E) (F)

(G) (H)

Figure 15-2 *(continued)*
(E) Six months after initial treatment skeletal positions of the metacarpals are exactly the same as those on the initial radiograph (Figure 15-2A). **(F)** Digital extension at this time noted on radial view. **(G)** Digital flexion. Grossly impaired function resulted because of non-unions, instability of metacarpal bases, and extension contractures of the MP joints. **(H)** Reconstruction of this mutilated hand included insertion of a massive iliac bone graft to provide stability for the central metacarpus and attempted reduction and fixation of the thumb unit. This case demonstrates the prolonged morbidity and grossly impaired hand function specifically because of improper inadequate initial treatment of extensive skeletal pathology.

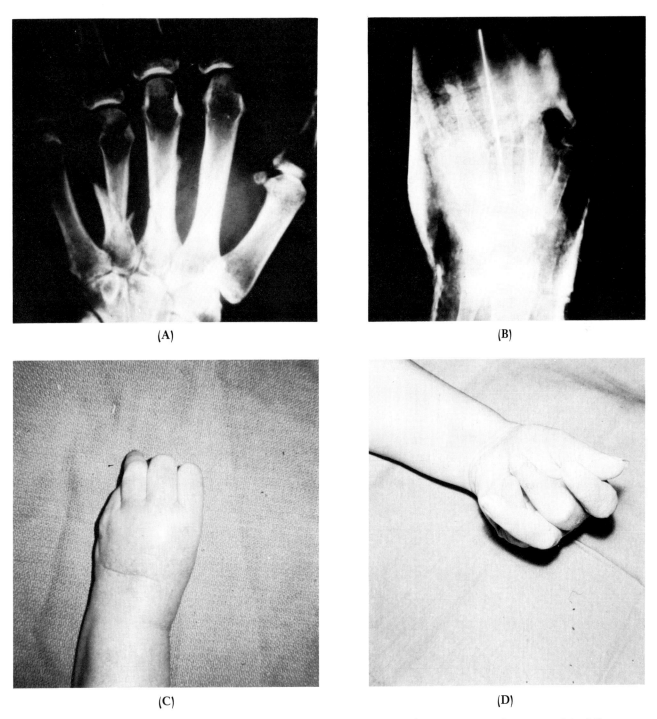

(A)

(B)

(C)

(D)

Figure 15-3 **(A)** Comminuted, impacted shaft fractures of long and ring finger metacarpals sustained in fall. **(B)** Unnecessary longitudinal Kirschner wire fixation of long finger metacarpal shaft fracture, with all MP joints incorrectly immobilized in complete extension. **(C)** Extension contractures of all MP joints, divergence of long and ring fingers, and gross edema persisted for 2½ months after the original injury and surgery. Attempt to make a fist shows minimal MP flexion due to improper surgical immobilization of long finger metacarpal shaft fracture and improper external cast immobilization of all MP joints in extension for a total of 5 weeks. **(D)** Attempt at flexion 3½ months later shows subsidence of edema and divergence of long and ring fingers, with impingement of little finger beneath ring finger.

(continued)

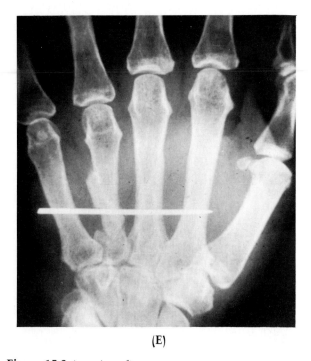

(E)

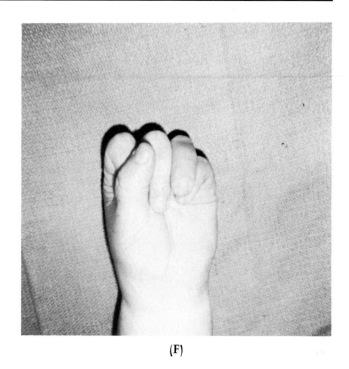

(F)

Figure 15-3 *(continued)*
(E) PA radiograph after reconstructive rotational osteotomy of ring finger metacarpal. **(F)** Complete digital extension attained 10 months after surgery. Acceptable flexion of all digits resulted with some residual crossover of little finger and incomplete MP flexion.

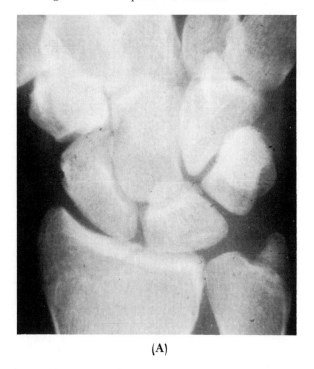

(A)

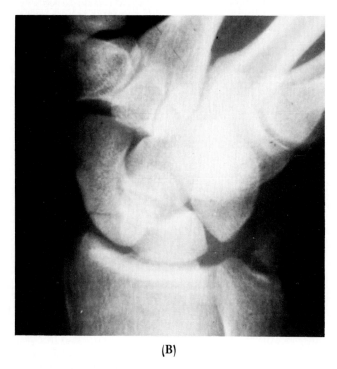

(B)

Figure 15-4 **(A)** High-pressure injection injury in palm thought to be due to leak in an air hose. However, symptoms of pain and tenderness were in area of wrist, *not* in area of laceration. PA radiograph disclosed fracture of ulnar styloid process and undisplaced fracture of distal radius, with possible undisplaced fracture of scaphoid. **(B)** Scaphoid view shows definite fracture through proximal third of scaphoid.

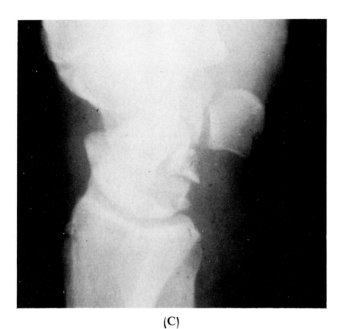

(C)

Figure 15-4 *(continued)*
(C) Lateral view shows displaced palmar lip fracture of anterior lunate articular surface. Hand actually had been blown against a metal stanchion by a loose high-pressure air hose which had suddenly developed a leak. Various views were necessary for accurate diagnosis. Scaphoid fracture treatment was 8 weeks of immobilization; no treatment necessary for displaced lunate fracture. Normal function resulted.

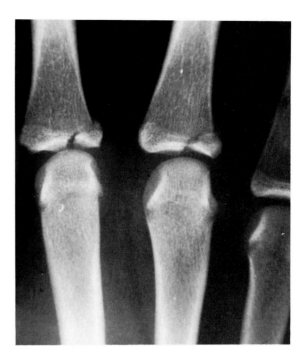

Figure 15-6 Minimally displaced articular fractures of index and long finger proximal phalangeal bases treated by 3 weeks of immobilization in functional position.

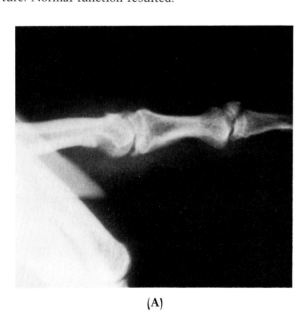

(A)

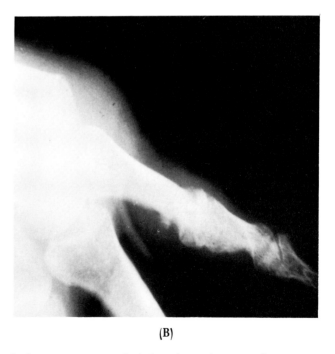

(B)

Figure 15-5 **(A)** Lateral radiograph of multiple injuries of little finger. Injuries included avulsion fracture of large articular fragment from dorsum of distal phalanx, palmar chip fracture of palmar plate attachment to middle phalanx, distal shaft fracture of proximal phalanx, and fracture of distal metacarpal metaphysis or neck. **(B)** Oblique view emphasizing metacarpal fracture, palmarly angulated approximately 60°, and distal shaft fracture of proximal phalanx. Successful closed treatment for all four fractures in finger.

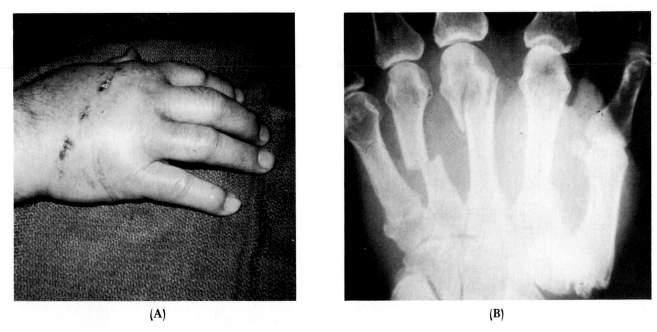

(A)

(B)

Figure 15-7 (A) Oblique view of massively edematous and congested hand resulting from a severe fall by a 64-year-old man in mild congestive heart failure. (B) PA radiograph shows relatively undisplaced oblique comminuted fracture of long finger metacarpal distal metaphysis, somewhat displaced transverse fracture of ring finger metacarpal midshaft, and undisplaced fracture of little finger metacarpal base. Grasp was nearly normal following therapy after 2½ weeks of physiologic immobilization and elevation. Thumb metacarpal base not fractured but shows evidence of severe degenerative and posttraumatic arthritic changes.

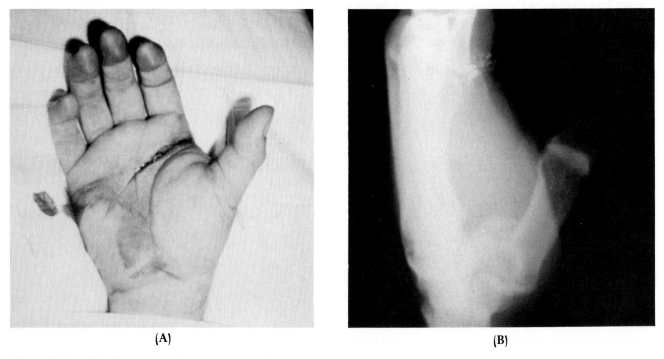

(A)

(B)

Figure 15-8 (A) Palmar view of open extensively contaminated crush injury with thumb MP joint dislocation and displaced Bennett's fracture of the thumb metacarpal base. (B) PA view of the thumb illustrates radial displacement of the thumb metacarpal base and skeletal overlapping at the MP joint area.

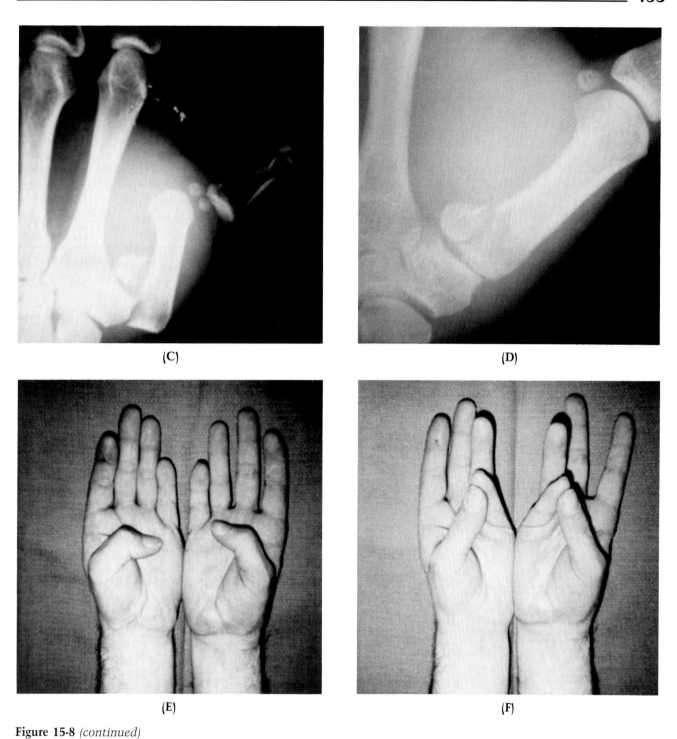

(C)   (D)

(E)   (F)

Figure 15-8 *(continued)*
(C) Lateral view of the thumb shows complete dislocation of both MP and carpometacarpal joints of the thumb. **(D)** Following meticulous wound toilet reduction of the fractures was achieved and splint immobilization provided with the thumb in abduction and opposition. Both the reduced MP joint and Bennett's fracture proved to be stable and healed without further treatment. **(E)** Three months later opposition of both thumbs is compared; the injured thumb on the right. **(F)** Thumb flexion.

(continued)

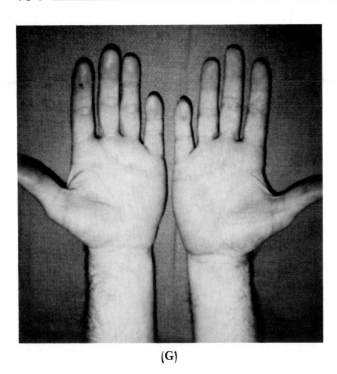

(G)

Figure 15-8 *(continued)*
(G) Thumb extension.

tion of a well-molded, snugly fitting plaster cast (Figures 15-8A–G).

Also, if open reduction is necessary for one or more of the fractures after subsidence of edema and congestion, the severely traumatized soft tissues will be less susceptible to possible bacterial invasion. If the physician suspects wound contamination, delayed primary closure should usually precede any open treatment of the fracture or fractures.

Often multiple varying methods of treatment are carried out for different fractures or dislocations of the same hand.[1] A combination of closed reduction, closed reduction and percutaneous fixation, open reduction and percutaneous fixation, and open reduction and internal fixation may be carried out for different wounds of the same hand (Figures 15-9A–G, 15-10A–D).

In the multiply injured elderly or chronically ill person, partial reductions with external immobilization at times may be accepted rather than subjecting the patient to surgery to attain anatomic reductions (Figures 15-7A,B).

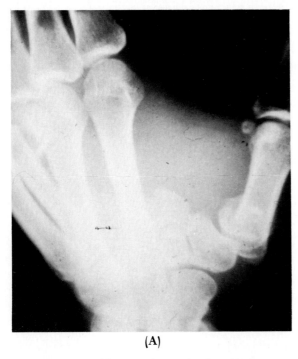

(A)

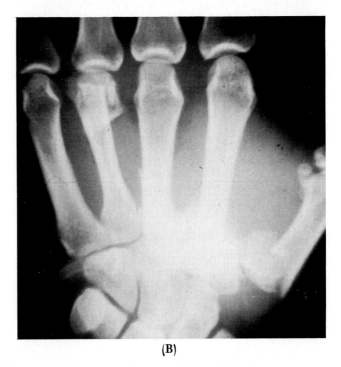

(B)

Figure 15-9 **(A)** Oblique radiograph of multiple metacarpal fractures: palmar angulation and dorsal displacement of proximal metaphysis of thumb metacarpal; dorsal displacement of proximal metaphyseal fractures of index and long finger metacarpals; and palmarly angulated displaced fracture of ring finger distal metaphysis or neck. **(B)** PA view shows displacement of ring finger metacarpal at distal metaphysis.

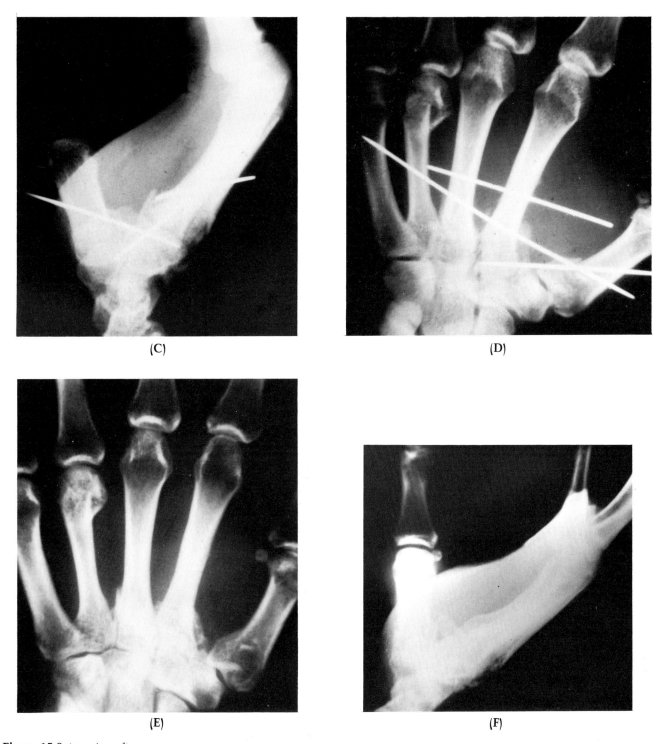

(C)

(D)

(E)

(F)

Figure 15-9 *(continued)*
(C) Lateral radiograph after open reduction of index and long metacarpal fractures with percutaneous Kirschner wire fixation, closed reduction of thumb metacarpal proximal metaphyseal fracture with percutaneous Kirschner wire immobilization, and closed manipulation and reduction of ring finger distal metaphyseal fracture. **(D)** Oblique radiograph. **(E)** PA radiograph 3 months after injury shows some shortening of ring finger metacarpal due to comminuted distal metaphyseal fracture. **(F)** Simultaneous lateral view.

(continued)

Figure 15-9 *(continued)*
(G) Ulnar view 8 months after injury shows MP and IP flexion. Note slight recession of ring finger metacarpal head. Complete extension of all digits was achieved, except little finger, which sustained large skin and partial extensor tendon loss over radial aspect of middle and distal phalanges, treated initially by split thickness skin graft coverage.

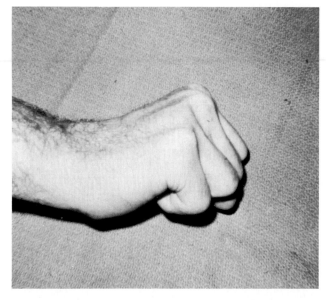

(G)

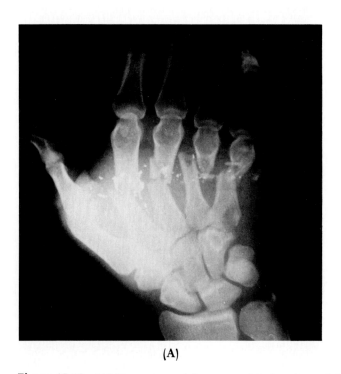

(A)

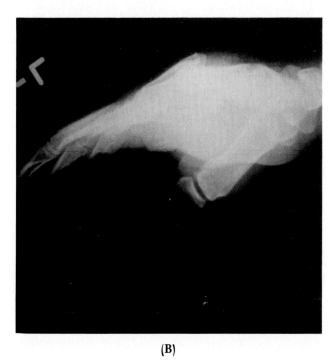

(B)

Figure 15-10 **(A)** Comminuted fractures of index through little finger metacarpals resulting from transverse passage of a .38 caliber bullet directly across the metacarpus. **(B)** Lateral view.

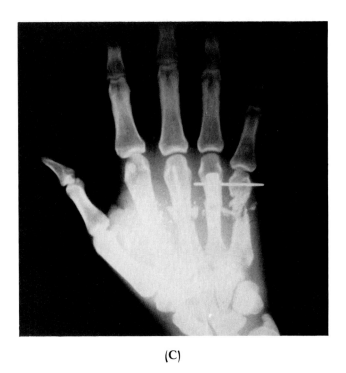

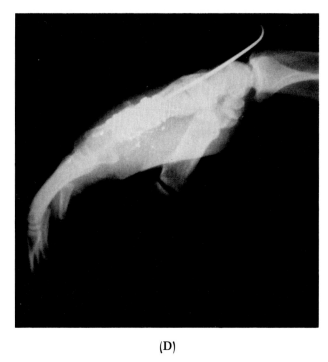

(C)   (D)

Figure 15-10 *(continued)*
(C) Combination of fixation techniques restored and maintained anatomic metacarpal architecture as well as possible. One additional transverse Kirschner wire was placed from the little finger metacarpal head into the ring and long finger metacarpals. **(D)** Corresponding lateral view.

In all patients, but particularly those suffering from or prone to develop degenerative joint changes, it is important to mobilize all joints not immobilized in the treatment of a multiply injured hand and to commence light active and passive motion in the injured digit or digits as soon as feasible (Figures 15-7A,B).

Certain general rules apply to multiple fractures in open injuries (Figures 15-4A–C, 15-8, 15-9, 15-10, 15-11A–E):

1. Meticulous wound toilet, including cleansing, irrigation and debridement, is vitally important
2. With precarious viability, additional surgical exposure of the wound and prolonged extensive surgical procedures are contraindicated
3. Internal fixation should be used with discretion

Temporary longitudinal Kirschner wire fixation is often very valuable to grossly align severely comminuted open fractures, particularly those with precarious viability (refer to Figures 11-34A–C in Chapter 11, Physeal Injuries). This initial treatment may yield excellent results with no necessary reconstructive surgery (Figures 15-11A–E). In the nearly amputated digit which survives but which lacks extensor and flexor tendons and has sustained joint damage, arthrodesis of appropriate joints may be the best solution.

In multiple digital injuries salvage of those digits with precarious viability is often successful (Figures 15-11A–E), although some distal necrosis may result. Reimplantation will not be discussed other than to mention that priorities for reimplantation include the thumb, any digit in a child, and as many digits as possible in multiple amputations. In an adult, reimplantation of a single digit other than the thumb is discouraged; even in the case of two amputated digits, the practicality of reimplantation is questionable. In general, reimplantation should not be performed for amputations at or distal to the DIP joint or in severe crushing type injuries in which massive soft tissue trauma occurs. Reimplantation demands anastamosis of one vein for each artery and, if necessary, arterial reconstruction by a free vein graft. Skeletal shortening of the digit or extremity may be necessary to enable anastamosis of potentially viable soft tissue after debridement proximally and distally.

Figure 15-11 (A) Multiple open severe injuries of thumb, index, long, and ring fingers from a ripsaw: near amputation of the index finger through PIP joint and long finger through middle phalanx; complete laceration of flexor tendons and palmar proper neurovascular bundle to ulnar aspect of index finger (noted during exploration); incomplete laceration of flexor tendons of long finger and palmar proper digital nerve to its ulnar aspect, and deep pulp laceration of thumb distal phalanx and ring finger distal phalanx. (B) Lateral radiograph after debridement, irrigation, cleansing, open reduction, and longitudinal fixation of long finger comminuted middle phalangeal fracture shown superiorly and of fracture dislocation of index finger PIP joint shown inferiorly. Loose primary skin closures were used. (C) PA radiograph 5 weeks after surgery following removal of temporary Kirschner wire fixations of index and long fingers shows good healing of long finger middle phalangeal fracture and good alignment of its PIP and DIP joints, and some ulnar displacement after reduction of index finger PIP joint fracture dislocation.

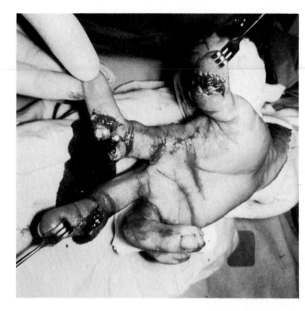

(A)

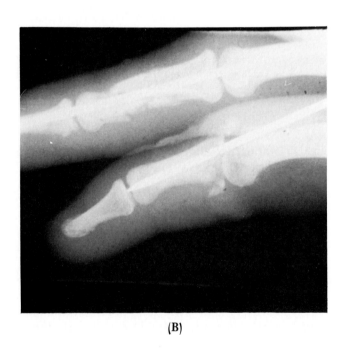

(B)

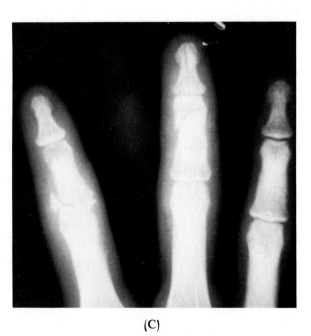

(C)

Since reimplantation is performed in few hospitals, the patient and the amputated segment(s) must be transported as quickly as possible to a suitably equipped institution with adequately trained surgeons. The amputated segment(s) should be wrapped in sterile gauze, saturated with normal sterile saline or other physiologic solution, and placed in a plastic bag which is put on the surface of ice in an ice chest, *not dry ice*. The specimen definitely should not be frozen or kept at room temperature.

Multiple injuries may involve areas of the same extremity (refer to Figures 2-28A–D and Figure 8-11B) or involve the contralateral upper extremity (Figures 5-5A–E). After satisfactory examination of the obviously injured area, attention should be directed to other areas of the upper extremity, particularly the wrist, elbow, and shoulder. Only in this way can fractures of the radial head and coronoid process at the elbow and fractures about the shoulder be diagnosed accurately. The patient who has sustained

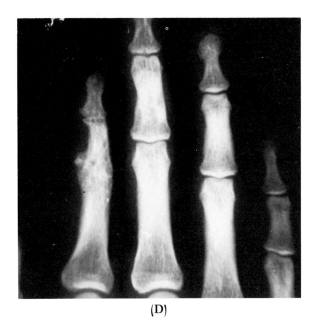

(D)

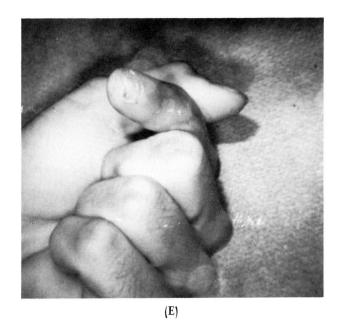

(E)

Figure 15-11 *(continued)*
(D) PA radiograph 2½ months after attempted arthrodesis of PIP and DIP joints of index finger shows fusion of PIP joint and a stable pseudoarthrosis of DIP joint, with excellent healing and remodeling of long finger middle phalangeal fracture. **(E)** Normal flexion of long finger PIP and DIP joints resulted. Strong, stable, sensible index finger pinch followed PIP joint fusion in physiologic flexion.

multiple injuries should be periodically reexamined and reevaluated to diagnose injuries initially occult or overlooked in the initial treatment of other massive injuries (Figures 2-28A–D in Chapter 2) or in life-threatening situations.

References

1. Sandzén SC Jr: Complex injuries of the wrist and hand, in Meyers MH (ed): *The Multiply Injured Patient With Complex Fractures.* Philadelphia, Lea & Febiger, 1984, pp 365–400.

CHAPTER 16

External, Percutaneous and Internal Skeletal Fixation

This chapter hopefully provides a commonsense approach to the use of Kirschner wires, plates, screws, "pins and plaster" fixation, external fixators, pull out wires, dynamic skeletal traction and intraosseous wiring techniques applicable to the distal forearm, wrist and hand.[1]

Open Fractures

As described elsewhere, immediate meticulous wound toilet is the principal concern in treating open fractures. Skeletal stability should be provided as soon as possible. The two principal considerations for primary internal fixation in an open wound are the degree of wound contamination and how precarious the blood supply is to tissues distal to an unstable fracture or dislocation.

If satisfactory wound toilet has been effected and neither the history, mechanism of injury nor the findings at debridement, cleansing and irrigation indicate excessive contamination, primary internal fixation is recommended. In the face of massive contamination, however, delayed primary fracture fixation is indicated (refer to Figure 3-1A in Chapter 3, Injuries to the Distal Radius and Ulna) at the time of redebridement if the wound remains clean with no evidence of infection or further tissue necrosis.

At the time of initial treatment, an alternative is the use of external percutaneous immobilization in the form of an external fixator or pins-and-plaster immobilization. With either method, particularly the former, frequent dressing changes and redebridements are easily carried out. Antibiotics should be employed with open wounds of any appreciable severity and certainly with contaminated wounds. An initial intravenous dose of 1 gm of a cephalosporin is given in the emergency room and a second gram intraoperatively prior to tourniquet inflation. Coverage continues 48 to 72 hours postoperatively unless infection becomes evident.

Radius and Ulna

Dynamic compression plate (DCP) fixation is strongly recommended for diaphyseal fractures of both the radius and ulna.[2,3] Technically, in treating a both bone fracture of the forearm, both fractures should be reduced simultaneously, the easier fracture first. Temporary fixation with bone holding clamps or with one screw on each side of the fracture site of each fracture precedes permanent plate fixations. If, instead one fracture is definitively plated first, the other shaft fracture may prove to be irreducible (Figure 16-1).

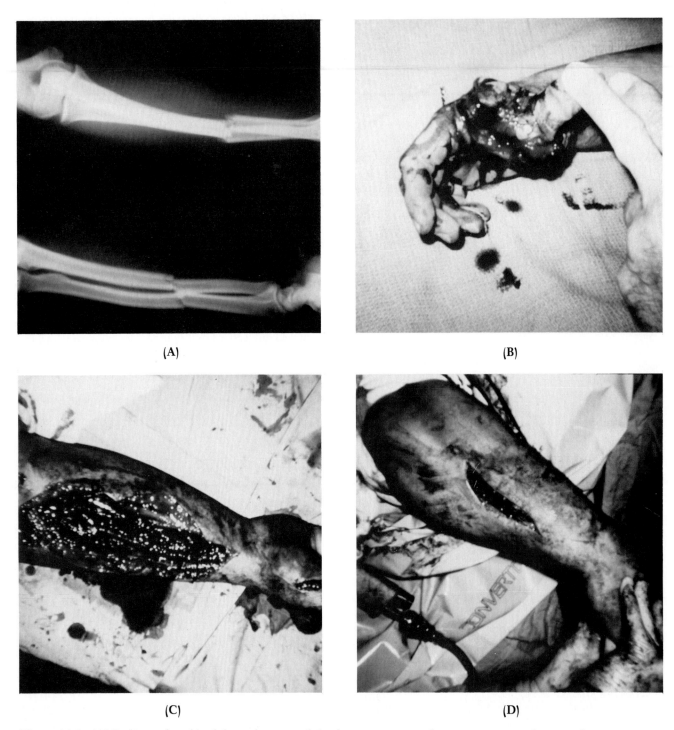

(A)

(B)

(C)

(D)

Figure 16-1 (**A**) Radiographs of both-bone fracture of the forearm sustained in a massive crush injury between a heavy engine suspended on a cable and a concrete pillar. (**B**) Simultaneous open near avulsion of the thumb at the MP joint level. (**C**) Because of the nature of the injury and all the physical findings of a closed compartment syndrome of the forearm radical-fascial lyses were effected at the time of primary reductions and plate fixations of both fractures. (**D**) Dorsal view showing incision for exploration of the dorsal forearm including fascial lyses and plate fixations.

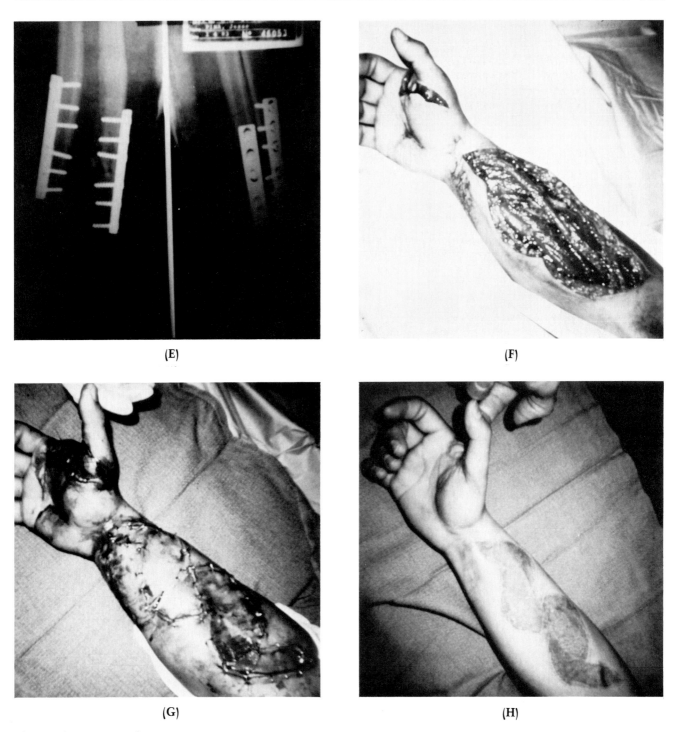

(E) (F)

(G) (H)

Figure 16-1 *(continued)*
(E) Stable plate fixations. **(F)** Status at the completion of second redebridement five days after the original wound shows all soft tissue of forearm clean with no evidence of infection or additional tissue necrosis. The thumb is viable. **(G)** Split thickness skin graft resurfacing of the forearm and multiple thumb defects. **(H)** Healed status prior to thumb reconstruction. All forearm muscles remained viable and fully functional after rehabilitation.

A minimum of three screws proximally and three screws distally when using a 4.5 mm plate and four screws proximally and distally with a 3.5 mm plate are recommended. A comminuted or "butterfly" fragment obviously necessitates a longer plate for secure fixation. The simultaneous introduction of an autogenous bone graft depends upon the personal preference of the treating physician but is recommended with comminuted fractures or with a bone deficit in a clean wound. To prevent radio-ulnar synostosis, the graft should be placed away from the interosseous membrane.

Though longitudinal intramedullary fixation of a diaphyseal fracture of either the radius or the ulna has been recommended in the past, this is generally contraindicated and plate fixation offers a much more stable fixation with impaction at the fracture site (Figure 16-2A).

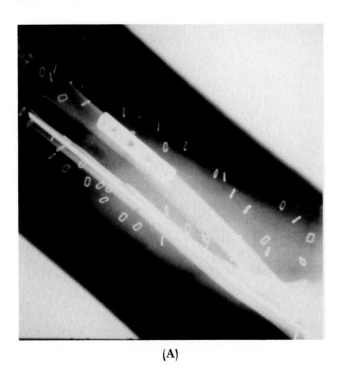

(A)

(B)

(C)

Figure 16-2 **(A)** Radiograph of skeletal fixation includes plate fixation of the radius and longitudinal intramedullary rod fixation of the ulna. A severe crush injury of the forearm was sustained with simultaneous distal radial and metacarpal fractures. The associated fractures were manipulated and reduced closed.
(B) Status two days after injury shows massive swelling and tense non-pitting edema with venous congestion of the palmar forearm. **(C)** Similar appearances noted on the dorsum with the open site of fracture of the radius and location of plate fixation. Note the massive edema of the dorsum of the hand and the intrinsic minus position of the digits.

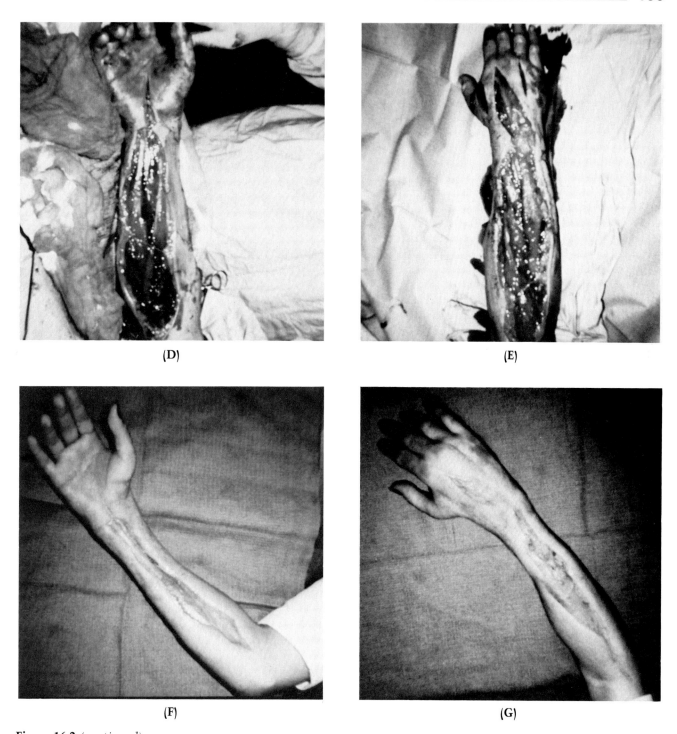

(D)

(E)

(F)

(G)

Figure 16-2 *(continued)*
(D) Radical fascial lyses of entire forearm and all palmar compartments of the hand revealed necrosis of the deep muscle bellies (flexor digitorum profundus, flexor pollicis longus and pronator quadratus). **(E)** Similar fascial lyses of the dorsal forearm and all interosseous compartments of the dorsum of the hand showed some necrosis of the extensor muscle mass. **(F)** Healed status after split thickness skin grafts, palmar aspect. **(G)** Simultaneous dorsal view. After multiple reconstructive procedures gross digital flexion and extension resulted.

A far greater concern, however, with the use of longitudinal internal fixation of a diaphyseal fracture of the radius or ulna is the possibility of developing a closed compartment syndrome since the operative approach for this technique does not include fascial lysis at exposure (Figures 16-2A–G).

Reconstructively for delayed or non-union debridement of bone ends down to clean viable appearing bleeding cortex after release of the tourniquet precedes interposition of a large iliac bone graft supplemented with cancellous bone combined with plate fixation. Plate removal should not be performed under one year following application to avoid stress fracture.

Fractures of the Distal Radius

First and foremost, differentiation of distal metaphyseal fractures from segmental articular fractures of the distal radius is essential for proper treatment (refer to Chapter 3, Injuries to the Distal Radius and Ulna). The majority of distal radial metaphyseal fractures can usually be managed by closed manipulation reduction and external splint or cast immobilization in the elderly population. However, a comminuted shortened and/or displaced fracture in a physiologically young person often is best treated by either pins-and-plaster or by external fixation technique.

The technique for pins-and-plaster fixation is presented in Chapter 3. It is important that the proximal pin be placed in the shaft of the radius proximal to the fracture site, *not the ulna* (Figure 16-3). The radial nerve and/or branches and adjacent soft tissues must be protected by open surgical exposure down to bone using a drill guide, and the segment of pin extending through the shaft of the radius should be threaded but the remainder extending through the soft tissue and skin smooth (e.g., modified Haggie pin). The distal pin (a smooth Kirschner wire) must not impinge upon the thumb-index web or the extensor tendons. Immobilization must continue for a minimum of eight to 10 weeks.

Use of the external fixator techniques demands appropriate expertise (Figure 16-4) to properly place the proximal and distal pins. As noted, the proximal pins are placed in the radius by open surgical exposure to protect the radial nerve and all soft tissues. If the Roger Anderson apparatus is used, pins must be sufficiently strong to prevent breakage (Figure 16-5).

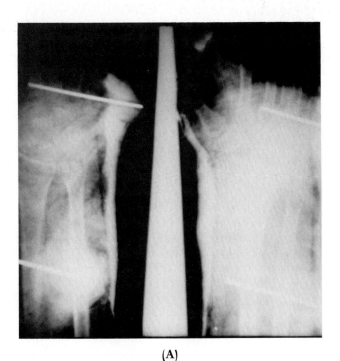

(A)

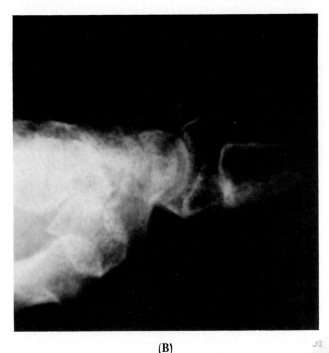

(B)

Figure 16-3 **(A)** Inappropriate use of pins and plaster fixation in which the proximal pin is placed in the ulna and the distal pin in the long and ring metacarpal bases. **(B)** Lateral radiograph after healing shows malunion with shortening of the radius and dorsal angulation of the distal radial articular surface with secondary rotational instabilities of the scaphoid and lunate.

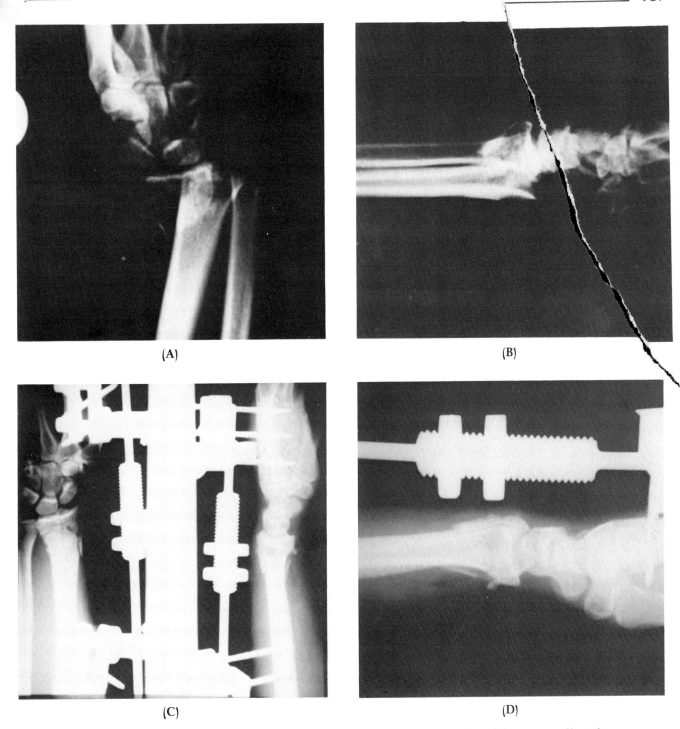

(A)

(B)

(C)

(D)

Figure 16-4 **(A)** Oblique view of comminuted unstable dorsal distal radial metaphyseal fracture (Colles's fracture). **(B)** Corresponding lateral view illustrates dorsal displacement and comminution. **(C)** External fixator technique following closed reduction shows acceptable length and position of the distal radial metaphysis ...stored. **(D)** Close-up of the lateral view shows excellent restoration of anatomy except for loss of palmar ...ulation of the distal radial articular surface. *(Figures 16-4A–D courtesy of O. Ogunro, M.D.)*

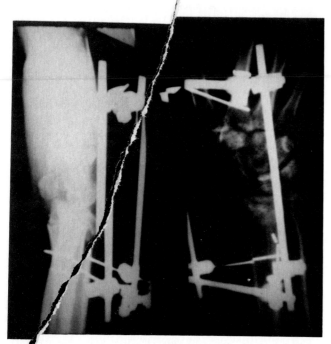

Figure 16-5 Roger Anderson external fixation with stress fracture of proximal pins which are of a too narrow caliber.

A buttress plate may be preferred to stabilize a palmarly displaced distal metaphyseal fracture and less commonly for similar treatment of the dorsal variant. A bone graft is usually necessary to fill the bony defect.

In the latter case, since the extensor tendons are subjected to chronic irritation causing attrition and possible rupture, removal of the dorsal buttress plate is necessary after fracture healing.

Treatment of a segmental articular fracture of the distal radius is often either by internal or percutaneous Kirschner wire fixation after anatomic reduction. A buttress plate may be preferred to immobilize the palmar segmental articular fracture (refer to Figure 3-24 in Chapter 3, Injuries to the Distal Radius and Ulna) and less commonly for the dorsal variant with the necessity for later plate removal as noted above. If anatomy of the distal radial articular surface can be restored by Chinese finger trap traction, pins-and-plaster immobilization may be preferred.

Wrist Joint

Restoration of the distal radial articular surface (comminuted distal metaphyseal fractures including the articular surface and segmental articular fractures of the distal radius) is necessary in acute injury to minimize posttraumatic arthritis and to restore functional wrist motion. Reconstructively for symptomatic posttraumatic arthritic changes of the wrist joint, the choice rests between arthroplasty (proximal row carpectomy with or without silastic hinged implant arthroplasty) or arthrodesis.

In the average person, wrist arthrodesis can be accomplished successfully by any number of methods (e.g., dorsal sliding graft, iliac bone graft, Kirschner wire fixation, screw fixation or plate fixation). However, in a spastic patient (e.g., postcerebral vascular accident or cerebral palsy patient) secure DCP fixation extending from the distal radius across the carpus and on to the third metacarpal is mandatory preferably with three screws proximally and distally combined with an iliac bone graft (Figure 16-6).[4]

Carpus

Anatomic reduction of fractures, dislocations and fracture/dislocations of the carpus is paramount prior to either internal or percutaneous Kirschner wire fixations with appropriate ligamentous repairs as indicated.

Arthrodesis of any single or multiple intercarpal or carpometacarpal joints mandates a similar precise technique using an autogenous bone graft from either ilium or distal radial metaphysis. Arthrodesis of the thumb or little finger carpometacarpal joint is best achieved by Kirschner wire fixation with bone graft. If plate fixation is used, the plate must not impinge upon adjacent joints and must provide adequate stability (Figure 16-7).

Kienböck's disease (avascular necrosis of the lunate) may be treated by various methods depending upon theoretical approach.

Watson's "tri-scaphe" arthrodeses (fusion of the distal scaphoid to the trapezium and trapezoid), arthrodesis of the lunate, scaphoid and capitate, osteotomy of either the radius (to shorten) or ulna (to lengthen) in an ulnar minus variant, and arthrodesis of the capitate to the hamate each has its advocates. Capitate hamate fusion is not recommended since the capitate and hamate with the trapezium and trapezoid and index and long metacarpals normally form the stable portion of the hand which therefore is basically an anatomically stable osseoligamentous unit.

Reconstructive treatment of carpal rotational instability (dorsal—DISI and palmar—PISI) lunate instability, scaphoid rotational instability and

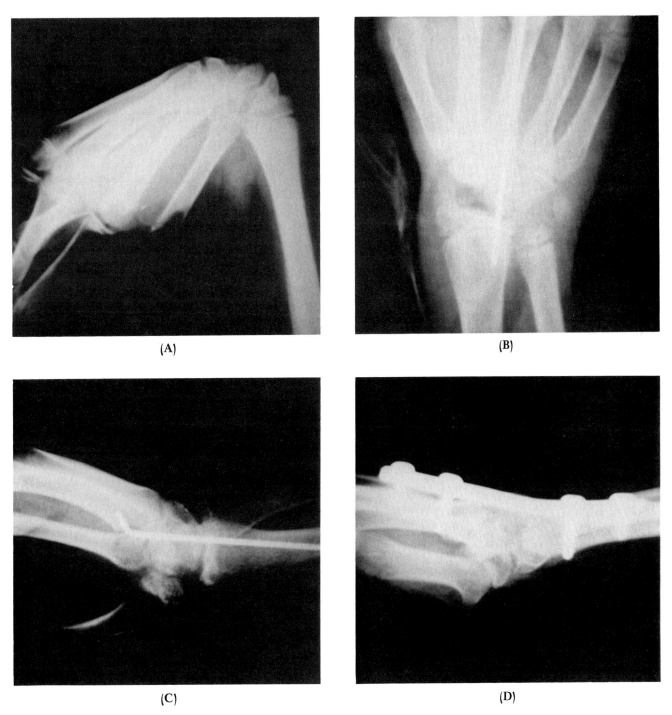

(A) (B)

(C) (D)

Figure 16-6 (A) Severe fixed flexion contracture of the wrist in a patient with cerebral palsy. (B) Proximal row carpectomy and temporary Kirschner wire fixation to resolve flexion contracture. (C) Recurrence of flexion contracture necessitated attempted arthrodesis of capitate to the distal radius with Kirschner wire fixation, an ill-advised and inadequate technique. (D) Painful pseudarthrosis between the capitate and distal radius, a result of the failed attempted arthrodesis, was treated successfully by compression plate fixation and iliac bone graft arthrodesis.

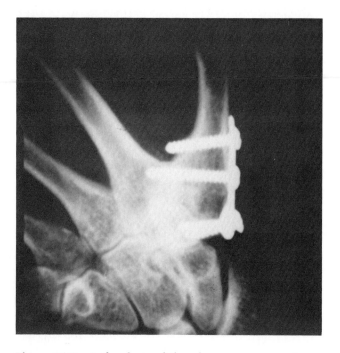

Figure 16-7 Arthrodesis of thumb carpometacarpal joint by plate fixation impinged upon the scaphoid-trapezium joint resulting in virtually no thumb metacarpal motion.

scapholunate diastasis may be treated by any of the above methods noted to treat Kienböck's disease except, obviously, for osteotomy of the radius or ulna. In addition, ligament reconstructions usually involving tendon grafts or transfers have been advocated but in the long run generally do not hold up.

Precise restoration of anatomy and arthrodesis using either internal fixation or percutaneous Kirschner wire fixation with bone graft is necessary for all intercarpal osseous procedures noted above.

Though acute scaphoid fracture may be treated by the AO or Herbert screw techniques specifically to allow early motion, these techniques are usually reserved to treat delayed or nonunions and each commands precise surgical technique for success (refer to Figures 4-26, 4-27 in Chapter 4, Wrist Injuries).

If injury to both the distal radius and the carpus has occurred, each area should be treated individually as a separate entity (Figure 16-8). However, if the wrist joint remains unstable, then and only then should temporary fixation extend across the wrist joint itself (Figure 16-9).

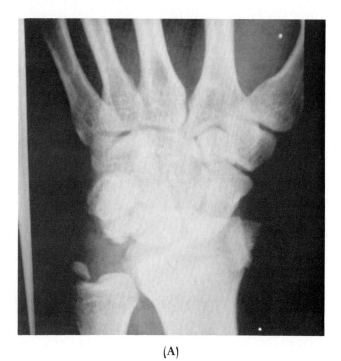

(A)

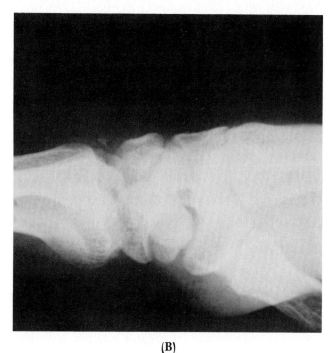

(B)

Figure 16-8 **(A)** Radial segmental articular fracture of the distal radius (Chauffeur's fracture) with dorsal transtriquetral perilunate fracture dislocation of the wrist and fractured ulnar styloid process. **(B)** Simultaneous lateral view of this complex injury.

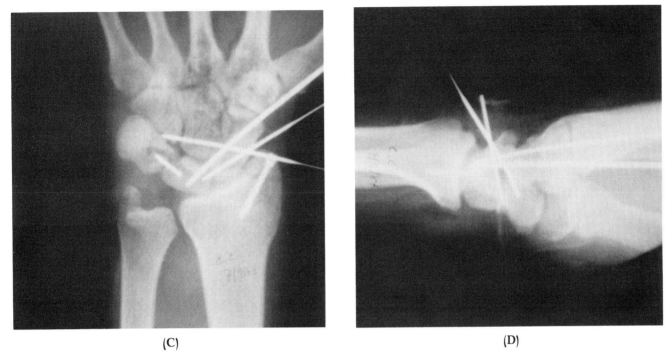

(C)   (D)

Figure 16-8 *(continued)*
(C) Anatomic reduction of the carpal anatomy was treated by multiple Kirschner wire fixation and the radial segmental articular fracture by Herbert screw fixation. No fixation extended across the wrist joint itself and the ulnar styloid process fracture was not fixed. **(D)** Corresponding lateral view shows excellent restoration of anatomy. *(Figures 16-8A–D courtesy of M. Ezaki, M.D.)*

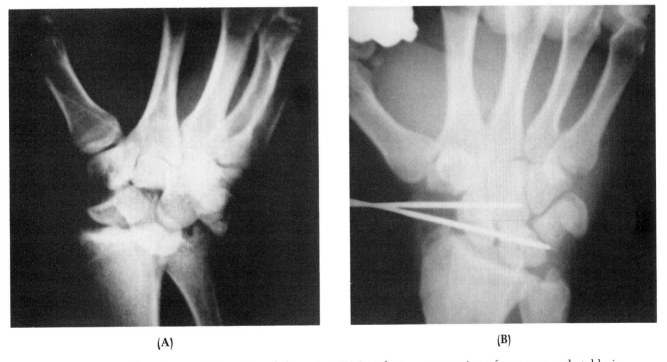

(A)   (B)

Figure 16-9 **(A)** Dorsal perilunate dislocation of the wrist. **(B)** Satisfactory restoration of anatomy and stable intercarpal Kirschner wire fixations provided.

(continued)

Figure 16-9 *(continued)*
(C) Lateral view shows acceptable carpal anatomy with some dorsal displacement of the proximal pole of the scaphoid. **(D)** Seven days later this PA radiograph shows complete distortion of the wrist joint with superimposition of the scaphoid proximal pole on the distal radius. **(E)** Lateral view in plaster again illustrates dorsal dislocation of the proximal scaphoid pole and recurrence of the dorsal perilunate dislocation. Despite the fact that carpal anatomy had been restored initially, temporary immobilization across the wrist joint should have been provided because of extensive ligamentous disruption and gross instability of the wrist joint itself.

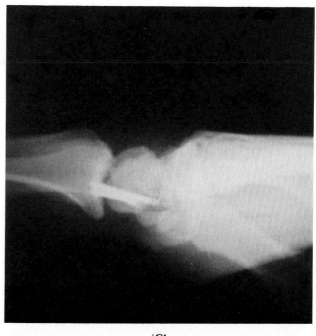

(C)

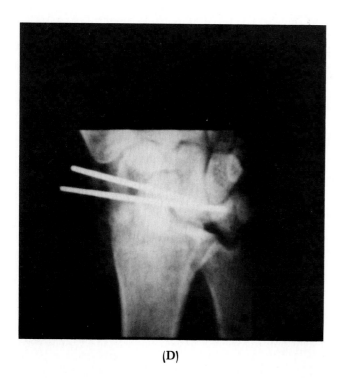

(D)

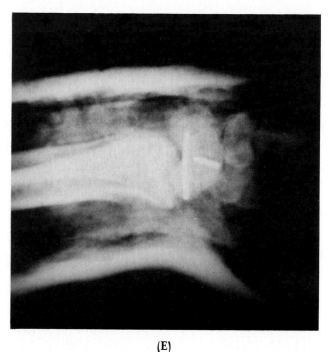

(E)

Metacarpals

Excellent fixation for either single or multiple metacarpal shaft fractures is achieved by either transverse Kirschner wire fixation of the fractured metacarpal(s) into adjacent intact metacarpals or by longitudinal intramedullary fixation which requires an operative approach. In the former, strict attention to prevent malrotation, angulation and distraction (Figure 16-10) is necessary, and in the latter, the Kirschner wire must not impinge upon the MP joint (Figure 16-11). Any immobilization which restricts

Figure 16-10 **(A)** Transverse ring finger metacarpal diaphyseal fracture with 50° palmar angulation. **(B)** Transverse percutaneous Kirschner wire fixation of the ring finger metacarpal distal metaphysis to the long finger metacarpal head. Distraction at the fracture site resulted in nonunion. **(C)** Ill-advised intraosseous wiring of the metacarpal shaft fracture combined with longitudinal Kirschner wire fixation impinging upon the MP joint. Prolonged healing time and restricted MP joint motion required aggressive persistent effort to regain acceptable MP joint flexion and extension after removal of hardware.

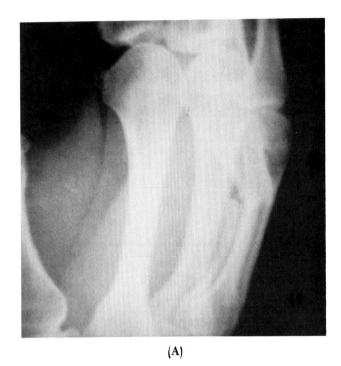

(A)

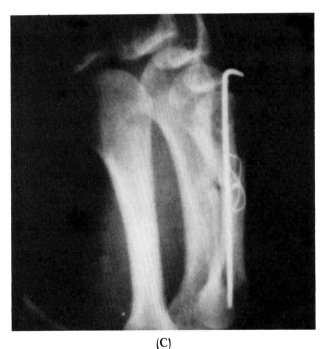

(B)

(C)

MP joint ranges of motion is improper and malrotation must be avoided. Occasionally, plate fixation of an acute fracture may be preferred if early light motion is necessary (e.g., bilateral hand injuries) and with massive periosteal damage (e.g., crush injury) if proper equipment and expertise are available.[5]

Other acceptable fixations include screw (Figure 16-12) or Kirschner wire fixation of oblique fractures. Intraosseous wiring of a transverse metacarpal shaft fracture is contraindicated because of the small diameter of the diaphysis and the sparcity of cancellous bone (Figures 16-10C, 16-13).

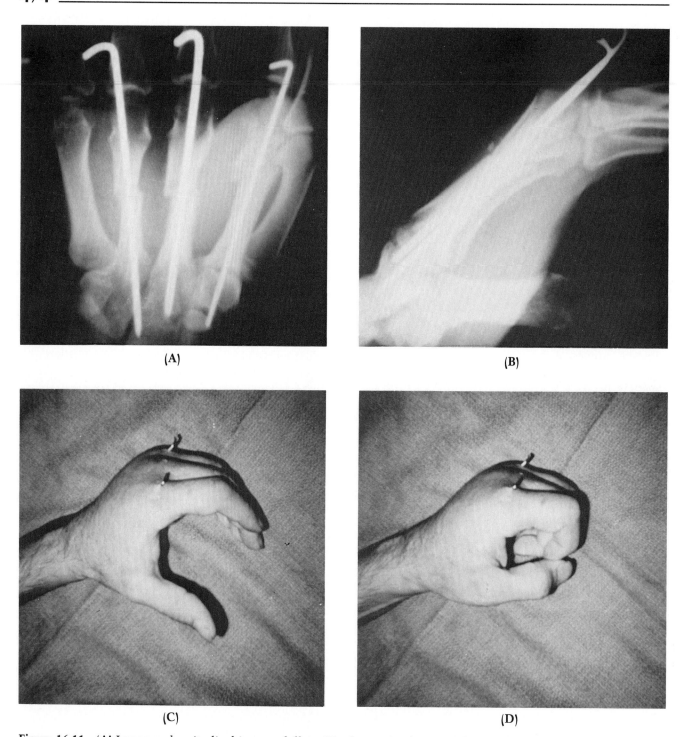

(A)　　　　　　　　　　　　(B)

(C)　　　　　　　　　　　　(D)

Figure 16-11 (A) Improper longitudinal intramedullary Kirschner wire fixation of index, long and ring metacarpal diaphyseal fractures. Not only are the fractures unreduced because the Kirschner wires are of too small diameter but the MP joints are restricted in motion. (B) Corresponding lateral view shows that in addition to restricting MP joint ranges of motion the Kirschner wires have been driven through the articular cartilage of the metacarpal heads. (C) Degree of MP joint extension. (D) Degree of MP joint flexion. Such misuse of this technique is unacceptable and permanent joint damage with restricted motion is inevitable.

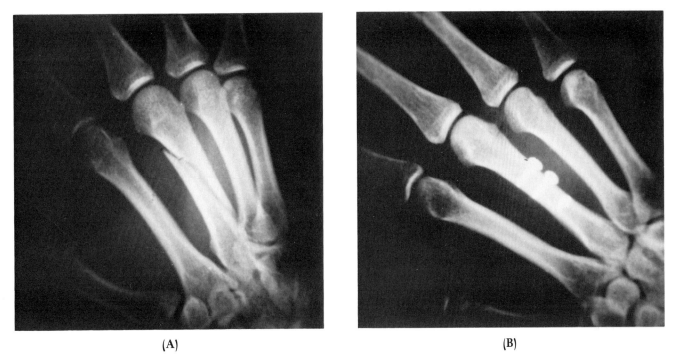

(A)   (B)

Figure 16-12 **(A)** Oblique long metacarpal diaphyseal fracture. **(B)** Anatomic reduction and secure fixation by three screws.

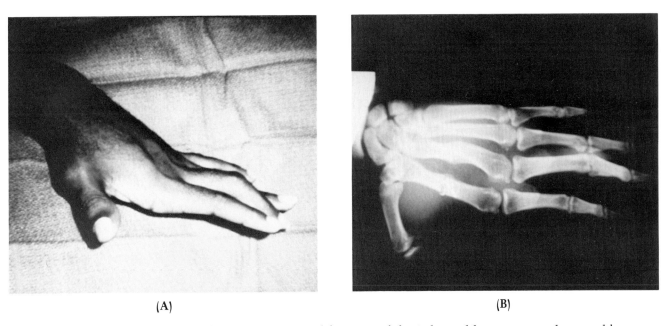

(A)   (B)

Figure 16-13 **(A)** Six months prior this patient sustained fractures of the index and long metacarpals treated by open reduction and internal fixation of the index metacarpal. At this time there is weak active radial and ulnar deviation of the index finger, weak thumb-index pinch, hyperextension of the long finger MP joint and flexion of the PIP joint. **(B)** Corresponding radiographs show delayed union of an intraosseous wiring of the index metacarpal fracture and malunion with palmar angulation of the long finger transverse metacarpal metaphyseal fracture. Ill-advised technique of index metacarpal fixation was complicated by damage to the motor branch of the ulnar nerve causing weakness of adductor pollicis, first dorsal interosseous, first palmar interosseous and second dorsal interosseous muscles. Also inadequate conservative treatment of the long finger metacarpal fracture resulted in palmar angulation causing MP joint hyperextension and PIP joint flexion.

(continued)

Figure 16-13 *(continued)*
(C) Debridement of the long finger metacarpal malunion, realignment and plate fixation with autogenous bone graft from the distal radius completed the reconstruction. **(D)** Long finger alignment was improved by correction of the palmar angulation and healing at the site of long finger metacarpal nonunion. **(E)** Acceptable MP joint flexion was restored.

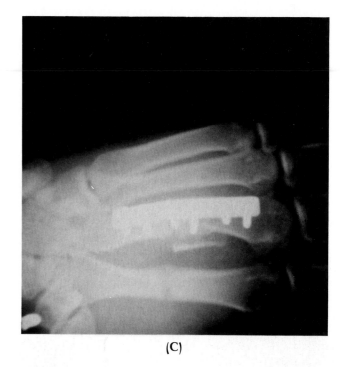

(C)

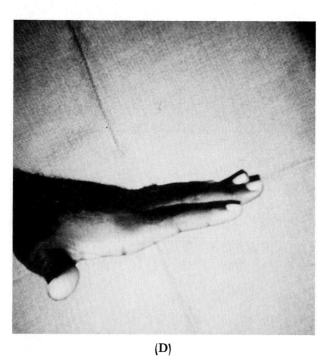

(D)

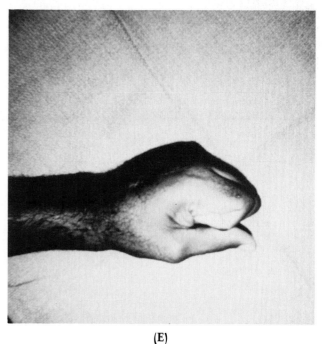

(E)

Though infrequently used, skeletal traction is occasionally excellent treatment, particularly for a comminuted unstable articular fracture or a comminuted proximal metaphyseal fracture of the thumb metacarpal base, and diaphysis only if properly applied and maintained. The thumb metacarpal must be immobilized in wide abduction and opposition and distraction at the fracture site, and malrotation must be prevented.

In reconstructive metacarpal surgery whether for nonunion or for an osseous defect, plate fixation with autogenous bone graft (either iliac or distal radial metaphysis) is strongly recommended (Figure 16-13, refer to Figure 13-8H Chapter 13, Crush Injuries).

Phalanges

Internal fixation of phalangeal fractures is similar to that for metacarpal fractures except that longitudinal intramedullary fixation is seldom used (Figure 16-14). However, for middle and distal phalangeal fractures it may be preferred with unavoidable violation of the DIP joint in the treatment of a middle phalangeal fracture. Oblique Kirschner wire fixation is the easiest and the most practical approach but, for an oblique fracture, screw fixation may be preferred (Figure 16-15) or intraosseous wiring for a transverse fracture. Technically, in intraosseous wiring (Figure 16-16) the transverse Kirschner wire must be placed dorsal to the flexion-extension axis. If placed palmar to that axis, compression is exerted palmarly and progressive flexion angulation will occur with malunion.[6]

Rarely, if ever, is plate fixation indicated for

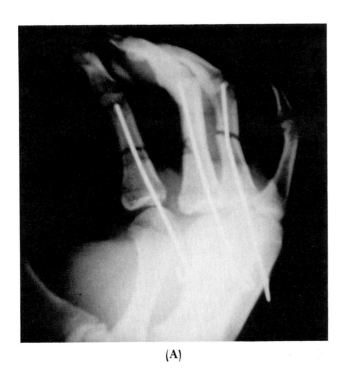

(A)

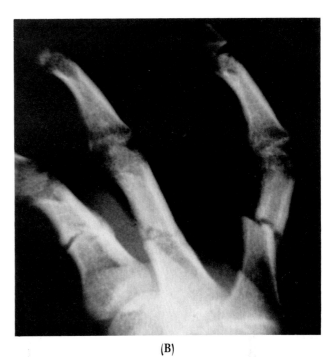

(B)

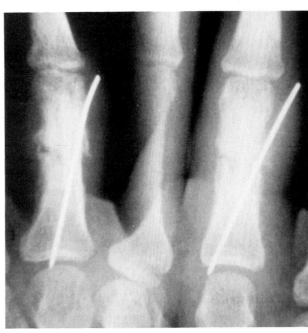

(C)

Figure 16-14 (A) Improper technique of longitudinal intramedullary fixation of index, long and ring finger proximal phalangeal diaphyseal fractures. Kirschner wires are of insufficient caliber and impinge on the MP joints. (B) Nonunion with angulation of the ring finger proximal phalanx occurred. (C) Intramedullary peg bone graft and Kirschner wire fixation solved this problem.

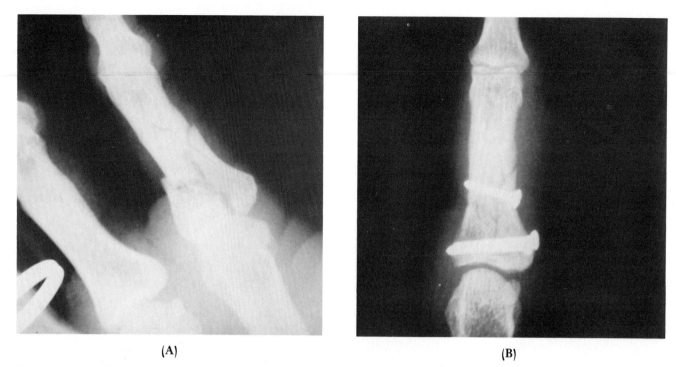

(A) (B)

Figure 16-15 (A) Comminuted proximal metaphyseal fracture of the index finger proximal phalanx with displaced articular component. (B) Anatomic reduction and secure fixation achieved by two screws.

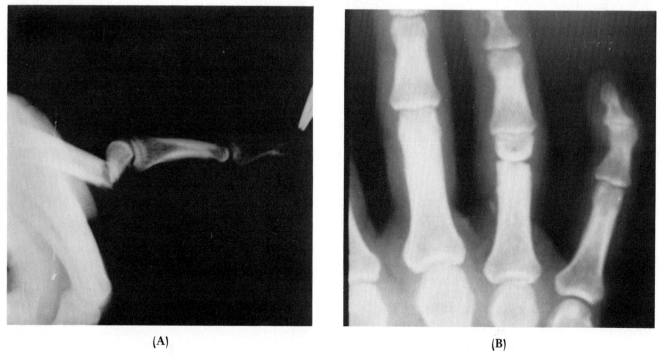

(A) (B)

Figure 16-16 (A) Nonunion of transverse fracture of proximal phalangeal distal metaphysis with 90° dorsal angulation. Lateral view. (B) PA view.

Figure 16-16 *(continued)*
(C) Surgical exposure of the nonunion. **(D)** Intraosseous wiring after anatomic reduction provided stable fixation. **(E)** Corresponding lateral view. *(Figures 16-16A–E courtesy of O. Ogunro, M.D.)*

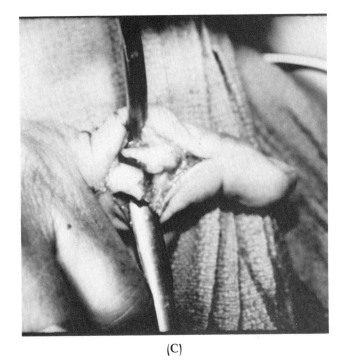

(C)

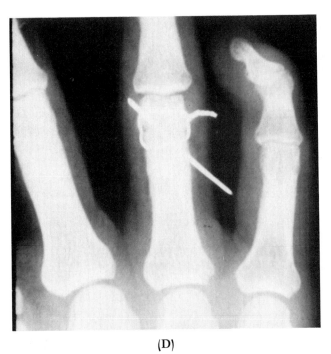

(D)

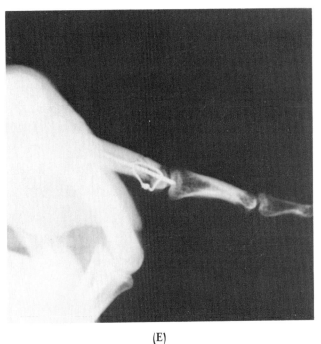

(E)

any phalangeal fracture except possibly for treatment of a nonunion of a proximal phalangeal fracture and more rarely for a middle phalangeal fracture, accompanied with simultaneous bone graft. Rarely, a comminuted unstable fracture of either the proximal or middle phalanx of other digits (index through little fingers) may be treated by dynamic skeletal traction but great care must be taken to prevent distraction and malrotation.

Most important in treatment of phalangeal fractures as with metacarpal fractures is prevention of malrotation and impingement of an oblique fracture on either MP, PIP or DIP joints.

Fracture Avulsions and Articular Fractures

Anatomic reduction is essential for an articular fracture avulsion or pure articular fracture (Figures 16-17, 16-18, 16-19) before internal fixation by either Kirschner wires, screw or pull out wire (Blalock technique is often valuable to accurately reduce and fix a fracture avulsion of either tendon or ligament insertion) (Figure 16-20, refer to Figures 8-51A–C in Chapter 8, Phalangeal Fractures). Temporary Kirschner wire fixation across a joint is often advisable to guarantee joint stability and prevent subsequent subluxation or dislocation, but a threaded Kirschner wire should never be used (Figure 8-51A).

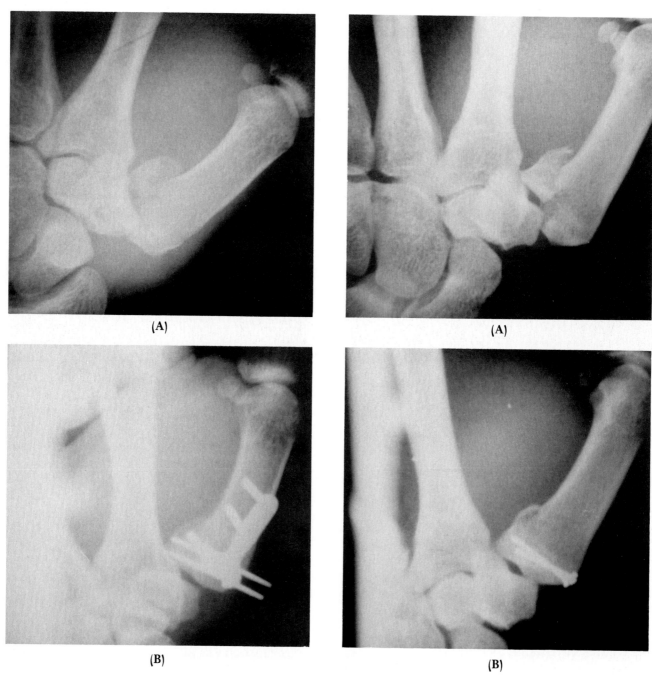

(A)

(B)

(A)

(B)

Figure 16-17 **(A)** Displaced Bennett's fracture of the thumb metacarpal. **(B)** Anatomic reduction and secure fixation provided by Kirschner wires and buttress plate.

Figure 16-18 **(A)** Similar displaced Bennett's fracture of the thumb metacarpal. **(B)** Acceptable reduction and good fixation provided by screw fixation.

Figure 16-19 (A) Reduction and attempted fixation of articular fracture of the base of the little finger proximal phalanx was inadequate and redisplacement occurred. (B) Dorsal displacement and rotation of a large articular fracture of the little finger metacarpal head. (C) Poor technique of attempted longitudinal Kirschner wire fracture fixation. The fracture, however, remains unreduced and the Kirschner wire improperly immobilizes the MP joint in extension. *Articular fractures must be anatomically reduced!*

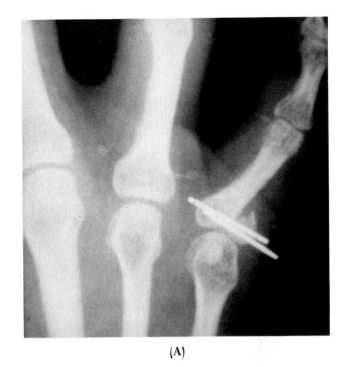

(A)

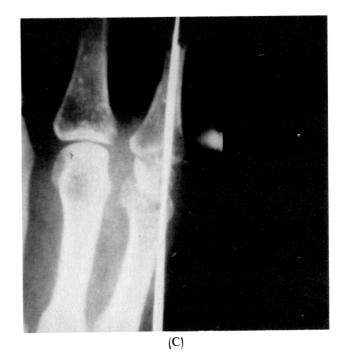

(B)   (C)

Physes

Though closed reduction of the majority of physeal injuries is usually simple, occasionally open reduction may be necessary to remove impinged capsule or tendon preventing reduction. In this situation and also for the unstable physeal separation, skeletal fixation is indicated for stability. Only smooth Kirschner wires should be used, as few as possible, placed through the center of the physis not the periphery

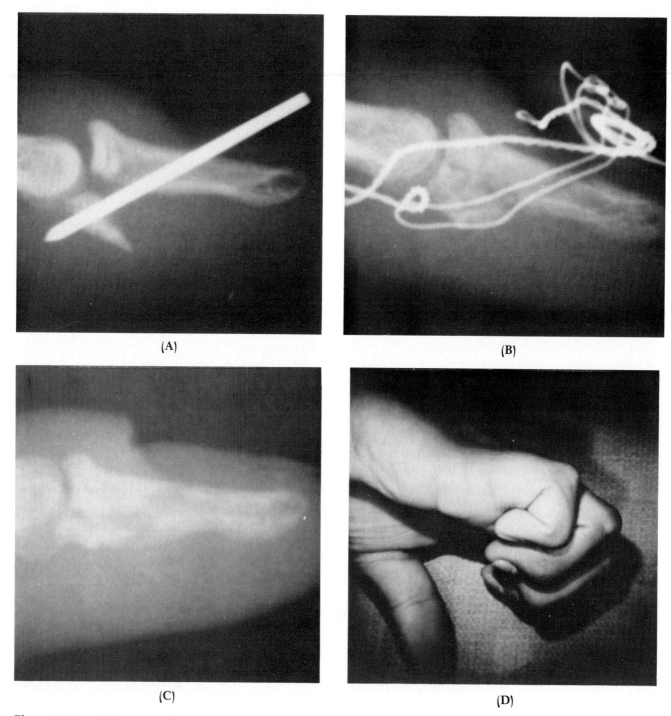

(A)

(B)

(C)

(D)

Figure 16-20 **(A)** Unsuccessful attempt at open reduction and fixation of a flexor digitorum profundus fracture avulsion. **(B)** Open reduction and the Blalock technique of fracture fixation solved this problem. **(C)** A congruent joint produced excellent profundus function. **(D)** Excellent powerful DIP flexion resulted.

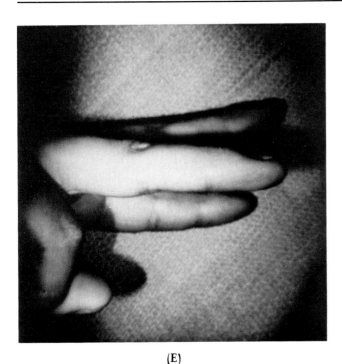

(E)

Figure 16-20 *(continued)*
(E) Nearly normal extension.

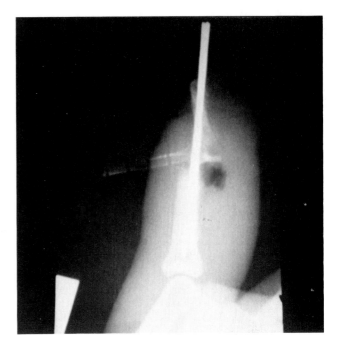

Figure 16-21 Massive soft tissue edema and osteomyelitis of middle and distal phalanges following pin tract infection of longitudinal Kirschner wires to treat fracture dislocation of the DIP joint.

since penetration of the periphery may cause premature cessation of growth in that area (refer to Figure 11-34).

Infection

Infection may occur with use of any percutaneous or internal fixation whether in the acute injury or later reconstruction. To minimize this possibility in an acute injury meticulous aseptic technique including hemostasis, copious irrigation of the wound with either physiologic saline or antibiotic preparation, and gentle handling of all soft tissues is paramount to prevent contamination, hematoma formation, dead space, tissue dessication and tissue necrosis.

If percutaneous Kirschner wires are allowed to protrude from the skin a few millimeters, fewer problems are caused than if these wires are buried subcutaneously unless they are cut flush with the bone. The patient must be instructed on proper hygiene to keep the protruding wires clean, protected and away from contaminated situations (Figure 16-21, refer to Figure 8-56 in Chapter 8, Phalangeal Injuries).

Summary

Kirschner Wires

Kirschner wire fixation is applicable in virtually all locations in the forearm, wrist and hand except for the treatment of diaphyseal fractures of the radius and ulna.

Percutaneous Kirschner wire fixation of fractures directly or with the use of pins and plaster or external fixator technique (Figure 16-22) is excellent if acceptable closed or open reduction is achieved and verified either by image intensifier or radiographs.

Transverse percutaneous Kirschner wire fixation is excellent for metacarpal diaphyseal fracture fixation, thumb metacarpal proximal metaphyseal and basilar articular fractures (Bennett's fracture and fracture of Rolando) and for proximal diaphyseal thumb metacarpal fractures.

Open reduction and Kirschner wire fixation is the easiest and the most versatile fixation available in the treatment of fractures of the wrist and hand. Crossed Kirschner wire fixation is the most commonly used. Longitudinal intramedullary Kirschner wire fixation works well for metacarpal diaphyseal

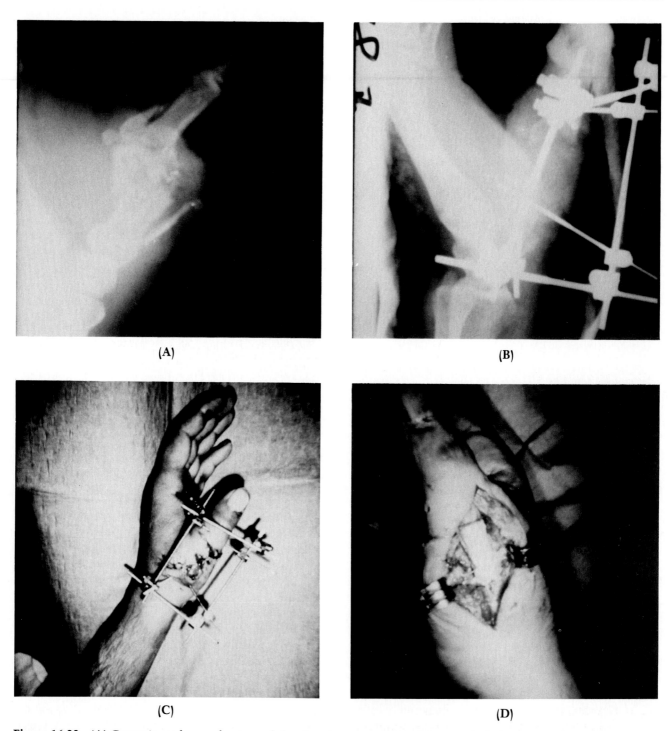

(A)

(B)

(C)

(D)

Figure 16-22 **(A)** Comminuted open fracture of the thumb metacarpal and proximal phalanx resulting from a gunshot wound. **(B)** External fixator was used to maintain thumb alignment and distraction at the site of bone loss from debridement. **(C)** Dorsal view of the external fixator. **(D)** Surgical exposure at the time of iliac bone graft.

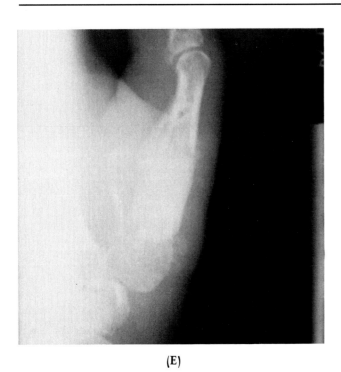

(E)

Figure 16-22 *(continued)*
(E) Healed iliac bone graft uniting the thumb metacarpal to the proximal phalanx in good position with restoration of acceptable length.

and distal metaphyseal fractures and for middle and distal phalangeal fractures.

Threaded Kirschner wires are rarely necessary and should never be placed across a joint unless arthrodesis is contemplated.

Plate Fixation

Dynamic compression plate (DCP) fixation is recommended for all diaphyseal fractures of the radius and ulna, occasionally for metacarpal transverse fractures and rarely for proximal phalangeal fractures.

A buttress plate may be useful to treat fractures of the distal radial metaphysis and segmental articular fractures of the distal radius, particularly the palmar manifestations (palmar distal metaphyseal fracture—Smith's fracture and palmar segmental articular fracture-palmar Barton's fracture).

In addition, buttress plates occasionally may be preferred for metaphyseal fractures adjacent to carpometacarpal, metacarpophalangeal or proximal interphalangeal joints, for large articular fractures and for arthrodesis fixation, particularly carpometacarpal joints.

Pull Out Wire Technique

Pull out wires will securely immobilize fracture avulsions and tendon and ligament avulsions. The Blalock technique may be particularly useful.

Intraosseous Wiring

Intraosseous wiring is applicable to treat transverse fractures of the proximal and middle phalanges and affords excellent fixation for MP and PIP joint arthrodesis[7] but is contraindicated in metacarpal transverse fractures.

Screw Fixation

Screw fixation may be chosen to treat oblique fractures of the metacarpals and proximal and middle phalanges and occasionally to fix a large oblique articular fracture or a large oblique fragment of tendon or ligament fracture avulsion. The Herbert screw and ASIF screw fixation are usually reserved to treat delayed or nonunion of scaphoid fractures and in selected cases of acute scaphoid fracture.

Skeletal Traction

Dynamic skeletal traction is excellent treatment for a comminuted unstable fracture of the thumb metacarpal base whether metaphyseal or articular. Occasionally, it may be useful to treat extensively comminuted unstable metacarpal proximal and middle phalangeal fractures. This technique must be limited to a reliable patient population to prevent distraction and malrotation of the fracture and infection.

References

1. Sandzén SC Jr: Complex injuries of the wrist and hand, in Meyers MH (ed): *The Multiply Injured Patient With Complex Fractures.* Philadelphia, Lea & Febiger, 1984, pp 365–400.
2. Anderson LD: Fractures of the shafts of the radius and ulna, in Rockwood CA Jr, Green DP (eds): *Fractures in Adults,* ed 2. Philadelphia, J.B. Lippincott Co., 1984, vol 1.
3. King RE: Fractures of the shafts of the radius and ulna, in Rockwood CA Jr, Wilkins KE, King RE (eds): *Fractures in Children.* Philadelphia, J.B. Lippincott Co., 1984, vol 3.
4. Louis DS, Hankin FM, Bowers WH: Capitate-radius arthrodesis: An alternative method of radiocarpal arthrodesis. *J Hand Surg* 1984;9A:365–369.
5. Heim V, Pfeiffer KM, Meuli HC: *Small Fragment Set Manual Technique Recommended by the ASIF Group (Swiss Association for Study of Internal Fixation).* New York, Springer-Verlag, 1974.
6. Lister G: Intraosseous wiring of the digital skeleton. *J Hand Surg* 1978;3(5):427–435.
7. Allende BT, Engelem JC: Tension-band arthrodesis in the finger joints. *J Hand Surg* 1980;5(3):269–271.

Index